Risk Adjustment for Measuring Health Care Outcomes

Third Edition

Risk Adjustment for Measuring Health Care Outcomes

Third Edition

Edited by
Lisa I. Iezzoni

Health Administration Press
Chicago, Illinois

Your board, staff, or clients may also benefit from this book's insight. For more information on quantity discounts, contact the Health Administration Press Marketing Manager at (312) 424-9470.

07 06 05 04 03   5 4 3 2 1

Library of Congress Cataloging-in-Publication Data

Risk adjustment for measuring health care outcomes / edited by Lisa I. Iezzoni.—3rd ed.
   p. cm.
    Includes bibliographical references and index.
    ISBN 1-56793-207-X (alk. paper)
   1. Health risk assessment. 2. Outcome assessment (Medical care) I. Iezzoni, Lisa I.
   RA427.3.R567 2003
362.1—dc21

                                 2003045292

Acquisitions manager: Audrey Kaufman; project manager: Joyce Sherman; book and cover design: Matt Avery.

Health Administration Press
A division of the Foundation
  of the American College of
  Healthcare Executives
One North Franklin Street
Suite 1700
Chicago, IL 60606
(312) 424-2800

Dedication

We dedicate this book to two wonderful men who died this year at the height of exemplary careers, John M. Eisenberg (1946–2002), who had directed the Agency for Healthcare Research and Quality (AHRQ) since 1997, and Douglas K. Richardson (1951–2002), associate professor of pediatrics at Harvard Medical School and associate professor of maternal and child health at the Harvard School of Public Health. Both shared deep insight into risk adjustment and conviction of its importance, but both also appropriately saw risk adjustment as only a means to the ultimate end of improving quality of care for all persons.

John was one of those rare individuals who taught volumes simply by being himself. As an academic clinical leader, he taught the primacy of respectful, compassionate, comprehensive care that considers all aspects of patients' lives. His teachings held, however, that care even of individual patients occurs within broader contexts of complex health care delivery systems. His research sought to explicate that complicated milieu, untangling its interwoven scientific, professional, organizational, financial, political, and societal forces. In his final years leading AHRQ, John taught the value of collaboration and understanding diverse viewpoints while remaining faithful to a laser-focused vision—ensuring the best quality care for everybody. John and I had evolved a predictable patter during our occasional meetings over the years. "Have you solved risk adjustment?" John would ask. "Not yet," I'd reply, "but we're working on it." "Keep it up," he'd smile, ever encouraging. We are, keeping our own faith with John's vision.

The first priority of Doug's professional life was "caring" for patients, in the fullest meaning of that word. As a superb neonatologist and associate chief in the Department of Neonatology at Beth Israel Deaconess Medical Center, Doug cared not only for the tiniest newborns, but also for their parents and extended families and for his professional colleagues who joined him at the bedside. Doug's vision, however, reached beyond his own patients. To improve quality of care for all neonates, he led the development of SNAP, the Score for Neonatal Acute Physiology. Using SNAP for risk adjustment, Doug worked openly, generously, and collaboratively with any and all who shared his goal of informing improvement of neonatal intensive care through meaningful information about patients' outcomes. I loved running into Doug in the hallway of our hospital. Even if we had only a few seconds together, I always left smiling, infected by Doug's joy, vigor, and unbridled enthusiasm. That joy remains central to his memory.

Lisa I. Iezzoni
December 20, 2002

CONTENTS IN BRIEF

Detailed Contents

Preface

Our book aims to introduce the issues underlying risk adjustment and to suggest important conceptual and methodological considerations in designing and evaluating a risk-adjustment strategy. As have prior versions, this third edition examines conceptual and methodological issues raised by risk adjustment for comparing outcomes of care, including costs, clinical, and patient-centered outcomes, broadly defined, in various settings of care. We update our methodological presentations, describing statistical techniques that are now used widely in risk-adjustment studies. We briefly address such topics as conducting surveys, measuring validity and reliability, general linear and logistic regression modeling, propensity scores and instrumental variables, and hierarchical modeling.

In prior editions, given the state of the art at the time, we relied largely on hospital-based examples. We now expand to outpatient settings and include new sections on pediatrics, mental health, long-term care, and care for persons with disabilities. The second edition also drew heavily from our study of hospital-based severity-of-illness measures. Some of the methods we examined then are no longer available or have changed substantially. Nevertheless, in this edition, we use selected findings from that study because the results effectively make particular points. Furthermore, since analysts have studied hospital-based severity measures for more than 20 years, numerous relevant publications are readily available.

Hundreds of public and private initiatives nationwide now examine risk-adjusted outcomes, and new efforts start almost weekly. In prior editions, I reviewed these activities, but in this edition, I do not: The field is too voluminous and changing too rapidly, driven by breathtaking advances in information technology barely envisioned before. Nevertheless, throughout this book, various authors cite examples from ongoing initiatives in the United States to make conceptual or practical points, with the caveat that details of methodologies described here may change. Specific issues relating to risk adjustment, especially data sources and capitation payment policies, differ in other countries.

We wrote this book for a multidisciplinary audience, realizing that some readers will concentrate only on certain chapters. Because of this, selected key concepts are repeated throughout the book. In addition, within each area, we emphasize issues most relevant to risk adjustment and do not duplicate detailed technical discussions found in statistical and methodological textbooks.

Acknowledgments

As will become clear, designing meaningful risk-adjustment methods is inherently multidisciplinary. At a minimum, it requires input from diverse clinicians as well as research methodologists and statisticians. This is obvious to us, a multidisciplinary team, as we have investigated risk adjustment for almost two decades and as we wrote this book. Although each chapter lists only one to three authors, much of this book represents a collaboration. Certain chapters reflect thoughtful and invaluable insight from other contributors, bringing knowledge and perspectives that are different from those of the designated author(s).

Our initial thanks go to readers of the prior two edition for their generous support and helpful comments. We sincerely appreciate their input and advice, which has resulted in this expanded third edition. In particular, we include four new chapters about risk adjustment for specific populations: children, persons with mental health problems, people with disabilities, and patients receiving long-term care. Another new chapter addresses two techniques—instrumental variables and propensity scores—which are used increasingly to address risk-adjustment concerns.

Given the current proprietary nature of risk-adjustment methods, we must declare potential conflicts of interest up front. All of us have received research funding to investigate risk adjustment at one or more points during our careers. Since 1984, I have served as a clinical coinvestigator with Arlene S. Ash, as she and other colleagues developed and refined the diagnostic cost group (DCG) methodology under cooperative agreements and contracts, first with the Health Care Financing Administration (HCFA) and now with the Centers for Medicare & Medicaid Services (HCFA renamed). Arlene became an equity partner in D_XCG, the Boston-based company that develops, supports, and markets the DCGs; I have not participated in any DCG commercial activities. Under a grant from the Agency for Health Care Policy and Research (subsequently renamed the Agency for Healthcare Research and Quality, or AHRQ), Jennifer Daley and I, along with others, developed the Complications Screening Program (CSP), which is mentioned at several points in this book. Neither she nor I have personal financial or intellectual interests in commercial applications of the CSP.

We thank Elinor Walker, our infallibly supportive project officer at AHRQ, which funded much of our research described in this book. Chapter 9 borrows extensively from the thoughts of John S. Hughes, M.D., our much-missed Yale University colleague who collaborated on the first two editions. Lori Goyette, my administrative assistant, patiently and with good humor dealt with almost 1,400 bibliographical citations and helped with other production tasks. Micaela Coady, a summer research assistant, comprehensively searched the Internet and local libraries to update our knowledge and find new insight. Developers and vendors of the risk adjusters summarized in tables in Chapter 2 endured numerous queries and requests for information. We appreciate their forbearance and assistance. The final content of this book remains our responsibility alone.

REASONS FOR RISK ADJUSTMENT

Lisa I. Iezzoni

Risks are everywhere. At all times, we each face some measurable—even if infinitesimal—likelihood of imminent calamity. Risks arise from myriad sources, from the molecular imperatives of genetics to the global uncertainties of geopolitical forces. Some risks defy our control, whereas others trace inexorably back to our own actions. Sometimes risks become evident only in retrospect, after disaster has struck.

Fortunately, however, most of us escape outright catastrophe, at least in the developed world. Nevertheless, we daily confront innumerable choices large and small, and we consciously or unconsciously weigh the risks of alternative actions before choosing our course. In making these choices, we usually seek the path that will yield the best outcome. Even for mundane, routine decisions, we typically aim to minimize our risks.

Risks are particularly relevant to health and health care. In the fullness of time, few of us ultimately dodge disease, discomfort, or disability, and none of us eludes death. Certain individuals and populations, however, do develop health problems earlier and more often than others: With rare exceptions, diseases are not distributed randomly across people or populations. This suggests that certain persons and populations carry higher likelihoods of experiencing health problems, for such diverse reasons as genetics, behavior (e.g., smoking, diet, exercise), socioeconomic status, and environmental milieu. Thus, some people and populations face higher risks of poor health outcomes than do others.

When ill or injured, most U.S. residents enter the health care system, seeking advice, intervention, and relief, variously defined. Given the personal stakes, health care decisions require explicit weighing of risks: Even the most benign-appearing therapies, like aspirin or lengthy bed rest, carry some measurable likelihood of harm (e.g., gastrointestinal hemorrhage, deep vein thrombosis leading to pulmonary embolism). Typically, people and their health care professionals delineate acceptable risks and choose therapeutic interventions within each individual context, with little outside oversight and follow-up. However, these myriad individual decisions have one virtually guaranteed outcome—an effect on health care costs.

U.S. health care costs are rising again, having shed the constraints of managed care and other temporizing measures from the mid-1990s. National health expenditures were expected to top $1.5 trillion in 2002, with projected outlays exceeding $2.8 trillion, or 17.0 percent of the gross domestic product, by 2011 (Heffler et al. 2002, 208). Governmental programs, like Medicare and Medicaid, pay nearly half of these costs (almost $700 billion in 2002, rising to $1.3 trillion in 2011), and individuals also spend significant amounts out-of-pocket, about $227 billion in 2002 (Heffler et al. 2002, 211).

Despite these enormous outlays, a 2002 national survey found that 22 percent of Americans have delayed seeking care, rising to 41 percent among persons (17 percent) without health insurance (National Public Radio 2002). Being uninsured, even for one to four years, may worsen general health status; persons without insurance for more than four years face higher risks of premature death than those with private coverage (Institute of Medicine 2002a). Looking ahead, almost half of survey respondents worry about affording health care, but only 23 percent support fundamental change, compared to 37 percent in 1992 before the fractious debate about President Clinton's health care reform plan (National Public Radio 2002).

Compounding problems with cost and access are concerns about what the nation is, in fact, purchasing for its health care dollar. In its seminal report *Crossing the Quality Chasm,* the Institute of Medicine (2001a, 2) concluded, "As medical science and technology have advanced at a rapid pace, . . . the health care delivery system has floundered in its ability to provide consistently high quality care to all Americans." Striking variations in care across small geographic areas, first noted three decades ago (Wennberg and Gittelsohn 1973), persist; expenditures per Medicare beneficiary vary more than twofold across regions, such as between Minneapolis ($3,341 in 1996) and Miami ($8,414; Wennberg, Fisher, and Skinner 2002). Fragmented, poorly coordinated, and ill-designed systems of care are particularly inadequate to the needs of people with chronic conditions—those who consume the most resources. Rates of errors in caring for individual patients are unacceptably high (Institute of Medicine 2000).

From a population perspective, other studies have identified large disparities in health between more privileged and disadvantaged subgroups, such as racial and ethnic minorities and persons with disabilities (U.S. DHHS 2000; Institute of Medicine 2002b). The responsibility of the health care system for disparities in mortality rates, for example, remains unclear. According to Adler and Newman (2002, 61), "The most fundamental causes of health disparities are socioeconomic disparities." Researchers have thus sought to explain health disparities by examining income, education, occupation, and social class (Mechanic 2002). Generally, however, accounting for socioeconomic factors only reduces, but does not eliminate, disparities in health outcomes.

Given this context, many compelling arguments support efforts to examine and better understand the health care system. For individual patients, more information could assist decision making not only about the value of specific clinical interventions but also about which providers offer high-quality care. Similarly, purchasers, payers, and policymakers would benefit from identifying providers and health care systems meriting attention and improvement. Once reforms are initiated, continued measurement could track successes and failures, practices to emulate, and those requiring heightened vigilance. As suggested by these varied purposes, productive examination of the health care system requires comparisons across different "units of observation"— subgroups of patients, treatments, providers, delivery systems, health plans, and populations. The goal is to answer such questions as the following:

- Which treatments are most effective?
- Which providers give the best care?
- Which health plans are most efficient?
- Which delivery systems provide the most patient-centered care?
- Who produces the best outcomes?

Purpose of Risk Adjustment

Meaningful comparisons within the health care system generally require risk adjustment—accounting for patient-associated factors before comparing outcomes across different patients, treatments, providers, health plans, or populations. The rationale is obvious. On average, sicker patients—or persons with more health-related risks—cost more to treat and do less well than their healthier counterparts. This virtual truism would not matter if individuals were randomly assigned to different comparison groups (e.g., treatments, providers, health plans), but they are not. Instead, many factors affect how persons find care, ranging from specific health concerns to financial considerations to geographic location to preferences and expectations for health outcomes and services.

Not surprisingly, therefore, the mix of persons treated by different clinical interventions, providers, or health plans varies. These differences have consequences. Higher-risk patients typically generate larger costs, even with efficient providers or health plans. Persons with complex illnesses, multiple coexisting diseases, or other significant risk factors generally develop more complications and experience worse outcomes, even with excellent care, than healthier individuals. Risk adjustment aims to account for differences in intrinsic health risks that patients bring to their health care encounters. For determining costs or comparing outcomes, it thus "levels the playing field," ensuring that "apples are compared to apples, not to oranges," like-to-like.

Risk adjustment is therefore essential to examining outcomes in the real world. In the artificial environment of randomized controlled trials (RCT)— where experts administer treatments following tightly specified protocols in closely monitored settings—randomization presumably sorts patients into comparison groups regardless of their baseline risks. Random assignment theoretically produces treatment (case) and nontreatment (control) groups with similar risk factors. RCTs thus yield the "gold-standard" evidence of treatment "efficacy." In examining routine care as practiced daily throughout communities, though, the focus shifts to quantifying "effectiveness." Risk adjustment is integral to calculating the so-called "algebra of effectiveness," which recognizes patients' outcomes as complex functions of intrinsic patient attributes and other factors:

$$\text{Outcomes} = f(\text{intrinsic patient-related risk factors,}$$
$$\text{treatment effectiveness, quality of care, random chance})$$

The specifics of this equation vary depending on the outcome of interest and the range of intrinsic patient attributes that must be considered. As suggested by Figure 1.1, these equations can become complex and far reaching: Many diverse attributes, clinical and nonclinical, contribute to health-related risks.

More than two decades of intensive research have produced credible risk-adjustment methods for certain outcomes in widely divergent contexts, such as the following:

- predicting in-hospital mortality for children and adults treated in intensive care units (ICUs); a web site sponsored by the French Society of Anesthesia and Intensive Care allows visitors to calculate risk scores using 25 different adult, pediatric, or specialty ICU risk-adjustment methods;[1]
- predicting in-hospital mortality and postoperative complications for coronary artery bypass graft (CABG) and other major surgeries;
- examining patient-reported satisfaction with health care or health plans;
- setting prospective payment levels for specific episodes of care (Medicare Payment Advisory Commission [MedPAC] 2002a), such as acute care hospital reimbursement based on diagnosis related groups (DRGs) and nursing home payments using resource utilization groups (RUGs; Table 1.1); and
- setting capitation payment levels for managed care organizations (MCOs) enrolling Medicare beneficiaries, Medicaid recipients, or other members.

Existing risk-adjustment methods are widely used by private and public payers, governmental and voluntary oversight bodies (e.g., for provider accreditation), quality-improvement organizations (QIO), health data organizations, media (e.g., magazines producing their "best hospitals" issues), clinicians, health services researchers, and others. However, risk-adjustment methods remain underdeveloped for many critical aspects of care, such as routine outpatient settings, nonsurgical inpatient care, and specific subpopulations (e.g., children outside ICUs, persons with mental health conditions or disabilities). In addition, although risk adjusters for setting capitation payments are substantially better than standard demographic approaches, questions remain about whether supplementary policies (e.g., partial capitation) are needed to improve fairness of payment for particularly costly enrollees (MedPAC 2000).

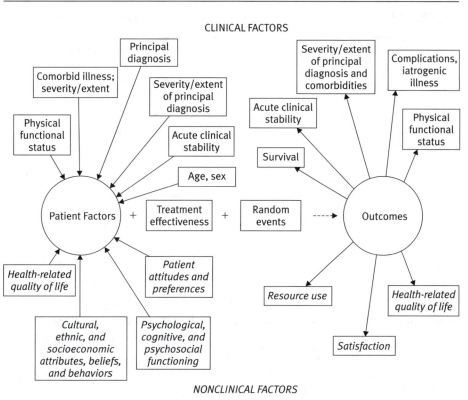

FIGURE 1.1

The Algebra of Effectiveness

CLINICAL FACTORS

Thus, the devil of risk adjustment is in the details. As described in Chapter 2, one cannot begin risk adjustment without first defining basic terms: risk of what? Nevertheless, failing to account adequately for patients' risks can prove embarrassing. A prime example was the first public release in March 1986 of Medicare's hospital mortality figures by the Health Care Financing Administration (HCFA, renamed the Centers for Medicare & Medicaid Services, or CMS, in 2001) (Brinkley 1986). According to HCFA's predictions, 142 hospitals had significantly higher death rates than predicted, whereas 127 had significantly lower rates. At the institution with the most aberrant death rate, 87.6 percent of Medicare patients died compared to a predicted 22.5 percent. This facility, however, was a hospice caring for terminally ill patients. HCFA's risk-adjustment model had not adequately captured patients' risks of death.[2]

Purpose of this Book and Updates

As have prior versions, this third edition examines conceptual and methodological issues raised by risk adjustment for comparing outcomes of care, including costs, clinical, and patient-centered outcomes, broadly defined, in various settings of care. We update our methodological presentations, describing

TABLE 1.1
Product Classifications (or risk adjusters) for Medicare Prospective Payment by Practice Setting: 2002

Practice Setting	Year Began[a]	Classification System
Acute care hospitals	1984	506 diagnosis related groups (DRGs)
Hospital outpatient departments	2000	750 ambulatory payment classifications (APCs)
Skilled nursing facilities	1998	44 resource utilization groups, version 3 (RUGs-III)
Home health agencies	2001	80 home health resource groups (HHRGs)
Inpatient rehabilitation facilities	2002	385 case-mix groups (CMGs)

SOURCE: Adapted from MedPAC (2002a, 6, 8, Table 1-1).
[a]Fiscal year prospective payment began.

statistical techniques that are now used widely in risk-adjustment studies. We briefly address such topics as conducting surveys, measuring validity and reliability, general linear and logistic regression modeling, propensity scores and instrumental variables, and hierarchical modeling. Within each area, we emphasize issues most relevant to risk adjustment and do not duplicate detailed technical discussions found in statistical and methodological textbooks.

In prior editions, given the state of the art at the time, we relied largely on hospital-based examples. We now expand to outpatient settings and include new sections on pediatrics, mental health, long-term care, and care for persons with disabilities. The second edition also drew heavily from our study of hospital-based severity-of-illness measures (Iezzoni 1997; Hughes et al. 1996; Iezzoni et al. 1995a, 1995b, 1995c, 1996a, 1996b, 1996c, 1996d, 1996e, 1997; Landon et al. 1996; Shwartz et al. 1996a). Some of the methods we examined then are no longer available or have changed substantially. Nevertheless, in this edition, we use selected findings from that study because the results effectively make particular points. Furthermore, since analysts have studied hospital-based severity measures for more than 20 years, numerous relevant publications are readily available. Over the last decade, prominent risk-adjustment methods have become increasingly proprietary, often preventing outsiders from completely reviewing their inner workings. Sometimes, commercial affiliations facilitate further development, user support, design and maintenance of applications software, and productive dissemination within practice settings (Knaus 2002).[3] Obtaining commercial risk adjusters for research studies is nonetheless frequently difficult, especially for projects comparing methodologies. Today, we could not replicate our mid-1990s study.

Despite these obstacles, the global health policy impetus for risk adjustment has grown. Since completing the second edition, the U.S. health care delivery system has continued its puzzling course at a dizzying pace. Fundamental structural problems, like the lack of universal coverage, remain. In many settings, capitated health plans co-opted the phrase "risk adjustment," despite questions about whether current risk-adjustment methods are entirely sufficient to direct payments (Newhouse 1998; MedPAC 2000). The 1997 Balanced Budget Act (P.L. 105-33) required Medicare to begin risk adjusting its capitated payments to MCOs by 1 January 2000, presumably to improve the fairness of payment. Historically, capitated plans had profited handsomely from enrolling members who were less costly than average beneficiaries: Medicare had overpaid capitated plans by 5 to 20 percent because of their healthier members (Greenwald et al. 1998). For its risk adjuster, Medicare chose the principal inpatient diagnostic cost groups (PIP-DCGs), which assign enrollees to payment levels based largely on their principal diagnosis from inpatient stays (Iezzoni et al. 1998; Pope et al. 2000a).[4] Since then, however, MCOs have left Medicare in droves, setting needy beneficiaries adrift. One real but rarely articulated impetus for this exodus is MCOs' fear of lower payments under risk adjustment.

Meanwhile, hundreds of public and private initiatives nationwide now examine risk-adjusted outcomes, and new efforts start almost weekly. In prior editions, I reviewed these activities, but in this edition, I do not: The field is too voluminous and changing too rapidly, driven by breathtaking advances in information technology barely envisioned before. Nevertheless, throughout this book, various authors cite examples from ongoing initiatives in the United States to make conceptual or practical points, with the caveat that details of methodologies described here may change. Specific issues relating to risk adjustment, especially data sources and capitation payment policies, differ in other countries (Rice and Smith 2001).

Some prominent initiatives, such as New York State's CABG mortality reports and Pennsylvania's use of MedisGroups to risk adjust hospital mortality and morbidity rates, both of which started in the mid- to late 1980s, continue today. In fact, other states, such as California and Massachusetts, are following New York's lead in publishing hospital "report cards" on CABG mortality rates. CABGs were a logical starting point for risk adjusting performance reports, as CABGs have undergone extensive study, including RCTs; risk factors are well characterized; a clearly defined outcome, mortality, is common enough for rigorous statistical modeling; and outcomes vary across facilities and surgeons. New York's risk-adjusted CABG hospital mortality report initially gained widespread credibility: The state worked closely with the clinical community to design the risk-adjustment method, and early results appeared in the *Journal of the American Medical Association* (Hannan et al. 1990). Controversy erupted in 1991, when New York *Newsday* published figures for individual surgeons by name. Further concerns arose with anecdotal claims of data manipulation and stories about cardiothoracic surgeons' declining high-risk cases to avoid tarnishing their outcomes. Nevertheless, New York's risk-adjusted mortality rate for isolated CABG surgery fell from 4.17 percent in 1989 to 2.45 percent in 1992, a decline of 41 percent (Hannan et al. 1994, 765). Some attribute this drop to quality improvement and other efforts motivated by publishing CABG mortality reports, although others credit secular trends (Chassin, Hannan, and DeBuono 1996). According to Mark R. Chassin (2002, 49), commissioner of health during the first release:

> The New York program has proved its durability, having lasted through the terms of four commissioners of health in governments administered by two governors of different political parties. I believe that its endurance is attributable to three factors: its integration into the routine processes of a governmental agency, the continuous commitment of those closest to the program to publishing in scientific journals a variety of analyses of its impact, and the vigorous involvement of the state's leading cardiac surgeons and cardiologists in the advisory committee process.

Meanwhile, one widely touted initiative to examine risk-adjusted hospital outcomes foundered because of risk-adjustment politics. The Cleveland Health Quality Choice (CHQC) program, a voluntary coalition of businesses, hospitals, and physicians, gathered detailed clinical data from medical records to risk adjust hospital outcomes on ICU death rates and in-hospital deaths and/or prolonged hospitalizations for general medical, surgical, and obstetrical care. Initial CHQC data were released privately to hospitals for internal improvement activities, with the first public report in April 1993. Since the outset, however, Cleveland Clinic officials had complained that the CHQC risk adjustment ignored special characteristics of their patient population (Vogel and Topol 1996). They also protested against paying $2 million annually for gathering the data. Finally, in February 1999, the CHQC announced that it would disband in July because nine Cleveland Clinic–affiliated hospitals refused to continue submitting their data voluntarily. As further justification for its withdrawal, the Cleveland Clinic noted, with some irony, that the CHQC data were not being used.

Nevertheless, current trends strongly suggest that risk-adjusted performance information will become even more important in coming years, as calls for value-based purchasing increase. In October 2002, questions about quality and the purchasing might of six federal health programs (Medicare, Medicaid, Department of Defense TRICARE programs, Veterans Health Administration, State Children's Health Insurance Program, and the Indian Health Service) prompted the Institute of Medicine (2002c, 1) to encourage

> . . . the federal government to take full advantage of its influential position to set the quality standard for the health care sector. Specifically, regulatory processes should be used to establish clinical data reporting requirements; purchasing strategies should provide rewards to providers who achieve higher levels of quality; health care delivery systems operated by public programs should serve as laboratories for the development of 21st century care delivery models; and applied

health services research should be expanded to accelerate the development of knowledge and tools in support of quality enhancement.

Governmental and private purchasers alike now chant the mantra "pay for performance." Undoubtedly, risk-adjusted outcomes information will assume center stage in pay-for-performance schemes. As the Institute of Medicine (2002c) concedes, however, more research is required to produce robust performance measures. Already, Internet web sites purportedly grade health care providers, ostensibly to help patients choose good-quality caregivers. Nevertheless, the utility of this information for individual patients remains murky (Krumholz et al. 2002; Naylor 2002). For purchasers, finding high-quality providers to reward through value-based purchasing must overcome such methodological barriers as small sample sizes and inadequate risk adjustment (Hofer et al. 1999; Greenfield et al. 2002; Eisenberg 2002). As MedPAC (2002b, 36) observed, "Without adequate risk adjustment, some institutions or clinicians could appear to have poorer outcomes simply because they see sicker patients."

Historical Precedents

We tend to think ourselves unusually enlightened in examining outcomes of care. In fact, historical precedents for this are noteworthy, not only because of the compilation and comparison of outcomes data but also because of vigorous efforts to discover the causes of variations and use this knowledge to improve care. Many motivations and consequent controversies uncannily anticipated today's discourse (Iezzoni 1996).

For centuries, Britain gathered data on population death rates, primarily to track epidemic illness. Overwhelmed by deaths from plague, royal authorities initiated weekly "Bills of Mortality" in the early 1500s (Walker 1929). Starting in the late eighteenth century, profound social upheavals of the industrial revolution spurred this interest. As populations shifted from the countryside, massing within congested industrial centers, statistics clearly depicted worsening public health. By the 1830s, civic and business leaders had founded statistical societies throughout England, aiming to quantify the effects of social changes. The archetypal member was "a liberal Whig, Unitarian, reform-minded" (Eyler 1979, 14). These early Victorian statisticians viewed facts as the scientific impetus for political change.

English hospitals, which were primarily charitable institutions serving the poor, had independently accumulated patient statistics since the 1600s. In the mid-nineteenth century, even England's registrar-general had trouble determining which facilities, or parts of facilities, were actually hospitals as opposed to workhouses: In 1861, workhouses contained 81 percent of beds for physically ill persons (Pinker 1966). Statistics quantified results of hospitals' charity for wealthy benefactors and encouraged new subscribers and donations. As today, those funding hospitals, and even philanthropists, wanted proof they were getting their money's worth. In addition, as noted in an 1863 report for the medical officer of the Privy Council, "The public as a rule still look to the death-rates of hospitals as the best indication of their relative healthiness" (Bristowe and Holmes 1864, 512).

Improving and Monitoring Outcomes

In 1863, Florence Nightingale (1820–1910; Figure 1.2) published the third edition of her *Notes on Hospitals*, recommending fundamental changes in the configuration, location, and operation of hospitals to reduce deaths caused by unsanitary conditions. Seven years earlier, Nightingale had returned from Crimean War service at British military hospitals as perhaps the first wartime celebrity ever created by the news media (Cohen 1984). Crafted by a *Times* correspondent, her image as the lone lady nursing sick solders lit by her hand-held lamp earned Nightingale an admiring lifelong audience. This gentle, ministering angel persona, however, belied her tough-minded, laser-focused administrative acumen. In 1855, six months after arriving at Barrack Hospital in Scutari, Turkey, she cut military hospital death rates from 42.7 to 2.2 percent (Cohen 1984).

Upon returning home, Nightingale continued targeting military installations, but needing statistical help, she turned to William Farr (1807–1883), a physician and prominent social reformer who had conducted analyses for the registrar-general since 1838. In 1856, they made a pact: Farr would assist her with army reforms, and Nightingale would aid his efforts to reduce civilian deaths (Eyler 1979). In her 1863 *Notes on Hospitals*, Nightingale concentrated primarily on civilian hospitals.

Farr and Nightingale viewed high hospital death rates as incontrovertible proof of the dangers of urban mid-nineteenth century hospitals; Table 1.2, taken from her book, shows the deaths at "106 principal hospitals of England" in 1861. Most startling was the 90.84 "mortality per cent on inmates" at 24 London hospitals, taken verbatim from Farr's *24th Annual Report of the Registrar-General*. These figures led Nightingale (1863, 4) to question the value of these inner-city hospitals:

> Facts such as these (and it is not the first time that they have been placed before the public) have sometimes raised grave doubts as to the advantages to be derived from hospitals at all, and have led many a one to think that in all probability a poor sufferer would have a much better chance of recovery if treated at home.

Nightingale warned that such figures did not adequately capture patients' risks, observing that, at a minimum, one must consider differences across hospitals in patients' ages and "state of the cases on admission" (Nightingale 1863, 2). Despite these caveats, she observed that deaths rates were lower at facilities with better sanitation and less crowding in cramped wards

FIGURE 1.2
Florence
Nightingale and
Ernest Amory
Codman

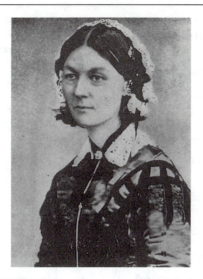 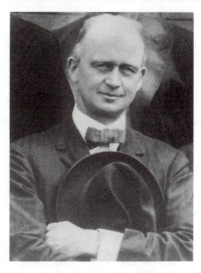

SOURCE: Codman photograph courtesy of the Boston Medical Library in the Francis A. Countway Library of Medicine.

and at sites away from raw sewage and urban congestion. These observations supported Nightingale's theory about miasmas—noxious vapors spreading disease—and led her to propose changes in ward configuration, sanitation, and hospital location that ultimately helped reduce hospital mortality. Nightingale introduced fresh air, light, and ample space into hospitals and apportioned patients to separate pavilions.

Nightingale continued to argue that compiling and disseminating outcome statistics for hospitals were critical to understanding and improving care. With an eerily modern ring, she lamented the state of this endeavor:

> Accurate hospital statistics are much more rare than is generally imagined, and at the best they only give the mortality which has taken place in the hospitals, and take no cognizance of those cases which are discharged in a hopeless condition, to die immediately afterwards, a practice which is followed to a much greater extent by some hospitals than by others. We have known incurable cases discharged from one hospital, to which the deaths ought to have been accounted, and received into another hospital, to die there in a day or two after admission, thereby lowering the mortality rate of the first at the expense of the second (Nightingale 1863, 2).

However, Nightingale (1863, 4) emphasized that numbers should not focus only on mortality, stating, "If the function of a hospital were to kill the sick, statistical comparisons of this nature would be admissible." She argued that, since hospitals ultimately aim to restore health, statistics should concen-

TABLE 1.2

Mortality Per
Cent. in the
Principal
Hospitals of
England: 1861

	Number of SPECIAL INMATES on the 8th April, 1861.	Average Number of INMATES in each HOSPITAL.	Number of DEATHS registered in the Year 1861.	MORTALITY per Cent. on INMATES.
IN 106 PRINCIPAL HOSPITALS OF ENGLAND	12709	120	7227	56·87
24 London Hospitals	4214	176	3828	90·84
12 Hospitals in Large Towns ...	1870	156	1555	83·16
25 County and Important Provincial Hospitals	2248	90	886	39·41
30 Other Hospitals	1136	38	457	40·23
13 Naval and Military Hospitals ...	3000	231	470	15·67
1 Royal Sea Bathing Infirmary (Margate)	133	133	17	12·78
1 Dane Hill Metropolitan Infirmary (Margate)	108	108	14	12·96

SOURCE: Nightingale (1863).

trate on recovery and its speed. Nevertheless, 140 years after Nightingale's observations, information on patients' health following medical encounters remains rarely available.

Publication of Nightingale's *Notes on Hospitals* unleashed several months of acerbic public debate between Farr and his methodological critics. The testy tone and issues raised parallel today's controversies surrounding releases of performance reports on physicians and hospitals. This tale therefore resumes as an epilogue to Chapter 17.

Focusing on End Results

The most articulate early American proponent of monitoring outcomes of care was Ernest Amory Codman (1869–1940; Figure 1.2), a Boston surgeon (Berwick 1989; Donabedian 1989; Mulley 1989; Neuhauser 1990). Although perhaps apocryphal, the story of how Codman first became interested in monitoring outcomes offers insight into not only his character, but also his future methods. Codman and his Harvard Medical School classmate Harvey Cushing (1869–1939), who became a renowned neurosurgeon, served together as clerks at the Massachusetts General Hospital (Neuhauser 1990). The role of the medical students was to provide anesthesia to surgical patients. After being anesthetized, Cushing's first patient vomited and died. Although this event troubled Cushing, the senior surgeon was unconcerned, stating that such deaths were fairly common. Cushing and Codman challenged each other to compare their patients' outcomes during the clerkship. Both students maintained intraoperative records on each anesthetized patient; Codman's charts graphed the patient's pulse and respirations every five minutes. These records represent the first intraoperative anesthesia charts, now standard practice. The winner of this challenge is unclear. In 1920, Cushing remembered that Codman had won, but in 1939, he wrote that Codman had lost (Neuhauser 1990).

This experience initiated Codman's lifelong interest—some might say obsession—with looking at surgical outcomes. He willingly compared his results with those of others, albeit acknowledging, "Comparisons are odious, but comparison is necessary in science. Until we freely make therapeutic comparisons, we cannot claim that a given hospital is efficient, for efficiency implies that the results have been looked into" (Codman 1934, xxiii). Codman's unique contribution was trying to link specific interventions with their effects on patients. He labeled this approach the "end-results idea,"

> . . . which was merely the commonsense notion that every hospital should follow every patient it treats, long enough to determine whether or not the treatment has been successful, and then to inquire "if not, why not" with a view to preventing similar failures in the future (Codman 1934, xii).

For operative patients, this could require monitoring for years after the surgery.

Codman tried putting his end-results idea into practice at Massachusetts General Hospital, tracking down patients a year after surgery and examining them. Some of his surgical colleagues viewed these activities as extreme. Nevertheless, Codman (1917, 137) argued that this approach was essential for improving the quality of care:

> So I am called eccentric for saying in public: that Hospitals, if they wish to be sure of improvement,
>
> • Must find out what their results are.
> • Must analyze their results, to find their strong and weak points.
> • Must compare their results with those of other hospitals. . . .
> • Must welcome publicity not only for their successes, but for their errors. . . .

Such opinions will not be eccentric a few years hence.

Discouraged about the prospects for fully implementing the end-results idea at Massachusetts General Hospital, in 1911 Codman opened his own ten-bed hospital on Pinkney Street in Boston's Beacon Hill, where two dozen other surgeons, including Cushing, assisted him (Neuhauser 1990). Codman completely installed his end-results tracking system, and he paid the Thomas Todd Co. to print annual volumes documenting the outcomes of each individual case treated during the year. When he felt an error in treatment or other failure had occurred, he categorized the cause, such as (Codman 1917)

• Errors due to lack of technical knowledge or skill
• Errors possibly due to lack of judgment
• Errors due to lack of care or equipment

- Errors due to incorrect diagnosis
- Cases in which the nature and extent of the disease were the main cause of failure
- Cases who refused to accept treatment

Thus, Codman linked specific outcomes to specific interventions or errors in a way that truly informed—going far beyond the information provided in today's performance reports on physicians and hospitals (see Chapter 12).

Codman fought doggedly against what he saw as laxity in the medical establishment, as suggested by the dedication of the circa 1917 publication of the Codman hospital's end results:

> This Volume is Dedicated to
> RICHARD C. CABOT
> because I respect his motives, admire his courage and energy,
> but heartily disapprove of some of his opinions and methods,
> for he seems to want to reform the bottom of the
> profession, while I think the blame
> belongs at the top.

In 1914, Codman resigned from Massachusetts General Hospital to protest against the seniority system of promotion, seeing it as antithetical to the end-results idea. The day his resignation was accepted he reapplied, asking to be appointed surgeon-in-chief because the end results of his cases for the last decade were better than those of other surgeons. Of course this request was ignored, but by 1916 Massachusetts General Hospital had abandoned its seniority system of promotion. Nonetheless, this candor made Codman unpopular. With few referrals, his hospital closed in 1918.

In discussing the end-results idea, Codman (1917, 93) clearly recognized the concept of risk:

> For the man who practices surgery, there are two kinds of mortality—chance and intentional.
>
> Chance mortality is the kind which occurs unexpectedly, and which no amount of foresight can prevent. It is caused by unanticipated Calamities or Catastrophes. Death from pulmonary embolism is a good example. . . . Is it not possible to determine what this percentage of danger is, just as easily as it is to compute fire risk? . . .
>
> Intentional mortality is incurred by the chief surgeon when he attempts cases in which the condition is acknowledged to be grave. It is speculative—like gambling against known chances in a game in which skill, judgment, and luck all count.

Surgeons in Codman's era, however, had a somewhat different perspective than today. Nowadays, publicly releasing mortality or other outcome information raises concerns that surgeons will avoid difficult cases, fearing that poor results will be held against them. In Codman's day,

. . . a certain number of deaths are necessary to the surgeon in his business. A surgeon whose cases always get well gets no reputation for "nerve." It is said that he will never take a chance when he ought to do so. A surgeon must be "fearless" and "bold," and the only way he can prove that he is, is by a death now and then in his practice (Codman 1917, 105).

Despite this, Codman's (1917, 106) attitude toward compensation is also rare today:

Shall I say in the future?:

1. You are too bad a risk; go to a first-class surgeon.
2. You are a bad risk; I must double my usual fee.
3. You are a bad risk; you need not pay unless you live.

All are logical. I like the last best.

Conclusions

Both Nightingale and Codman viewed outcomes information as a means to the end of improving patient outcomes and quality of care. Their work holds an important lesson: Simply knowing rates of events is insufficient. Knowing why these events occurred is essential. Risk adjustment aims to isolate one potential cause: patients' intrinsic attributes that inherently increase likelihood of poor outcomes.

Although the remainder of this book concerns measurement of risk, we acknowledge that this is only a first step in examining costs and quality. Risk adjustment is simply a tool for identifying what is really important, such as inefficiencies or substandard quality. Other methods and approaches are required for the more important next step—understanding how to improve outcomes.

Notes

1. The web site (http://www.sfar.org/scores2/scores2.html) is maintained by the Société Française d'Anesthésie et de Réanimation. Among adult general ICU risk adjusters are the Acute Physiology, Age, and Chronic Health Evaluation (APACHE II), the Simplified Acute Physiology Score (SAPS II), the Mortality Probability Model (MPM), and the Sequential Organ Failure Assessment (SOFA). Among methods for children are the Pediatric RISK of Mortality (PRISM) and the Score for Neonatal Acute Physiology (SNAP).
2. In June 1993, newly appointed HCFA administrator Bruce Vladeck halted production of the Medicare hospital mortality reports, concerned that they unfairly penalized inner-city public institutions, which routinely

had higher-than-expected death rates. The administrative data used for the HCFA reports did not allow adjustment for critical risk factors associated with poverty and medical indigence.

3. In a thoughtful and introspective article, William A. Knaus (2002) reflects on the development of APACHE—from his 1978 observations at the bedside of a dying patient, which first planted the idea—to the sale of APACHE Medical Systems, Inc., to Cerner Corp. in 2001. Knaus makes a compelling argument that moving from a research to commercial setting allowed further development of APACHE and facilitated its dissemination to hospitals throughout the country, with the goal of improving the quality of ICU care.

4. The reliance of the PIP-DCGs on principal inpatient diagnoses is ironic given the context (Iezzoni et al. 1998; Pope et al. 2000a). One way health maintenance organizations (HMOs) and now MCOs have controlled costs is by keeping their enrollees out of hospitals. The decision to use PIP-DCGs was driven completely by data concerns. Medicare had not previously required HMOs or MCOs to report diagnostic data on their patients as happens routinely in billing fee-for-service Medicare (see Chapter 5). Newly requiring diagnostic information to set health-based capitated payments would necessitate considerable investments by health plans, which at the time were also confronting expensive Y2K computer system upgrades. Medicare decided to start by requiring MCOs to report only information from hospitalizations, hence the choice of PIP-DCGs.

GETTING STARTED AND DEFINING TERMS

Lisa I. Iezzoni

The first step in risk adjustment is defining terms. Clinicians constantly use words such as "risk" assuming that their colleagues share common definitions. Starting in the 1980s, however, others within the health care marketplace adopted similar terms, spurred initially by Medicare's DRG-based prospective hospital payment. "Risk adjustment" joined other poorly defined but oft-used words and phrases—"case mix," "severity," "sickness," "intensity," "complexity," "comorbidity," "health status"—employed not only by clinicians and researchers but also by payers, policymakers, managers, regulators, quality assessors, performance profilers, and health insurance actuaries. These diverse groups often assign fundamentally different meanings to terms such as risk, thus complicating productive debate about critical health care issues.

Throughout this book, we use the phrase risk adjustment broadly: a generic reference to accounting for patient-related factors before examining outcomes of care, regardless of the context. We quickly become specific, though. Defining and then devising appropriate risk-adjustment strategies require answers to four major questions:

1. Risk of what outcome?
2. Over what time frame?
3. For what population?
4. For what purpose?

Other questions soon follow, such as, Considering what risk factors? Using what data source? Employing which analytic methods?

This chapter begins sketching answers to these questions, and the remaining chapters fill in more details. Throughout this book, we use examples from existing risk-adjustment methods. As described in Chapter 8, developing risk adjusters *de novo* is complicated and often frustrating. Therefore, we generally recommend taking methods "off the shelf" if their attributes match a project's goals reasonably well. Although some risk-adjustment methods are widely used for highly public purposes, such as setting payments or publishing performance reports, many more have been developed for disease-specific research projects. In this chapter, I draw examples from 11 diverse methods, well represented in the peer-reviewed, scholarly literature (Table 2.1). In later chapters, we introduce other risk-adjustment methods also described in research publications. We cannot exhaustively review existing approaches—the field is too big and grows almost daily—and details of many risk adjusters frequently change. Numerous commercial methods that are not reported in the scholarly literature are available. Primarily intended for managerial or administrative purposes, their complete logic is rarely open to external scrutiny.

Risk of What?

As stated in Chapter 1, the notion of risk permeates daily life. The word portends negative consequences: "1. The possibility of suffering harm or loss; danger. 2. A factor, thing, element, or course involving uncertain danger; a hazard" (*American Heritage Dictionary* 2000). However, the phrase risk adjustment is meaningless without first answering the question, Risk of what? Replies fall broadly into three camps: clinical outcomes of care, such as deaths, complications, and physical and mental functional status; resources used, such as costs or lengths of stay; and patient-centered outcomes, such as satisfaction that care met patients' preferences and expectations.

Two brief vignettes demonstrate differences among definitions of risk. Mr. A had an adenocarcinoma of the lung detected on a routine chest radiograph taken during an employment physical examination. Radiographically, the tumor looked like an isolated lung nodule. Mr. A had an extensive diagnostic evaluation to determine whether the disease had metastasized elsewhere. He received computed tomography (CT) scans of his chest and abdomen, nuclear medicine scans of his bones and liver, and eventually a needle biopsy of the nodule to make a tissue diagnosis. Finding no metastases, Mr. A underwent a lobectomy, a major operation to remove the tumor; he experienced no complications. Mr. A, a nonsmoker, is otherwise healthy, and his physicians believe he has a high likelihood of a surgical cure.

In contrast, Mr. B had widely metastatic adenocarcinoma of the lung. He had exhausted current aggressive therapies, and he desired to be kept comfortable as he neared death. He asked for "comfort measures only," avoiding even routine blood tests. Mr. B also wanted "do not resuscitate" (DNR) status: If his respirations or heart stopped, clinicians would not intervene. At home under hospice care, he was placed on a patient-controlled analgesia (PCA) pump, an intravenous line with a button Mr. B could push to administer medications to maintain his comfort. With loved ones at his bedside, Mr. B died.

Both scenarios involve lung adenocarcinoma. Mr. A had a high risk of incurring high costs (extensive diagnostic work up, major surgery), but he had a low risk of imminent death. In contrast, Mr. B's care was relatively inexpensive (home-based pain control), but he had a high risk of dying soon. Mr. A expected aggressive treatment; Mr. B desired to maintain comfort without intensive intervention. Mr. A and Mr. B chose clinicians and institutions that

Acronym	Name of Risk Adjuster; Vendor or Source	Internet Web Site
ACGs[a]	Adjusted Clinical Groups (formerly Ambulatory Care Groups); The Johns Hopkins University, Baltimore, MD (academic users), and CSC's Healthcare Group, Southfield, MI	http://www.acg.jhsph.edu http://www.csc.com/industries/ healthservices/offeringdetails/ 18.shtml
APACHE[b]	Acute Physiology and Chronic Health Evaluation	
I[c]	Original version (1981)	
II[d]	Second version (1985)	
III[e]	Third version (1991), with updates in 1998 (III-I) and 2002 (III-J); Cerner Corp., Kansas City, MO	http://www.cerner.com
APR-DRGs[b,f]	All Patient Refined Diagnosis Related Groups, 3M Health Information Systems, Wallingford, CT	http://www.3m.com/us/ healthcare/his/products/ coding/refined_drg.jhtml
CDPS[g]	Chronic Illness and Disability Payment System (formerly Disability Payment System); University of California San Diego	http://www.medicine.ucsd.edu/ fpm/cdps/
Medicaid Rx[h]	Prescription drug–based model	
CSI[®i]	Comprehensive Severity Index (formerly Computerized Severity Index); International Severity Information Systems, Salt Lake City, UT	http://www.isisicor.com/CSI
DCG/HCC[j]	Diagnostic Cost Groups/Hierarchical Condition Category; D_xCG,® Inc., Boston	http://www.dxcg.com
RxGroups®	Prescription drug–based model	
PIP-DCGs[k]	Principal Inpatient Diagnostic Cost Groups; D_xCG and CMS	http://www.cms.gov/ healthplans/rates/
DRGs[l]	Diagnosis Related Groups; CMS and 3M Health Information Systems, Wallingford, CT	
DS[b,m]	Disease Staging; The MEDSTAT Group, Ann Arbor, MI, part of the Thomson Corp.	http://www.medstat.com
Clinical	Clinical criteria version	
Coded Staging	Computerized version calculating disease categories and stages from discharge abstract data	
Scale	Computerized version calculating patient-level severity scales from discharge abstract data	
MedisGroups[®b,n]	Atlas 3.7; Cardinal Health—Clinical Information Management, Marlborough, MA (formerly MediQual)	http://www.mediqual.com
NSQIP[o]	National Surigical Quality Improvement Program; Department of Veterans Affairs, Washington, DC	http://www.nsqip.org
PRISM[p]	Pediatric Risk of Mortality Score	http://www.picues.org

TABLE 2.1

Examples of Risk Adjusters

[a]Starfield et al. (1991); Weiner et al. (1991, 1996a, 1996b, 1998); Tucker et al. (2002).
[b]Hughes et al. (1996); Iezzoni (1997); Iezzoni et al. (1995a, 1995b, 1996a, 1996b, 1996c, 1996d, 1996e, 1997); Landon et al. (1996); Shwartz et al. (1996a).

TABLE 2.1
Continued

[c]Knaus et al. (1981); Knaus (2002).

[d]Knaus et al. (1985, 1986); Knaus (2002); Société Française d'Anesthésie et de Réanimation (2002).

[e]Knaus et al. (1991, 1993); Knaus, Wagner, and Lynn (1991); Shortell et al. (1994); Knaus (2002).

[f]Edwards et al. (1994); Goldfield and Boland (1996); Chen et al. (1999); Romano and Chan (2000); Goldfield and Averill (2000).

[g]Kronick, Zhou, and Dreyfus (1995); Kronick et al. (1996, 2000); Payne et al. (2000).

[h]Gilmer et al. (2001).

[i]Horn et al. (1991, 2002); Averill et al. (1992); Iezzoni and Daley (1992); Horn, Sharkey, and Gassaway (1996); Willson et al. (2001).

[j]Ellis and Ash (1995); Ellis et al. (1996); Ash et al. (2000, 2001).

[k]Iezzoni et al. (1998); Pope et al. (1998, 2000a).

[l]Fetter et al. (1980); Vladeck (1984); *Federal Register*, Vol. 67, No. 148, 1 August 2002, pp. 49985–50248.

[m]Gonnella, Hornbrook, and Louis (1984); Conklin et al. (1984); Gonnella et al. (1990); Louis et al. (1999); Carpenter et al. (1999); Rattner et al. (2001).

[n]Brewster et al. (1985); Iezzoni and Moskowitz (1988); Steen et al. (1993); Steen (1994); Silber et al. (1997, 1999).

[o]Khuri et al. (1995, 1997, 1998, 2001); Khuri, Daley, and Henderson (1999); Daley et al. (1997); Daley, Henderson, and Khuri (2001).

[p]Pollack, Ruttimann, and Getson (1987, 1988); Pollack et al. (1994, 2000); Pollack, Patel, and Ruttimann (1996); Ruttimann, Pollack, and Fiser (1996).

best met their personal goals and clinical needs. Mr. A sought care at a major academic medical center, whereas Mr. B obtained care in his community, close to family and friends. Thus, comparisons of cost and mortality outcomes for lung cancer patients across different hospitals must account for differences in their patient mixes: Some institutions treat more Mr. As, whereas others see more Mr. Bs. Mr. As have high risks of incurring costs and low risks of dying, whereas Mr. Bs present the opposite scenario.

The selected risk-adjustment methods define risks differently, using either cost or clinical outcomes (Table 2.2).[1] Some methods offer multiple versions, targeting different outcomes. For example, APR-DRGs have two versions, one predicting hospital costs and the other predicting in-hospital mortality. When analysts obtain risk adjusters from a family of methods (like APR-DRGs, with its two versions), they must carefully use the appropriate version.

As suggested by the scenarios of Mr. A and Mr. B, risk adjusters designed to predict costs do less well at predicting deaths than methods derived specifically for mortality analyses. For example, when refining DRGs to improve their sensitivity to illness severity, researchers found that medical inpatients who died within two days of admission generated relatively low costs (Freeman et al. 1995). Risk-adjustment methods for one outcome may not work well for another. For instance, New York's risk adjustment for CABG mortality (see Chapter 1) is irrelevant for examining obstetrical complications; DRGs are suitable for acute care hospital payments but inappropriate for reimbursing rehabilitation hospitals or setting capitation levels. Therefore, the best strategy involves choosing a risk-adjustment method designed specifically for the target outcome. In other words, analysts and their risk adjusters should offer identical—or similar—answers when asked, Risk of what?

Method	Risk of What?	Pertinent Populations
ACGs	Resource consumption over the course of time based on morbidity profile; risk of high cost; disease markers	All persons within a general population
APACHE		
I	In-hospital mortality	Adults in ICUs
II	In-hospital mortality	Adults in ICUs
III	Multiple risk equations: in-hospital and ICU mortality and LOS, risk of active treatment, days on mechanical ventilation	Adults in ICUs
APR-DRGs	Two versions: resource use (also called "severity of illness") and in-hospital mortality	All hospitalized patients, including pediatric populations
CDPS	Total expenditures over the next year (prospective model) or present year (concurrent model)	Medicaid recipients (Temporary Aid to Needy Families and disabled); another version for Medicare beneficiaries
Medicaid R_x	Total expenditures over the next year for typical benefit package of an acute care HMO	Medicaid recipients
CSI	Physiologic complexity comprising the extent and interactions of patients' diseases presented to medical personnel	Separate componernts for: adult inpatients; pediatric inpatients; adult outpatients; pediatric outpatients; long-term care; hospice care; and rehabilitation care
DCG/HCC	Total expenditures over the next year (prospective model) or present year (concurrent model); several options, including truncating costs at $25,000, $50,000, and $100,000 and excluding pharmacy costs.	All persons within a general population (including versions for Medicare, Medicaid, and commercially insured)
RxGroups	Total expenditures (medical and pharmacy) over the next year (prospective model) or nonpharmacy expenditures this year (concurrent model)	All persons in a general commercial (privately insured, age < 65) population
PIP-DCGs	Total Medicare expenditures over the next year	Medicare managed care enrollees
DRGs	Total hospital charges or LOS	All hospitalized patients
DS		
Clinical	Complexity, etiology, and extent of organ system involvement	All patients with one or more of 600+ diseases covering all clinical conditions
Coded Staging	Complexity, etiology, and extent of organ system involvement	All patients
Scale	Definition depends on individual scale: total charges/costs, LOS, and in-hospital mortality	All hospitalized patients
MedisGroups	Admission-based mortality risk Midstay mortality risk	All hospitalized patients

TABLE 2.2

Definitions of Risk and Pertinent Populations

TABLE 2.2
Continued

Method	Risk of What?	Pertinent Populations
	Admission-based LOS	
	LOS outlier status	
	Preoperative CABG mortality risk	
	C-section risk (1° nulliparous)	
	C-section risk (2° multiparous)	
	C-section risk (repeat)	
NSQIP	Death within 30 days of major surgery; postopertive complications within 30 days of major surgery	Veterans undergoing major surgery in eight surgical specialities (general, cardiac, noncardiac thoracic, orthopedic, vascular, urology, otolaryngology, plastic)
PRISM	PICU mortality	Patients in PICUs

Over What Time Frame?

Risks must be framed within specific time windows. As an extreme example, calculating risks of death is moot if the time window involves lifetimes: Everybody faces a 100 percent risk of dying. Mr. A may not die for decades, whereas Mr. B's death occurred in a few weeks. Similarly, costs are typically measured within explicit time frames, such as a hospitalization or year of care. Time frames thus clarify the outcome of interest as well as suggest which risk factors are most important.

Chapter 4 addresses in detail the issues raised by different time frames. Perceptions of outcomes can change substantially with even small shifts in the window of observation. A pointed example comes from the CHQC program described in Chapter 1. The program existed from 1991 through 1997, during which Cleveland's absolute, risk-adjusted, in-hospital mortality rates declined by up to 4.8 percent (Baker et al. 2002a). Had quality of care actually improved, yielding such dramatic results? Probably not. When Baker and colleagues (2002a) looked instead at mortality 30 days after hospital admission (a fixed time window), relatively few changes had occurred. Between 1991 and 1997, deaths shifted from Cleveland hospitals to other settings soon after discharge.

The time frame generally determines the data sources and vice versa. For example, as described in Chapter 5, many studies rely on computerized hospital discharge abstracts; their diagnosis and procedure codes represent the entire hospitalization. Thus, the window of observation for discharge-abstract-based risk adjusters is, by definition, the complete hospital stay. In contrast, risk adjusters modeling hospital outcomes to identify quality shortfalls try to capture risk factors that predate care. Otherwise, serious clinical findings (potential risk factors) could become confounded or confused with substandard care (which can itself cause severe clinical derangements; see Chapter 4). For quality assessment, the time window for extracting risk factors helps determine the "attributional validity" of the risk-adjusted outcomes information—the likelihood that poor risk-adjusted outcomes reflect poor care rather than high patient risks (see Chapter 9). Narrower pretreatment time windows presumably have superior attributional validity to those with wider windows.

Table 2.3 shows the time windows for the selected risk adjusters alongside the timing of the data used to score risk and the classification approach (either a continuous rating, like a relative weight, or a category, like level 1, 2, 3, or 4). Risk adjusters predicting costs over a year often have two versions, both derived from computerized claims or encounter records filed during a year (see Chapter 5). "Concurrent" models use data from a particular year to predict costs for that same year, whereas "prospective" models predict costs for the following year. Obviously, predicting future costs is more difficult than modeling current costs. The preferred approach depends on the purpose.

For What Population?

By definition, the U.S. population is remarkably diverse. Many of us live daily exquisitely aware of this diversity. From the earliest moments of self-recognition, we learn our age, sex, skin color, language, and immediate world around us. As we grow, our interpretation of these basic dimensions modulates, and their meanings expand. Age becomes generation; sex becomes gender; skin color becomes race; language becomes ethnicity; and immediate world, with its myriad complexities, becomes culture. We develop other, sometimes shifting associations—with economic class, religion, occupational group, and political ideology.

These many dimensions, alone or in combinations, help delineate populations or subpopulations that often have very different risks for various health-related outcomes (see Chapter 3). Some distinctions are self-evident: Children, on average, face lower risks of imminent death than do persons in extreme old age. Women and men have different risks for certain diseases. As described in Chapter 3, troubling risks arise not from intrinsic individual factors (i.e., not from biological or physiological differences), but from disparities in the way people are treated within our health care system or society at large because of their characteristics.

Thus, the population of interest helps determine the range of risk factors required for assessing the specified outcome within the pertinent time frame. For example, when examining ICU mortality rates, the relevant physiologic parameters vary somewhat among neonates, children, and adults, although immediate acute findings are particularly relevant. Depending on how populations are defined, some outcomes are more pertinent than others. As noted in Chapter 1, this third edition of our book adds four chapters on specific populations: children (see Chapter 13); persons with mental health conditions (see

TABLE 2.3
Role of Diagnosis and Major Procedure in Quantifying Risk

Method	Role of Diagnosis	Role of Major Procedures
ACGs	Diagnosis from all patient encounters (inpatient and outpatient) used to assign persons to 1 of 32 ADGs	Procedure codes not used
APACHE		
I	Calculates APACHE score independent of diagnosis; calculates probability of death	Independent of major surgery
II	Calculates APACHE score independent of diagnosis; calculates probability of death using 50 disease categories	Distinguishes postoperative patients from others
III	Calculates APACHE score independent of diagnosis; calculates predictions using 78 disease categories; III-I and III-J use 434 diagnosis codes and 95 diagnostic categories	Distinguishes postoperative patients from others; does not predict outcomes for burn patients and most transplants
APR-DRGs	Subclasses within DRGs based largely on secondary diagnoses	Starts with DRG assignment (grouping major surgery cases by type of operation)
CDPS	Assignments based on patterns of outpatient and inpatient diagnoses	Independent of major surgery
Medicaid R_x	Diagnoses are proxied by prescription drugs	Independent of major procedures; uses codes for prescription drugs
CSI	Each diagnosis generates specific criteria used to calculate diagnosis-specific severity for each disease present (> 6,000 criteria sets); overall scores consider severity of all diagnoses	Independent of major surgery and other treatments; some criteria derived from diagnostic tests
DCG/HCC	Assignment based on patterns of outpatient and inpatient diagnoses	Independent of major procedures
RxGroups	Inpatient diagnoses using DCG/HCC classification in one version	Independent of major procedures; uses codes for prescription drugs
PIP-DCGs	For most persons, uses principal diagnosis only from acute care hospitalizations	Independent of major procedures
DRGs	Groups medical cases by diagnosis	Groups major surgery cases by type of operation
DS		
Clinical	Clinical criteria within diagnosis categories	Independent of major procedures
Coded Staging	Diagnosis specific	Generally independent of ICD-9-CM procedures, except for C-sections
MedisGroups	Diagnosis specific	Independent of major procedures
NSQIP	Diagnoses important as comorbid conditions	Risk-adjustment models specific to surgical specialty or major surgery type (e.g., abdominal aortic aneurysm)
PRISM	Includes diagnosis in calculating mortality risk	Operative status is a risk factor

Chapter 14); persons with disabilities (see Chapter 15); and individuals receiving long-term care in institutional and home-based settings (see Chapter 16). Especially relevant outcomes vary across these populations. Although children experience similar life-and-death outcomes as adults, albeit at different rates, specific functional outcomes differ (e.g., school performance and developmental milestones for children; productive employment for working-age adults). Important outcomes for persons with psychiatric disorders emphasize mental and emotional health and ability to perform routine social roles. For persons with disabilities and long-term-care populations, functional abilities and performance of daily activities are key outcomes.

Table 2.2 lists the populations targeted by selected risk adjusters. Obviously, the target population reflects the underlying purpose of the developers of the risk-adjustment method: For example, the designers of PRISM were explicitly interested in children treated in ICUs. The purpose often helps determine the data source and thus sometimes defines the population. The developers of CDPS, for example, wanted to create a method to capitate payments specifically for Medicaid recipients. By using Medicaid databases, they thus created a risk adjuster calibrated to poor persons, primarily impoverished women and their children, and persons with disabilities.

For What Purpose?

Answers to the three previous questions (risk of what, time frame, and population) are obviously driven by the purpose of using risk adjustment—or of assessing outcomes at all. As described in Chapter 1, the underlying motivation of risk adjustment is comparison: contrasting outcomes or performance for individual patients, groups of patients, or populations to those of their counterparts. Potential purposes include

- setting payment levels for individual patients (e.g., DRGs for hospitalizations) or health plan enrollees (e.g., capitation payments);
- encouraging providers or health plans to treat or accept high-cost or potentially high-risk patients;
- comparing efficiency and costs of care across providers or health plans;
- producing public report cards about performance of individual providers, as in Cleveland and New York state (see Chapters 1 and 12); and
- internal comparisons of patient outcomes across physicians within an individual practice setting to motivate quality improvement (see Chapter 8).

The purpose dictates how well the risk adjuster must itself perform to succeed (i.e., to produce valid comparisons; see Chapter 9). For example, methods designed to predict costs over one year rely on administrative data, which are often messy and contain limited clinical information (see Chapter 5);

these risk adjusters typically explain less than 10 percent of the variation in future costs. Nevertheless, this performance is far superior to adjustments using only demographic information (e.g., age, sex), and it meets the needs of important purchasers like Medicare and Medicaid. In contrast, another purpose for risk adjustment is to motivate quality improvement. Without this adjustment, providers with poor outcomes could argue that they are treated unfairly: "My patients are sicker; that's why my results are worse." Most clinicians stipulate that risk adjusters must be clinically credible before they will believe and act on the results. Meeting these expectations can require additional data collection and in-depth review of the clinical logic underlying the risk-adjustment model (see Chapter 8).

No risk adjuster is ever perfect. Adjusting for all patient characteristics is neither necessary nor possible. Therefore, efforts shift to identifying those that are sufficiently valid for the explicit purpose. Statistical measures of model performance (e.g., percentage of variation explained; see Chapter 10) cannot determine validity alone. Such statistical measures reveal little about whether systematic errors in predictions occur for selected subpopulations or whether important risk factors are included appropriately. Complicating matters, risk adjusters with similar predictive abilities can give different answers about whether outcomes are statistically different from expected values for particular comparison groups, such as hospitals (Iezzoni et al. 1995a, 1996a, 1996e; Poses et al. 2000). Our study of hospital-based severity measures (see Chapter 1) found that DS had the highest statistical performance for predicting in-hospital deaths for acute myocardial infarction (AMI), APR-DRGs for CABG, and MedisGroups for pneumonia and stroke (Iezzoni 1997). Different severity measures predicted different probabilities of death for many patients, and they frequently disagreed about which hospitals had particularly low or high risk-adjusted death rates. Agreement in identifying low- and high-mortality hospitals between severity-adjusted and unadjusted death rates was often better than agreement between severity measures.

For some purposes, ethical concerns raise questions about whether and how to risk adjust. This happens when persons with certain attributes (e.g., gender, race, socioeconomic status) that might be potential risk factors for given outcomes simultaneously face the likelihood of receiving substandard care precisely because of those attributes. An example involves performance reports comparing rates of routine screening tests or preventive services for enrollees of different health plans. Outcomes (here, technically processes of care[2]) that require positive actions by patients (e.g., obtaining a mammogram, bringing an infant for immunization) raise special concerns. Education, motivation, wherewithal (e.g., transportation, child care, time off from work), preferences for care and outcomes, cultural concerns, and a host of other factors affect these actions. Different health plans and providers see different mixes of patients along these critical dimensions. Therefore, from a purist's perspective, risk adjustment is indicated. After all, evidence suggests that racial and ethnic minorities and persons with low socioeconomic status obtain these services at lower rates. However, as Romano (2000, 978) observed:

> Before instituting case-mix adjustment of health plan or provider per-formance measures, we must consider both the hidden assumptions and the potential consequences. One assumption is that persons of lower socioeconomic status *inherently* use preventive services less than persons of higher socioeconomic status. If culturally sensitive, readily accessible systems of care can eliminate or substantially reduce sociodemographic disparities . . . , then adjusting for case mix would implicitly "excuse" health plans for failing to implement disparity-reducing innovations. . . . [Plans might also find that] it is easier to boost [their] scores by focusing on better educated, easier-to-reach members. A related implication is that we should accept lower performance, or set lower performance targets, for plans that enroll diverse populations.

Therefore, risk adjusting for these attributes seems inappropriate, given the ultimate purpose of using outcomes data to motivate improvement for all patients. Risk stratification, described in Chapter 3, offers a simple solution that could also yield useful insight about how different subpopulations fare.

Additional Considerations

Answering these four major questions is simply the beginning; many important issues remain. The most crucial practical consideration is the data source. Will the risk adjuster rely on standard, coded administrative data (see Chapter 5), clinical information from medical records (see Chapter 6), or responses directly from patients (see Chapter 7)? Table 2.4 lists the data sources for selected risk adjusters. The nature of the database helps shape how the risk-adjustment method will be designed: With large data sets, analysts can develop and test risk adjusters empirically, whereas without such data, measures must rely on clinical judgment. As described in Chapter 8, the most statistically and conceptually robust risk adjusters generally result from interactions between clinicians and statistical modeling.

The data also delimit the range of candidate risk factors (see Chapter 3). Especially when predicting costs, one important distinction involves whether the risk adjuster considers procedure use (Table 2.5). Methods aiming to predict short-term costs (e.g., DRGs) rely heavily on procedural information, particularly the presence and type of major surgery: The costs of operations generally overwhelm costs of medical or recuperative care. Not surprisingly, DRGs overall are poor risk adjusters for hospital mortality, although they per-form slightly better within surgical DRGs (Hofer and Hayward 1996). Because the use of many procedures is highly discretionary, risk adjusters targeting clin-ical outcomes generally eschew procedures in rating risk (see Chapter 3). As

TABLE 2.4

Data Requirements and Development of Methods

Method	Data Requirements	Development Approach
ACGs	ICD-9-CM diagnosis codes, age, sex	Clinical judgment to create basic framework; commonly occurring morbidity patterns and empirical modeling used to categorize individuals
APACHE		
I	Values of 34 acute physiologic parameters and limited other clinical information	Clinical judgment
II	Values of 12 acute physiologic parameters and limited other clinical information	Clinical judgment with some empirical modeling
III	Values of 17 acute physiologic parameters and limited other clinical information (including age, chronic health conditions)	Empirical modeling with some clinical judgment
APR-DRGs	Computerized discharge abstract data, birthweight	Clinical judgment to create basic framework, then empirical modeling
CDPS	Diagnosis codes taken from hospital or physician claims or encounter records	Clinical judgment to create basic framework, then empirical modeling
Medicaid R$_x$	NDCs on pharmacy claims from Medicaid administrative data	Review of literature, consultation with clinical experts to create basic framework, then empirical modeling
CSI	Disease-specific clinical factors; identifies diseases using groupings of > 19,000 ICD-9-CM diagnosis codes; each code matched to disease-specific criteria set	Clinical judgment; in some instances, final calibration based on data concerning LOS, cost, and mortality
DCG/HCC	Diagnosis codes taken from hospital or physician claims or encounter records	Clinical judgment to create basic framework, then empirical modeling
RxGroups	NDCs from outpatient pharmacy claims, either alone or in conjunction with inpatient diagnoses	Clinical judgment, then empirical modeling
PIP-DCGs	Computerized hospital discharge abstracts and Medicare enrollment and eligibility information	Clinical judgment to create basic framework, then empirical modeling
DRGs	Computerized discharge abstract data	Clinical judgment to create basic framework, then empirical modeling
DS		
Clinical	Clinical information, including diagnostic test results	Clinical judgment and peer-reviewed literature
Coded Staging	Computerized discharge abstract data	Clinical judgment
Scale	Computerized discharge abstract data	Empirical modeling using DRGs, diseases, and stages
MedisGroups	250+ "key clinical findings" (KCFs)	Empirical modeling: logistic regression for mortality and C-section outcomes; multiple linear regression for LOS

Method	Data Requirements	Development Approach	**TABLE 2.4** Continued
NSQIP	Information from clinical data systems on 60 preoperative risk factors, 17 intraoperative characteristics, and 33 outcome variables	Literature review, clinical judgment, and empirical modeling; final models reviewed for clinical credibility	
PRISM	14 acute physiologic variables and limited clinical information	Clinical judgment to create framework, then empirical modeling	
PRISM III	17 acute physiologic variables and limited clinical information	Empirical modeling	

pharmacy data become increasingly available, some risk adjusters employ that information to proxy disease burden.

Finally, choosing appropriate and reasonable analytic techniques raises important questions. As described in Chapter 11, risk adjustment is often used to examine results within observational studies—where patients are not assigned randomly to various treatments or care plans. Sample sizes are frequently small. Often, there is no single "right" way to analyze the data. Nevertheless, analytic choices can carry important implications, as suggested in Chapters 10 through 12. Keeping these implications in mind is essential for meaningful interpretation of risk-adjusted outcomes information.

Even after risk adjustment, questions frequently remain about what comparative outcomes information really means. For example, even with optimal risk adjustment, do risk-adjusted mortality rates provide meaningful clues about hospital quality (Thomas and Hofer 1999)? Answering this question in a meaningful fashion may prove even more vexing than designing the risk-adjustment methodology. As Nightingale and Codman might say (see Chapter 1), however, this question about quality finally highlights the ultimate purpose of gathering and analyzing the data: to motivate and guide improvements.

Notes

1. Initiatives comparing patient satisfaction have not used risk adjusters like those in the Chapter 2 tables to risk adjust satisfaction rates. Instead, a few well-selected questions about potential risk factors are included in the satisfaction survey. For example, most satisfaction measures risk adjust using respondents' self-reported overall health status. Chapter 7 examines this in greater detail using the Consumer Assessment of Health Plans Study (CAHPS) as an example.
2. Performance measures are often sorted into two types—outcomes and processes. Outcomes, or how patients do, generally have a clear rationale for requiring risk adjustment (see Chapter 1). Process measures, or what is done for patients, can also warrant risk adjustment, although

TABLE 2.5
Window of
Observation
and
Classification
Approach

Method	Window of Observation	Classification Approach
ACGs	Typically one year	ADGs: all ICD-9-CM codes are assigned to 32 categories based on the expected effect of diagnosis on health service use ACGs: 81–93 (depending on chosen options) mutually exclusive actuarial cells based on morbidity patterns and recursive partitioning algorithm
APACHE	Hospital admission	
I	Admission scores taken from worst value over first 32 hours after ICU admission	Integer scores from 0 to 50
II	Admission scores taken from worst value over first 24 hours after ICU admission	Integer scores from 0 to 71
III	Admission scores taken from worst value over first 8–32 hours after ICU admission; scores, mortality, and active treatment can be computed for every ICU day	Integer scores from 0 to 299
APR-DRGs	Discharge abstract: entire hospitalization	Divides most DRGs into four complexity subclasses: minor, moderate, major, or extreme
CDPS	Current year or next year: uses claims or encounter records from entire year	Diagnoses assigned to clinically homogeneous CDPS subcategories; 57 subcategories recommended for use in prospective risk-adjustment models; individuals assigned relative weight based on age, sex, patterns of CDPS subcategories, and category of Medicaid assistance
Medicaid R_x	Uses claims from base year	NDCs assigned to 48 categories; individuals assigned relative-weight-based on NDC categories and other characteristics
CSI	For hospitalizations: admission review covers first 24 hours, discharge review covers last 24 hours, maximum severity score covers entire hospital stay; scores can be computed for any time window depending on purpose For outpatients: clinical findings from encounter generate severity score; long-term and hospice care can use varying time windows; severity score based on most abnormal clinical findings during window	Scores 1, 2, 3, or 4 for each individual disease; scores 1, 2, 3, or 4 for all diseases combined; "continuous scores" (integer $\geq$ 0) for all diseases combined
DCG/HCC	Current year or next year: uses claims or encounter records from entire year	Diagnoses assigned to 781 DxGroups; DxGroups assigned to 184 Condition Categories (CCs); CCs grouped into clinically

TABLE 2.5
Continued

Method	Window of Observation	Classification Approach
		homogenous hierarchies (HCCs); individuals are assigned relative weight based on age, sex, and pattern of CCs and HCCs
RxGroups	Current year or next year; claims from entire year recommended	NDCs grouped into 155 RxGroups based on therapeutic functionality; individuals assigned relative weights based on age, sex, and pattern of RxGroups (and, when available, HCCs based on inpatient diagnoses)
PIP-DCGs	Next year; uses claims or encounter records from entire year	Persons are sorted into 15 PIP-DCGs; payments are determined by age, sex, PIP-DCG, originally disabled Medicare eligibility, and Medicaid status
DRGs	Discharge abstract: entire hospitalization	For FY 2003, 510 DRGs within 25 major diagnostic categories (MDCs); each DRG assigned a relative payment weight
DS	Depends on purpose	
Clinical	Determined by user; could encompass any period	Within 600+ conditions, assigns stages 0, 1.0, 2.0, or 3.0, with substages
Coded Staging	Computerized abstract: entire hospitalization or ambulatory period	Stages 0, 1.0, 2.0, or 3.0, with substages possible; number of substages varies across diseases
Scale	Discharge abstract: entire hospitalization	Relative weight with 100 as an average (e.g., a weight of 115 is 15 percent more than average)
MedisGroups	Hospital admission: Review 1—days 0–1; review 2—days 2–5; selected KCFs allowed up to 30 days preadmission	Mortality predicted as probability (0–1) and classified nonlinearly into one of five score groups (0–4); LOS predicted in hospital days; mortality and LOS modeled for 73 disease groups (MedisGroups); C-section predicted as probability (0–1)
NSQIP	Preoperative information prior to major surgery; intraoperative data; postoperative surveillance for 30 days; all data either directly downloaded from computerized clinical information systems or abstracted	Predictions based on multivariable logistic regression models
PRISM	PICU admission day data	Integer score from 0 to 76
PRISM III	Data for initial 12 hours or 24 hours of PICU care	Integer score from 0 to 74

the conceptualization of the measures dictates the extent of adjustment required. Some observers increasingly blur the semantics distinguishing outcome from process measures: For example, is obtaining a mammogram an outcome or process of care? Many quintessential process measures build in explicit information about patient characteristics that are essentially risk factors for obtaining the service. For example, use of beta-blockers after an AMI is a widely accepted process measure, but with the stipulation that patients not have any of a list of contraindications. Risk adjustment involving contraindications becomes moot.

RANGE OF RISK FACTORS

Lisa I. Iezzoni

Human beings are complex and multidimensional. We function on innumerable levels within multiple spheres—as biological organisms powered by miraculously engineered physiologic forces; as thinkers and communicators who shape and are shaped by our environments; as members of families, communities, and cultures; and as individuals with goals, preferences, and expectations about our lives and futures. From the mundane to the existential, these varied dimensions hold implications for our health, some directly, others more circuitously. As such, each could become a patient-specific risk factor in a risk-adjustment methodology!

Perhaps the most important feature of any risk-adjustment approach involves its set of risk factors—which risk factors are included and how they are represented and handled analytically. The scope of risk factors determines whether risk-adjusted results are credible and valid (see Chapters 8 and 9). The risk factors dictate the "medical meaningfulness" of a risk adjuster: "the extent to which knowledge of a patient's case type alone—without other information about the individual patient—conveys clinical expectations and enables clinicians to exchange information about those expectations" (Wood, Ament, and Kobrinski 1981, 249). Given that the ultimate goal of risk-adjusted information is frequently to affect clinicians' behavior or gain their cooperation, medical meaningfulness is crucial.

No risk-adjustment method can ever account for all relevant risk factors. As described in Chapters 5 through 7, data limitations pose immutable constraints: Gathering information on all potential risk factors is logistically and practically infeasible. Because risk-adjustment methods will never be perfect, the question becomes, how credible and trustworthy are our findings when we use risk-adjustment method X in the following way to answer question Y (see Chapter 9)? Addressing this question requires an *a priori* conceptual model of which risk factors should be in a risk-adjustment method for a given outcome, time window, population, and purpose. Then, one can identify those risk factors not considered by the risk-adjustment method. Understanding which risk factors are conceptually important but excluded (generally for practical reasons) suggests how cautiously or confidently one can interpret risk-adjusted results. Are the findings believable? Do differences in outcomes result from unmeasured risk factors or from variations in therapeutic effectiveness, quality of care, efficiency, or another aspect of care?

This chapter enumerates and describes selected human attributes that might be important risk factors in specific settings. Table 3.1 lists risk factors by broad category, and Table 3.2 presents brief clinical synopses reflecting these risk factors. Implied distinctions among these attributes are artificial: Concepts often overlap and are seldom clinically separable, especially for individual patients. I discuss them individually to organize a systematic review of wide-ranging, intertwined characteristics, recognizing that the relevance of particular risk factors varies by outcome, time window, population, and purpose of risk adjustment. Chapter 4 considers how the window of observation affects the role of various risk factors. Chapter 8 describes how researchers might choose conceptually among risk factors and how to use risk factor information empirically to derive risk-adjustment methods.

Age

A patient's age cannot change regardless of the effectiveness, efficiency, or quality of care. For epidemiologic studies across populations, accounting for age is essential. Aging is closely linked to significant chronic conditions, such as cardiovascular disease, certain cancers, diabetes, and osteoarthritis. Surveys of older persons suggest that rates of serious functional limitations have declined importantly over recent years (Manton, Corder, and Stallard 1997; Manton and Gu 2001; Cutler 2001). Nevertheless, if disease prevalence patterns remain unchanged, the number of older Americans with functional limitations largely caused by chronic conditions will rise by at least 311 percent by 2049 (Boult et al. 1996, 1391).

The physiology of aging remains elusive, likely related to complex interplays among genetics, environment, and biological aging processes (Perls 2002). On average, however, older persons have worse clinical outcomes than younger persons. Symptoms and signs of disease can differ between older and younger patients. For example, as age increases, pneumonia patients become less likely to report nonrespiratory and respiratory symptoms, despite having active infections (Metlay et al. 1997). The cost of acute care for older persons can exceed that for younger patients because of prolonged recuperative periods and greater incidence of complications. On the other hand, since elderly patients frequently receive less aggressive treatment, their care can be less expensive than that for younger adults.

In assessing overall patient risk, age can have an independent effect regardless of other risk factors. Even for gravely ill patients in ICUs, age independently predicts imminent death regardless of the extent of organ system failure. APACHE III, designed to predict in-hospital mortality for ICU patients, assigns separate points for age to its score, ranging from 0 points for those younger than 45 years old to 24 points for persons at least 85 years old (Knaus et al. 1991, 1624).[1]

Depending on the clinical setting, other dimensions of risk should be viewed within the context of patients' age. One obvious distinction is

TABLE 3.1

Range of Risk
Factors

Demographic characteristics
- Age
- Sex
- Race and ethnicity

Clinical factors
- Acute physiologic stability
- Principal diagnosis ("case mix")
- Severity of principal diagnosis
- Extent and severity of comorbidities
- Physical functional status
- Cognitive status
- Mental health

Socioeconomic factors
- Familial characteristics and household composition
- Educational attainment, health literacy
- Economic resources
- Employment and occupation
- Housing and neighborhood characteristics
- Health insurance coverage
- Cultural beliefs and behaviors

Health-related behaviors and activities
- Tobacco use
- Alcohol use
- Use of illicit drugs
- Sexual practices ("safe sex")
- Diet and nutrition
- Obesity and overweight

Attitudes and perceptions
- Overall health status and quality of life
- Religious beliefs and behaviors
- Preferences and expectations for health care services

among newborns, children, and adults. The Pediatric Risk of Mortality Score (PRISM) uses 14 physiologic variables to predict in-hospital mortality for PICU patients. In assigning points, PRISM employs different ranges for systolic blood pressure, heart rate, and respiratory rate depending on the patient's age, for example, 7 points for systolic blood pressures of less than 40 mm Hg for infants and less than 50 mm Hg for children (Pollack, Ruttimann, and Getson 1988, 1113). Calculations of the probability of in-hospital mortality include not only PRISM scores but also patient age in months. Thus, PRISM weights certain physiologic risk factors differently by patient age but also treats age as an independent predictor of death.

Neonatal populations present special dilemmas for capturing age effects. Developers of the Score for Neonatal Acute Physiology, Perinatal Extension, Version II (SNAPPE-II) wanted to use gestational age rather than birthweight as a risk factor for neonatal ICU (NICU) mortality; they viewed gestational age as a more clinically valid indicator of neonatal physiology

TABLE 3.2
Ten Clinical Synopses: Adenocarcinoma of the Colon

Patient	Clinical Synopsis
A	No symptoms. Microscopic nidus of well-differentiated adenocarcinoma found in polyp during a routine screening colonoscopy. Considered a surgical cure. Otherwise in good health.
B	No symptoms. Microscopic nidus of well-differentiated adenocarcinoma found in polyp during a routine screening colonoscopy. Considered a surgical cure. History of stroke one year ago. Partially paralyzed on right side of body; has difficulty speaking.
C	No symptoms. Microscopic nidus of well-differentiated adenocarcinoma found in polyp during a routine screening colonoscopy. Considered a surgical cure. Patient refused medication to treat serious depression; recently lost job. No known family or friends.
D	Patient septic with *Clostridium perfringens* bacteria. Polyp found on colonoscopy; microscopic nidus of well-diferentiated adenocarcinoma found in polyp. Otherwise in good health.
E	Large adenocarcinoma with invasion deep into wall of colon. No evidence of distant metastases. Otherwise in good health.
F	Large adenocarcinoma with invasion deep into wall of colon. No evidence of distant metastases. History of poorly controlled essential hypertension, with routine blood pressure readings of 164/94 mm Hg.
G	Large adenocarcinoma causing bowel obstruction. No evidence of distant metastases. Patient acutely septic and in shock.
H	Widespread metastatic disease. Patient desires active intervention, including ICU admission and intubation if necessary.
I	Widespread metastatic disease. Patient requests DNR status, desiring "comfort measures only."
J	Patient doing well during admission but dies unexpectedly.
K	Patient doing poorly during admission and dies as expected.

(Richardson et al. 2001). However, difficulties collecting accurate gestational age data led them to use birthweight instead.

Standard statistical measures, such as c and R^2 values (see Chapter 10), quantifying how well age explains various outcomes are typically unimpressive. In a study of 30-day postadmission mortality for elderly Medicare patients, age and sex explained only 1 to 3 percent of variation in deaths (Keeler et al. 1990, 1967). In another study, age and sex produced modest c-statistics for predicting in-hospital mortality: 0.69 for AMI (Iezzoni et al. 1996e), 0.67 for pneumonia (Iezzoni et al. 1996a), and 0.60 for stroke (Iezzoni et al. 1995a). Among gravely ill patients, age added little to predictions of six-month survival after adjusting for illness severity and baseline functional status (Hamel et al. 1999a).

The importance of age may depend on the age ranges within the study populations and the outcome of interest. When examining "adults" defined as over 17 years of age, separating patients into younger and older strata may offer insight. For instance, we compared illness severity among roughly 4,500 adult inpatients at teaching and nonteaching hospitals in metropolitan Boston (Iezzoni et al. 1990). Severity patterns by hospital teaching status varied by age strata across different disease groups. Only younger patients appeared sicker at teaching compared to nonteaching hospitals for coronary artery disease and low back pain; AMI severity was higher at teaching facilities for both younger and older patients. We hypothesized that patient preferences and practice patterns may cause certain differences: Younger and older patients may vary in their willingness to travel to distant, inner-city hospitals or to seek intensive, high-technology care.

Increasing numbers are joining the "oldest old," variably defined as age above 80 or 85 years. Many believe that these persons differ physiologically from younger patients, even holding constant other factors like disease severity. Very old patients have lower "physiologic reserves," or ability to rebound from the physical assaults of acute illness, and are more likely to develop complications. Despite this, carefully selected oldest old patients benefit significantly from major surgery, with improved postoperative functional status. Between 1987 and 1995 for men age 85 and older, the average annual rates of procedures grew 15 percent for CABG, 22 percent for angioplasty, 11 percent for carotid endarterectomy, and 26 percent for hip replacement (Fuchs 1999, 14).[2] Centenarians, a special subclass of oldest old patients, frequently remain in good health until the very end of their lives (Perls et al. 2002).

Nonetheless, when adjusting for age in observational studies, the possibility of "ageism" merits consideration. Although increasing numbers of elderly patients get sophisticated invasive treatments, older patients sometimes receive less intensive therapy than younger patients with similar clinical presentations and preferences (Hamel et al. 1999b, 2000). Ageism may cause undertreatment or mistreatment of elderly compared to younger patients (Greenfield et al. 1987; Bennett et al. 1991; Montague et al. 1991). Disentangling ageism from varying preferences among older patients is, however, important. Accounting for detailed clinical findings and other patient factors (e.g., refusal of therapy) can explain differences in treatment between older and younger cancer patients (Guadagnoli et al. 1997; Velanovich et al. 2002). One study found that, although elderly cancer patients received less aggressive care, they spent more time discussing limitations of treatments with their physicians (Rose et al. 2000). Older patients may have different expectations of health care services and are often more satisfied than younger patients. Among major elective surgery patients, elderly persons had similar global health perceptions to younger patients, despite worse role and physical function, energy, and fatigue (Mangione et al. 1993).

Age is simple and straightforward, with good face validity as an important risk factor. Information on age is almost always available, and users expect age to appear in risk-adjustment models. While often statistically insignificant, age is easy to understand and explain. Including age is therefore standard in risk adjustment.

Sex and Gender

Women and men differ chromosomally, anatomically, physiologically, and hormonally. Men and women also face divergent risks for certain diseases and death by age strata, with longer average life spans for women than men. In the United States in 2000, among persons age 65 years and older, men had higher crude death rates than women for heart disease, malignant neoplasms, chronic lower respiratory disease, influenza and pneumonia, and diabetes mellitus, whereas cerebrovascular disease death rates were higher for women (Anderson 2002, 17, 19). Identical patterns pertained to persons age 85 years and older. Controlling for sex is therefore crucial for epidemiological studies of long-term population outcomes.

However, differences between men and women transcend biological considerations. As Gesensway (2001, 936) observed:

> Research now shows that sex matters beyond the hormonal, anatomic, physiologic, and reproductive differences that make men men and women women. Socioeconomic circumstances that influence women's lives differently from men's—such as parenthood, poverty, or violence—can lead women to develop or react to diseases and treatments differently from men. Well-documented differences in the communication and human interaction styles of men and women affect how each sex uses the health care system, describes illnesses, or participates in decision-making with a physician.

The distinction between "sex" and "gender" is emblematic. Sex typically refers to the chromosomally mediated distinction between men and women as physical beings, whereas gender introduces concepts relating to social roles.

The historical exclusion of women from efficacy trials of new treatments hinders creation of *a priori* hypotheses about sex as a clinical risk factor.[3] The National Institutes of Health Revitalization Act, passed in 1993, aimed to remedy this problem by requiring inclusion of women and racial and ethnic minorities in clinical research, as methodologically appropriate. However, reviews of journal articles through 1998 and 1999 suggest that women remain outside clinical studies; only roughly one-fifth of published studies included women (Vidaver et al. 2000; Ramasubbu, Gurm, and Litaker 2001). Among studies that did include women, relatively few analyzed results by the sex of study subjects.

Sex only modestly predicts many short-term outcomes. Neither APACHE III (Knaus et al. 1991) nor PRISM (Pollack, Ruttimann, and Getson 1988) includes sex in its predictive model. A large study of Medicare beneficiaries found that sex significantly predicted 30-day posthospitalization mortality for only one of five conditions—hip fracture—with men having higher risks of death than women (Keeler et al. 1990). A study of almost 90,000 patients admitted for one of six common medical diagnoses controlled for risk using clinical findings abstracted from medical records (Gordon and Rosenthal 1999).[4] Adjusting for clinical risk factors, including DNR status, men were significantly more likely to die in hospital than women for four conditions and equally likely for two.

A growing literature raises questions about disparities in treatment between men and women, especially for cardiovascular interventions. Heart disease is the leading cause of death for women, although many women fail to recognize this. Women and men appear equally willing to undergo invasive cardiovascular procedures (Saha, Stettin, and Redberg 1999). Nevertheless, many studies suggest that women with coronary artery disease receive fewer invasive diagnostic and therapeutic procedures and have higher in-hospital death or complication rates than men (Steingart et al. 1991; Ayanian and Epstein 1991; Udvarhelyi et al. 1992; Krumholz et al. 1992; Bickell et al. 1992; Shaw et al. 1994; Capdeville, Lee, and Taylor 2001; Watanabe, Maynard, and Ritchie 2001). In contrast, other studies failed to find significant sex differences in coronary artery procedures or outcomes after controlling for important risk factors (O'Connor et al. 1993; Mark et al. 1994; Hannan et al. 1999; Jacobs et al. 2002; Rathore et al. 2002).

We examined in-hospital death and use of coronary angiography, CABG, and percutaneous transluminal coronary angioplasty (PTCA) for 14,083 AMI patients admitted in 1991 (Iezzoni et al. 1997). Our study examined ten risk adjusters, six based on administrative data and four derived from clinical information. The severity measures differed about whether women were sicker than men,[5] although women frequently had severe clinical findings on admission (Table 3.3). After adjusting for severity and age, women were significantly more likely than men to die in hospital and less likely to receive coronary angiography and CABG; PTCA was similar by sex. All ten risk adjusters produced comparable odds ratios reflecting sex differences in procedure utilization and death rates.

As with age, sex is a simple, routinely available, easily measured variable with reasonable face validity as a risk factor in certain settings. Nonetheless, suspicions about gender bias in treatment decisions need further exploration and could confound risk-adjusted outcome assessments. Stratifying analyses—examining risk-adjusted results separately for men and women—could allay this concern.

TABLE 3.3

Percentage of Patients with Clinical Findings on Admission

| Clinical Finding | Percent with Clinical Findings by Case Type and by Sex | | | | | |
| | Medical Cases | | CABG Cases | | All Cases | |
	Men	Women	Men	Women	Men	Women
CHF on admission	11.0	17.1*	5.8	8.0	9.2	15.4*
Pulmonary edema on admission	5.5	7.3*	2.9	6.2+	4.6	6.6*
Coma on admission	3.5	4.6**	0.7	1.1	2.8	4.1*
Low systolic blood pressure ($\leq$ 60 mm Hg) on admission	3.4	5.0*	1.0	2.2	2.8	4.5*
Low left ventricular ejection fraction ($\leq$ 35%)	6.2	5.5	9.2	6.9	6.5	5.6+
Elevated blood urea nitrogen (BUN $\geq$ 31) on admission	14.3	19.8*	4.1	6.9	11.8	17.8*

SOURCE: Adapted from Iezzoni et al. (1997).
*$p \leq 0.0001$; **$0.0001 < p \leq 0.001$; + $0.01 < p \leq 0.05$.

Race and Ethnicity

Several parallels with sex arise when viewing race and ethnicity as risk factors. As with sex, well-documented differences exist in disease prevalence and leading causes of death by race and ethnicity. The high prevalence of accidents, human immunodeficiency virus (HIV) infection, and suicide in some subpopulations defined by race and ethnicity (Anderson 2002) suggests that social forces drive many of these patterns—differences are not genetic or biological. As with sex, generating *a priori* hypotheses about the clinical effect of racial or ethnic differences is hampered by the historical exclusion of minorities from therapeutic trials (Svensson 1989). Pointed and unresolved ethical questions, notably those raised by the horrific Tuskegee Syphilis Study, chill efforts to recruit black persons as experimental subjects (Corbie-Smith et al. 1999). A review of heart failure clinical trials from 1985 through 1999 showed no improvement in the involvement of black men and women (Heiat, Gross, and Krumholz 2002).

Unlike sex, however, race and ethnicity are hard to capture in a clear, consistent, and meaningful fashion. Race, ethnicity, and other ancestral identifications are not scientifically credible categories. "Race is a social category, not a biological concept. . . . What is actually measured by the race variable is skin color" (LaVeist 1994, 2, 11). The U.S. Bureau of the Census has collected data on race since the first decennial census in 1790, which counted three racial categories: "whites, blacks as three-fifths of a person and only those Indians who paid taxes" (Williams 1999, 121).[6] Since 1977, Statistical Policy Directive No. 15, promulgated by the Office of Management and Budget (OMB 2002), has set federal standards for gathering racial and ethnic data. Extensive study following the 1990 census examined strategies to allow persons to self-identify more than one race and led the OMB to significantly revise Directive No. 15. Beginning with the 2000 census, Directive No. 15 stipulated that two separate questions be asked, one about race, another about ethnicity. Data on race involve at least five categories: American Indian or Alaska Native, Asian, Black or African American, Native Hawaiian or Other Pacific Islander, and White. If persons wish to self-identify more than one race, they may do so, but a single "multiracial" category is not included. Ethnicity is captured through two categories: Hispanic or Latino and Not Hispanic or Latino. All federal programs were to have implemented OMB Directive No. 15 standards by 1 January 2003.

Gathering consistent and accurate data on race and ethnicity is impeded by important practical considerations (Hahn 1992; McKenney and Bennett 1994; LaVeist 1994; Hahn and Stroup 1994; Williams 1996, 1999). Survey respondents often misunderstand the intended distinction between race and ethnicity or feel that a dichotomous response about Hispanic origin ignores important cultural distinctions among ancestral countries (e.g., Cuba, Mexico, Puerto Rico, Argentina). How people reply to questions about race and ethnicity changes over time or across surveys because of "fuzzy group boundaries" (ambiguities about what constitutes group membership) and "shifting identity" (Hahn 1992). Shifting identification prompted by political and social trends partially caused a 72 percent increase in the reported American Indian population between the 1970 and 1980 censuses (McKenney and Bennett 1994, 22).

The accuracy of racial or ethnic identification depends on the data source—self-reports versus external observers (Williams 1996, 1999). Hospital discharge abstracts (see Chapter 5) can obtain racial information from either patients or completely unrelated persons, such as intake receptionists or admitting clerks (LaVeist 1994). Instructions for birth registrations stipulate that personal information be obtained from mothers, fathers, or other knowledgeable persons (Hahn, Mulinare, and Teutsch 1992). In contrast, death certificates typically use statements from the next of kin to funeral directors, although funeral directors sometimes independently assign race based on their views of the decedent's appearance. Relying on funeral directors or sources unrelated to the decedents yields highly suspect data on race. Studies have found startling changes in death rates by racial group (e.g., among American Indians) when racial misclassifications are corrected (Williams 1999, 127).

Some advocate abandoning collection of racial data because of such ambiguities. Others counter that these data are crucial precisely because of social, economic, and political dynamics inextricably linked to race by our nation's history and persisting racism. After controlling for various demographic factors, one study found that experiences of discrimination because of race or socioeconomic status were strongly associated with poor self-reported health status (Ren, Amick, and Williams 1999). LaVeist (2000) argues that, instead of giving up on gathering these data, we need to do better at understanding the complex roles of race and ethnicity in health and health care.

Health services researchers often include race in their analyses as a proxy for the unmeasured quantities of socioeconomic status, discrimination, culture, and unspecified but presumed biological differences (LaVeist 1994). Williams (1994) examined 192 studies published between 1966 and 1990 in the journal *Health Services Research*, finding that 63.0 percent included race and ethnicity. However, 54.5 percent made black-white distinctions only (most including this binary variable as a dummy in regression equations), and only 13.2 percent defined or justified the use of race in their research. Using racial variables in regression analyses may obscure important relationships, such as those involving education, socioeconomic class, culture, and health beliefs (Schulman et al. 1995). Observing higher unadjusted mortality rates among black compared to white adults, one study teased apart the causes using detailed clinical information (Otten et al. 1990). About 31 percent of the unexplained mortality differential disappeared after adjusting for smoking, systolic blood pressure, cholesterol level, body mass index, alcohol intake, and diabetes mellitus. Another 38 percent vanished after adjusting for income. Nonetheless, 31 percent of the higher mortality of blacks versus whites remained unexplained.

Causes of these discrepancies in health and health outcomes are complex and poorly understood (Williams 1996, 493, 495–97).

> Traditional explanations for health status differences between the races have focused on biological differences between racial populations . . . [but] available scientific evidence suggests that race is a social and not a biological category. . . . Adjusting racial (black-white) disparities in health for SES [socioeconomic status] sometimes eliminates, but always substantially reduces, these differences. However, a frequent finding is that within each level of SES blacks still have worse health than whites . . . irrespective of race, there are large disparities in health by income and education. . . . While there is considerable overlap between race and SES, race reflects more than SES and . . . fully understanding racial differences in health will require researchers to move beyond the traditional approaches.

Consideration of race and ethnicity is further complicated by disparities in the quality of health care between racial and ethnic minorities and white populations, as extensively documented in *Unequal Treatment* (Institute of Medicine 2002b). Reviewing the voluminous literature on health care use and outcomes across racial and ethnic groups is beyond my scope here, but examples give a flavor of these findings. Some studies find that racial and ethnic minorities receive fewer acute care services or experience worse outcomes than white patients, although the strength of these associations sometimes varies by procedure, varies by racial or ethnic group, or is attenuated by risk adjustment (Phillips et al. 1996; Hannan et al. 1999; Collins et al. 2002). Other studies fail to find consistent racial or ethnic differences after controlling for patient risk factors (Williams et al. 1995; Collins et al. 2001; Horner et al. 2002; Petersen 2002). Yet other studies have identified disparities in service use, with blacks receiving less intensive interventions, but no differences in survival (Peterson et al. 1994, 2002). Sometimes differences in appropriateness of services partially explain observed racial discrepancies, but questions about differential use persist (Epstein et al. 2000; Schneider et al. 2001a). Finally, some studies find racial differences in use of screening or preventive services, sometimes partially explained by other patient attributes (Burns et al. 1996; Schneider et al. 2001b; Schneider, Zaslavsky, and Epstein 2002).

These concerns raise serious questions about adjusting for race or ethnicity in examining outcomes of care: Such adjustment could hide significant racial disparities or confuse interpretation of the results. Some data collection systems, especially among private health insurers, do not collect information on race or ethnicity, arguing that gathering such data perpetuates discriminatory attitudes. However, as Williams (1994) observed, evidence of persisting racial bias in the health care system demands continued scrutiny. To understand fully the effect of this important patient attribute, looking explicitly at outcome differences by race and ethnicity is critical. The best strategy is to examine results separately for patients grouped into strata by race and ethnicity.

Acute Clinical Stability

Acute clinical stability reflects patients' current physiologic functioning as indicated by basic homeostatic measures. This dimension examines the most general and fundamental indicators of bodily function, such as vital signs (heart rate, respiratory rate, blood pressure, temperature), serum electrolytes, hematologic findings (e.g., hematocrit, white blood cell count, clotting indices), arterial oxygenation, and levels of consciousness or neurologic functioning. The goal is to assess whether patients face an imminent risk of death. For example, although patient E's colon cancer is more extensive than patient D's (see Table 3.2), patient D faces immediate, life-threatening risks from sepsis.

Assessing acute clinical stability is crucial for studying outcomes of acutely ill patients in short time frames, such as death during an acute care hospitalization or within a brief time window (e.g., 30 days from admission). The physiologic risk factors represent basic organ functions required to keep patients alive (e.g., cardiac, respiratory, renal, neurologic function). Concentrating on core physiologic functions makes this dimension "generic" or independent of specific diagnoses: At the level of the "whole person," a "final common pathway" of physiological functions reflects patient risk. This independence derives from the concept of "homeostasis" expounded by Walter B. Cannon in 1929: "The body's major physiologic systems interact to maintain internal balance and rapidly correct disturbances" (Wagner, Knaus, and Draper 1986, 1389). In other words, regardless of whether the patient develops shock because of sepsis, heart failure, or hemorrhage, the same measures (e.g., heart rate, blood pressure) become deranged in similar ways.

Several comments about the indicators of acute clinical stability are pertinent. First, a relatively small set of variables encompasses the most important predictors across both children and adults (Table 3.4). The first version of APACHE contained information on 34 physiologic parameters (Knaus et al. 1981), but in producing APACHE II, Knaus and colleagues (1985) found that 12 physiologic parameters retained acceptable statistical performance. APACHE III added several variables to the core group (Knaus et al. 1991). SAPS II uses fewer variables (Le Gall, Lemeshow, and Saulnier 1993), whereas the MPM is even more economical (Lemeshow et al. 1993, 1994). PRISM also uses few variables to predict outcomes in pediatric ICUs (Pollack, Ruttimann, and Getson 1988). SOFA, developed by the European Society of Intensive Care Medicine, contains only six variables (Vincent et al. 1996, 1998; Ferreira et al. 2001).[7]

Second, because these physiologic parameters serve as clinical guideposts for physicians treating acutely ill patients, most are measured routinely and with minimal technological intervention (e.g., venipuncture). Since relatively few values are unmeasured, analysts avoid vexing questions about handling missing values (see Chapter 8). Many ICUs now monitor routine physiologic parameters using automated probes and other devices, and credible acute physiology scores can be computed using data downloaded directly from monitoring equipment (Junger et al. 2002). Gathering ICU information on paper abstraction forms is almost obsolete, replaced by automated systems (see Chapter 6).

Third, measures of acute clinical stability are used most commonly to predict risk of imminent death for gravely ill patients. However, knowing only acute physiologic status may not sufficiently predict imminent death. The MPM also considers the presence of metastatic cancer, chronic renal failure, or cirrhosis (Lemeshow et al. 1993); SAPS II incorporates age and metastatic cancer, hematologic malignancy (lymphoma, acute leukemia, multiple myeloma), and acquired immunodeficiency syndrome (AIDS) (Le Gall, Lemeshow, and Saulnier 1993). APACHE III adds an age category and points for seven comorbid conditions in calculating scores (Knaus et al. 1991). So-called long-term acute care hospitals—specialized centers caring for critically ill persons needing long-term ventilatory support or other intensive treatment and monitoring—raise special questions. Standard ICU measures (e.g., APACHE II, MPM II, SAPS II) may not perform well in such settings (Carson and Bach 2001).

Clinical Variable	APACHE II[a]	III[b]	PRISM[c]	MPM II Admission[d]	MPM II At 24, 48, and 72 hours[e]	SAPS II[f]
A-a gradient	x	x				
Albumin		x				
Arterial carbon dioxide		x	x			
Arterial oxygenation	x	x	x		x	
Arterial pH	x	x				
Blood pressure	x	x	x	x		x
BUN		x				x
Bicarbonate			x			x
Calcium			x			
Glucose		x	x			
Heart rate	x	x	x	x		x
Hematocrit	x	x				
Level of consciousness, Glasgow Coma Score	x	x	x	x	x	x
PaO$_2$/FiO$_2$						x
Prothrombin time/partial thromboplastin time (PT/PTT)			x		x	
Respiratory rate	x	x	x			
Serum creatinine	x	x			x	
Serum sodium	x	x				x
Serum potassium	x		x			x
Temperature	x	x				x
Total bilirubin		x	x			x
Urine output		x			x	x
Pupillary reactions			x			
White blood cell count	x	x				x

TABLE 3.4 Physiologic Variables Included in Different Measures of Acute Clinical Stability

[a] Knaus et al. (1985).
[b] Knaus et al. (1991).
[c] Pollack, Ruttimann, and Getson (1988).
[d] Lemeshow et al. (1993).
[e] Lemeshow et al. (1994).
[f] Le Gall, Lemeshow, and Saulnier (1994).

Finally, today's acute physiology-based risk-adjustment methods are developed empirically with clinical conceptual guidance (see Chapter 8). This raises various questions. Because empirically derived methods inevitably reflect treatment patterns and outcomes from their underlying databases, developers should periodically update the weights assigned to different risk factors. Especially in intensive care, where therapies change over time, periodic recalibration seems essential. Users must consider whether their practices and care settings differ significantly from those within the developmental database; if so, the empirically derived weights may not apply equally well to their patients. Another question is whether weights assigned to acute physiologic variables should vary depending on patients' diagnoses. For example, should blood pressure receive different weights for patients admitted for CHF versus gastrointestinal hemorrhage? Empirical modeling allows developers to consider such inter-relationships in various ways (Lemeshow and Le Gall 1994). For simplicity, many developers retain generic weighting of physiologic risk factors, noting that disease-specific weightings provide only marginally better predictions.

The value of acute physiologic parameters in assessing patient risk for imminent clinical outcomes is undisputed. Acute clinical stability is obviously central to evaluating risk for imminent death and complications, such as respiratory failure or shock. Its utility for predicting resource use is less apparent.

Principal Diagnosis

> The diagnosis is a hypothesis regarding the nature of the patient's illness. . . . Because the diagnosis is such a focal point in the physician's interaction with the patient, this concept is fundamental to measurement of hospital output: the diagnosis establishes the relevant technology of care and, hence, the types and levels of resources required to treat the illness. (Hornbrook 1982, 74)

Few argue that risks for many outcomes—from resource use to clinical events—differ dramatically by diagnosis. However, older patients in particular rarely have single diagnoses. Disentangling the leading disease process from coexisting conditions is frequently difficult. Nevertheless, for the discussion here, I focus first on risks associated with the "principal diagnosis" and then consider "comorbid" disease.

Defining and Delineating Diseases and Diagnoses

For hospitalized patients, the principal diagnosis is defined administratively (e.g., by Medicare) as the leading disease that brings a patient into contact with the health care system and for which services are sought (see Chapter 5). This distinction belies the complexity of designating diagnoses. Defining diagnoses has preoccupied medicine since Hippocratic times, spawning volumes of nomenclatures and commentary. As Feinstein observed (1967, 73):

> Diagnosis is the focal point of thought in the treatment of a patient. From diagnosis, which gives a name to the patient's ailment, the thinking goes chronologically backward to decide about pathogenesis and etiology of the ailment. From diagnosis also, the thinking goes chronologically forward to predict prognosis and to choose therapy. As the main language of clinical communication, diagnostic labels transmit a rapid understanding of the contents of the package . . .

However, even with new diagnostic technologies, making a diagnosis can be complicated and requires multiple steps. "Each disease should be defined in terms of some specific organ or organ system involved . . . some characteristic pathophysiological change . . . [and] an etiologic factor or set of factors causing the pathophysiological changes" (Gonnella, Hornbrook, and Louis 1984, 638). Sometimes, designating diagnoses along these multilevel dimensions is straightforward (e.g., *Streptococcus pneumoniae* infections of the lung). Other times, definitive diagnoses are impossible. For example, despite fiberoptic studies, angiography, radionuclide scans, and barium enemas, the source and causes of lower gastrointestinal tract bleeding may remain elusive. Clinicians assign a "diagnosis" of gastrointestinal hemorrhage, reflecting a sign of underlying disease rather than the disease itself. The demands of acutely managing a potentially cataclysmic event can divert attention from precise diagnosis. Later, after stabilizing the patient, clinicians can investigate the exact cause.

In certain situations, the dividing line between the presence and absence of disease is blurred. For example, dysplasia of the cervix, an abnormal finding on a Pap smear, can presage cervical cancer. Subtle morphologic differences between dysplastic and normal cells compromise the reliability of dysplasia identification, and the condition generally vanishes spontaneously. Even while present, dysplastic cells do not cause pain or disability (Eddy 1984). Numerous examples exist of "diseases . . . being defined by an abnormal result on some test, leaving uncertainty about its real meaning to a patient and the appropriate treatment" (Eddy 1984, 76).

Some vague diagnostic terminology reflects habit, sloppiness, or situations where specifying the cause is clinically unimportant. CHF—a common term—is generally caused by long-standing hypertension or coronary artery disease but occasionally results from such diverse etiologies as viruses, alcohol, or disordered iron metabolism. Some causes require specific interventions. Once CHF is present, however, exacerbations are often treated similarly. Therefore, physicians may not specify the cause of CHF when listing the patient's diagnosis codes.

Finally, certain specific diagnoses produce widely varying manifestations, whereas very different diseases lead to similar problems. For example, diabetic complications range from blinding retinopathy to chronic renal failure. These varying complications require different diagnostic approaches and therapeutic interventions. Depending on their purpose, analysts may group together all patients with specific serious complications regardless of underlying etiology. For example, a study of end-stage renal disease may encompass patients with hypertension, diabetes, lupus, and certain infections—all causes of kidney failure. Chronic renal failure from any cause necessitates renal transplantation or lifelong dialysis.

Thus, using comprehensive criteria to specify diagnoses is sometimes infeasible. Nevertheless, when using diagnosis as a risk factor, having a definitive diagnosis that meets rigorous standards may not be essential, depending on the context. Such vagaries often reflect the realities of today's clinical practice.

However, if diagnostic information is questionable (e.g., diagnoses are not definitively established), this may affect the utility of diagnosis as a risk factor.

Severity or Extent of Principal Diagnosis

In some contexts, knowing principal diagnosis alone is insufficient; analysts must also understand the severity or extent of the diagnosis. For example, persons with colon cancer isolated to a polyp (patients A to C; see Table 3.2) have different prognoses and therapeutic needs than persons with widely disseminated malignancy (patients H and I). Many studies of medical effectiveness and patient outcomes focus on a single principal diagnosis, thus making it unnecessary to separate patients by diagnoses. Nevertheless, determining severity levels within the diagnostic category often remains important.

The concept of severity has many layers, often organized around prognosis—expectations about patients' clinical outcomes relating to the extent and nature of disease. Prognoses, obviously, vary depending on the time frame: months or years versus hours, days, or weeks (see Chapter 4). Long- and short-run assessments of severity may differ. For example, patient D (see Table 3.2) presents with sepsis from a dangerous bacteria. The patient needs immediate, aggressive treatment. Later, on colonoscopy, physicians find an adenomatous polyp containing a small nidus of adenocarcinoma. Patient I's colon cancer has metastasized widely. The patient needs treatment to alleviate pain and appears cachectic but not acutely ill, not at immediate risk. The short- and long-term prognoses of these patients differ. The first has an immediately life-threatening condition; if treated, the patient could live for years. The second patient's condition is not immediately life threatening but portends a very poor long-term prognosis.

However, the term "prognosis" generates the same question as does "risk": Prognosis for what? As noted in Chapter 2, many studies target death. Death, however, is most relevant for diagnoses where deaths are relatively common and imminent regardless of intensive therapeutic intervention. Imminent death is irrelevant for assessing most outpatient conditions. For instance, the Framingham study and other investigations suggest that the risk of cardiovascular death associated with hypertension doubles as diastolic blood pressure rises into the range of 80 to 89 mm Hg (Working Group on Risk and High Blood Pressure 1985). Does this mean that patients with diastolic pressures of 90 mm Hg are twice as "sick" as those with pressures of 80 mm Hg? Because death is often years away, this may make little difference in the immediate assessment of the patient.

For those many diagnoses where death is uncommon or distant, precisely defining severity becomes more complicated. Diseases with protean presentations introduce special complexities. Which is the most severe manifestation of diabetes: blindness, end-stage renal disease, or debilitating peripheral vascular disease? Quality-of-life considerations enter this equation, albeit tied to personal values (e.g., one person may adapt to blindness, whereas another may find it intolerable). Contrasts are muddied further when comparing acute with chronic manifestations of single diseases. For example, is a patient whose sickle-cell anemia is marked by multiple painful crises sicker than one whose disease caused renal failure? Comparing severity among diseases is even more treacherous, often amounting to "comparing apples with oranges." Colon cancer seems more serious than psoriasis, for example, but the truth depends on the extent of each disease. Early, asymptomatic colon cancer is less severe (e.g., in terms of imminent death, discomfort, disability) than psoriasis with diffuse erythroderma and infection with antibiotic-resistant bacteria.

Complete measurement may require observing patients over time. For example, suppose three patients presented acutely with identical, severe, neurological deficits from cerebrovascular disease. Patient 1's symptoms resolve fully in 24 hours, patient 2's deficits slowly improve over a week but never vanish completely, and patient 3's debilities persist without change. The severity of illness clearly differs across patients 1, 2, and 3, but focusing only on their initial deficits would miss these distinctions. As discussed in Chapter 4, one pitfall with longitudinal examinations is possible confounding with substandard care.

Finally, the principal diagnosis may affect how analysts rate other risk factors. For the CSI, specific diagnoses dictate the importance assigned to various risk factors (Horn et al. 1991; Iezzoni and Daley 1992). The CSI, for example, views a temperature of 102°F as very severe for patients with leukemia but only moderately severe for patients with pneumonia.

Extent and Severity of Comorbidities

"Comorbidities," or coexisting diagnoses, are diseases unrelated in etiology or causality to the principal diagnosis. Comorbidities differ from "complications"—sequelae of the principal diagnosis. For example, for colon cancer patients (see Table 3.2), cerebrovascular disease (patient B) is a comorbidity, whereas bowel obstruction (patient G) is a complication. The prototypical comorbidity is a chronic condition, such as diabetes mellitus, chronic obstructive pulmonary disease, or chronic ischemic heart disease (Table 3.5). In 2000, an estimated 125 million Americans had at least one chronic condition, and chronic conditions generated 75 percent of health spending (Anderson and Knickman 2001, 147). Depending on the context, however, comorbid illnesses can be acute (e.g., an AMI following admission to treat colon cancer).

In most instances, compared to persons without chronic conditions, patients with comorbidities have higher risks of death and complications, have higher rates of functional impairments and disability, and often require additional diagnostic testing and therapeutic interventions. Most RCTs exclude these patients because of concerns that comorbid disease might confound perceptions of treatment efficacy. Observational and medical effectiveness studies, however, examine outcomes in the real world, where chronic conditions are

TABLE 3.5
Variables
Included in
Three Measures
of Comorbid
Illness

Comorbid Condition	Points Assigned		
	Charlson Index	RAND Index	APACHE III
Myocardial infarction	1		
CHF	1	1	
Peripheral vascular disease	1		
Cerebrovascular disease	1	2	
Dementia	1	2	
Chronic pulmonary disease	1		
Connective tissue disease	1		
Ulcer disease	1		
Mild liver disease	1		
Diabetes without end-organ damage	1	1	
Hemiplegia	2		
Moderate or severe renal disease	2	3	
Diabetes with end-organ damage	2		
Any tumor, cancer	2	3	
Leukemia	2		10
Lymphoma	2		13
Moderate or severe liver disease	3		
Cirrhosis		2	4
Hepatic failure			16
Metastatic solid tumor	6		11
AIDS	6		23
Immunosuppression		2	10
Multiple myeloma		2	10[a]
Valvular disease, angina, myocardial infarction, or heart surgery		2	
Arrhythmias		2	
Swallowing disorders (e.g., aspiration, dysphagia)		2	
Use of nasogastric tube		3	
Hospitalization in the last month		2	
Thoracic or abdominal surgery in the last month		2	
Disease of the thorax		3	
Splenectomy		2	
Smoking		2	
Alcoholism		2	
Morbid obesity		2	
Hypoalbuminemia or malnourishment		3	

NOTE: Definitions of comorbid conditions vary across measures. See Charlson Index (Charlson et al. 1987); RAND Index (Keeler et al. 1990); APACHE III (Knaus et al. 1991).
[a] APACHE III considers leukemia/multiple myeloma as a single comorbid condition.

common, especially as patients age. Therefore, comorbidities are potentially important risk factors.

As for principal diagnoses, the extent or severity of a chronic condition determines its importance as a risk factor. For example, the effect of patient F's hypertension (see Table 3.2) depends on its complications, such as renal insufficiency or heart failure. The effect of comorbidities often varies by time frame; chronic conditions strongly influence long-term survival and functioning (see Chapter 4). Charlson and colleagues (1987) examined the one-year survival of 559 patients admitted to the medical service at New York Hospital during a one-month period in 1984. They used information on coexisting illnesses, taken from medical records, to create a comorbidity index (Table 3.5).[8] Greenfield and colleagues (1993) developed the Index of Coexistent Disease (ICED) to quantify risk from comorbid illness. ICED aims to capture quality of life by answering the question, "If a patient is rated as 'severe,' will he or she have poor quality of life or be unable to tolerate rigorous therapy over the next 2 or so years?" (Greenfield et al. 1994, 300). ICED melds physiologic derangements and impairments related to comorbid illness in computing overall levels of risk.

Comorbidities also are important in examining shorter-term outcomes, such as hospital mortality rates. For example, a study of 201 ICU patients found that the Charlson comorbidity index significantly predicted in-hospital death, even controlling for APACHE II scores (Poses et al. 1996). A study of more than 27,200 heart surgery patients in northern New England adjusted for specific cardiac risk factors but found that chronic conditions added significantly to predictions of in-hospital mortality (Clough et al. 2002).[9] Especially significant comorbidities were dialysis-dependent renal failure, chronic obstructive pulmonary disease, and vascular disease. The RAND study of the effect of Medicare's prospective hospital payment system also considered comorbidity (Keeler et al. 1990), using broad definitions of coexisting conditions (Table 3.5), including smoking, obesity, and certain procedures (use of a nasogastric tube, thoracic or abdominal surgery in the last month, use of home oxygen). The researchers assigned weights to each of 16 conditions using clinical judgment and logistic regression predictions of 30-day mortality. The comorbidity index significantly predicted 30-day mortality for only two of the five study conditions (pneumonia and hip fracture) when added to a model containing acute physiologic variables.

APACHE III's developers explored the influence of comorbid disease for imminent death in ICU patients. After investigating 34 candidate chronic conditions, they found that seven independently predicted in-hospital mortality (Table 3.5). Total APACHE III scores range from 0 to 299, and the contribution for comorbid illness varies from 4 points for cirrhosis to 23 for AIDS (Knaus et al. 1991, 1624). Among elective postoperative ICU admissions, however, these conditions were uncommon and did not enhance predictive power of the model. Therefore, points for chronic disease are not included for elective postoperative ICU cases.

Acute comorbidities (e.g., pneumonia, AMI) may be iatrogenic, raising questions about quality of care and medical errors. The exact semantic distinctions among acute comorbidities, complications, iatrogenic illnesses, adverse events, and other similar terms are often unclear. Although conceptually important, distinguishing acute comorbidities related to underlying disease from those caused by iatrogenic events is often difficult (Brailer et al. 1996). One practical problem is determining the timing of events; some data sources offer little or unreliable insight into when events occurred.

Some approaches quantify the overall burden of patients' conditions in a single rating. An example is the Physical Status Classification of the American Society of Anesthesiologists (ASA), used in preoperative evaluations of surgical patients. ASA scores rate risks of perioperative death on a global, subjective, five-point scale encompassing all aspects of a patient's presentation (level 5 indicates patients expected to die within 24 hours). ASA scores often perform well in observational studies of surgical mortality, complications, and LOS (see Chapter 8). Similarly, although the CSI assigns specific severity scores to each individual diagnosis, it also computes an overall severity score combining the effects of all diagnoses.

Incorporating all diagnoses is especially important in risk adjustment for capitating payment. The ACGs consider the combined effect of all outpatient diagnoses over a year in using branching logic to assign patients to one of 51 mutually exclusive, terminal ACGs (Starfield et al. 1991). The DCG/HCC model considers all inpatient hospital, outpatient hospital, and physician diagnoses, but within hierarchies: If a patient has multiple diagnoses related to the same underlying disease process, only the single most influential of these interrelated diagnoses is considered (Ellis et al. 1996).

Functional Status

As with acute clinical stability, functional status represents a final common pathway. For instance, difficulty walking results from diverse causes, such as arthritis, back problems, stroke, amputation, and injury. Functional limitations thus reflect numerous factors—congenital or acquired, permanent or transient, sensory or motor, systemic or localized, physical or psychosocial. According to the U.S. DHHS (2000), 54 million Americans have some form of disabling condition (see Chapter 15). Mobility impairments are the leading reason for functional limitations among adults, affecting an estimated 19 million persons living in communities (Iezzoni et al. 2001a). Depending on one's purpose, specifying the exact cause of a functional deficit is less important than describing the extent of impairment.

In comprehensive risk assessments, functional status is distinguishable from the concepts of health status or quality of life described below. Some find such distinctions spurious, however, preferring global measures of well-being that cut across various dimensions. Nonetheless, an important distinction is that functional status typically captures observable behaviors rather than individuals' perceptions of health (Rubenstein et al. 1989, 563):

> Functional status . . . encompasses the more limited areas of physical, mental, and social functioning in daily life. Functioning is observable; it consists of everyday behaviors as they occur in a person's home and community life. Measures of functioning include items about daily activities such as eating, dressing, bathing, walking, handling finances, or visiting friends and relatives. Functional status is the end result of a person's health (absence of disease), well-being (capacity to participate fully in life), and coping (capacity to overcome health problems).

Over the last few decades, developing conceptual models relating functional impairments to medical disorders and disability has generated considerable interest, and hundreds of measures now exist to quantify functional status within specific clinical conditions or generically across diagnoses (see Chapter 7). New computerized techniques, such as those using item response theory, allow surveyors to elicit specific information by asking small numbers of well-targeted questions. Historically, functional-status measures have typically included basic activities of daily living (ADLs; e.g., feeding, bathing, dressing, toileting, walking) and instrumental ADLs (IADLs; e.g., shopping, cooking, doing housework, using public transportation, using the telephone, balancing a checkbook). Most comprehensive measures of functioning also address cognitive abilities (e.g., level of alertness, orientation, long- and short-term memory, capacity for learning and computation), affective health (e.g., happiness, anxiety, depression), and social activities (e.g., visiting friends, sexual relationships).

The measurement context can affect perceptions of functional ability. For example, "capability" indicates what persons can do in controlled settings, whereas "performance" assesses what a person does in everyday life. Capability typically exceeds performance (Young et al. 1996). In addition, patients and clinicians frequently hold discordant views about patients' functioning (see Chapters 7). About 1,400 participants in the Framingham study, for example, completed a mailed disability questionnaire before their biennial physical examination, during which nurses tested their functional abilities (Kelly-Hayes et al. 1992). Most of the roughly 7 percent of differences found between self-reported and observed performance pertained to walking and stair climbing; for at least 89 percent of discrepancies, respondents reported significantly worse functioning than study nurses observed.

In contrast, a study of 620 women who had recent strokes found that the women reported considerably better functioning than was found on physical testing; self-reports and examination results disagreed substantially for

19.3 percent of women and slightly for 55 percent (Owens et al. 2002, 806). The researchers suggested that physicians consider conducting a physical performance test rather than rely on patients' self-reports. Many physicians, however, are themselves poor at assessing patients' functional limitations (Hoenig 1993). A study of 408 outpatients found that 22 percent reported difficulties walking one block or climbing one flight of stairs; 31 percent had trouble walking several blocks. The 118 physicians underestimated or failed to recognize roughly two-thirds of these problems (Calkins et al. 1991).

Baseline functional status strongly predicts subsequent functional status. Functional status also significantly predicts other outcomes, such as imminent death, complications, resource consumption, and satisfaction with care. Among Medicare beneficiaries with pneumonia, baseline walking difficulties significantly predicted mortality 30 days following hospitalization (Daley et al. 1988; Keeler et al. 1990). Functional status may predict annual health care costs, although research findings are somewhat contradictory (see Chapter 7). Some analysts advocate adding functional-status measures to diagnostic information in determining capitation payment levels (Hornbrook 1999). Medicare beneficiaries with various functional impairments report significantly higher rates of dissatisfaction with their health care experiences along a range of dimensions (Iezzoni et al. 2002; Jha et al. 2002).

Head-to-head comparisons of functional-status measures with physiologic findings have yielded interesting results. Using forward stepwise logistic regression to predict in-hospital death for pneumonia and stroke patients, Davis and colleagues (1995) found that nursing assessments of patients' functional status were stronger predictors than most laboratory test values and comorbid diseases.[10] A global assessment by nurses of patients' needs for ADL assistance better predicted in-hospital death among AIDS patients than three validated AIDS mortality measures (Justice et al. 1996).

Clinical and functional status dimensions probably convey different information. For example, we studied 185 patients admitted for AMI and 111 admitted for pneumonia by conducting detailed medical record reviews and patient interviews with the 36-item Health Status Questionnaire (HSQ) developed during the Medical Outcomes Study (MOS, similar to the short form, or SF-36; Stewart and Ware 1992). As expected, the eight HSQ dimensions showed highly positive correlations (Iezzoni 1995; Stewart, Hays, and Ware 1988). In contrast, some, but not all, of the medical record measures were significantly correlated with HSQ dimensions (Table 3.6). An ADL measure abstracted from nursing notes displayed significant positive correlations with each HSQ dimension. In contrast, the acute physiology score (APS) component of APACHE II showed an important correlation only with physical functioning. APACHE II scores were also negatively correlated with several dimensions, possibly because age is used in calculating complete APACHE values. The presence of chronic conditions was strongly negatively linked to four dimensions (physical, role-physical, energy, and overall health); as the

TABLE 3.6

Correlation Among the HSQ Functional Status Dimensions and Other Attributes

Other Patient Attributes or Findings	HSQ Functional Status Dimensions							
	Physical	Social	Role— physical	Role— emotional	Mental	Energy	Pain	Health
Age	−0.51*	−0.02	−0.20[+]	−0.02	−0.01	−0.23*	−0.05	0.12[‡]
LOS	−0.12[‡]	−0.12[‡]	−0.10	0.06	0.00	−0.11	−0.14[‡]	−0.14[‡]
ADLs[a]	0.50*	0.24*	0.23*	0.18[§]	0.14[‡]	0.26*	0.13[‡]	0.28*
APS (APACHE II)	−0.17[§]	−0.08	−0.14[‡]	0.00	0.04	−0.11	−0.06	−0.12[‡]
APACHE II score	−0.40*	−0.14[‡]	−0.26*	−0.04	0.01	−0.26*	−0.12[‡]	−0.23*
Presence of chronic conditions[b]	−0.38*	−0.15[§]	−0.22*	−0.07	−0.08	−0.28*	−0.09	−0.21[+]

SOURCE: Iezzoni, L. I. 1995. "Risk Adjustment for Medical Effectiveness Research: An Overview of Conceptual and Methodological Considerations." *Journal f Investigative Medicine* 43 (2): Table 7, p. 143.
* $p \leq 0.0001$.
[+] $p \leq 0.001$.
[§] $p \leq 0.01$.
[‡] $p \leq 0.05$.
[a] The purpose of the ADL scale was to assess the patients' ability to care for themselves. Scale included feeding, bathing, dressing, bed mobility, ambulation, and bladder and bowel function.
[b] Chronic conditions included AMI within three months prior to admission; CHF prior to admission; cancer with a poor prognosis; diabetes mellitus; stroke; cirrhosis, portal hypertension, or ascites; chronic renal failure; chronic obstructive pulmonary disease; peripheral vascular disease requiring bypass of leg, arteries or amputation of leg, foot, or toes; psychosis or depression; prior hospitalization within six months; and dementia.

number of chronic conditions increased, patients reported worse functioning.

Measuring functional status raises several additional issues. First, functional status is not determined by basic demographic or clinical characteristics alone. The MOS found that controlling for sociodemographic characteristics (age, sex, income, education) and medical illnesses explained only a fraction of the variation in functional status (Stewart et al. 1989).[11] Second, specific functional-status measures may not perform equally well across the entire spectrum of impairment or within selected patient populations. For example, Bindman, Keane, and Lurie (1990) used the MOS general health survey (MOS-20), an instrument largely designed and tested among outpatients, on 414 patients in poor health admitted to public hospitals. Six months later, patients were asked if their health had changed. At baseline, the patients had much lower functional status than did MOS participants; these poor functional levels changed little over six months. Nonetheless, more than half of the public hospital patients reported that their health status had actually declined. In-depth evaluation suggested that the MOS-20 failed to detect declining health among very sick patients, the so-called "floor effect." The opposite concern—a "ceiling effect"—arises when instruments fail to detect improvements among persons with higher functioning (Bindman, Keane, and Lurie 1990; Andresen et al. 1995).

Third, the mode of administration of the functional-status measure (e.g., face-to-face interview, mail with self-administration, telephone interview, Internet) requires consideration. In face-to-face interviews, respondents may hesitate to reveal their extent of dysfunction. A study of 172 veterans administered the SF-36 found significant differences in patients' reports over the course of a week depending on the mode of administration. For four of the eight SF-36 dimensions, face-to-face administration elicited a more optimistic view of health than did self-administration (Weinberger et al. 1996). More research is needed to evaluate whether Internet administration produces comparable results to other modes of administration.

Fourth, although many functioning measures are generic (i.e., independent of diagnoses or underlying condition), disease-specific approaches are more appropriate in some contexts. For instance, the Arthritis Impact Measurement Scale (Meenan 1986) and McMaster Health Index Questionnaire (Chambers et al. 1982) aim to assess patients with arthritis; the Visual Analogue Pain Scale (McDowell and Newell 1987) addresses situations where pain predominates; the Tinetti Balance and Gait Evaluation (Tinetti, Williams, and Mayewski 1986) applies to patients with gait abnormalities; and the Activities of Daily Vision Scale quantifies the functional effect of low vision (Mangione et al. 1992). These condition-specific scales are more sensitive to change in specified functions (e.g., vision) than are generic measures.

Fifth, tension exists between single, composite, summary scores of function versus multiple scales capturing different dimensions of functional status. Single numbers may prove inadequate. "How can an overall health score be assigned to a person with a serious chronic disease, such as diabetes, who feels well and functions as a productive person with no role or social limitations?" (Stewart and Ware 1992, 22). The SF-36, for example, produces two summary measures, the Physical Component Summary (PCS) and the Mental Component Summary (MCS) scales. Survey researchers continue to explore the implications of creating composite measures.

Psychological, Cognitive, and Psychosocial Functioning

Psychological, cognitive, and psychosocial functioning encompass such attributes as patients' abilities to appreciate and interact with their surroundings and other people, their capacity to understand information about their health and health care needs and to act productively on this information, and having others who can provide care or social support. These factors particularly affect outcomes outside controlled institutional environments. In hospitals, the staff oversees all patient needs, like giving medications on schedule in proper dosages. In the community, however, psychological and cognitive problems can compromise patients' activity levels, self-care, motivation, and perceptions, with negative effects on outcomes. According to one study, patients with depressive symptoms are less likely than others to comply with their antihypertensive medication regimens (Wang et al. 2002). Patient C (see Table 3.2), who refused treatment for depression, faces greater risks of poor outcomes than patient A, who has identical colon cancer.

Scales of overall functioning often contain measures of these attributes (e.g., the MCS of the SF-36). However, Applegate, Blass, and Williams (1990, 1210) warned, "Because many elderly persons with mild-to-moderate cognitive impairment often maintain their social skills in terms of superficial interactions, clinically important impairment may remain undetected." Scales of cognitive functioning suffer many of the drawbacks mentioned above, such as floor and ceiling effects (inability to detect small changes in cognitive functioning at either end of the scale). In addition, patients' level of education affects most cognitive functioning scales. Older people in particular may feel threatened when asked to complete cognitive evaluations, such as the Mini-Mental State Examination; they may try to memorize basic recall words to maximize their scores (Kutner et al. 1992).

The MOS developed a scale explicitly to measure social support, including 19 "support items," such as having someone to show love and affection, confide in, hug, understand problems, have a good time with, prepare meals, and turn to for suggestions (Sherbourne and Stewart 1991). Persons with low social support reported much worse physical functioning and emotional well-being at the start of the study than persons with high social support, and this difference persisted over two years (Sherbourne et al. 1992).

Even without detailed interviews or data collection, basic facts about how patients live offer important insight. After adjusting for many clinical factors, AMI patients living alone had worse outcomes than patients living with others—relative risks of 1.54 for recurrent cardiac events and 1.58 for cardiac death (Case et al. 1992). Another study followed patients treated medically for coronary artery disease, tracking the occurrence of cardiac death over five years (Williams et al. 1992). Despite controlling for "all known medical prognostic factors," social variables remained important predictors of death. Having a spouse or confidant was the strongest predictor; unmarried persons without confidants had a relative risk of 3.34 for cardiac death compared to other patients. One study followed patients for 36 months after their heart attack, finding that high life stress and social isolation independently predicted mortality (Ruberman et al. 1984).

Often, these various mental health and psychosocial attributes are highly interrelated. Using data from the National Health Interview Survey, we produced multivariable logistic regression models to predict self-reports of feeling depressed or anxious (Iezzoni 2003). Adjusted odds ratios were significantly higher for persons who lived alone or were divorced, widowed, or never married. Thus, psychological functioning (depression or anxiety) was closely linked to social factors (household composition and marital status). Close associations among such risk factors might affect how analysts should use these variables in models to predict outcomes.

Health Behavior, Sociocultural, and Environmental Attributes

Especially for long-term prevention of premature death and debility, health behaviors play a crucial role. Important behavior-related risk factors include tobacco use, nutritional practices, physical activity levels, alcohol consumption, illicit drug use, sexual practices, societal and domestic violence, and seat belt use. In addition, although often considered outside the medical mainstream, cultural, socioeconomic, and environmental attributes significantly affect a wide variety of short- and long-term patient outcomes.

The negative effects of certain health-related behaviors are well known. Smoking attracts the greatest attention. Annually in the United States, tobacco use precipitates at least $50 billion in health care costs, before accounting for income lost by illness and premature death, according to the CDC (2000, 3). Cigarette smoking contributes to 20 percent of deaths, or 400,000 deaths annually; adult smoking rates vary nationwide, from 13 percent in Utah to 31 percent in Kentucky (CDC 2002, 37). Obesity has risen to "epidemic proportions" in all age groups: In 2000, an estimated 30.5 percent of adult Americans were obese, and 64.5 percent were overweight (Flegal et al. 2002, 1723). Direct and indirect U.S. costs of overweight and obesity were $117 billion in 2000, and obesity causes roughly 300,000 premature deaths yearly (CDC 2002, 55). Despite proven health benefits from physical activity, more than 28 percent of American adults report no physical activities during their leisure time (CDC 2002, 43). Various risky health behaviors thus contribute to diverse outcomes, including mortality, morbidity, and health care costs.

Rates of high-risk health behaviors are typically higher among lower-income persons than to higher-income persons. This prompts some to argue that risky behaviors produce the worse health care outcomes observed among poorer persons. Recent research dispels that notion. Even after analysts control for health behaviors, health status remains worse among lower- than higher-income persons (Lantz et al. 1998, 2001).

Numerous publications have documented socioeconomic disparities in health status in the United States and worldwide (Braveman and Tarimo 2002). Explaining why some people are healthy and others are not (Evans, Barer, and Marmor 1994) has generated considerable interest and prompted various theories, several with an increasingly convincing evidence base. Some proposed causes are obvious consequences of poverty. One study estimated that 1.3 million Americans with disabilities did not take their prescribed medications because they could not afford the drugs (Kennedy and Erb 2002, 1120). The Institute of Medicine (2002a) noted that being without health insurance, even for one to four years, might worsen general health status (see Chapter 1). Living in substandard housing heightens morbidity, including respiratory infections, asthma, lead poisoning, injuries, and mental health problems (Krieger and Higgins 2002).

Other causes for the social gradient in health status are subtler, reflecting complex dynamics among genetic, biological, environmental (physical and social, in childhood and at older ages), and other factors. One example involves higher rates of low-birthweight babies among poor compared to other women (Starfield 1992, 18).

> The chain of events is complex. Predisposing factors involve environmental conditions, social conditions, and genetic risk factors. Some of these operate directly (such as housing with lead-based paint), and some operate indirectly through mediating factors involving induced behaviors, stress, social isolation, and decreased access to medical care. All risks interact in unknown ways in their effect on health.

People's jobs also affect their risks. Occupational exposures cause or heighten susceptibility to certain illnesses, such as respiratory conditions resulting from exposure to dusts, gases, or fumes. Exposure to coal dust, asbestos, silica, talc, and animal proteins can cause pulmonary fibrosis; coal dust, welding fumes, and other compounds can precipitate bronchitis; and toluene diisocyanate, chromium, grains, animal products, and cotton can produce chronic airway disease. Many such conditions are exacerbated further by smoking. Jobs also affect mental health. For instance, stresses associated with air traffic control and front-line law enforcement are well documented.

Poor or marginal health literacy heightens risks for poor outcomes. One study among English- and Spanish-speaking diabetes patients over age 30 found that 38 percent had inadequate health literacy and 13 percent had marginal literacy (Schillinger et al. 2002, 478). Compared to people with adequate health literacy, those with inadequate literacy were significantly less likely to experience tight glycemic control and more likely to have poor glycemic control and retinopathy. A study among Medicare beneficiaries found that persons with inadequate health literacy experienced significantly more hospitalizations than persons with adequate health literacy, even accounting for differences in age, sex, race and ethnicity, education, income, smoking, alcohol use, chronic diseases, and self-reported physical and mental health (Baker et al. 2002b).

Culture and religion may affect compliance with prescribed therapy, diet and other daily life activities, and attitudes toward health and medical care. A prominent example is Jehovah's Witnesses' prohibition against blood transfusions regardless of clinical circumstances. Another example involves the dietary cravings of pica, particularly during pregnancy—women may desire substances such as earth or clay (geophagia), laundry starch (amylophagia), or ice (pagophagia). Pica is particularly common in the South and is associated with maternal anemia and poor birth outcomes. Churches can help define community perceptions toward health and health care services, sometimes encouraging parishioners to seek care and other times raising cautionary notes (Markens et al. 2002).

Thus, socioeconomic characteristics may be particularly relevant to studies of service use—to risk adjusting processes of care. For example, in both the United States and Canada (which has universal health insurance), women with higher education and higher incomes were more likely than other women to receive screening mammograms (Katz, Zemencuk, and Hofer 2000). One study examined the performance of 568 physicians caring for more than 600,000 managed care patients, looking at physician-specific rates of mammograms, diabetic eye checks, and Pap tests (Franks and Fiscella 2002). The researchers adjusted their physician profiles for patients' socioeconomic status based on information related to their zip codes (median household income, percentage white, percentage who had at least graduated high school, and percentage white-collar workers). This adjustment largely diminished the number of physicians seen as outliers (i.e., poor performers): "Without socioeconomic adjustment physicians caring for on average lower socioeconomic patients have profiles reflecting lower prevention compliance" (Franks and Fiscella 2002, 720).

Overall Health Status and Health-Related Quality of Life

Health status and quality of life reflect patients' points of view about their overall health and how their health and other factors affect their lives. Unlike functional status, which can be measured by outsiders, only patients (or perhaps proxies) can assess health status and quality of life. Thus, these measures provide critical insight into the outcomes of care. They also are significant risk factors for a variety of outcomes, especially such patient-centered outcomes as future overall health status and quality of life, satisfaction with care, and mental and physical functional status.

Tools to measure health status and quality of life can be brief: How do you rate your overall health: excellent, good, fair, or poor? Other instruments include dozens of questions, encompassing specific markers of disease, general physical capabilities, psychosocial and emotional functioning, and sense of well-being. As described in Chapter 7, the published literature addressing health status and quality-of-life measures has grown tremendously over the last decade, and hundreds of measurement tools now exist for different populations and purposes. Table 3.7 summarizes ten widely used general health surveys "considered generic to the extent that they assess health concepts that represent basic human values relevant to functional status and well-being" (Ware 1995, 329).

Despite the growing number of articles addressing health status and quality of life, the exact goals of measurement can remain unclear. A review of 75 articles purporting to discuss quality-of-life measurement found references to 159 different instruments (Table 3.8), with a mean of 3 instruments (range 1 to 19) per article (Gill and Feinstein 1994, 622). However, only 15 percent of articles contained a conceptual definition of quality of life, and just 17

TABLE 3.7

Summary of Information About Widely Used General Health Surveys

	QWB	SIP	HIE	NHP	QLI	COOP	EURO-QOL	DUKE	MOS FWBP	MOS SF-36
Concept[a]										
Physical functioning	x	x	x	x	x	x	x	x	x	x
Social functioning	x	x	x	x	x	x	x	x	x	x
Role functioning	x	x	x	x	x	x	x	x	x	x
Psychological distress		x	x	x	x	x	x	x	x	x
Health perceptions (general)			x	x	x	x	x	x	x	x
Pain (bodily)		x	x	x		x	x	x	x	x
Energy/fatigue	x		x	x				x	x	x
Psychological well-being			x					x	x	x
Sleep		x		x				x	x	
Cognitive functioning		x						x	x	
Quality of life			x			x			x	
Reported health transition						x			x	x
Characteristics										
Administration method (S = self, I = interviewer, P = proxy)										
	I, P	S, I, P	S, P	S, I	S, P	S, I	S	S, I	S, I	S, I, P
Scaling method (L = Likert, R = Rasch, T = Thurstone, U = utility)										
	U	T	L	T	L	L	U	L	L	L, R
Number of questions	107	136	86	38	5	9	9	17	149	36
Scoring options (P = profile, SS = summary scores, SI = single index)										
	SI	P, SS, SI	P	P	SI	P	SI	P, SI	P	P, SS

SOURCE: Ware, J. E., Jr. 1995. "The Status of Health Assessment 1994." *Annual Review of Public Health* 16: 330.
NOTE: QWB = Quality of Well-Being Scale; SIP = Sickness Impact Profile; HIE = Health Insurance Experiment surveys; NHP = Nottingham Health Profile; QLI = Quality of Life Index; COOP = Dartmouth Function Charts; EUROQOL = European Quality of Life Index; DUKE = Duke Health Profile; MOS FWBP = MOS Functioning and Well-Being Profile; MOS SF-36 = MOS 36-Item Short-Form Health Survey.
[a] Rows are ordered in terms of how frequently concepts are represented; only concepts represented in two or more surveys are listed. Analyses of content were based on published definitions (Ware 1987). Columns are roughly ordered in terms of date of first publication.

percent had invited patients to rate their global quality of life. Thus, "while professing to measure quality of life, many researchers are really measuring various aspects of health status. . . . Quality of life is something that is perceived by each patient individually. The need to incorporate patients' values and preferences is what distinguishes quality of life from all other measures of health" (Gill and Feinstein 1994, 624).

Eliciting patients' own values is essential to measuring quality of life because the value that each of us places on a given health state may differ from the values held by others. Evidence suggests that "old people tend to be health optimists, having more favorable health perceptions than their levels of physical functioning objectively allow" (Kutner et al. 1992, 534). The health

TABLE 3.8

Names of Quality-of-Life Instruments from 75 Articles

Ability to Work
Activities of Daily Living (ADLs)
Activity Index
Additive Daily Activities Profile Test (ADAPT)
Anamnestic Comparative Self-Assessment Instrument (ACSA)
Angina Pectoris Quality of Life Questionnaire (APQLQ)
Arthritis Categorical Scale
Arthritis Ladder Scale
Attitude Towards Warfarin
Body Satisfaction Scale
Bradburn Affect-Balance Scale
Cancer Instrument (ad hoc)
Cancer Rehabilitation Evaluation System (CARES)
Center for Epidemiologic Studies Depression Inventory (CES-D)
Chronic Disease Assessment Tool (CDAT) Quality of Life Scale
Chronic Disease Count
City of Hope Medical Center Quality of Life Survey
Cognitive Impairment
Colorectal Cancer Quality of Life Interview
Daily Activities
Digit Symbol Substitution Test
Disease Symptoms
Eastern Cooperative Oncology Group (ECOG) Performance Score
Eating Behavior (adapted from Sickness Impact Profile)
Emotional Experience (developed from RAND)
Emotional State (ad hoc)
Employment Status
EORTC GU Group's Quality of Life Form
Feelings About Present Life (Hard/Easy)
Feelings About Present Life (Tied Down/Free)

Functional Disability
Functional Living Index—Cancer (FLIC)
Functional Status (adapted from Sickness Impact Profile)
General Health Index
General Health Perceptions (GHP MOS-13)
General Health Perceptions (five-point scale)
General Symptoms
General Well-Being Adjustment Scale
General Well-Being Index
Geriatric Depression Scale (GDS)
Geriatric Mental State Schedule
Global Perceived Health (adapted from GHP MOS-13)
Good Days Last Week
Hand Grip Strength
Happiness
Health Assessment Questionnaire (HAQ)
Health Index
Health Satisfaction
Hearing Handicap Inventory for the Elderly (HHIE)
Home Parenteral Nutrition Questionnaire
HR—Quality of Life Instrument (using Multitrait-Multimethod Analysis)
Index of General Affect
Index of Overall Life Satisfaction
Index of Psychological Affect
Index of Well-Being
Inflammatory Bowel Disease Symptoms Questionnaire (ISQ)
Intellectual Function (ad hoc)
Jenkins Sleep Dysfunction Scale
Karnofsky Performance Index
Katz Adjustment Scale—Relatives' Form (KAS-R)
Keitel Assessment
Kidney Disease Questionnaire

Ladder Scale (Cantrell) for Quality of Life
Lee Functional Index
Life Events
Life Satisfaction (four domains)
Life Satisfaction (Global with Cantrell Ladder)
Life Satisfaction (Likert—seven-point scale)
Life Satisfaction (ten-item scale)
Life Satisfaction Index
Life Style Questionnaire
Linear Analogue Self-Assessment (LASA)
Locus of Control of Behavior (LCB)
McGill Pain Questionnaire
McMaster Health Index Questionnaire (MHIQ)
McMaster–Toronto Arthritis (MACTAR) Patient Function Preference Questionnaire
Medical Outcomes Study (MOS)-36
Mental Health Index
Mental Status
Metastatic Breast Cancer Questionnaire
Minnesota Multiphasic Personality Inventory (MMPI)
National Institute of Mental Health Depression Questionnaire
Need for Control
Nominal Group Process Technique
Nottingham Health Profile
Other Symptoms
Overall Current Health (adapted from RAND)
Overall Health (Global with Cantrell Ladder)
Overall Health Scale (10 cm)
Overall Life Satisfaction
Pain Index
Pain Ladder Scale
Pain Line (10 cm)
Patient Diary
Patient Utility Measurement Scale (PUMS)

TABLE 3.8

Continued

Perceived Health Questionnaire (PHQ)
Perceived Health Status
Perceived Quality of Life Scale (PQOL)
Performance Status Classification
Physical Sense of Well-Being
Physical Status
Physical Symptoms (Standard Questionnaire)
Physical Symptoms Distress Index
Present Pain and Discomfort
Profile of Mood States (POMS)
Psychological Adjustment to Illness Scale (PAIS)
Psychological General Well-Being Schedule (PGWB)
Purpose Designed Questionnaire
QL-Index
Quality of Life Checklist
Quality of Life Index
Quality of Life Index
Quality of Life Index (QALI)
Quality of Life Questionnaire
Quality of Life Questionnaire in Severe CHF (QLQ-SHF)
Quality of Life Scale
Quality of Well-Being (QWB)

Quantified Denver Scale of Communication Function (QDS)
RAND Current Health Assessment
RAND General Health Perceptions Questionnaire
Rey Auditory Verbal Learning Test
Rey-Osterreith Complex Figure Test
Rotterdam Symptom Checklist (RSCL)
Satisfaction with Life Domain Scale (SLDS)
Self Assessment Scale
Self-Evaluation of Life Function (SELF)
Self-Perceived Overall Quality of Life
Sentence Writing (timed)
Serial 7's
Sexual Function
Sexual Symptoms Distress Index
Short Portable Mental Status Questionnaire (SPMSQ)
Sickness Impact Profile
Side Effects and Symptoms (Hypertension)
Side Effects of Chemotherapy (ad hoc)
Sleep, Energy, and Appetite Scale (SEAS)

Social Activity
Social Difficulty Questionnaire
Social Participation (Global with Cantrell Ladder)
Social Participation Index
Standard Gamble Questionnaire
Subjective Rating Scale
Subjectively Appraised Work Load
Symptom Checklist (SCL)-90
Symptom Experience Report (SER)
Taylor Complex Figure Tests
Time Trade Off
Toronto Activities of Daily Living Questionnaire
Unfavorable External Working Conditions
Unfavorable Interpersonal Difficulties
Uniscale
Uremia Quality of Life Questionnaire (ad hoc)
Visual Analogue Scale for Global State of Well-Being
Walking Test
Well-Being Ill-Being Clinical Observation Scale
Willingness to Pay Questionnaire
Word Recall
Work/Daily Role Well-Being Scale

SOURCE: Gill, T. M., and A. R. Feinstein. 1994. "A Critical Appraisal of the Quality of Quality-of-Life Measurements." *Journal of the American Medical Association* 272 (8): 622. Copyrighted 1994, American Medical Association.

values of gravely ill patients vary widely and cannot be clearly predicted based on patients' current states of health (Tsevat et al. 1995). Hearing from patients is especially important for persons with disabilities (Dolan 1996, 559):

> . . . Those in what others may perceive to be "poor" health place a relatively high value on their own health since they have adjusted their life styles and expectations to take account of their condition. This may be particularly true of young disabled men and women, since one-quarter of this group of respondents describe their health as "poor" yet value it as "good." Conversely, young people who describe themselves as "healthy" . . . may be reluctant to value their

> health near the top . . . because they have high expectations about what being in the "best imaginable health state" involves. . . . More than one-fifth of respondents [without disabilities] describe their health as "good" yet value it as "poor."

Specific notions of health status and quality of life also differ for children and adolescents compared to adults (Starfield et al. 1993).

Despite the obvious appeal of quantifying patients' perspectives, several caveats arise. Efforts to be inclusive frequently produce "megavariable" indices (Feinstein 1992). Numerous items of lesser importance can overwhelm potentially critical variables (e.g., particularly troubling symptoms). Some health status and quality-of-life measures relate specifically to persons with particular conditions, whereas others are generic (see Table 3.8). No single method suits all research needs. Choosing an approach depends on the specific research question. Mosteller, Ware, and Levine (1989) recommended routinely using both condition-specific and generic methods; Patrick and Deyo (1989) suggested using standardized, generic instruments with disease-specific supplements.

Relationships between health status or quality of life and various outcomes may be complex or counterintuitive. One complexity is that perceived health status and quality of life change; especially in acutely ill patients, perceptions of overall health can shift over short periods, if not daily. Therefore, questions arise about whether to capture absolute health status at one time point or its trajectory as health status worsens, improves, or remains unchanged (Covinsky et al. 1998). Another example involves using health status to predict resource needs (Steinwachs 1989, S14).

> The relationship of health status to needs for care is not necessarily simple since not all deficits in health status will require health services. The need for care may depend on the severity of the deficit and the potential for timely and appropriate health services to maximize return to the highest level of attainable function. Similarly, individuals with high levels of health status may also have needs for care, including periodic preventive care and counseling on health behaviors that may contribute to future decrements in health status.

Another important question is what to do when patients themselves cannot respond for whatever reason (e.g., poor health, cognitive impairment, logistical considerations). Family members or close friends are often used as proxy respondents. As discussed in Chapter 7, however, proxies may not accurately reflect patients' views. The direction of potential bias—whether proxies report better or worse views than would patients—is unclear. The research evidence is contradictory. To complicate matters, the direction of bias may vary for different subpopulations (e.g., young versus elderly persons).

In the end, however, analysts may need to live with some imperfection in their measures (Bergner 1989, S153–S154).

The terms quality of life, health status, and functional status are often used interchangeably and without specific definition. . . . Quality of life, just as health or illness, must be assessed specifically. . . . Somewhere in the process of deciding on the domains and choosing measures, clinical investigators often start the futile search for the measure, the gold standard that everyone will find appropriate and credible. The bitter truth is that there is no gold standard, there is unlikely ever to be one, and it is unlikely to be desirable to have one.

Patients' Attitudes and Preferences for Outcomes

Finally, patients' attitudes and preferences often affect their clinical outcomes and thus become putative risk factors. Some patients, for example, seek more aggressive care than others. Aggressive interventions may delay death or impairment but may also cause treatment-related complications.

Studies suggest that about one-third of patients do not follow their physicians' recommendations, especially for preventive and outpatient care. The reasons relate largely to patients' health beliefs (especially personal views of vulnerability and seriousness of their condition), health-related motivations, and perceptions of the psychological and other costs of following recommendations. More than one-third of adult Americans annually seek alternatives to traditional allopathic medicine, especially for chronic conditions, but many do not tell their doctors (Eisenberg et al. 1993, 1998). Patients' goals and preferences influence not only clinical outcomes but also costs of their care.

Patients' attitudes and preferences distill a lifetime of experiences, beliefs, goals, health status, quality of life, and understanding about prognosis and treatment options. By definition, this process is uniquely personal. Categorizing patients' attitudes and preferences for care is complex. In addition, these views may change over time as patients weigh their clinical course and personal circumstances. One study tracked preferences of 2,073 patients over two years and found that preferences for such interventions as cardiopulmonary resuscitation, artificial respiration, and tube feeding frequently altered over time (Danis et al. 1994). Because of these complexities, are attitudes and preferences appropriate risk factors? Are attitudes and preferences distributed randomly across populations, making it unnecessary to consider them?

Evidence suggests that patients' preferences and attitudes and how providers address patients' desires are distinctly nonrandom. Adherence rates are especially poor among patients of low socioeconomic status. Highly educated, wealthier patients are more likely to obtain recommended preventive services, such as mammograms. Patients who participate more actively in decision making about their care may do better (Kaplan and Ware 1989). Based on audiotaped interactions between patients and physicians during outpatient visits, Kaplan, Greenfield, and Ware (1989) rated patients' conversational styles. Patients who assumed control of conversations (e.g., asking more questions, directing the flow of discussions and their physicians' behavior) during a base-line office visit reported fewer days lost from work, fewer health problems, lower functional limitations because of health, and higher health status at a follow-up visit. Physiologic outcome measures were also linked to patients' conversational control: At follow-up visits, patients seeking more control had lower blood glucose and blood pressure levels.

DNR orders clearly aim to reflect patients' goals and preferences. Not surprisingly, admission orders of DNR strongly predict 30-day mortality for stroke, pneumonia, and AMI beyond physiological severity indicators (Daley et al. 1988). However, physicians and hospitals vary in their DNR practices. After adjusting for patient and hospital characteristics, analysts found that DNR orders were assigned more frequently to women and less often to black patients, Medicaid recipients, and rural hospital patients (Wenger et al. 1995). Discordance about DNR preferences is common between patients and physicians. For 56.9 percent of patients desiring cardiopulmonary resuscitation, physicians' perceptions agreed, but when patients preferred DNR status, only 47.0 percent of physicians' perceptions agreed (Teno et al. 1995, 182).

The Patient Self-Determination Act, implemented in 1991, requires health care institutions to notify patients about advance directive provisions. Nevertheless, one study found that use of advance directives and living wills did not significantly affect clinical decision making for seriously ill patients (Teno et al. 1994). Preferences for comfort care rather than life-sustaining therapies were frequently disregarded, even among persons age 80 and older (Somogyi-Zalud et al. 2002). On the other hand, although older patients often eschewed aggressive care, some desired cardiopulmonary resuscitation and care to extend life; nonetheless, these patients received less aggressive care than younger patients (Hamel et al. 2000). Even after controlling for patients' prognoses and preferences, older age significantly predicted decisions to withhold ventilator support, surgery, and dialysis (Hamel et al. 1999b).

Patient preferences can affect report cards on provider performance using risk-adjusted outcomes. State analysts informed one hospital in Pennsylvania that its MedisGroups severity-adjusted mortality rate for cancer patients was much higher than expected. Even more worrisome, patients with admission scores of 0 (indicating mild if any clinical instability) had high death rates. Upon investigating, the oncologists found that patients who died with scores of 0 had entered the hospital for pain control and explicitly terminal care. Physicians had actively talked with these patients about whether they wanted even routine testing (e.g., phlebotomy to monitor basic serum chemistries), but the patients had requested comfort measures only. Thus, the standard blood tests used by many severity measures (e.g., serum sodium, potassium, hematocrit, white blood cell count) were not performed. Without measurement, no KCFs were identified, hence producing severity scores of 0. In this circumstance, the 0 scores represented the desire of terminally ill patients to maximize their comfort at the end of life, not the absence of severe disease.

Additional Issues

Several loose ends relating to risk factors remain.

Role of Processes of Care

As noted throughout this book, risk factors aim to capture attributes patients bring to health care encounters that might affect their risks for particular outcomes. Typically, the goal of risk adjusting outcomes is to isolate the effectiveness or quality of care from the patient-related risk factors. Therefore, analysts generally avoid using processes of care, such as specific treatments or procedures, as risk factors. Practice pattern variations could confound efforts to isolate effectiveness or quality and lead to manipulation or gameability of the risk adjuster.

However, in designing their risk adjuster for congenital heart disease surgical mortality in pediatric populations (see Chapter 13), Jenkins and colleagues (2002) argued that little if any discretion exists in the operations performed for various heart defects. Working extensively with panels of physicians, they repeatedly returned to specific operations as crystallizing patients' clinical risk factors for surgical outcomes. Their Risk Adjustment for Congenital Heart Surgery (RACHS-1) measure used expert consensus and empirical methods to determine relative risks of in-hospital death based on specific surgical procedure and other clinical characteristics. In this highly technical area, Jenkins and collaborators (2002) believe that surgeons cannot manipulate the operative approach for pediatric heart surgery patients simply to game or manipulate their risk-adjusted outcomes.

Other investigators have developed risk adjusters based on pharmacy claims, using prescription information to indicate patients' burden of disease (Johnson, Hornbrook, and Nichols 1994; Gilmer et al. 2001). The CDPS and DCG developers have recently released versions based on pharmacy claims—Medicaid R_x and RxGroups, respectively (see Table 2.3). Not surprisingly, these models significantly predict annual costs of care. However, pharmacy claims reflect not only patients' conditions but also practice patterns. In many instances, the decision to prescribe any drug or a specific type of drug is discretionary or highly variable across physicians. Depending on their use, these risk adjusters could have counterproductive effects: "Pharmacy-based risk adjustment may reward those plans and providers that prescribe drugs liberally, and punish those that have adopted more conservative prescribing practices" (Gilmer et al. 2001, 1201).

Nature of the Intervention

Beyond risks arising from patient attributes, the nature of the intervention being studied is also important—the treatment itself may present its own risks. For example, major surgery requiring general anesthesia typically raises more immediate risks than surgery using local or spinal anesthesia. In some instances, complications (e.g., idiosyncratic but deadly reactions to anesthetic agents) result from the intervention itself rather than the underlying disease or patient risk factors. In many circumstances, surgery is contraindicated for patients with extensive disease in major organ systems, such as the lungs and heart. Thus, the decision to forgo surgical intervention because of serious coexisting diseases could confound observational comparisons of surgical and medical therapies.

Similarly, certain medical therapies pose immediate inherent risks. The express goal of most chemotherapeutic regimens is to destroy malignant cells; this process may result in well-anticipated and defined physiologic derangements. Chemotherapy side effects may be particularly problematic for patients with certain comorbid illnesses (e.g., cardiomyopathy, renal failure). Therefore, among chemotherapy patients, certain acute physiologic derangements (low white blood cell counts, high uric acid or potassium levels because of tumor lysis) may indicate the presumed effectiveness of treatment. Persistence of such abnormalities, however, generates concern. The nature and timing of these "intentional" abnormalities resulting from treatment must be considered in assessing risks.

Random Chance

Finally, despite comprehensive efforts to capture risk factors, some important attributes inevitably elude detection or quantification. Nevertheless, even with comprehensive risk adjusters, prediction is imperfect. Although analysts can sometimes predict, with some assurance, individual outcomes, other patients' outcomes are unexpected. Outcomes can result from random chance or "noise." "Whenever the focus is on outlier events, the group of outliers will be composed of 'normals' who experienced bad outcomes by chance and true 'abnormals' who actually had a high risk of bad outcomes. This problem arises particularly when patient populations are small and poor outcomes are rare" (Luft and Romano 1993, 336). One study found that randomness caused the majority of the differences in mortality rates across hospitals (Park et al. 1990). Concerns about interpreting findings based on small sample sizes are particularly pressing when looking at provider-specific, risk-adjusted outcomes (see Chapter 12).

Notes

1. Point scores across all age ranges for APACHE III are as follows: ≤44 years, 0 points; 45–59 years, 5 points; 60–64 years, 11 points; 65–69 years, 13 points; 70–74 years, 16 points; 75–84 years, 17 points; and ≥85 years, 24 points (Knaus et al. 1991, 1624).
2. For women age 85 and older, the average rates of change per year from 1987 through 1995 for major procedures were as follows: 11 percent for CABG; 20 percent for angioplasty; 12 percent for carotid endarterectomy; and 29 percent for hip replacement (Fuchs 1999, 14).

3. A study by the U.S. General Accounting Office (1992) found that 60 percent of clinical trials for new drugs underrepresented female subjects. Of 53 drug trials studied, only 25 (47 percent) specifically assessed whether men and women responded differently to the medication being tested. Female representation was particularly poor for trials involving new cardiovascular drugs: For 7 of 13 cardiovascular medication trials examined, the proportion of female subjects was more than 20 percent below the percentage of women in the population with the disease in question. Similar underrepresentation of women in federally funded research studies prompted the creation of the National Institutes of Health, Office of Research on Women's Health.

4. The six conditions were AMI, congestive heart failure (CHF), obstructive airway disease, gastrointestinal hemorrhage, pneumonia, and stroke. Patients admitted as interhospital transfers were excluded. After controlling for risk factors, men died in hospital significantly more often than women for all conditions except AMI and CHF.

5. The severity measures provided somewhat different views about whether women were sicker than men. Regardless of treatment, the Comorbidity Index and DS stage uniformly suggested that women and men had comparable severity ($p > 0.05$). In contrast, APR-DRGs, Body Systems Count, the Patient Management Categories (PMC) severity score, and Physiology Score 2 always viewed women as significantly more severely ill than men ($p \leq 0.05$). The clinical-data-based measures did not always agree. For all cases, for example, the two MedisGroups measures rated women as having comparable severity as men, whereas the two physiology scores saw women as significantly sicker. These differences across severity measures thus left contradictory impressions about whether women were more severely ill than men. We could not go back to medical records to determine which severity measures were "right." As a preliminary exploration of this question, we identified six clinical findings thought to represent severe illness in AMI and then used admission KCFs to see whether men or women were more likely to have the indicator. For medical and all cases, women were generally significantly more likely than men to have the finding. An exception involved low left ventricular ejection fraction, but we could not determine whether this represented detection bias (i.e., men were more likely to have it measured). The only KCF with significant sex differences for CABG cases was pulmonary edema (6.2 percent of women, 2.9 percent of men). PTCA cases exhibited no significant sex differences.

6. The Thirteenth Amendment abolished the three-fifths rule, and American Indians were only fully counted starting in 1924 (Williams 1999).

7. SOFA variables are a respiratory indicator (Pa_{O_2}/Fi_{O_2} mm Hg), coagulation (platelets $10^3/mm^2$), bilirubin, hypotension, Glasgow

Coma Score, and creatinine.

8. For each candidate comorbidity, Charlson and colleagues (1987, 377) calculated adjusted relative risks from a Cox proportional-hazards model. Based on these findings, comorbidities were assigned weights ranging from 1 (adjusted relative risk ≥ 1.2 and < 1.5) to 6 (adjusted relative risk ≥ 6). The weighted index significantly predicted one-year mortality ($p < 0.0001$).

9. The logistic regression models controlled for age, sex, prior heart surgery, priority of surgery (elective, urgent, emergency), extent of left main coronary artery disease, number of diseased coronary arteries, and left ventricular ejection fraction, in addition to 11 comorbid conditions (hypertension, diabetes, obesity, severe obesity, vascular disease, chronic obstructive pulmonary disease, peptic ulcer, cancer, end-stage renal disease, liver disease, and dementia) (Clough et al. 2002).

10. Needing total assistance with bathing produced an adjusted odds ratio (95 percent confidence interval [CI]) for dying of 6.69 (2.89–15.49), for stroke patients, and 4.98 (2.74–9.08) for pneumonia patients (Davis et al. 1995, 913, 915).

11. As measured by R^2, the amount of variation explained was 24 percent for physical functioning, 20 percent for role functioning, 14 percent for social functioning, 12 percent for mental health, 29 percent for health perceptions, and 14 percent for pain (Stewart et al. 1989, 910).

WINDOWS OF OBSERVATION

Amy K. Rosen

T he importance of specific risk factors depends on the time frame. Is the outcome of interest imminent, within minutes or hours, or years away? For example, today's blood glucose level indicates whether patients with diabetes are at immediate risk of ketoacidosis or hyperglycemic coma. For more distant outcomes, such as retinopathy, peripheral vascular disease, or lower extremity amputation, indicators of longer-term glycemic control (e.g., hemoglobin A_{1c}) are more relevant risk factors. When developing or assessing risk-adjustment methods, specifying the time window is therefore crucial: risk of what outcome, over what time frame, for what population, and for what purpose?

Most risk adjusters focus on specific time periods, such as hospital admissions or one year of health care utilization (see Table 2.5). This chapter examines the implications of these time windows for conceptualizing risk and identifying risk factors. It also takes an in-depth look at three specific time frames: hospitalizations, one-year periods, and episodes of care.

Conceptual Framework

Windows of observation are the time periods or events circumscribing the outcome of interest. The definition of the windows of observation typically derives directly from the targeted outcome. For example, for assessing hospital mortality rates, the window of observation is the time from admission to discharge (alive or dead) or some short, fixed time frame triggered by hospitalization (e.g., 30 days after admission).

Fixing the time window, such as specifying the number of days or months, reduces concerns about comparing outcomes across pertinent units of observation, such as hospitals, with varying practice patterns. For example, Jencks, Williams, and Kay (1988) found that Massachusetts hospitals had systematically higher in-hospital mortality rates for Medicare beneficiaries than did California hospitals. At the time, almost 20 years ago, California hospitals had dramatically shorter lengths of stay than did Massachusetts facilities. The longer the time window, the more deaths were detected. Fixing the window of observation at 30 days following admission caused differences in hospital death rates across the two states to disappear.

As suggested above, some risk factors are more or less useful depending on the window of observation. For example, extremely high or low blood pressure is an acute physiologic derangement that portends imminent death. Extreme hypertension or hypotension can result from acute pathophysiologic processes (e.g., an idiosyncratic drug reaction, severe bleeding, or shock from trauma) that, if successfully treated, may have few long-term consequences. While such extreme blood pressure readings heighten risk of death within hours or days, they may not predict longer-term outcomes, such as mortality a year or two hence. A lower level of persistent hypertension may, however, raise risks of future events, such as stroke or CHF. Many sociodemographic, economic, lifestyle, and cultural attributes are risk factors for important health care outcomes. Some hold implications for short-term outcomes, such as Jehovah's Witnesses' prohibition against blood transfusions (see Chapter 3). Most, however, like smoking and poverty, are linked to longer-term outcomes years or even decades in the future.

The window of observation relates directly to the outcome of interest. However, the time window from which risk factor information is drawn may be different depending on the purpose of the analysis and on the available database. For instance, if the purpose of a hospital mortality analysis is to isolate potential quality-of-care problems, using risk factors only from the period shortly after admission is essential; otherwise, the risk factors could become confounded with quality problems, the very quantity of interest. For example, although low blood pressure following admission for pneumonia will strongly predict death, hypotension could result from failure to carefully monitor the patient and recognize sepsis or septic shock. Including low blood pressure readings from several days into the hospitalization would mask problems at hospitals that fail to adequately monitor their pneumonia patients.

Characteristics of databases could also affect the time frame from which analysts draw risk factors. Information from before a hospital admission could provide important insight into risk factors for hospitalization outcomes. For instance, routine preoperative testing is often now performed up to two weeks before patients are admitted for elective surgery; medical records may contain little information from the preadmission evaluation. With longitudinal administrative records (see Chapter 5), looking back to claims or encounter records from six months to a year prior to admission offers information about chronic conditions that could be important for risk adjusting hospitalization outcomes.

Some risk factors may be important for the current time period but not for the future. For example, algorithms to predict costs over one year of care often have two versions, one predicting costs in the year in which the predictor variables (typically diagnoses) occur, so-called "concurrent models," and one predicting costs in future years, generally the year following that from which the diagnoses are drawn. Sometimes, significant predictors from the concurrent model are not predictive of next year's costs (i.e., the prospective model). A clear example is appendicitis. Appendicitis increases costs in the current year because of the surgery and hospitalization required to treat the condition. Once the appendix is removed, however, patients can never again have appendicitis; the condition cannot increase future costs.

Risk factor information from surveys (see Chapter 7) can carry its own time window. For example, functional-status questionnaires often ask people about functional abilities within specific time frames, such as the prior 30 days. When using such time-sensitive information, linking the date of the survey with the date of the index event (e.g., a hospitalization) or outcome of interest (e.g., mortality) may be important. As noted in Chapter 3, the best predictor of future functional status is previous functional status (e.g., some designated "baseline"), but analysts must take care not to create a tautology. For example, using current self-reported functional status to predict functioning in the short term may become, in essence, circular reasoning. Determining the appropriate timing for measuring baseline and future functional status will depend on the analytic questions and context.

Finally, in conjunction with the outcome of interest, the purpose of the project or study will help define the appropriate time window. For example, to profile providers, looking at an episode of care for managing a specific disease or condition may offer important insight. Here, the unit of observation is the episode. The goal of risk adjustment might be to improve the clinical homogeneity of episodes, accounting for differences in patient characteristics that would affect the services received (e.g., procedures, treatments, and tests) and expected resource utilization. If the analysis focuses on characterizing the nature of the episode rather than the patient, risk factors such as patients' psychosocial functioning and health-related behaviors may be less important than in other contexts.

If the goal is to predict resource needs of a given population, a fixed period (e.g., a year) is appropriate. Within this time frame, analysts would account for the cumulative effect of patients' various conditions. Here, a variety of patient attributes might be important risk factors, including demographic characteristics, diagnoses, health-related behaviors, functional status, and self-reported global health status.

Therefore, when designing a risk-adjustment strategy, one must answer questions about time window: risk of what outcome over what time frame? The window of observation has important implications for which risk factors are most relevant as analysts develop their conceptual model of risk (see Chapter 8). Depending on the purpose, database, setting, and context, the options of windows of observation are almost infinitely varied. Here, I describe in greater depth three common time windows, focusing especially on episodes of care.

Acute Care Hospitalization

Within health care settings, acute care hospitalizations provide perhaps the most obvious window of observation. Certainly, hospitalizations have generated extensive study. For almost three decades, researchers have used increasingly sophisticated risk-adjustment approaches to examine costs, lengths of stay, and outcomes potentially related to quality of care. Therefore, many risk adjusters exist for evaluating outcomes of acute care hospitalizations. DRGs, used to adjust prospective Medicare payments for acute care hospitalizations, remain the best known and most widely adopted risk-adjustment method. Although DRGs are inextricably linked to payment, they originated through efforts at Yale University to develop LOS norms for utilization review based on groupings of patients that were "interpretable medically" (Fetter et al. 1980).

Defining when windows start and end is essential for identifying both relevant risk adjusters and outcomes. The beginning and ending of acute care hospitalizations seem obvious: the window starts when patients are admitted and closes at discharge. Often, though, these time points are unclear. Especially over the last several years, administrative and local environmental concerns have sometimes blurred the exact time of admission. Because of complex insurance coverage issues, some hospitals keep certain patients in "observation beds" rather than formally admitting them to the facility; such patients may eventually be admitted if they fail to recover quickly. With overcrowded emergency rooms and full hospitals, patients can wait many hours before being admitted for an acute illness. These practices vary across hospitals. Crowded inner-city teaching hospitals are typically more likely to experience delays in their emergency rooms than are suburban facilities.

Determining the endpoint of acute hospitalizations can also be complicated. One obvious concern involves transfers, not only to other acute care hospitals but also increasingly to such settings as acute rehabilitation hospitals and nursing homes. In the past, poststroke rehabilitation, for example, generally began during lengthy acute care hospitalizations. Now patients are usually transferred quickly to so-called "post acute care" facilities. Transfer practices vary by hospital type (e.g., academic teaching versus community facilities) and by services available in the local community.

The impetus for speedy discharges also varies by hospital ownership. For instance, hospitals run by the VA often allow longer stays than private facilities. One study compared in-hospital mortality for ICU patients admitted to a VHA hospital to 27 private-sector hospitals in 1994–95 (Kaboli et al. 2001, 1014). Average LOS was much higher at the VA compared to private hospitals (28.3 versus 11.3 days), and unadjusted mortality was similarly higher (14.5 percent versus 12.0 percent). These differences disappeared after adjusting for severity. More importantly, a higher proportion of VA deaths occurred after 21 days in hospital. After Kaboli and colleagues (2001, 1014) applied proportional-hazards regression models, censoring patients at hospital discharge, the VA patients actually had a lower risk of death (hazard ratio 0.70, $p < 0.001$).

Therefore, factors affecting the timing of hospital admission and discharge vary widely across hospitals, potentially biasing comparisons using hospitalization as the window of observation. Perceptions of outcomes can shift dramatically after accounting for varying time windows. To deal with differing discharge practices, analysts often define hospitalization windows using fixed periods following admission, such as 30, 90, or 180 days. A fascinating study examined mortality trends at local hospitals from 1991 through 1997, the period during which the CHQC program was in place (Baker et al. 2002a). This initiative required collection of extensive clinical data to support risk adjustment of mortality rates (see Chapter 1). During this period across the six study conditions, absolute rates of risk-adjusted in-hospital mortality did decline significantly, from 2.1 percent for chronic obstructive pulmonary disease to 4.8 percent for pneumonia (Baker et al. 2002a, 886). When the researchers instead examined 30-day mortality, however, relatively few changes had occurred. Between 1991 and 1997, deaths had shifted from Cleveland hospitals to other settings soon after discharge. For stroke, the absolute rates of risk-adjusted 30-day mortality had actually significantly increased (by 4.3 percent).

Virtually by definition, important risk factors for acute care hospitalizations include acute clinical stability and acute attributes of principal diagnoses and comorbid conditions. However, depending on the outcome of interest, chronic conditions can also significantly predict acute care results (Charlson et al. 1987; D'Hoore, Bouckaert, and Tilquin 1996; Rosen et al. 1992, 1995; Elixhauser et al. 1998). Physical functional status is a critical risk factor for in-hospital mortality for some conditions (Davis et al. 1995; Justice et al. 1996). Therefore, longer-term risk factors can significantly predict outcomes even within short time windows.

Fixed, Longer-Term Windows

Another way of specifying time windows is to look at the calendar. If one aims to capture outcomes for populations within a system of care regardless of where, when, or how services are provided, focusing on a fixed block of time makes sense. In today's health policy context, for example, counting total costs expended in caring for a particular population (e.g., enrollees of a health plan) is often important. In this setting, analysts typically choose one year (12 months based on calendar or fiscal years) for this accounting.

Most of the early interest in one-year time windows focused on costs. Quantifying risk over a year is now used to adjust capitation payments to managed care plans, profile expenditures by provider, and assist allocation of resources. More recently, year-long risk adjustment has expanded to other applications, such as identifying persons with particular medical problems for disease management programs or potentially high-cost persons for case management. As noted above, two types of models differing by the time frame of the outcome are typically employed. Concurrent (same-year) models are often used to understand how disease burden affects historical costs or to produce provider profiles. Prospective models use information from the current, or base, year to predict future (next year's) costs or identify next year's high-cost patients.

Although specifying the beginning and ending of 12-month periods is clear, identifying who belongs within the target population can become complicated. Especially when populations are defined by insurance status, analysts generally use enrollment dates for insurance coverage to identify those within the target population. Insurance coverage can come and go during year-long periods. Fluctuating insurance status is particularly common among Medicaid recipients, whose coverage depends largely on their income. For example, one study examined more than 42 million Medicaid-eligible individuals in 1999 using data from the Medicaid State Information System (MSIS). The researchers found that 47 percent were eligible for all 12 months of the year; however, 5 percent had at least a one-month interruption in their Medicaid coverage during the year (Gilden 2002).[1]

In these instances, analysts often look at each month of coverage, reweighting information for individuals without a full year of data by how many twelfths of a year they were actually covered. DCGs, for example, annualize the costs for individuals with less than one full year of entitlement in the prospective year based on their observed cost per month; in analyses, these data are treated as "fractional observations" (Ellis and Ash 1995). Thus, a person with costs of $10,000 who has entitlement through the third month has annualized costs of $40,000. Similarly, using the CDPS to analyze residuals from unweighted regression models for Medicaid beneficiaries, Kronick and colleagues (2000, 34) found that one method of reducing the influence of shorter entitlement periods was to weight each observation by $(1 - 0.067 \times [12 - \text{number of eligible months}])$.

Longer windows of observation are typically used to examine outcomes for populations regardless of the setting of care. Therefore, risk factors are often drawn from various sources, including not only acute care hospitalizations but also outpatient visits. As noted above, acute physiologic stability is probably not a significant risk factor for longer-term outcomes, but virtually all other dimensions of risk are potential candidates—depending on the outcome of interest, specific population, and purpose of the evaluation.

As shown in Chapter 2, various risk-adjustment tools focus on predicting total costs (or expenditures) for one year of care for insured populations. Taking one of these methods "off the shelf" may be appropriate in some settings, recognizing that risk-adjustment methods developed for one population may not perform as well in populations with differing characteristics. Researchers sometimes supplement these off-the-shelf models with additional disease-specific indicators relevant to their own populations as well as sociodemographic variables (e.g., marital status, race/ethnicity, socioeconomic status) to improve the predictive ability of these models (Rosen et al. 2002; Ettner et al. 1998, 1999; Ash et al. 2000). Pharmacy data are increasingly used as proxies for disease burden in predicting health care resource use within a 12-

month period (Gilmer et al. 2001; Fishman and Shay 1999; Roblin 1998; Zhao et al. 2001). Models combining pharmacy claims and inpatient data have performed significantly better than either model alone and "provided a more complete picture of the distribution of illness in the population" (Zhao et al. 2001, 190).

Although most risk adjusters for one-year outcomes have focused on predicting resource use, important exceptions include the comorbidity index developed by Charlson and colleagues (1987) and the ICED (Greenfield et al. 1993). These two comorbidity indices were derived from medical records of hospitalized patients to predict risks of one-year mortality and one-year health-related quality of life, respectively (see Chapter 3). Although primarily used to predict clinical outcomes within a 12-month period, the indices may predict outcomes over longer time frames, such as five-year survival (Krousel-Wood, Abdoh, and Re 1996). Conversely, the Charlson index may also predict short-term mortality (Poses et al. 1996), and it has frequently been used in studies of acute hospitalization outcomes.

Episodes of Care

An episode of care is a "series of temporally contiguous health care services related to treatment of a given spell of illness or provided in response to a specific request by the patient or other relevant entity" (Hornbrook, Hurtado, and Johnson 1985, 171). An episode framework relates health care inputs (e.g., specific events, primary care and specialist services, time required to produce particular outcomes) to health care outputs (e.g., duration and course of illness). In truth, many persons, especially elderly patients, have concurrent chronic conditions that wax and wane, with fuzzy boundaries around putative episodes. Erecting strict perimeters specifying the start and finish of a health problem defies this reality. Nevertheless, an episode approach facilitates analysis of both processes and outcomes of care and has recently become a popular management tool.

Determining which risk factors to incorporate into an episode is complicated. To specify episodes, analysts must first identify the clinical trigger that starts the episode, such as a particular procedure or visit for a certain diagnosis. That trigger could be defined in detailed clinical terms, perhaps making risk adjustment unnecessary. Patients in the same episode should be reasonably clinically homogeneous with respect to the specific health problem addressed by the episode and experience similar patterns of resource use (Rosen and Mayer-Oakes 1998, 1999). Nevertheless, other clinical attributes, such as severity of illness and comorbidities, may need consideration to compare episodes across patients with varying clinical complexity. Therefore, meaningful comparisons of episodes usually require risk adjustment.

Episodes may involve one or more encounters over time and have varying lengths. Risk factors relevant to episodes of short duration may not apply to those covering longer periods. Beginning and ending points of episodes are defined differently in different contexts. For example, episodes may commence with the initial contact with the health care system or when a diagnosis is confirmed. Episodes may end within predetermined intervals (e.g., 30 days after the index visit) or when the condition is cured or resolves. "Clean periods" (Rosen et al. 1998, 28) are time intervals without service use and are often employed to define when an episode ends; new episodes begin when services resume after the clean period. Using the clean-period approach means that endpoints represent varying outcomes. For example, episodes can end when patients no longer seek care for whatever reason, when they leave a particular system of care, or when treatment is no longer necessary. Short episodes typically provide "snapshots" of care and can be tightly defined to isolate the effect of specific conditions. Episodes with longer windows of observation allow more extensive insight but may reflect the influence of comorbid diseases or factors outside the targeted condition.

The episode framework is generally better suited to acute diseases with definite starting and stopping points, where the course is well defined. In contrast, chronic diseases often have indeterminate beginnings and endings; their courses typically last 90 days or more, often spanning years or even lifetimes (Hornbrook, Hurtado, and Johnson 1985). One strategy for defining chronic disease episodes (e.g., for diabetes) involves subdividing their course into subepisodes or phases, such as a diagnostic phase (when diabetes is first recognized), a maintenance phase (routine management of glycemic control), an acute flare-up phase (when metabolic disturbances like ketoacidosis develop), and a chronic complication phase (for conditions resulting from end-organ damage, such as foot ulcers) (Hornbrook, Hurtado, and Johnson 1985; Rosen et al. 1998; Rosen and Mayer-Oakes 1999). Each phase can have its own set of risk factors. Another approach is dividing chronic disease episodes into fixed-length intervals, such as one-year periods.

Implementing Episode Algorithms

Episodes of care are generally easy to operationalize using administrative data (see Chapter 5), such as claims or encounter databases containing diagnosis codes, codes for each service, and service dates. Using these dates, analysts can array services in chronologic order. Various commercial software products called "episode groupers" (Rosen and Mayer-Oakes 1999, 113) use retrospective computerized algorithms to cluster services into discrete episodes to support provider profiling, quality assessment, and outcomes measurement. The most important risk factors include inpatient and outpatient primary and secondary diagnosis codes and patients' demographic characteristics. Some groupers also include pharmacy claims and procedural information.

Commercial episode groupers vary in how they define the target conditions, the episodes themselves (i.e., start- and endpoints), and the complexity of risk adjustment, if any (Rosen and Mayer-Oakes 1999). Some episode groupers explicitly consider comorbidities, whereas others do not. Figures 4.1 and 4.2 illustrate the conceptualization of an acute episode of pharyngitis by two episode groupers. Episode treatment groups (ETGs) are conceptually similar to DRGs, except that they classify an entire episode of care rather than a hospitalization (Figure 4.1). Risk adjustment is based on age, sex, comorbidities, and complications indicating severity of illness, such as the surgical procedure used for treatment. Each of the 558 ETGs has its own clean period that is marked by the absence of treatment; therefore, episodes have no predetermined length. In contrast, the physician review system (PRS; Figure 4.2) builds episodes from 200 clinical conditions that are rated according to three levels of severity and three levels of comorbidity (mild, moderate, and high). These ratings create a three-dimensional matrix (severity, comorbidity, and type of condition). Each condition has a predefined episode length depending on whether the condition is chronic or acute.

Several features of episode approaches suggest which risk factors should be considered (Hornbrook, Hurtado, and Johnson 1985). First is the target outcome of the episode: the question, risk of what? Beyond capturing patient-specific information, episode groupers targeting resource utilization may also incorporate provider- and system-level factors. In contrast, episode algorithms targeting health status when the episode ends focus on such concerns as pre-episode risk (i.e., patients' baseline health status) and patients' health-related behaviors. A second feature is episode duration. With longer time windows, patient-level risk factors become more important. As in other settings, the more time that elapses, the more likely that factors outside providers' control (e.g., specific processes of care) will influence outcomes. Longer time frames increase the potential of confounding quality of care with risk factors.

Third is episode course—the rate of progression or natural history of the targeted condition. Some conditions have very rapid onsets and progress quickly, whereas others may advance or recede more slowly. However, variability of the rate of progression within conditions is also important. Patients with identical diagnoses can experience widely varying courses of illness, perhaps because of inherent physiologic variations or perhaps related to other factors, such as comorbid conditions or physical frailty. Finally, disentangling processes of care for persons with multiple conditions is complicated. One strategy is creating separate episodes for each disease; another is to combine all diseases into a single episode, risk adjusting outcomes (e.g., overall resource utilization) for comorbid conditions.

An Episode Approach for Asthma Patients

My colleagues and I adopted an episode methodology to evaluate the quality of care delivered to patients with asthma (Rosen et al. 1998; Rosen and Mayer-Oakes 1999). Our experiences illustrate how risk adjustment might be incorporated into episodes of care. We constructed the episodes using several iterative steps. Episodes began with an index clinical event (e.g., a provider

FIGURE 4.1

Episode
Treatment
Groups (ETGs)

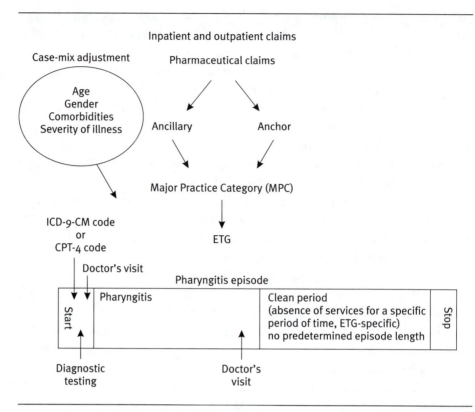

encounter) with a specific diagnosis code for asthma. We identified episodes using only principal diagnoses on claims; we did not include cases when claims listed asthma as a secondary diagnosis. We applied DS, which examines all diagnoses, to rate the severity of asthma episodes. For example, DS assigns stage 1.1 to cases of asymptomatic bronchial asthma or clinically mild asthma. In contrast, stage 3.0 or greater includes codes for severe asthma or status asthmaticus as well as asthma with respiratory failure.

We defined clean periods based on the peak asthma severity level within the episode. For example, stage 1.1 asthma episodes involved a cluster of services related to treatment of stage 1.1 asthma (i.e., asymptomatic bronchial asthma or clinically mild asthma), which had a clean period of 15 days. As the stage of the episode increased, the length of the clean period also increased, with a maximum clean period of 45 days. Figure 4.3 illustrates our asthma episode construction.

We also considered patients' health status before their asthma episodes (i.e., a "pre-episode risk period"), as this may influence the course and outcome of the episode. Variables used as proxies of severity in this six-month time frame included number of comorbidities, defined by diagnosis codes, and number and type of asthma-related services. We classified services as asthma related based on the principal diagnosis associated with the service claim. We further divided these services into three categories based on asthma-related

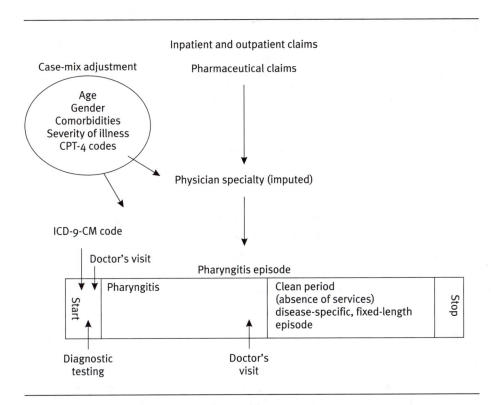

FIGURE 4.2
Physician
Review System
(PRS)

procedure codes to create a "treatment intensity" variable: (1) pulmonary function testing, (2) treatment of bronchial spasms with bronchodilators, and (3) all other treatments for asthma management.

Because asthma is a chronic disease, we created two types of asthma episodes—acute and maintenance episodes. Acute episodes exhibited clear-cut start- and endpoints, with a relatively obvious clinical course, as defined by an acute care hospitalization, interventions commonly used to manage acute flare-ups (e.g., nebulizer treatments), an emergency room visit, or DS stage 2.2 or higher. We considered all other episodes to be maintenance episodes, where treatment aimed toward preserving stability and preventing deterioration.

Conclusions

Different windows of observation affect the range of risk factors that should be considered in developing risk-adjustment methods. Risk factors vary in their importance, depending on the time frame. The time interval also holds significant implications for the meaning of risk-adjusted outcomes information, especially for calculating the "algebra of effectiveness"—the extent to which risk factors contribute to outcomes as opposed to the health care interventions, the quality of that care, and random chance.

Just as the United States performs a decennial census to count its population, assessments of population health often extend over years, even decades.

FIGURE 4.3

Asthma
Episode
Construction

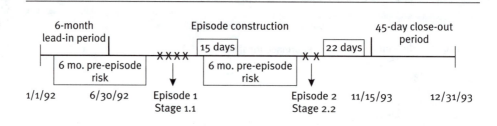

The National Center for Health Statistics (NCHS) reports yearly a detailed cross-sectional view of population health, but these reports include tables noting trends (e.g., in death rates by conditions) across years, even decades. When taking this long view, many factors beyond specific clinical interventions become critically important, including health-related behaviors (such as smoking), sociodemographic characteristics, and environmental attributes (Institute of Medicine 2001b; Williams 1996; Marmot 2002).

Note

1. The latter estimate was calculated by evaluating differences between an individual's number of Medicaid-eligible months and the duration in months between an individual's first and last Medicaid-eligible month in the year. If the length of months between an individual's first and last eligible months in the year was greater than his or her total Medicaid-eligible months in the year, he or she was identified as having an interruption in coverage.

CODED DATA FROM ADMINISTRATIVE SOURCES

Lisa I. Iezzoni

Administrative data result from running the health care system—enrolling people in health plans, paying claims, determining reimbursement amounts, certifying coverage, approving expenditures, tracking service utilization, and monitoring costs and performance. Although not produced explicitly to examine the health or health care of populations, administrative data nonetheless offer important advantages for this purpose:

- They include large numbers of people, sometimes entire populations (e.g., all persons hospitalized in a state).
- They represent care practiced throughout the community rather than in specialized settings.
- When records for individuals are linked, they can track persons over time and across settings of care.
- Federal regulations standardizing data content and formats make certain administrative data comparable throughout the public and private health care delivery systems.
- Large numbers help hide personal identities, thus protecting confidentiality after individual identifiers are removed.
- They already exist, are relatively inexpensive to acquire, and are computer readable.

Administrative data have offered profound insights into health care practices. Three decades ago, Wennberg and Gittlesohn (1973) used hospital discharge data to expose wide variations in rates of expensive medical interventions across small geographical areas with ostensibly similar populations. In the 1980s, administrative data were tapped to assess community-based care. The law authorizing the federal Agency for Health Care Policy and Research (AHCPR, now the Agency for Healthcare Research and Quality, or AHRQ), Section 6103 of the Omnibus Budget Reconciliation Act of 1989 (P.L. 101-239), mandated use of large administrative databases to examine the "outcomes, effectiveness, and appropriateness" of health care services. AHCPR's flagship projects, the patient outcomes research teams (PORTs), began with administrative data (Clancy and Eisenberg 1997).

Administrative data, however, inherit two significant limitations from the fragmented American health care delivery system. First, to produce claims or encounter records, people typically must have public or private health insurance. Most person-level administrative databases do not include uninsured individuals, estimated at 42 million (15 percent of the population) in 1999 (Institute of Medicine 2001c, 23). Uninsured persons represent a particularly vulnerable subpopulation (Institute of Medicine 2002a; see Chapter 1). Additionally, many enrollees stay relatively briefly in needs-based public insurance (Medicaid) and specific private, employment-based plans. High turnover, common among Medicaid recipients and within rapidly changing work forces, impedes efforts to create longitudinal, population-based databases.

Second, health insurance must cover specific services for claims or encounter records to be submitted and enter the database. However, many important services, particularly for chronic conditions, are not covered, especially by Medicare and private health plans (Institute of Medicine 2001a). Insurers often set annual limits on mental health services or "carve out" their coverage to other organizations (Gitterman, Strum, and Scheffler 2001; see Chapter 14). Even insured people can spend thousands of dollars annually out of pocket for health-related services (Foote and Hogan 2001). Thus, the services and medical conditions represented by claims or encounter records do not fully reflect health care experiences or needs.

Administrative data have other limitations. Most importantly, their primary clinical insight comes from diagnoses coded with questionable accuracy, completeness, clinical scope, and meaningfulness. Furthermore, administrative data can be cumbersome to handle and somewhat out of date. These and other problems led the former Office of Technology Assessment (1994, 6) to conclude: "Contrary to the expectations expressed in the legislation establishing AHCPR and the mandates of the PORTs, administrative databases generally have not proved useful in answering questions about the comparative effectiveness of alternative medical treatments."

Despite these problems, administrative data provide important information about health services utilization, expenditures, selected clinical outcomes, and quality of care. Managers, policymakers, and researchers rely heavily on these data sets to examine important outcomes of care, and many risk-adjustment methods were designed specifically for administrative databases. This chapter examines major U.S. administrative databases, describes their clinical content, briefly discusses data systems internationally, offers ways to augment the usefulness of administrative data, and suggests issues that will shape future administrative databases.

Overview of Administrative Databases in the United States

Administrative data are the by-product of operating and overseeing the health care system. In some administrative databases, the unit of observation is a specific service, typically acute care hospitalizations. As of the late 1990s, 42 states systematically collected information about hospital discharges, primarily using the UB-92 format (see below). With some exceptions, patients do not have unique statewide identification numbers, preventing tracking of admissions for individuals across hospitals. Furthermore, these databases generally cannot link with other settings of care. Nevertheless, AHRQ's Healthcare Cost and Utilization Project (HCUP; 2001) has compiled states' hospitalization information since 1988 and now includes 29 states, representing more than half of all U.S. general acute care admissions. HCUP data offer analysts a powerful database to explore inpatient stays.[1]

In health insurance databases, persons are usually the unit of observation.[2] Individuals receive unique identifiers, allowing tracking of their services across settings covered by the insurer. Most health insurance databases contain two types of files: enrollment files, indicating eligibility for the health plan and demographic information; and claims (in fee for service) or encounter records (in managed care plans), representing individual services or sets of services. We focus here on person-level administrative data produced by public (e.g., Medicare, Medicaid, VA) and private health insurers. Persons outside the organizations producing these databases (such as CMS) can sometimes gain access to these data after meeting specific confidentiality and security requirements.

Most clinical insight from administrative data comes from records for individual services. Here, I sort these files into two types: "standard" and "enriched," reflecting the clinical content of the data. In standard administrative data, the most helpful clinical information comes as

- diagnoses coded using ICD-9-CM;
- procedures or services coded using ICD-9-CM for claims submitted by institutional providers such as hospitals, the American Medical Association's CPT-4 for individual physician services, or the *Healthcare Common Procedure Coding System* (HCPCS) for nonphysician services not in CPT-4, including durable medical equipment; and
- prescription drugs often coded using NDCs (U.S. Food and Drug Administration 2003) on pharmacy claims from insurance plans (including Medicaid) offering drug coverage.[3]

Standard administrative data are submitted when billing for care (fee for service) or when capitated plans must report health care encounters. Medicare MCOs currently must submit encounter records only for hospitalizations, although additional reporting requirements for specific health conditions are pending (to assist with risk adjusting capitation payments). Over the next several years, major administrative records throughout the entire health care system must comply with transaction standards specified pursuant to Title II of the 1996 Health Insurance Portability and Accountability Act (HIPAA; P.L. 104-191). As described below, HIPAA mandates standardized content, formats, and code sets for various computerized records. These new requirements should make the content of standard administrative databases comparable across public and private payers.

Because law or regulation requires it, some clinically detailed information is technically administrative. However, because of the extensive clinical content, I view these data as enriched—offering substantial clinical insight despite routine collection by regulatory or programmatic fiat. Well-known examples come from Medicare and include the Minimum Data Set (MDS), administered quarterly in nursing homes (see Chapter 16); the Outcome and Assessment Information Set (OASIS), collected during home health care visits (see Chapter 16); and the Patient Assessment Instrument (PAI) for inpatient rehabilitation facilities (IRF), or IRF-PAI, which contains the Functional Independence Measure (CMS 2002a, 2002b; see Chapter 15).

The MDS supports nursing home prospective payment using RUGs, while OASIS underlies home care prospective payment (HHRGs). IRF-PAI data elements funnel rehabilitation hospital patients into one of 85 clinical or five administrative CMGs for prospective payment. Finding multiple data-gathering tools for populations with roughly similar clinical concerns, Med-PAC (2001, 94) recommended development of a single "patient classification system that predicts costs within and across post-acute settings." My discussion below concentrates on standard administrative data; Chapters 15 and 16, respectively, address the IRF-PAI and MDS.

Sources of Administrative Data

The three major sources of administrative data are the federal government (U.S. DHHS, VA), state governments, and private insurance companies. Initially, administrative data files concentrated primarily on acute care hospitalizations, with the Uniform Hospital Discharge Data Set (UHDDS) serving as the prototype. The National Committee on Vital and Health Statistics, U.S. Department of Health, Education, and Welfare (U.S. DHEW; 1980), formulated the UHDDS in 1972. Its intent was to create a uniform but "minimum" data set to facilitate investigation of the costs and quality of short-term hospital services at both local and national levels. In 1974, following initial testing, DHEW required submission of UHDDS data for all acute hospital discharges paid through Medicare and Medicaid. In 1979, a committee convened by DHEW revised the directions for completing the UHDDS while retaining the original 14 data elements (Table 5.1). The basic content of the UHDDS has changed little over the last three decades.

The UHDDS forms the core of most administrative hospital reports. In the mid-1980s, the UB-82 (Uniform Bill introduced in 1982) became the most widely used format, required for hospitals submitting reimbursement claims to Medicare, Medicaid, Blue Cross, and many commercial health insurance carriers. UB-82 contained more than 90 data fields, including patient identifiers, hospitalization descriptors (e.g., admission type: emergent, urgent,

No. and Item	Definition and Comments
1. Personal identification	"The unique number assigned to each patient within a hospital that distinguishes the patient and his or her hospital record from all others in that institution" (p. 8). Social Security number was not recommended because it is not always unique to an individual. The guidelines recommend using the hospital-assigned medical record number.
2. Date of birth	Date of birth was requested because it was perceived as more accurate than age.
3. Sex	
4. Race and ethnicity	American Indian or Alaskan Native, black, hispanic, white, other.
5. Residence	Zip code of patient residence. Zip code was viewed as preferable to street address because of lesser concerns about patient confidentiality and because no coding of the information is required.
6. Hospital identification	Medicare provider or some other unique number.
7. Admission date	"An inpatient *admission* begins with the formal acceptance by a hospital of a patient who is to receive physician, dentist, or allied services while receiving room, board, and continuous nursing services" (pp. 10–11).
8. Discharge date	"An inpatient *discharge* occurs with the termination of the room, board, and continuous nursing services, and the formal release of an inpatient by the hospital" (p. 11).
9. Attending physician identification	A unique number within each hospital for "the clinician who is primarily and largely responsible for the care of the patient from the beginning of the hospital episode" (p. 11).
10. Operating physician identification	A unique number within each hospital for "the clinician who performed the principal procedure" (p. 11).
11. Diagnoses[*]	The 1979 recommendation was that a maximum of five diagnoses be recorded, including "all diagnoses that affect the current hospital stay." The following definitions were provided (p. 12): a. "Principal diagnosis is designated and defined as: the condition established after study to be chiefly responsible for occasioning the admission of the patient to the hospital for care." b. "Other diagnoses to be designated and defined as associated with the current hospital stay are: all conditions that coexist at the time of admission, that develop subsequently, or that affect the treatment received and/or the length of stay. Diagnoses that relate to an earlier episode which have no bearing on the current hospital stay, are to be excluded."
12. Procedures and dates[*]	The 1979 recommendation was that all "Class 1, 2, and 3" procedures ("surgery" and "significant procedures") be recorded along with their dates of performance. One procedure was to be designated the principal procedure using the following criteria: "(1) The principal procedure is one that was performed for definitive treatment rather than one performed for diagnostic or exploratory purposes, or was

TABLE 5.1

Contents of the Uniform Hospital Discharge Data Set

No. and Item	Definition and Comments
	necessary to take care of a complication. (2) The principal procedure is that procedure most related to the principal diagnosis" (p. 12). Until 1992, Medicare allowed only three positions for listing procedures.
13. Disposition of the patient	Discharged to home (routine discharge), left against medical advice, discharged to another short-term hospital, discharged to a long-term institution, died.
14. Expected principal source of payment	Self-pay, workers' compensation, Medicare, Medicaid, maternal and child health, other government payments, Blue Cross, insurance companies, no charge (free, charity, special research, or teaching), other.

TABLE 5.1
Continued

SOURCE: Adapted from the National Committee on Vital and Health Statistics, U.S. DHEW (1980).
* Coded using ICD-9-CM.

elective), insurance coverage (e.g., deductibles and coinsurance), charge and billing amounts, and slots for five diagnoses (principal plus four others) and three procedures with dates (principal plus two others). In 1992, HCFA increased the number of coding slots to nine diagnosis fields and six procedure fields. The electronic version of the 1992 Uniform Bill (UB-92) has become the institutional claim standard. Today, Medicare receives more than 98 percent of hospital claims electronically. UB-02, the 2002 update, will be available shortly. CMS has accumulated hospital billing data since 1983 and now has computer files representing well over 100 million hospital discharges and billions of other claims.

Medicare

Congress established Medicare in 1965 as Title XVIII of the Social Security Act, with benefits for eligible beneficiaries 65 years of age and older beginning 1 July 1966. The 1972 amendments extended coverage to younger persons with disabilities and persons with end-stage renal disease. Traditional Medicare includes two distinct parts: Part A, hospital insurance (coverage for services provided in institutional settings, including hospitals, skilled nursing facilities, hospices, and some home health services), and Part B, supplemental medical insurance (coverage for physician services, outpatient hospital services, certain medical equipment, and other services). Part B enrollment is voluntary. Since the late 1990s, the Medicare+Choice program (also called Part C) has allowed beneficiaries living in certain regions to enroll in private managed care plans. As of 2000, Medicare covered 39.9 million persons, including 34.4 million elderly people (De Lew 2000, 88). With the aging population, Medicare enrollment should exceed 77 million by 2030, with almost 69 million elderly.

In administering Medicare, CMS processes massive quantities of beneficiary, institutional, billing, and other administrative data. In FY 1999, Medicare received more than 850 million claims, processing 97 percent of Part A and 80 percent of Part B claims electronically (De Lew 2000, 84). Medicare's administrative records are compiled into huge, computerized data files reflecting CMS's three primary functions: (1) enrolling and tracking beneficiaries, each of whom receives a unique identification number; (2) designating and monitoring providers and institutions approved to accept Medicare payments; and (3) reimbursing health plans and individual services. Since 1991, all institutional provider and physician/supplier claims have been entered weekly into the National Claims History (NCH) file, containing approximately 375 variables and billions of records. Researchers inside and outside CMS have used NCH extracts linked with other administrative databases (e.g., beneficiaries' dates of death) to investigate the experiences of Medicare beneficiaries.

Processing this enormous volume of information is complex. Briefly, no claims are submitted directly to CMS. In 1991, HCFA partitioned the country into nine distinct processing sectors, each with a designated contractor or "host" producing a Common Working File (CWF). Each beneficiary is uniquely assigned to a CWF host, which maintains information on that beneficiary's eligibility status and Part A and B utilization records (the Health Insurance Master Records). Institutional provider claims (UB-92) arrive at the CWF host from a local fiscal intermediary, while physician and supplier claims (HCFA Form 1500) come through a local carrier.

Prior to 1991, HCFA stored claims (then called "bills") within separate files (e.g., inpatient, home health, outpatient, physician) that were then used to derive other files for analysis. Since 1991, all institutional provider and physician/supplier claims submitted daily by the nine CWF hosts are entered weekly into the NCH 100% Nearline File. This file is now the only file containing all claims submitted for Medicare beneficiaries, including adjustments, interim claims, and denials. Claims are processed through the NCH quality assurance systems, which apply routine edits for completeness and internal consistency as well as in-depth examination of providers whose billing patterns appear unusually inconsistent or unreliable.

The NCH 100% Nearline File is enormous, containing more than 6 billion records and about 375 variables. Each record type has two parts: a "fixed portion," consisting of items that occur only once per record (e.g., beneficiary demographics, claim transaction history, diagnosis, payment amounts), and "trailer groups," which vary by record type and can be repeated multiple times. The NCH 100% Nearline File includes six record types: four for institutional claims (inpatient/skilled nursing facility, outpatient, home health agency, and hospice), one for physicians or other suppliers, and another for durable medical equipment (DME).

Because of this complexity, working with the NCH requires skill and extensive knowledge. The NCH is not a standard "public-use" file because of beneficiary confidentiality and logistical concerns, although under carefully controlled circumstances some researchers can access the NCH. More often, researchers use data extracted from the NCH and configured into analytic files available for public purchase. These files protect beneficiary confidentiality, and they represent the "final action" for a given event, after all administrative adjustments are finalized (i.e., instead of containing multiple interim claims for a single event).

One such extract is the Medicare Provider Analysis and Review (MEDPAR) file, containing information on inpatient stays (in hospitals and skilled nursing facilities) from 1984 onward. MEDPAR contains data elements from the UB-92 hospital claim, including demographic information, principal and other diagnosis codes, procedure codes and dates, charges for a variety of cost centers, and reimbursement information. Public-use MEDPAR files have encrypted patient identifiers. For about $3,655 per year of data, analysts can purchase MEDPAR files containing 100 percent of hospital discharge records for Medicare beneficiaries after meeting certain data use requirements.[4] Researchers can also obtain files containing final claims from other institutional providers, physicians and other suppliers, and DME vendors.

Various files, such as the Provider of Service (POS) File and the Hospital Cost Report Information System (HCRIS), maintain information on providers eligible for Medicare reimbursement. The POS File includes information from Medicare certification applications and surveys from hospitals, skilled nursing facilities, home health agencies, independent laboratories, and a range of other facilities. The file, continually updated from recertification applications, has 2,400 data elements, including information on facility location, bed size, services offered, staff size and professional configuration, and ownership. The POS File contains about 228,000 records. The HCRIS contains information extracted from the Medicare cost reports submitted annually by participating hospitals, providing fiscal information, data on services rendered, and patient volume during the preceding year. The cost report asks about basic structural characteristics, such as ownership, number of beds, and staff size, as well as about capital expenditures, depreciation expenses, and costs for salaries, malpractice, and activities within various cost centers.

Because they were previously absolved of reporting requirements, Medicare's HMOs and MCOs have heretofore produced little administrative data. While more than 80 percent of beneficiaries remain in traditional Medicare, 6.2 million were enrolled in MCOs in 2000 (De Lew 2000, 101). In 1999, MCOs started submitting hospitalization encounter records, which are used to set capitation payments as mandated by the 1997 Balanced Budget Act (Iezzoni et al. 1998; Pope et al. 2000a). Without information, MCO enrollees—possibly a healthier subset of Medicare beneficiaries (Riley et al. 1996; Morgan et al. 1997)—are thus excluded from studies using Medicare administrative data.

The VA

Other federal agencies also collect data while administering health services programs. Both the departments of Defense and VA oversee provision of health care to large, albeit selected, populations—employees of the uniformed services and their families and military veterans. The Department of Defense, Office of Civilian Health and Medical Program of the Uniformed Services (CHAMPUS) and affiliated TRICARE health plans maintain an automated information and reporting system primarily to manage their health care delivery system. CHAMPUS and TRICARE information is available on a limited special-request basis to support service or command projects, not for general health services research.

In contrast, the VA maintains an active health services research program, drawing extensively from the computerized files created through administering VA hospitals and clinics. To obtain VA care, persons must be veterans (more than 180 days of military service); be honorably discharged; and either have a service-connected illness, injury, or disability or meet specified poverty levels. In 2001, more than 4.2 million persons obtained health care at a VA facility, with almost 440,000 patients admitted to acute care hospitals, 45,000 long-term care stays, and 43 million outpatient visits (VA 2002). The VHA supports a variety of institutions ranging from tertiary medical centers to domiciliaries and nursing homes. Unlike Medicare, the VA does not maintain a computerized file identifying all persons eligible for VA benefits.

For decades, the VHA information systems had foundered, but in the 1990s, the VHA devoted considerable resources to improving information content and flow. Now the VHA is nationally recognized for its advanced electronic health data systems. As described by Dr. Daley, who helped develop the VA NSQIP (see Chapter 8), VHA computerized information systems now support routine collection of even detailed clinical data. The NSQIP derives much of its clinically sophisticated risk-adjustment models from electronic data. Some attribute substantial improvements in VHA health care quality to the oversight facilitated by these new information systems (Fihn 2000).

In late 1993, beta testing concluded on the VA's Event Driven Reporting (EDR) system. Through this system, computerized data maintained at each health care facility (e.g., on hospital admissions, clinic visits, procedures) are automatically extracted, transmitted, and entered into the national EDR database every 24 hours (Meistrell and Schlehuber 1996). The Patient Treatment File (PTF), a core analytic file, had previously lagged 2 to 14 months but with EDR is virtually contemporaneous. The PTF contains information on all persons receiving inpatient care at a VHA facility, nursing home, or domiciliary or who obtain inpatient care elsewhere at VA expense (Lamoreaux 1996). The PTF includes the following types of information: demographic (Social Security number [SSN], age, gender, race, residence, means test), administrative (hospitalization dates, hospital identifier, number of stays on different clinical "bedsections," number of trips to the operating room), clinical (DRG, primary and secondary diagnoses, nonoperating room procedures), and surgical procedures. Another file contains information on inpatient stays at non-VA facilities.

VHA leadership is integrating its four national databases—EDR, PTF, Outpatient Clinic System, and Integrated Patient Database—into the new National Patient Care Database. Housed at the Austin Automation Center, this combined database uses health care industry standards for data definitions and further improves the efficiency of data transmission from VHA sites nationwide. To gain access to VHA data, analysts must be VA employees, work closely with VA employees, or receive special permission.

The VHA has historically retained slightly different information than other public and private health care systems. The VHA defines the first-listed hospital diagnosis differently than does UHDDS. Medicare and the UB-92 adopted the UHDDS instructions that the "principal diagnosis is designated and defined as: the condition established after study to be chiefly responsible for occasioning the admission of the patient to the hospital for care" (see Table 5.1). In contrast, the VHA uses a "primary diagnosis"—the condition that was primarily responsible for the length of the hospitalization.[5] Although principal and primary diagnoses are generally identical, differences can hamper comparisons of diagnosis data between the VHA- and UHDDS-based data systems.

Furthermore, unlike most other health data systems, VHA data do not contain dollar claims for various services (doing so is unnecessary given global budgeting). Therefore, analyses of costs within the VHA must find proxies. In an analysis of ACGs and DCGs within the VA, Rosen and colleagues (2001a) used two proxies for costs: ambulatory provider encounters and service days (the number of ambulatory visit days plus the number of inpatient days) over one year.

Medicaid

Medicaid is a joint state and federal program enacted as Title XIX of the Social Security Act amendments of 1965. Although details vary by state, Medicaid covers three broad areas: (1) health insurance for low-income families and persons with disabilities, (2) long-term care for older persons and those with disabilities who meet income standards, and (3) supplemental coverage for low-income Medicare beneficiaries for services not covered by Medicare (such as outpatient prescription drugs) and costs of Medicare premiums and deductibles. In FY 1998, roughly 12 percent of the U.S. population had Medicaid coverage, an estimated 32.5 million persons (Provost and Hughes 2000, 145). Medicaid recipients with disabilities are growing at roughly twice the rate of other eligible populations, with approximately 6.6 million people in FY 1998. The Personal Responsibility and Work Opportunity Act of 1996 "effectively decoupled Medicaid from cash assistance for low-income families," with early evidence suggesting that "many such families did not retain their Medicaid benefits" (Klemm 2000, 110).

Specific Medicaid eligibility, benefits, and coverage standards vary across states, as do the databases. Since FY 1999, all Medicaid claims must be submitted electronically through the MSIS. Although the MSIS contains a data dictionary defining required variables, states can use their own coding schemes, especially for procedures. Medicaid administrative databases are currently available for 31 states and contain claims for all services (including prescription drugs) in the form of State Medicaid Research Files (SMRF; Research Data Assistance Center 2002). SMRF enrollment information can be linked to claims, creating person-level records. Unlike Medicaid files obtained directly from states, SMRF data have been extensively cleaned and purged of duplicate and interim claims.

In addition, as for Medicare, Medicaid MCOs do not consistently submit encounter information. Managed care penetration varies across states, with two states having 0 percent and 12 states having 76 percent to 100 percent MCO enrollment (Provost and Hughes 2000, 150). Some states link the State Children's Health Insurance Program (SCHIP), created by the 1997 Balanced Budget Act, directly to their Medicaid programs (Hakim, Boben, and Bonney 2000). In FY 2001, 4.6 million children were enrolled in SCHIP, a 38 percent increase over the prior year (CMS 2002c). Plans for generating comprehensive data about SCHIP enrollees and experiences are evolving.

Inconsistencies across states in how populations are defined, differences in code sets, large size and complexity, and lower visibility than Medicare files "have caused some analysts to despair and decide that Medicaid data are hopeless" (Ku, Ellwood, and Klemm 1990, 35). Furthermore, because of the huge volume of claims and fluctuations in eligibility of many Medicaid recipients, these files are generally massive and cumbersome to manipulate (Bright, Avorn, and Everitt 1989). Our recent work using SMRF data from California, Georgia, New Jersey, and Wisconsin repeatedly unearthed vexing differences in code sets and variable definitions. SMRFs contain much less coded information than Medicare files, limiting their clinical content. The SMRF inpatient file contains two diagnosis and two procedure code fields; the outpatient file has one diagnosis and one procedure slot; and the long-term-care file has one diagnosis but no procedure fields.

Steinwachs and colleagues (1998) looked at whether Medicaid fee-for-service providers even submit claims. A comparison of 1988 Medicaid administrative files with medical records found that 89.7 percent of billed visits were documented in records with corresponding dates. Seventy-nine percent of claims contained one diagnosis, whereas 21 percent had two (the maximum number allowed). Most worrisome, discordance between administrative files and records seemed biased by important provider and patient characteristics. Among providers classified as having low risk-adjusted costs, medical records identified 25 percent more visits than did the administrative data. Patients identified as low users based on claims had 40 percent more visits documented in their medical records.

Despite this, Medicaid data offer important opportunities. One particularly significant contribution concerns children, 51 percent of FY 1998

Medicaid recipients (Provost and Hughes 2000, 162). Few other publicly available data sets contain large numbers of children. Given the nature of Medicaid recipients, these studies often emphasize effects of poverty and chronic illness (Kuhlthau et al. 1998; Perrin et al. 1998a, 1998b, 1999; Ettner et al. 2000). Although Medicaid findings have limited generalizability, they provide important information about children who are potentially vulnerable because of poverty and disability.

Prescription drug information offers another advantage. Medicaid's computerized pharmacy data file contains information on all prescriptions dispensed by pharmacies, including the beneficiary's identification number, prescription date, specific drug (often the NDC code), quantity, prescribing physician, and reimbursement information. Data on drug prescriptions in the Medicaid file are reasonably reliable. One study found that 94 percent of pharmacy records matched claims in the Medicaid data set (Bright, Avorn, and Everitt 1989). The Medicaid pharmacy data represent prescriptions that were filled (not prescriptions written but never obtained). Information not required for reimbursement, such as outpatient diagnoses indicating the indication for a drug, is often questionable (Ray and Griffin 1989).

Medicaid data represent health care experiences of indigent persons, whose risk factors may differ from those of wealthier individuals (see Chapter 3). Risk-adjustment methods derived for other populations may not apply equally well to Medicaid recipients. Nonetheless, detailed information on this vulnerable population is an important strength of Medicaid data.

Private Insurance

As part of processing claims and encounter records, private health insurers also create administrative databases (Garnick et al. 1996; Hornbrook et al. 1998a). These files are structured for insurers' business purposes, not outside investigators, and they can be complicated. Nonetheless, certain companies have structured their files for analytic use, including by outside investigators. Some insurers submit their data sets to companies (e.g., Mercer, Medstat) that produce physician practice profiles or other comparative reports. These businesses sometimes sell these large, multiorganizational databases to external parties after ensuring confidentiality.

Private insurance claims offer information on services used by younger, employed adults and their children—populations not represented in public administrative databases. Insurance files typically include details about plan enrollment and each covered service; some include interesting additional information, like worker attendance and specifics about plan design. Apart from the technical and logistical hurdles of using private insurance claims files for population-based studies, however, questions arise concerning the scope and content of these files (Garnick et al. 1996; Hornbrook et al. 1998a). Claims files do not reflect utilization of services for which enrollees do not submit claims. Some plans require enrollees to pay high deductibles; patients may not submit claims until they meet the deductible limit (Hornbrook et al. 1998a). Some insurers retain information only on paid claims, deleting data on services below the deductible or above the maximum benefit levels. Thus, HMOs, with their own provider networks, may have information only on services rendered by outside providers who submit claims. Information on prescription drugs and mental health care is often incomplete, especially if these services are carved out of the insurance plan.

The content of private insurance claims reflects the mechanism for claims submission and payment (Garnick et al. 1996). For instance, providers may submit "bundled bills" for a series of services, possibly provided on different dates. Dates retained in the claim file may represent the date of payment or payment adjustment, not the date of service. Depending on billing procedures, the provider number listed on the claim can represent various entities—an individual physician, a group of doctors, or an institution.

Private insurers typically do not collect information on race or ethnicity of their enrollees. Health plans can restrict access to certain data because of confidentiality concerns. A survey of six HMOs found that some plans keep information on certain topics (e.g., HIV, AIDS, mental health, alcohol, substance abuse) in separate files with tighter security (Hornbrook et al. 1998a). Private insurers frequently require fewer diagnoses on claims than do public programs; HMO physicians typically report fewer diagnoses than do physicians within fee-for-service settings (Hornbrook et al. 1998a). In addition, insurers sometimes assign their own idiosyncratic diagnosis and procedure codes. Certain inconsistencies in administrative data across private insurers may disappear when HIPAA-mandated transaction standards take effect.

Because of these problems and difficulties gaining access to private insurance files, relatively few outsiders have used them. Nevertheless, creative use of these claims files can produce useful information. Few other data sources provide insight into health care experiences of employed, working-age adults and their children.

Diagnosis Codes

For examining health care outcomes, administrative data must contain credible clinical information about risk factors (see Chapter 3). According to skeptics, this is where administrative data fall short (Donaldson and Lohr 1994). Beyond age and sex, most clinical information in administrative files comes from diagnoses coded using ICD-9-CM. Many administrative data supplied by hospitals, including UB-92 and outpatient claims, also use ICD-9-CM to code procedures. Given its central role, I next explore the strengths and limitations of ICD-9-CM-coded data. The Internet web site of NCHS (http://www.cdc.gov/nchs/icd9.htm) offers extensive information on ICD-9-CM.

Origins of ICD-9-CM

ICD-9-CM traces its roots to the First Statistical Congress in Brussels in 1853 and a multinational agreement on the need for consistent coding of causes of death. Two years later in Paris, the congress adopted general disease classification principles proposed by William Farr (introduced in Chapter 1), grouping conditions primarily by anatomical site (Israel 1978). Following this basic schema, in 1893 the International Statistical Institute (the successor to the congress) produced the *Classification of Causes of Death*, urging revisions every ten years. This lexicon evolved into the *International Classification of Diseases* (ICD), maintained by the World Health Organization (WHO) since the 1940s. WHO convened the International Conference for the Ninth Revision in Geneva in 1977, and ICD-9 emerged in January 1979.

The ninth revision contained more than three times as many codes as the eighth. Nonetheless, some Americans believed that ICD-9 provided insufficient detail for U.S. uses (Slee 1978). Professional and provider associations therefore worked with NCHS staff to tailor ICD-9 for broadly defined clinical purposes. The resultant ICD-9-CM contains more than 14,000 codes and achieves much of its detail by adding fifth digits to many diagnosis codes (see below). ICD-9 was used for mortality reporting (i.e., to specify cause of death; ICD-10 replaced ICD-9 on 1 January 1999 for this purpose). ICD-9-CM became the major U.S. coding classification for morbidity.

In the United States, official coding guidelines are promulgated by the Central Office on ICD-9-CM after approval by the four Cooperating Parties for ICD-9-CM (Sheehy 1991)—the ICD-9-CM Coordination-Maintenance Committee at NCHS, CMS, the American Hospital Association (AHA), and the American Health Information Management Association. NCHS retains primary responsibility for diagnosis codes, ensuring that any changes comply with WHO policies and reflect technical or scientific advances in medical knowledge. ICD-9-CM procedure codes are used primarily by the United States; therefore, changes in procedure coding need not pass through WHO. Instead, CMS has authority for procedure coding revisions and updates, responding to technological advances and reimbursement concerns. The NCHS posts coding guidelines for ICD-9-CM on its web site (see above). The *AHA Coding Clinic for ICD-9-CM*, a quarterly publication, provides the official coding guidelines promulgated by the four Cooperating Parties.

ICD-9 was used by nations worldwide; since 1 January 1999, ICD-10 has superseded ICD-9 in many countries (see below). ICD-9-CM codes collapse neatly into ICD-9 categories, but difficulties may arise when fitting ICD-9 data into a grouping like DRGs developed for the more detailed ICD-9-CM codes. An Australian study found that some DRGs were missing from data sets containing only ICD-9 codes (e.g., DRG 27, traumatic stupor and coma with coma greater than one hour, required five-digit ICD-9-CM codes indicating the duration of coma) (Reid 1991). Data comparisons between the United States and other countries are thus complicated by different ICD coding schemes.

Organization and Format of ICD-9-CM

ICD-9-CM has three volumes: Volume I, Diseases, Tabular List; Volume II, Diseases, Alphabetic Index; and Volume III, Procedures, Tabular List and Alphabetic Index. Volume I presents diagnosis codes in a tabular list, organized into 17 broad categories. Some categories hearken back to the original grouping by anatomical locations, whereas others represent pathophysiological perspectives (e.g., infectious and parasitic diseases, neoplasms) and wide-ranging conditions (e.g., "symptoms, signs, and ill-defined conditions"). ICD-9-CM achieves its diagnostic detail by using fifth digits. All codes do not require five digits: three-, four-, and five-digit codes are used as necessary, representing increasing levels of specificity. For example, the code for pneumococcal pneumonia has only three digits (481), indicating that further detail is not needed. In contrast, the coding of diabetes mellitus spans all five digits, representing complications and type of diabetes.

Two "supplementary classifications" represent various factors affecting health and other needs. Codes up to five digits starting with the letter V portray factors influencing health status and contact with health services, such as personal history of penicillin allergy (V14.0), noncompliance with medical treatment (V15.81), outcomes of delivery (such as single liveborn, V27.0), and unemployment (V62.0). Other V codes indicate that services rather than diagnoses prompted the health care encounter, such as routine infant or child health check (V20.2), chemotherapy (V58.1), and examination for medicolegal reasons (blood alcohol tests, V70.4).

A second supplementary classification lists environmental events, circumstances, and conditions that have caused injury, poisoning, or other adverse events. These codes, up to five digits starting with the letter E, aim to provide details about patients' conditions, but they cannot be listed as the reason for admission or principal diagnosis under current UHDDS guidelines.[6] E codes convey detailed descriptive information, as suggested by the following examples: crew of commercial aircraft involved in accident at take-off or landing (E840.2), accidental poisoning by benzodiazepine tranquilizer (E853.2), excessive cold due to weather conditions (E901.0), child abuse by parent (E967.0), and bite by centipede or venomous millipede (E905.4).

The portion of the tabular list of diseases devoted to "symptoms, signs, and ill-defined conditions" portrays a broad array of conditions. Coding rules stipulate that signs or symptoms linked definitively to a specific diagnosis generally should not be coded—codes for definitive diagnoses should supersede them. Signs and symptoms should be listed, however, when a definitive diagnosis is not established or when the symptom represents "important problems in medical care." These codes also include abnormal results from various diagnostic tests. Examples are alteration of consciousness (780.0), abnormality of gait (781.2), anorexia (783.0), precordial chest pain (786.51), elevated sedimentation rate (790.1), and abnormal electrocardiogram (ECG) (794.31).

An interesting set of codes depicts complications resulting from medical care (codes 996–999). Many of these codes specify the nature of the problem but not its causality (e.g., "bad luck" versus negligence). Examples include mechanical complication due to a heart valve prosthesis (996.02), postoperative shock (998.0), accidental puncture or laceration during a procedure (998.2), postoperative infection (998.5), foreign body accidentally left during a procedure (998.4), and ABO blood type incompatibility reaction (999.6).

Thus, ICD-9-CM contains codes for many conditions that are technically not diseases (Table 5.2)—the name *International Classification of Diseases* is a misnomer. Given this diversity, putting together ICD-9-CM codes creatively and with clinical understanding can produce a fairly comprehensive picture of risk factors and patients' clinical status. Figure 5.1 shows discharge abstract information taken from a patient admitted to a California hospital in 1987 (Iezzoni et al. 1994a), suggesting the following story:

> A 64-year-old woman with a history of bowel resection came to the emergency room and was admitted emergently for surgical repair of a malfunctioning enterostomy. On the first hospital day, she underwent repair of a pericolostomy hernia and lysis of peritoneal adhesions. She developed postoperative gastrointestinal complications, and on the sixth hospital day again had surgery for lysis of adhesions. She developed a postoperative infection and became acutely unstable. Starting on the seventh hospital day, she required monitoring of her central venous pressure and pulmonary artery wedge pressures. She finally needed endotracheal intubation and mechanical ventilation. By the 23rd hospital day, she had recovered sufficiently to go home with home health care.

The detail of ICD-9-CM can become overwhelming. HCUP investigators at AHRQ (Elixhauser, Andrews, and Fox 1993; Elixhauser and McCarthy 1996) created their Clinical Classifications for Health Policy Research (now called the Clinical Classifications Software, or CCS) by grouping numeric diagnosis codes, V codes, and procedure codes and eliminating codes that were exceedingly general (e.g., V15.81, noncompliance with medical treatment; 780.7, malaise and fatigue). Using the 1987 version of ICD-9-CM, they first grouped diagnosis codes into 18 body systems and 650 "detailed diagnosis categories"; these were further combined into 185 mutually exclusive "summary diagnosis categories." They grouped the 3,500 procedure codes into 172 mutually exclusive procedure categories. These groupings yielded adequate sample sizes using hospital discharge data and a manageable number of categories for analysis. Analysts can download the CCS software from the AHRQ HCUP Internet web site (http://www.ahrq.gov/data/hcup/ccs.htm).

Type of Information	No.	Code Name
Clinical diagnosis	250.53	Type I diabetes mellitus with ophthalmic manifestations, uncontrolled
	410.01	AMI of anterolateral wall, initial episode of care
Pathological process	414.01	Coronary atherosclerosis of native coronary artery
	324.0	Intracranial abscess
Symptoms	569.42	Anal or rectal pain
	780.7	Malaise and fatigue
Physical findings	342.0	Flaccid hemiplegia
	786.7	Abnormal chest sounds
Laboratory or other test findings	794.31	Abnormal electrocardiogram
	790.2	Abnormal glucose tolerance test
Severity indicators	427.5	Cardiac arrest
	518.81	Respiratory failure
Potential quality indicators	968.3	Poisoning by intravenous anesthetics
	998.7	Acute reaction to foreign substance accidentally left during a procedure
Psychological factors	308.0	Acute reaction to stress, predominant disturbance of emotions
	V15.4	Psychological trauma
Cognitive factors	290.0	Senile dementia, uncomplicated
	290.13	Presenile dementia with depressive features
Substance abuse	304.21	Continuous cocaine dependency
	303.93	Chronic alcoholism in remission
Personal social factors	V61.1	Marital problems
	V62.0	Unemployment
	V60.0	Lack of housing
Functional status	344.1	Paraplegia
	V53.8	Wheelchair
External environmental factors	E900.0	Excessive heat due to weather conditions
	E965.0	Assault by a handgun

TABLE 5.2
Type of Information Contained in ICD-9-CM Codes

Clinical Content of ICD-9-CM Codes

Despite the detail implied by ICD-9-CM, questions remain about the clinical definitions of specific ICD-9-CM codes. Neither the Tabular List (Volume I) nor the Alphabetic Index (Volume II) offers clinical descriptions of the conditions represented by ICD-9-CM codes. For example, ICD-9-CM includes about 40 four- and five-digit codes for different types of anemia, such as iron deficiency anemia secondary to inadequate dietary iron intake (280.1), thalassemia (282.4), autoimmune hemolytic anemia (283.0), and constitutional aplastic anemia (284.0). Nowhere, however, does it specify what level of

FIGURE 5.1

Discharge Abstract Information for a Patient Hospitalized in California in 1987

Patient Data	Hospital Data	Admission Data	Disposition Data
ID: XXXXX	Hospital ID: XXXXX	Length of stay: 23 days	Disposition: home health service
Age: 64	Zip code: XXXXX	Admission type: emergency	DRG: 150 (peritoneal adhesiolysis with complication or comorbidity)
Sex: female		Source: emergency room	
Race: white		Total charges: $35,201	
Residence zip code: XXXXX		Payer: Medicare	

DIAGNOSIS AND PROCEDURE CODES AND DAYS FROM ADMISSION TO PROCEDURE

Diagnosis Codes		Procedure Codes		Days
5696	enterostomy malfunction	4642	pericolostomy hernia repair	0
56081	intestinal adhesion with obstruction	545	peritoneal adhesiolysis	0
311	depressive disorder NEC	9112	culture—peritoneum	0
9974	surgical complication—gastrointestinal tract	545	peritoneal adhesiolysis	6
9985	postoperative infection	9608	insert (naso-)intestinal tube	6
		9112	culture—peritoneum	6
		8964	pulmonary artery wedge monitor	7
		8962	central venous pressure monitoring	7
		8763	small bowell series	6
		8744	routine chest x-ray	6
		8819	abdominal x-ray NEC	6
		9604	insert endotracheal tube	6
		9392	mechanical respiratory assistance NEC	0
		9052	culture—blood	0
		9043	culture and sensitivity—lower respiratory tract	0
		8952	electrocardiogram	0

hematocrit justifies an anemia diagnosis. Similarly, the respiratory failure code (518.81) does not indicate what level of arterial oxygenation, respiratory rate or pattern, or other clinical abnormality merits that diagnosis.

Coders assign ICD-9-CM diagnoses based on what physicians document in medical records. Therefore, coding inevitability reflects the vagaries of physicians' documentation patterns and terminology. Furthermore, the absence of clear clinical definitions raises questions about what, exactly, different ICD-9-CM codes mean. We reviewed 485 medical records of elderly Medicare beneficiaries hospitalized in 1994 in California and Connecticut looking for the clinical evidence that supported assignment of specified ICD-9-CM diagnosis codes (McCarthy et al. 2000a). All codes were secondary diagnoses used by our Complications Screening Program (CSP) to identify potential in-hospital complications of care (Iezzoni et al. 1994a, 1994b).[7] Based on extensive literature reviews, we specified explicit clinical criteria confirming the presence of particular diagnoses and trained nurses to abstract these criteria from medical records. If nurses failed to find explicit criteria, they looked for whether physicians had simply noted that the condition existed. As shown in Table 5.3, the percentage of records containing explicit criteria confirming coded diagnoses varied across conditions and surgical versus medical cases. Across all surgical cases and all diagnoses, 68.8 percent had explicit clinical evidence supporting the coded diagnoses, compared to 43.7 percent of medical cases. In 19.4 percent and 29.9 percent of surgical and medical cases, respectively, neither clinical criteria nor physicians' notes were present (McCarthy et al. 2000a, 870).[8] Table 5.4 shows details of our findings for surgical patients with secondary diagnoses of pneumonia.

Despite the large number of codes, ICD-9-CM does not include certain patient characteristics that are significant risk factors. For example, the anemia codes do not specify the hematocrit level or how rapidly anemia developed. ICD-9-CM also fails to capture clinical concerns typically encountered in routine outpatient primary care. For 45 percent of ambulatory care visits, physicians at Group Health Cooperative of Puget Sound expressed dissatisfaction with the ICD-9-CM codes representing their patients' problems (Payne, Murphy, and Salazar 1992, 654). Best and colleagues (2002, 262) could find ICD-9-CM code proxies for 37 of 61 preoperative risk factors used by the VA's NSQIP (see Chapter 8).

In fairness, ICD-9-CM does contain many codes suggesting comorbid disease. Using these ICD-9-CM codes, researchers have developed comorbidity indices applicable to administrative data (Deyo, Cherkin, and Ciol 1992; Romano, Roos, and Jollis 1993; Ghali et al. 1996; Elixhauser et al. 1998). ICD-9-CM offers potential severity indicators, such as toxic diffuse goiter with thyroid storm (242.01), intrinsic asthma with status asthmaticus (493.11), and hepatic coma (572.2). However, ICD-9-CM offers few codes representing functional status. Code 344.9, paralysis unspecified, for example, depicts conditions from complete paralysis to generalized weakness. No codes indicate performance of ADLs or basic physical actions, like walking or climbing stairs. Without valid information about physical, sensory, cognitive, or emotional functioning, one cannot accurately identify people with potentially disabling conditions or track meaningful outcomes of care. Although the *International Classification of Functioning, Disability, and Health* (ICF), approved by the WHO in 2001 (see Chapter 15), classifies functional abilities and social and environmental contexts, ICF is not used routinely for administrative data collection in the United States.

Therefore, while ICD-9-CM contains numerous codes representing wide-ranging conditions, the clinical meaning of specific codes is often elusive. The lack of precise clinical definitions permits unreliable ICD-9-CM coding. Inconsistencies and imprecision in the terms physicians use to document the medical record certainly further increase coding variability. Physicians are not trained in ICD-9-CM, and "many medical record practitioners would say physicians' documentation is the true source of coding problems" (Sheehy 1991, 46). Concern also arises from the current context of diagnosis coding and questions about motivations for assigning ICD-9-CM codes.

TABLE 5.3

Type of Evidence Confirming Specified ICD-9-CM Diagnosis Codes

Secondary Diagnosis Codes for	Sample Size	Type of Evidence (%)		
		Explicit Clinical Evidence	Physicians' Notes Only	No Evidence
Pneumonia	40	50.0	30.0	20.0
Aspiration Pneumonia	32	53.1	37.5	9.4
AMI	37	81.1	8.1	10.8
Deep-vein thrombosis and pulmonary embolism				
Surgical cases	36	66.7	8.3	25.0
Medical cases	42	54.8	11.9	33.3
Gastrointestinal hemorrhage	39	69.2	7.7	23.1

SOURCE: Adapted from McCarthy et al. (2000a, Table 2). The ICD-9-CM codes defining each condition appear in Table 1 of McCarthy et al. (2000a).

Context of ICD-9-CM Diagnostic Coding and Sources of Error

According to Weigel and Lewis (1991, 70):

> Until very recently, the coding function was largely ignored by all but the technical experts and a few scholarly researchers. It was a function of the medical record department; and lacking any evidence to the contrary, it was considered to be a clerical task equivalent to typing and filing.

For more than 100 years, vital statistics systems have used ICD codes to specify causes of death; since UHDDS arrived in 1974, ICD has supported review and planning for hospitals. But the entire context of diagnosis coding in the United States changed with the 1983 enactment of Medicare's prospective payment system based on DRGs. In 1981, a prescient warning appeared in the *New England Journal of Medicine* (Simborg 1981, 1602, 1604):

> This article is intended to provide a case report of "DRG creep," a new phenomenon that is expected to occur in epidemic proportions in the 1980s. DRG creep may be defined as a deliberate and systematic shift in a hospital's reported case mix in order to improve reimbursement. . . . Minor diagnostic nuances and slight imprecisions of wording have little practical clinical importance, yet under DRG reimbursement they would have major financial consequences. . . . It is hoped that hospitals will refrain from disseminating the more virulent forms of DRG creep; however, the potential for a broad spectrum of manifestations certainly exists.

DRGs suddenly vested ICD-9-CM with powers for which it was never designed—determining hospital reimbursement (Vladeck 1984). Under

Clinical Factors	Presence of Clinical Factor, n (%)	Type of Clinical Evidence, n (%)
If preoperative chest radiograph, CT scan, or chest examination normal or respiratory symptoms are new or worsened from preoperative status, new infiltrate found on chest radiograph, AND new purulent sputum documented postoperatively within 48 hours of abnormal chest examination, or pneumonia pathogen documented postoperatively AND patient had fever, leukocytosis, or respiratory signs/symptoms	15 (37.5)	—
If preoperative chest radiograph, CT scan, or chest examination normal, new infiltrate found on chest radiograph, AND new purulent sputum documented postoperatively within 48 hours of abnormal chest examination, or pneumonia pathogen documented postoperatively	19 (47.5)	—
If preoperative chest radiograph, CT scan, or chest examination normal, new abnormal chest examination, AND new purulent sputum documented postoperatively within 48 hours of abnormal chest examination, or pneumonia pathogen documented postoperatively AND patient had fever, leukocytosis, or respiratory signs/symptoms	14 (35.0)	—
Had at least one objective clinical factor	—	20 (50.0)
Physician note but no objective clinical factor	—	12 (30.0)
No clinical factor or physician note	—	8 (20.0)

TABLE 5.4
Presence of Clinical Factors Confirming a Complication of Postoperative Pneumonia ($n = 40$)

SOURCE: McCarthy, E. P., L. I. Iezzoni, R. B. Davis, R. H. Palmer, M. Cahalane, M. B. Hamel, K. Mukamel, R. S. Phillips, and D. T. Davies, Jr. 2000. "Does Clinical Evidence Support ICD-9-CM Diagnosis Coding of Complications?" *Medical Care* 38 (8): 868–76.

DRG-based payment, ICD-9-CM codes translate directly into dollars. New words, such as "optimization" and "maximization," entered the coding vocabulary. Providers now eagerly focus on coding practices, hoping to maximize their reimbursement. Some hospitals reorganized, moving medical record departments from general administration to financial divisions (Waterstraat, Barlow, and Newman 1990). As of 1 April 1989, Medicare also required physicians to list ICD-9-CM diagnosis codes on their claims. Thus, concerns about diagnosis codes stem not only from the clinical content of ICD-9-CM but also from how it is applied. Are diagnosis codes complete, reliable, and accurate?

Steps in Coding

Researchers and analysts using administrative data often think that ICD-9-CM coding is easy and straightforward: Just take ICD-9-CM off the shelf, peruse the index for the desired code, and *voilà*. Nothing could be further from the truth. Like medicine, coding is both a science and an art form, but since coding is inextricably bound to medicine, it inevitably magnifies the vagaries of clinical practice, judgment, and documentation. Becoming an accredited record technician requires extensive training, and coders must keep up to date with new codes and guidelines. As noted earlier, NCHS posts coding guidelines for ICD-9-CM on its web site, and the quarterly *AHA Coding Clinic for ICD-9-CM* publishes official coding rules.

As described below, coding inpatient and outpatient diagnoses follows somewhat different rules. Often, outpatient claims or encounter records contain only one or two coding slots, while hospital discharge formats can accommodate up to 25 codes. Therefore, coding hospital discharge diagnoses is typically more time consuming and complicated than coding diagnoses on outpatient claims. The two major steps in coding discharge diagnoses are first, specifying the pertinent ICD-9-CM diagnosis codes, and second, determining their order—sequencing the codes. With few exceptions, the principal (first-listed) diagnosis drives DRG assignment and thus hospital reimbursement.

Deciding which diagnoses to code requires complete review of medical records, searching for diagnoses established or entertained by the physicians treating the patient. Coding guidelines note that achieving complete and accurate coding of discharge diagnoses requires a "joint effort" between physicians and coders. ICD-9-CM coding guidelines for the UHDDS demand coding of "all diagnoses that coexist at the time of admission, that develop subsequently, or that affect the treatment received and/or the length of stay. Diagnoses that relate to an earlier episode which have no bearing on the current hospital stay" are excluded. The NCHS coding guidelines (http://www.cdc.gov/nchs/data/icd9/icdguide.pdf, accessed 16 October 2002) indicate that secondary diagnoses should include conditions that affect patients' clinical evaluation, therapy, or diagnostic procedures or that extend hospital stays or increase nursing care or monitoring.

One highly technical step—sequencing—can cause considerable confusion. As Table 5.2 showed, ICD-9-CM contains codes representing diverse aspects of patients' clinical presentations. In particular, some ICD-9-CM codes depict specific diseases (or "etiologies"), whereas others indicate manifestations of these etiologies. Coding guidelines hold that etiology codes be sequenced (appear in a list) before related manifestation codes. Sometimes individual codes will instruct coders when to pair the code with another code. For instance, manifestation codes contain the notation "in diseases classified elsewhere"; such codes must always be sequenced following the specified disease.

After all codes and sequences are established, coders must choose which code to list in the first coding slot. Certain codes can never be listed first, such as E codes and codes for signs and symptoms (with few exceptions). The order of codes varies somewhat across data sets. For UHDDS and Medicare, ordering involves designating the principal diagnosis, the condition responsible for hospitalization. The principal diagnosis assigns most cases to MDCs and then to medical DRGs. In situations where two codes meet the definition of principal diagnosis, either may be selected.

As noted above, the VHA PTF lists first the primary diagnosis, the condition most responsible for the LOS. If a patient dies during a hospitalization, the cause of death could be the principal or primary diagnosis, but this is not necessarily so. Cause of death is determined based on mortality classification guidelines from ICD's original use (O'Gara 1990). For Medicare and UHDDS, no specific rule stipulates ordering of the other diagnoses, although guidelines indicate that "the more significant ones should be sequenced early in the list if there is any likelihood that data entries will be limited" (Brown 1989, 23).

This technical discussion of sequencing and ordering highlights the complexities of ICD-9-CM coding and suggests why sometimes physicians are confused. Physicians are generally unaware of arcane coding guidelines and may wonder why one code should be listed before another. Table 5.5 provides five brief clinical scenarios that, from a purely clinical viewpoint (ignoring coding rules), could be coded in various ways. However, the choice of codes carries financial consequences.

Not surprisingly, therefore, anecdotal reports suggest that physicians and coders rarely engage in productive dialog, although that may change with looming HIPAA compliance requirements (e.g., the need to guard against civil penalties from upcoding; Averill 1999). Especially as hospitals face financial crises, they try to enlist physicians' assistance in coding. Some hospitals periodically post notices in the physicians' lounges documenting the financial ramifications of coding. One hospital distributed an e-mail message to its medical staff urging them to use specific terminology rather than vague phrases that cannot sustain codes (e.g., to write "blood loss anemia" rather than "low HCT"). To prevent DRG creep, from the mid-1980s until September 1995, federal regulations required that physicians "attest" in writing to the accuracy of the discharge diagnoses of Medicare patients before hospitals' could submit bills for payment. In 1995, however, Vice President Al Gore eliminated the attestation requirement as part of his broader "reinventing government" initiative simplifying federal paperwork. Nonetheless, within a year, worries resurfaced about potential upcoding. Federal regulators found consultants hired by hospitals explicitly to maximize reimbursement through "enhancing" coding. Not surprisingly, in 1996 HIPAA stipulated that upcoding would merit strict civil penalties.

Coding Certainty and Specificity

A major difference between coding of inpatient and outpatient diagnoses involves the level of certainty. In outpatient settings, the term "first-listed" replaces the word "principal," and codes representing signs and symptoms are acceptable for reporting when a specific diagnosis is not yet established. In other words, outpatient codes are assigned to the highest level of certainty. If all that is known at the time of an outpatient visit is a patient's complaints or symptoms, those may be coded first. Contradicting the guidelines, however,

TABLE 5.5

Examples of Clinical Overlap Among ICD-9-CM Codes

Clinical Presentation	Symptom, Health Problem, or Severity of Illness	Clinical Diagnosis or Pathologic Process
Patient brought into emergency room with weakness of right arm and leg and aphasia; history suggestive of cerebrovascular thrombosis	ICD-9-CM code 342.9 (hemiplegia not otherwise specified) leading to DRG 12 (degenerative nervous system disorders); RW, 0.8918	ICD-9-CM code 434.00 (cerebral thrombosis) leading to DRG 14* (specific cerebrovascular disorders except transient ischemic attack); RW, 1.2943
Patient presents to outpatient clinic complaining of fatigue and weight loss; examination shows occult blood in stool and low hematocrit; patient is admitted and found to have colon cancer	ICD-9-CM code 280.0 (iron deficiency anemia secondary to chronic blood loss) leading to DRG 395 (red blood cell disorders age > 17); RW, 0.8156	ICD-9-CM code 153.6 (malignant neoplasm of ascending colon) leading to DRG 172* (digestive malignancy with complication or comorbidity); RW, 1.3624
Patient brought into emergency room unresponsive and with depressed respirations; gastric aspirate shows traces of barbiturates	ICD-9-CM code 780.01 (coma) leading to DRG 23 (nontraumatic stupor and coma); RW, 0.8220	ICD-9-CM code 967.0 (barbiturate poisoning) leading to DRG 449* (toxic effects of drugs age > 17 with complication or comorbidity); RW, 0.8267
Patient brought into emergency room in respiratory failure; sputum culture yields *Staphylococcus aureus*, and chest radiograph shows pneumonia	ICD-9-CM code 518.81 (respiratory failure) leading to DRG 87 (pulmonary edema and respiratory failure); RW, 1.3658	ICD-9-CM code 482.4 (staphylococcal pneumonia) leading to DRG 79* (respiratory infections and inflammations age > 17 with complication or comorbidity); RW, 1.6193
Patient is brought into emergency room in shock; evaluation shows bleeding esophageal varices; history confirms alcohol abuse	ICD-9-CM code 785.50 (shock not otherwise specified) leading to DRG 127* (heart failure and shock); RW, 1.0039	ICD-9-CM code 456.0 (esophageal varices with bleeding) leading to DRG 174 (gastrointestinal hemorrhage with complication or comorbidity); RW, 0.9952

SOURCE: Adapted from Iezzoni and Moskowitz 1986. DRG represents Version 10.0 (October 1, 1992–September 30, 1993). DRG relative weights (RW) from *Federal Register,* August 1, 2002, 67 (148): 50231–80.
*DRG with higher relative weight.

some insurers require clinicians to report presumptive diagnoses to justify tests or services. This inconsistent application of coding guidelines confuses the meaning of diagnoses listed on outpatient claims.

Sign, symptom, and ill-defined condition codes are typically not allowed as principal diagnoses for hospitalizations. If uncertainty exists, coders are instructed to follow the physician's reasoning about what specific condition underlies the patient's complaints. This instruction is colloquially called the rule-out rule, described by the NCHS guidelines as follows:

If the diagnosis documented at the time of discharge is qualified as "probably," "suspected," "likely," "questionable," "possible," or "still to be ruled out," code the condition as if it existed or was established. The bases for these guidelines are the diagnostic workup, arrangements for further workup or observation, and initial therapeutic approach that correspond most closely with the established diagnosis.

The rule-out rule has interesting analytic consequences, especially as hospital LOSs shrink and patients leave without established diagnoses.[9] Analysts cannot be certain that discharge diagnoses actually existed, especially if patients are admitted specifically for diagnostic workups. In June 1992, the committee examining revisions of the UHDDS proposed dropping the rule-out rule, suggesting its elimination would yield more accurate information (National Committee on Vital and Health Statistics 1992). Furthermore, eliminating the rule-out rule would make diagnosis coding for hospitalizations consistent with that for ambulatory visits. Nevertheless, because the rule-out rule is still promulgated by WHO, it remains in effect in the United States. Coding experts hope to eliminate the rule-out rule when ICD-10-CM is finally implemented for morbidity reporting (see below).

The Accuracy and Reliability of Coded Data

As early as the 1970s, studies questioned the accuracy of diagnostic coding (Institute of Medicine 1977a, 1977b). A review of 1,974 hospital discharge abstracts found nearly 100 percent accuracy for basic information, such as admission and discharge dates, patient age and sex, and payer. However, for principal diagnosis, the researchers and hospitals agreed on only 65.2 percent of the principal diagnosis codes (Institute of Medicine 1977a). Many problems related to vagaries of ICD-8 (the ICD of that time) and its diagnosis codes, coding guidelines, and sequencing rules. For 10.7 percent of cases reviewed, discrepancies between the researchers' and hospitals' principal diagnoses were irreconcilable because of legitimate professional disagreements in interpreting the medical record and pertinent coding guidelines, particularly sequencing (76.5 percent of indeterminate cases).[10] The investigators concluded, "One must assume that abstracted hospital data contain errors and use them with caution. The seriousness of the error depends on the purpose to which the data are applied" (Institute of Medicine 1977a, 49). Nevertheless, within a few years, Medicare made diagnosis codes the basis of hospital payment.

One barometer reflecting the effect of coding practices is the Medicare case-mix index (CMI). The CMI reflects the average relative weight of DRGs assigned to hospitalized patients. Watchdog groups and Medicare annually track the CMI for individual hospitals, looking for targets to investigate. Higher CMIs represent higher aggregate hospital reimbursements caused by a shifting DRG mix of patients.

The CMI rose 32.4 percent cumulatively from the first year of prospective payment through 1996 (ProPAC 1996, 61). The largest increases occurred in the two years after prospective payment arrived (FYs 1984 and 1985): Expenditures per hospital discharge rose 18.5 percent and 10.5 percent, respectively, with payments rising by 5 percent to 6 percent annually up to the ninth year. These higher CMIs suggested that Simborg's 1981 prophecy of DRG creep had come true, but the exact causes of CMI changes proved difficult to untangle. The central question was whether coding changes represented "creep" or "optimization." Creep implied willful disregard of coding rules, whereas optimization suggested taking lawful advantage of the vagaries of coding and DRG assignment described above. Although code creep caused some portion of the CMI growth, other influential factors included changes in practice patterns (e.g., shifting inpatient to outpatient care, substituting surgical for medical services, developing and diffusing new technologies), heightened oversight of admissions to acute care facilities, aging of the population, hospital structural changes, and changes in the Medicare hospital payment program (Goldfarb and Coffey 1992).

Soon after Medicare instituted DRGs for hospital payment, two studies attempted to disentangle the roots of CMI increases.[11] The first found that two-thirds of the 2.4 percent increase in the CMI between 1986 and 1987 was real, with one-third resulting from coding practice changes and modifications in the DRG classification system (Carter, Newhouse, and Relles 1990). A subsequent study examined a 3.3 percent increase in the CMI between 1987 and 1988, finding that half of the increment was real (Carter, Newhouse, and Relles 1991). Goldfarb and Coffey (1992) dissected real from coding changes in the CMI by looking at shifts in practice patterns and aging of the population. They found that hospitals had largely completed efforts to "improve" their coding practices by 1986. In the tenth and eleventh years of DRG-based payment, the CMI experienced the smallest two-year growth since the reimbursement change (3.6 percent and 3.5 percent, respectively) (ProPAC 1996, 64–65).

Although coding changes have contributed significantly to increases in Medicare's CMI, changes may not reflect willful errors, blatant inaccuracies, or fraud. Some changes represent more complete—and therefore accurate—coding of secondary diagnoses and procedures (MedPAC 2000, 103).[12]

> Upcoding does not necessarily indicate abusive billing practices; it may also result from improvements in medical record documentation and coding technique, which are natural outgrowths of providers learning to classify their patients or adopting [sic] to changes in the structure of the classification system.

Nevertheless, despite the legitimacy of many of these coding changes, the linkage of ICD-9-CM codes to hospital payment leaves a lingering uneasiness about their clinical credibility. Medicare now monitors every participating hospital's CMI annually, posting this information on its web site (http://cms.hhs.gov/medicare/ippswage.asp). Auditors use this information to target hospitals for in-depth reviews of their coding practices and potential monetary sanctions.

Studies of Coding Accuracy

The Office of the Inspector General (OIG) at U.S. DHHS has conducted the major nationwide studies of coding accuracy, explicitly focusing on coding for DRG assignment. The first OIG study sampled Medicare admissions between 1 October 1984 and 31 March 1985 from 239 hospitals nationwide (Hsia et al. 1988). An OIG contractor reviewed photocopied medical records and compared DRGs originally assigned by the hospitals to those from the reabstracted data. Of 7,050 cases, the OIG reabstraction changed DRG assignment for 1,374—an average of 20.8 percent changes after reweighting results by hospital size. Most importantly, regardless of size, 61.7 percent of discrepancies financially favored the hospitals. Given errors in DRG assignment, Medicare overpaid hospitals by $300 million in FY 1985.

The OIG repeated its DRG validation study using 2,451 patient records from 1988 admissions of Medicare beneficiaries (Hsia et al. 1992). In this sample, 14.7 percent of records contained errors that changed DRG assignment. Importantly, however, coding errors did not disproportionately favor the hospitals: 50.7 percent of errors financially benefited the hospital. Misspecification remained the most common cause of errors (62.9 percent), but the proportion of mis-specifications that financially favored the hospitals decreased significantly from the 1985 level. In contrast, mis-sequencing continued to overreimburse hospitals. Since the elimination of the physician attestation requirement (see above), concerns about coding accuracy have returned.[13]

The California Office of Statewide Health Planning and Development (OSHPD) has actively monitored hospital coding (Meux, Stith, and Zach 1990). In one study, OSHPD reabstracted 2,579 records from 1988 discharges from 30 randomly selected hospitals across a variety of conditions (e.g., obstetrics, newborn, and psychiatric conditions). The study found that coding accuracy varied by condition, ranging from 54.5 percent for old myocardial infarction to 97.9 percent for pneumonia and acute cerebrovascular disease (Romano and Luft 1992). Another California investigation involving reabstraction of 974 inpatients coded as having AMIs also found problems with coding even important secondary diagnoses. Coding quality was particularly "poor" for hypotension, pulmonary edema, other valve disease, nutritional deficiency, chronic liver disease, and late effects of cerebrovascular disease (Wilson, Smoley, and Werdegar 1996, 15–20).[14] California stopped adjusting for these poorly coded conditions in its report card on hospitals' AMI mortality rates.

Lawthers and colleagues (2000) examined secondary diagnosis (and some procedure) coding by reabstracting more than 1,200 medical records from California and Connecticut, but their reabstractions had a twist. After trained coding technicians completed their reviews using specially designed software, they pressed a button to display the codes originally assigned by the hospital; the coders then decided whether they wished to add other codes. Although about 85 percent of cases had their codes confirmed during the initial (blinded) review, the abstractors added new codes after seeing the hospitals' codes for the other 15 percent. Furthermore, interrater reliability among the coders was only moderate. Some codes (e.g., AMI, stroke, hemorrhage, pulmonary embolism) were more likely than others to be identified during the initial review and to demonstrate excellent interrater reliability.

Researchers have used longitudinal data to examine the completeness of coding of chronic, incurable conditions. Of Medicare beneficiaries coded with an inpatient or outpatient diagnosis of dementia in 1994, only 59 percent had dementia coded in 1995; for patients coded with paraplegia or quadriplegia in 1994, only 52 percent had these codes in 1995 (MedPAC 1998, 17). Using Medicaid data from seven states, the following percentages of people had specific diagnoses coded in the next year after having had the code the previous year: 80 percent for schizophrenia, 68 percent for diabetes, 58 percent for multiple sclerosis, 57 percent for quadriplegia, and 34 percent for cystic fibrosis (Kronick et al. 2000, 60). As these conditions do not disappear, their absence in the subsequent year highlights the incompleteness of coding.

Some conditions are rarely reported even if they exist. Coding guidelines stipulate that unless conditions are actively addressed, they should not be coded. Although codes exist for blindness, deafness, and hard of hearing, for example, hospitals and physicians infrequently list these conditions on claims for services unrelated to the eyes or ears. Mental retardation is rarely coded for adults or children, perhaps because few health interventions directly treat this condition (Perrin et al. 1999; Kronick et al. 2000). Sometimes physicians intentionally withhold coding potentially stigmatizing diagnoses (e.g., HIV, AIDS, mental health disorders) when they can legitimately list other conditions.

Coding of cause of death on death certificates is also suspect, although this was ICD's original role. The NCHS provides multimedia educational materials about coding cause of death, but few physicians see them. One study compared coding of six cases supplied in NCHS training materials and found only 56.9 percent agreement among 12 internists on listing cause of death (Messite and Stellman 1996, 795). Another study estimated that the nation overestimates coronary heart disease mortality by 7.9 percent to 24.3 percent because of inaccurate coding of death certificates (Lloyd-Jones et al. 1998).

Little information exists about the quality of coded diagnosis data in other inpatient facilities (e.g., psychiatric or rehabilitation hospitals) or outpatient settings. A comparison of Medicare Part B claims with physicians' office records for 1,596 Maryland patients from 1990 to 1991 produced worrisome results. The Part B claims and office records matched on only 40.3 percent of zip codes and 58.5 percent of birthdates (Fowles et al. 1995, 192). The kappa statistics (see Chapter 9) indicating the level of agreement ranged from 0.0 (ketoacidosis) to 0.72 (diabetes mellitus) for the 26 diagnoses examined and were greater than 0.40 for only six diagnoses. Claims frequently did not indicate diagnoses noted in the record.

Limitations of Coding Slots and Potential Undercoding

Administrative data are submitted in formats that limit diagnosis and procedure coding slots. For example, Medicare's UB-82 allowed coding of only five ICD-9-CM diagnoses and three procedures prior to 1992. While five diagnoses may suffice to describe an uncomplicated admission, they are often inadequate to portray complicated admissions or patients with multiple comorbidities. By 1987, almost half of Medicare discharges had all five diagnosis slots filled (Steinwald and Dummit 1989). Jencks, Williams, and Kay (1988) found that coding of secondary diagnoses was possibly biased by limitations in the number of coding spaces. Using Medicare data, they examined mortality 30 days following admission for stroke, pneumonia, acute myocardial infarction, or CHF, and discovered the following (Jencks, Williams, and Kay 1988, 2244):

> Patients with recorded [secondary] diagnoses of diabetes mellitus, unspecified anemia, essential hypertension, hypertensive heart disease, old myocardial infarction, angina, ischemic heart disease, mitral valvular disease, ventricular premature beats, and unclassified arrhythmias are significantly less likely to die within 30 days than patients without these recorded diagnoses. . . . These findings are so counterintuitive as to require explanation. The explanation most consistent with the data is a recording bias that reduces the likelihood of a chronic diagnosis being reported if the patient dies. . . . Medicare's limit of reporting five diagnoses would then be more likely to truncate chronic diagnoses from the diagnosis list.

Clinical explanations for the counterintuitive findings have been sought.[15] However, even those advancing these clinical hypotheses admitted reservations—these conditions generally do increase patients' risks. The possibility of coding bias because of limited secondary diagnosis slots prompted pressure for increasing the number of coding spaces. In response, in the UB-92 (also known as CMS-1450), HCFA expanded coding slots to nine discharge diagnoses (principal and eight other) and six procedures (principal and five other) as of 1 April 1992. UB-92 also contains one slot for the admitting diagnosis (the condition identified by the physician when the patient is admitted). Figure 5.2 shows the number of diagnoses listed for persons 65 years of age and older admitted to California hospitals in FY 1994 using MEDPAR data; Figure 5.3 shows the number of procedures coded in MEDPAR. For

FIGURE 5.2

Number of
Diagnoses
Listed per Case
in 1994
MEDPAR and
California Data

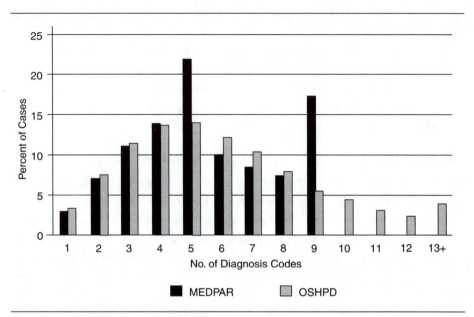

DATA SOURCES: FY 1994 MEDPAR data for California; 1994 hospital discharge abstract database from
California OSHPD.

comparison, both figures show the number of coding slots filled for persons 65 years of age and older taken from the 1994 California hospital discharge abstract database. California's data set contains space for 25 diagnosis and procedure codes.

Does expanding the number of diagnosis slots, such as in California, improve the coding completeness for comorbid and chronic conditions?[16] We examined this question using 1988 computerized hospital discharge abstract data from California with their 25 diagnosis and procedure coding slots (Iezzoni et al. 1992a), then updated our study using 1994 California data.[17] The 1994 findings were similar to those from 1988 and to the findings of Jencks, Williams, and Kay (1998). Some secondary diagnoses significantly decreased the adjusted odds of death (Table 5.6), whereas others had little effect (e.g., type I diabetes mellitus, unspecified anemia, coronary atherosclerosis, unspecified ischemic heart disease). Urinary tract infection significantly increased the adjusted odds of dying for pneumonia (1.34) and CHF (1.46) but decreased the adjusted odds for stroke (0.88) and AMI (0.88).

Coding of secondary diagnoses may be particularly problematic for conditions that could represent complications of care. Romano et al. (2002) examined results from reabstraction of 991 diskectomy cases admitted to California hospitals in 1990–91. The original hospital codes displayed only 35 percent sensitivity for identifying any complication determined by the "gold-standard" reabstraction. Most worrisome, underreporting was markedly worse at hospitals calculated to have lower risk-adjusted complication rates (see below). Undercoding extended beyond serious complications to more mild con-

FIGURE 5.3
Number of
Procedures
Listed per Case
in 1994
MEDPAR and
California Data

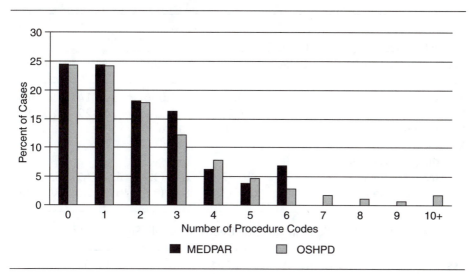

DATA SOURCES: FY 1994 MEDPAR data for California; 1994 hospital discharge abstract database from
California OSHPD.

ditions, such as atelectasis, posthemorrhagic anemia, and hypotension (Romano, Schembri, and Rainwater 2002). One study from Alberta, Canada,
examined the concordance between medical records and administrative data
for the conditions included in the Charlson comorbidity index (see Chapter
3). Administrative data underreported ten comorbidities but slightly overreported diabetes, mild liver disease, and rheumatologic disease (Quan, Parsons,
and Ghali 2002, 678).

Therefore, undercoding is an important problem. With discharge-
abstract-based risk adjusters, clinically appropriate ratings of individual cases
depend on coding of all relevant diagnoses. We abstracted detailed clinical
information on 27 patients, including verbatim the information listed on the
hospital's face sheet. We asked vendors to rate each case using this information
and performed scoring for APACHE II (Hughes et al. 1996; Iezzoni et al.
1995c). For the case shown in Table 5.7, the hospital assigned only two
codes—pseudomonas pneumonia and multiple myeloma. Given the extent
of the patient's acute derangements, additional codes, including sepsis, septic
shock, and respiratory failure, could have been listed. Several vendors informed
us that such codes would have changed their severity ratings. For example,
by adding sepsis, the Acuity Index Method (AIM) severity class (range 1–5)
would have risen from 1 to 3 and the predicted LOS from 7.3 to 12.6 days. By
adding septicemia and shock, the PMC severity score (range 1–7) would have
risen from 4 to 7, the PMC Relative Intensity Score (RIS; weight with 1.0 =
average) from 1.66 to 3.011, and the LOS prediction from 8.4 to 13.0 days.
In contrast, because they do not rely on diagnosis coding, the clinically based
measures assigned fairly severe scores, representing the range of physiological
derangements present on admission.

TABLE 5.6

Sample Characteristics and Odds Ratio Adjusted for Age and Sex of In-Hospital Death for Patients with Specified Secondary Diagnoses: 1994 California Hospital Discharge Abstract Data

Sample Characteristics and Secondary Diagnosis	ICD-9-CM Code	Condition			
		Stroke	Pneumonia	AMI	CHF
No. of cases		35,837	60,066	32,714	54,362
No. of deaths		4,290	7,575	4,329	3,192
Percent died		12.0	12.6	13.2	5.9
Mean (SD) no. of diagnosis codes					
Discharged alive		6.3 (2.9)	6.8 (3.2)	6.5 (3.2)	6.7 (2.9)
Discharged dead		6.7 (3.4)	8.6 (3.6)	8.0 (3.6)	8.3 (3.6)
Adjusted Odds Ratio of In-Hospital Death Generally Significantly <1.0					
Essential hypertension	401.9	0.70*	0.69*	0.59*	0.52*
Hypertension with heart disease	402.90	0.70[+]	0.71[+]	0.61[+]	0.49
Old myocardial infarction	412	0.99	0.91	0.78[+]	0.85[#]
Angina pectoris	413.9	0.50*	0.56*	0.37*	0.53*
Adjusted Odds Ratio of In-Hospital Death Generally Significantly >1.0					
Dehydration	276.50	1.27*	1.61*	1.77*	3.29*
Paroxysmal ventricular tachycardia	427.1	2.38*	2.26*	2.11*	2.03*
Atrial fibrillation	427.31	1.36*	1.48*	1.25*	1.12[+]
Cardiac arrest	427.5	47.98*	52.39*	21.64*	58.75*
Pneumonia, organism unspecified	486	2.60*	2.10[+]	2.04*	2.58*
Chronic obstructive pulmonary disease	496.00	1.16[+]	0.93[+]	1.13[#]	1.17[+]
Chronic renal failure	585	2.32*	1.98*	2.34*	2.32*
Cardiogenic shock	785.51	24.44*	22.61*	14.20*	23.60*
Respiratory failure	799.1	12.78*	7.95*	8.87*	10.82*

* $p \leq 0.0001$.
[+] $0.0001 < p \leq 0.01$.
[#] $0.01 < p < 0.05$.

Retrospective Nature of Discharge Diagnoses

Hospital discharge abstract information is retrospective—diagnoses and their sequences are assigned after patients leave the hospital. Discharge diagnosis codes thus reflect conditions diagnosed or treated during the entire admission. Knowing the timing of diagnoses is, however, crucial for distinguishing risks

Case Presentation	TABLE 5.7

A 54-year-old woman with a five-year history of multiple myeloma was admitted with dyspnea and diffuse bilateral infiltrates on chest x-ray. She had experienced recurrent paraspinal masses and cord compressions from the multiple myeloma, as well as pathologic fractures, and had received both chemotherapy and radiation therapy. At the time of admission, she was bedbound, cared for at home by her husband, and not receiving active myeloma treatment. On exam, her temperature was 98.6°F, pulse 120, respirations 36, and blood pressure palpable at 92. Arterial blood gas on room air: pH 7.45, pCO_2 39, pO_2 63. Leukocytes were 8.0 k, with 87 percent segmented forms and no bands. Sputum grew *pseudomonas*, and pleural fluid contained malignant cells. The patient initially requested maximal treatment, including intubation and mechanical ventilation. She was treated with intravenous antibiotics but deteriorated rapidly. On day 3 she became hypoxic, was intubated, and was transferred to the ICU with respiratory failure, necrotizing pneumonia, sepsis, and septic shock. Her respiratory failure worsened, and on day 5 she became unresponsive. At the family's request, orders for DNR status and comfort measures only were written on day 5, and she died the next day.

TABLE 5.7
Case Presentation, Discharge Abstract Data, and Severity Scores: Effect of Undercoding

Discharge Abstract Information

Age: 54 years

DRG 475, respiratory system
   diagnosis with ventilator support

LOS: six days

Total charges: $13,800

Discharge status: expired

Procedures:
   96.04, endotracheal intubation

Diagnoses listed by hospital:
   482.1, pneumonia due to
   pseudomonas
   203.0, multiple myeloma

Severity Ratings

Severity Measure	Patient's Score	Range of Scores
Clinically Based Measures		
APACHE II (worst values from day 1)		
APS	8	0–60
Total APACHE II score	10	0–71
CSI		
Admission score (days 1 and 2)	3	1–4
Maximum score (worst values from entire stay)	4	1–4
MedisGroups empirical version		
Admission score (days 1 and 2)	0.129	0–1.0
Midstay score (days 3–7)	0.415	0–1.0

TABLE 5.7
Continued

Severity Measure	Patient's Score	Range of Scores
Discharge Abstract–Based Measures		
AIM	1	1–5
APR-DRGs	2	1–4
DS mortality probability	0.054	0–1.0
PMCs severity score	4	1–7
PMC RIS	1.66	Base = 1.0
PMC LOS prediction (days)	8.4	> 0
R-DRGs	B	D,C,B

SOURCE: Adapted from Hughes et al. (1996).

caused by intrinsic patient factors from those caused by substandard inpatient care. For instance, suppose a patient had the following discharge diagnoses:

820.21	Closed intertrochanteric fracture of neck of femur
482.4	Staphylococcal pneumonia
599.0	Urinary tract infection, site not specified
250.70	Type II diabetes mellitus with peripheral circulatory disorders, not stated as uncontrolled

The type II diabetes is obvious preexisting, but either the pneumonia or urinary tract infection could have occurred in hospital, perhaps as nosocomial infections. The inability to differentiate the timing of diagnoses seriously hampers the utility of discharge abstracts for identifying patients' risk factors prior to medical intervention.

Lawthers and colleagues (2000, 789) looked at the timing of secondary diagnoses by reabstracting more than 1,200 medical records from California and Connecticut. To select cases to review, they attempted to maximize the likelihood that the secondary diagnoses occurred in hospital as complications of care (see Note 7). Among surgical cases, the percentages of secondary diagnoses present on admission included aspiration pneumonia, 15 percent; gastrointestinal hemorrhage, 15 percent; hip fracture or fall, 21 percent; deep-vein thrombosis or pulmonary embolism, 22 percent; and shock or cardiorespiratory arrest, 29 percent.

In our work on hospital-based severity measures, discharge-abstract-based risk adjusters were sometimes equal or better predictors of in-hospital mortality than measures derived from admission clinical findings (Iezzoni 1997; Iezzoni et al. 1995a, 1995b, 1996a, 1996e; Landon et al. 1996). For example, for AMI patients, discharge-abstract-based APR-DRGs and DS produced slightly higher c-statistics than either empirical MedisGroups or the physiology score that approximates APACHE III's APS (Table 5.8). When examining CABG mortality in New York state using MEDPAR versus clini-

Severity Measure	Condition				TABLE 5.8
	AMI	CABG	Pneumonia	Stroke	
Clinically Based Measures					
MedisGroups empirical version	0.83	0.74	0.85	0.87	
Physiology score 2	0.83	0.73	0.82	0.84	
Discharge-Abstract-Based Measures					
APR-DRGs	0.84	0.83	0.78	0.77	
DS mortality probability	0.86	0.78	0.80	0.74	
PMCs severity score	0.82	0.81	0.79	0.73	

TABLE 5.8 c-Statistics for Predicting In-Hospital Death

SOURCE: Adapted from Iezzoni et al. (1995b, 1996a, 1996c); Landon et al. (1996).

cal data, Hannan and colleagues (1997) found similar results: c-statistics for models fell when they eliminated ICD-9-CM codes representing complications rather than comorbidities. One hypothesis about why discharge-abstract-based risk adjusters performed well in predicting in-hospital deaths is their reliance on ICD-9-CM codes for conditions, such as cardiac arrest, arising late in the hospital stay. In contrast, the clinically based measures use findings from only the first two hospital days. Thus, we hypothesized that discharge-abstract-based measures benefited from a virtual tautology—using near-death experiences to predict death.

Anecdotal evidence supports this hypothesis. As described above, we abstracted detailed clinical and discharge abstract information on 27 patients and scored each case (Hughes et al. 1996; Iezzoni et al. 1995c). Several cases suggested that discharge-abstract-based measures rely heavily on codes representing serious conditions that might arise late during the hospital stay. The example in Table 5.9 involves an 81-year-old woman admitted for hip fracture repair. She was fairly stable on admission; the clinically based admission severity measures rated her as mildly to moderately severe. Postoperatively, however, she experienced serious complications—Gram-negative septicemia and respiratory failure. PMCs, APR-DRGs, and R-DRGs assigned her high severity scores. The two measures producing predicted probabilities of in-hospital death are particularly illustrative: The admission MedisGroups probability was 0.009, while DS's probability was 0.284.

To examine our hypothesis empirically, we used ICD-9-CM diagnosis codes to define variables similar to the MedisGroups KCFs. Given the limitations of ICD-9-CM, this was possible for only selected KCFs (Iezzoni et al. 1996b). Our analyses generally supported the hypothesis that discharge-abstract-based severity measures rely heavily on ICD-9-CM codes representing grave conditions potentially arising later in the hospital stay. Nevertheless, strategies exist for dealing with timing of diagnoses. Analysts could concentrate solely on ICD-9-CM codes representing chronic conditions, such as diabetes mellitus, malignancy, chronic obstructive pulmonary disease, and chronic renal failure. Shapiro and colleagues (1994) used this approach to compare mortality rates at municipal and voluntary hospitals in New York City. They specified two risk-adjustment models: "full other diagnoses," including 17 categories of other diagnoses, and "limited other diagnoses," eliminating all acute conditions that could potentially represent substandard care (e.g., septicemia, pulmonary embolism, pneumonia, acute tubular necrosis, cardiogenic shock, respiratory arrest). Perceptions about whether municipal and voluntary hospitals had different death rates generally varied across the two risk-adjustment methods.

When analysts use longitudinal files, they can identify comorbid diagnoses present during some period before hospitalization. For example, if patients have outpatient visit claims listing pneumonia from several days prior to hospitalization, a secondary discharge diagnosis of pneumonia probably represents a preexisting condition. This strategy must recognize that coding of outpatient diagnoses obeys different rules than inpatient coding and is often incomplete (see above). The predictive power of diagnoses identified from prior services varies depending on the research context. One study looking at in-hospital mortality found little benefit from adding diagnoses from prior hospitalizations (Stukenborg, Wagner, and Connors 2001).

Another approach involves combining items from the discharge abstract to draw inferences about the timing of diagnoses. One useful item is the date of major procedures (or LOS prior to major procedures). For instance, surgeons typically avoid operating on patients with acute pneumonia. Suppose patients have surgery on day 1 or 2 of their hospital stays and also have secondary diagnoses of staphylococcal pneumonia. The pneumonia is more likely to represent a postoperative nosocomial infection than a condition present on admission. In designing the CSP, we used this approach with administrative data to flag probable in-hospital complications (Iezzoni et al. 1994a, 1994b). Although playing these probabilities could differentiate preoperative from postoperative conditions across groups of patients, it may not work for individuals. In addition, this strategy is not useful for conditions that are not serious operative risks (e.g., urinary tract infection).

Some states (e.g., California, New York) have added slots to their hospital discharge abstracts indicating whether diagnoses were preexisting or arose during the hospitalization. Although significant questions remain about the accuracy of these flags, this information could considerably benefit risk adjusters designed to track quality-of-care outcomes: Risk adjusters could use only those diagnoses listed as present on admission. Motivated by HIPAA standardization activities, efforts are underway to include coding slots for timing of discharge diagnoses nationwide (see below).

Case Presentation	TABLE 5.9

<table>
<tr><td>

An 81-year-old widow, previously ambulatory and residing at a home for the aged, was admitted after she broke her hip. She had a history of hypertension, a previous syncopal episode with negative diagnostic workup, mitral regurgitation, and aortic regurgitation. Repair of her hip was delayed until day 4 by a syncopal episode that occurred in the emergency room on admission and by a urinary tract infection. Her postoperative course was complicated by persistent fever, a pleural effusion, and a probable urinary tract infection. Antibiotic coverage was broadened on day 10, and she was transferred to the ICU on day 11 due to hypotension (systolic pressure = 80 mm Hg), hypoxia (pO_2 = 66), and possible sepsis. She was intubated and mechanically ventilated but became more hypotensive despite intravenous dopamine and neosynephrine drugs. She died on day 12.

</td><td>

Case Presentation, Discharge Abstract Data, and Severity Scores: Comparison of Discharge-Abstract-Based and Clinically Based Measures

</td></tr>
</table>

Discharge Abstract Information

Age: 81 years

DRG 210, hip and femur procedures with complication or comorbidity

LOS: 12 days

Total charges: $20,900

Discharge status: expired

Procedures:
  79.35, open reduction of femur fracture with internal fixation

Diagnoses:
  820.21, pertrochanteric femur fracture, closed, intertrochanteric section

  780.2, syncope and collapse

  401.9, essential hypertension

  599.0, urinary tract infection

  038.40, Gram-negative septicemia

  518.5, pulmonary insufficiency following trauma and surgery

Severity Ratings

Severity Measure	Patient's Score	Range of Scores
Clinically Based Measures		
APACHE II (worst values from day 1)		
APS	1	0–60
Total APACHE II score	7	0–71
CSI		
Admission score (days 1 and 2)	1	1–4
Maximum score (worst values from entire stay)	4	1–4
MedisGroups empirical version		
Admission score (days 1 and 2)	0.009	0–1.0
Midstay score (days 3–7)	0.013	0–1.0

TABLE 5.9
Continued

Severity Measure	Patient's Score	Range of Scores
Discharge-Abstract-Based Measures		
APR-DRGs	3	1–4
DS mortality probability	0.284	0–1.0
PMCs severity score	7	1–7
R-DRGs	A	D,C,B,A

SOURCE: Adapted from Hughes et al. (1996).

Coding Differences Across Hospitals

Hospitals and other providers code with different levels of thoroughness and accuracy. Without additional information, one cannot tell whether these coding differences reflect true differences in the patient mix. Good circumstantial evidence suggests systematic biases in institutional coding practices. For example, using 1988 discharge abstract data for patients age 65 and older, we arrayed the 441 California hospitals by increasing average number of diagnoses per case (Iezzoni et al. 1992a). The mean number of diagnoses per case ranged from 2.5 for the lowest-coding hospital to 11.7 for the heaviest coder. Hospitals listing more codes per case were disproportionately large and private.

The reabstraction study of 974 AMI and 991 diskectomy patients admitted to California hospitals in 1990–91 described above was prompted by the state's initiative to produce hospital report cards on AMI mortality and diskectomy complication rates using administrative data (Wilson, Smoley, and Werdegar 1996). Not surprisingly, these reports attracted criticism because of their data source; in response, California reviewed medical records to validate coding accuracy. Analysts sampled cases within hospitals stratified into three groups—hospital risk-adjusted AMI mortality better than expected, neither better nor worse, and worse than expected.

Overall, 65.0 percent of discharge abstracts for AMI cases were missing at least one clinical risk factor, whereas 30.9 percent missed two risk factors (Wilson, Smoley, and Werdegar 1996, 14–16). Hospitals varied from 45 percent to 87 percent in the fraction of uncoded risk factors. The percentage of missing risk factors did not vary across the three hospital mortality categories. In contrast, 31.5 percent of the discharge abstracts contained at least one "unsupported risk factor." This overcoding was much more common at low-mortality hospitals than at intermediate- or high-mortality hospitals (36.7 percent versus 29.2 percent and 29.0 percent; $p = 0.04$). Overcoding rates ranged from 10 percent at one high-mortality hospital to 74 percent at a low-mortality hospital. Variation in coding accuracy explained part of the differences between high- and low-mortality hospitals. Similarly, under-reporting of diskectomy complications was much higher at hospitals with lower-than-expected complication rates (Romano et al. 2002).

Information About Procedures

Most risk adjusters do not incorporate procedures as risk factors; adjusting for procedure use becomes confounded with concerns about technical quality, appropriateness of care, and differences in physicians' practice patterns (see Table 2.3). Nonetheless, procedural information is obviously an essential component of outcomes studies.

Procedural Nomenclatures

Unlike for diagnoses, no single procedure classification scheme is used in the United States. Procedure classification and coding differ by context and setting. Hospitals report procedures using the ICD-9-CM for Medicare payment, while physicians employ CPT and HCPCS (see above; HCPCS is largely based on CPT). The codes in ICD-9-CM and CPT do not readily link. Health insurers frequently create their own idiosyncratic procedure codes to supplement CPT, further compromising efforts to obtain consistent information about procedures. HIPAA standardization of code sets leaves ICD-9-CM, HCPCS, and CPT intact within particular contexts but should presumably ease problems relating to plan-specific codes.

The ICD-9-CM procedural nomenclature generates serious reservations. One key "is that the outcome of surgery is coded and the approach is often ignored" (McMahon and Smits 1986, 563). As one example, ICD-9-CM fails to distinguish the approach for gastrointestinal procedures that today often involve endoscopy: Code 42.32 (local excision of other lesion or tissue of esophagus) describes what was done but not how. ICD-9-CM procedure codes do not identify the side of the body for procedures that could be bilateral. Despite these problems, ICD-9-CM procedure codes sometimes permit more insight into patients' experiences than do CPT and HCPCS, even about possible quality problems (Hannan et al. 1989). For example, ICD-9-CM contains a code for suture of laceration of the uterus; neither HCPCS nor CPT contain such codes. With their bundled billing, surgeons do not charge individually for services that are part of complete therapy. Patients are not billed for surgical treatments of operative complications. Therefore, regardless of the procedure coding system, no bill is available marking the event (Mitchell et al. 1994).

CPT provides thousands of codes detailing the approach taken for surgical and diagnostic procedures. One area that generates significant controversy involves coding of outpatient "evaluation and management" visits and inpatient consultations (Lasker and Marquis 1999). Physician billing and coding practices remain continually in flux as CMS changes Medicare physician reimbursement policies (e.g., the resource-based relative value scale).

Medicare prospective fee-for-service payment for outpatient services provided by hospitals, driven by the APCs, the outpatient analogue to DRGs, was implemented in mid-2000 and will affect coding practices. Diagnoses do not define APCs. Instead, APC assignment derives from the CPT evaluation and management codes and CPT and HCPCS codes for other services. Because the APC initiative aims to bundle billing (i.e., paying for packages of services rather than requiring claims for each separate service), the detail of outpatient hospital procedure coding will inevitably decrease.

Quality of Procedure Coding

Hospitals have been reimbursed by diagnoses (i.e., DRGs) only since 1983, but physicians have long been paid for specific procedures by submitting claims with relevant procedure codes. Coding of procedures should therefore be more complete and accurate than diagnosis coding. Indeed, the report from the 1970s on the accuracy of hospital discharge abstract data found better accuracy for procedure than diagnosis coding (Institute of Medicine 1977a). For principal diagnoses, hospitals' reports were only 65.2 percent accurate, but principal procedures showed 73.2 percent accuracy. Determining who coded correctly—the hospital or the reabstractors—was surprisingly more difficult for principal procedure than for principal diagnosis. Coding was indeterminate for 10.7 percent of principal diagnoses, compared to 16.3 percent of principal procedures.

In reanalyzing data collected by the OIG (Hsia et al. 1988), Fisher and colleagues (1992) found 76.2 percent agreement for principal procedures at the two-digit ICD-9-CM code level and 73.8 percent at the three-digit level. When they ignored the order of procedure codes, agreement rose considerably and was much higher for procedures than for diagnoses. The proportion of agreement ranged from 0.88 for cardiac catheterization to more than 0.95 for 10 of the 15 procedures examined. ICD-9-CM procedural data may therefore be more clinically meaningful and less difficult to interpret than diagnostic data (Fisher et al. 1992, 247).

Romano and Luft (1992) reanalyzed findings from the California study described above (Meux, Stith, and Zach 1990) to examine the accuracy of coding-specific procedures. Procedures coded originally by the hospital were virtually 100 percent specific (i.e., if the patient had not had the procedure, the procedure was not listed). However, sensitivity (i.e., the percentage of patients with the procedure who had the procedure coded) varied widely by procedure. Procedures coded with lower sensitivity were associated with lower costs or risks to patients.

As suggested above, one problem with procedure coding is the practice of "unbundling"—physicians submitting claims for multiple specific procedures that are all really part of a single procedure. Unbundling is facilitated by the massive detail of CPT: For example, numerous codes for various angiographic procedures and the associated injection of radiographic contrast materials are listed separately. HCPCS, with CPT at its core, contains more than 12,000 codes. At least for Medicare, the National Correct Coding Initiative (http://cms.hhs.gov/medlearn.asp, accessed 29 July 2002) aims to improve coding and reduce unbundling for claims from physicians' offices. CMS views roughly 175,000 pairs of codes as representing unacceptable unbundling. Separate claims for these services are denied, producing a powerful incentive to meet Medicare's coding standards.

Aggressive auditing of procedure claims lessens concerns about their accuracy. Because of this (Romano and Luft 1992, 61):

> Procedures also may be used as surrogates for diagnoses when the diagnoses are apt to be coded imprecisely. For example, preoperative use of an intra-aortic balloon pump can be used as a surrogate for severe ventricular dysfunction. . . . Obviously, this strategy works only if the date of a secondary procedure relative to the primary procedure is known. Any procedure used as a surrogate for a diagnosis should have relatively clear indications. . . .

Nevertheless, because of differences in practice patterns and discretion in use of even potentially life saving interventions, few analysts feel comfortable using procedures as surrogate risk factors for diagnoses.

The quality of coding for laboratory and low-cost procedures is more questionable than for more expensive interventions that attract the scrutiny of auditors. One study compared Medicare Part B claims with physician office records for almost 1,600 Maryland patients and found that coding of tests was less accurate than diagnosis coding. Many laboratory tests and procedures were missing from physicians' records. The kappa statistic indicating the agreement between the Part B claims and physician office records ranged from –0.02 for nuclear medicine scans to 0.73 for hemoglobin A_{1c} testing (Fowles et al. 1995, 195).

Pharmacy Data

Administrative databases from insurers offering prescription drug benefits, including Medicaid, generally contain pharmacy claims. Pharmacy data represent prescriptions that were filled (instead of prescriptions written but never obtained by the patient). Most public and private insurance files use NDCs to represent pharmaceuticals purchased from pharmacies. Coding of drugs within inpatient settings is more varied and often does not rely on NDCs.

Obviously, administrative files do not indicate whether people took medications as prescribed. Pharmacy data can identify people with specific conditions, such as diabetes, bipolar disorder, asthma, and AIDS (Johnson, Hornbrook, and Nichols 1994; Fishman and Shay 1999; Lamers 1999). These data suggest the severity of some medical conditions: For example, people receiving insulin presumably have more intractable diabetes mellitus than those taking oral hypoglycemic agents. However, as with procedure codes, pharmacy data identify only selected subgroups of people, varying practice patterns compromise the generalizability of findings, and drugs not covered by insurance plans escape detection.

Structural Attributes of Administrative Data

The principal question about administrative database structure is whether information from different sources can be linked for individual persons. Linking data across settings (e.g., hospitals, private doctors' offices, nursing homes, homes) and over time requires a unique personal identification number regardless of payer or provider, raising serious concerns about confidentiality and privacy (Donaldson and Lohr 1994, 141). Unique personal identifiers are generally available for Medicare, VA, and Medicaid databases but few others. Although a Medicare beneficiary's identification number can change, CMS has cross-referenced such numbers for some researchers (e.g., the PORTs) (Lave et al. 1994). To protect patient confidentiality, administrative databases obtained for research almost never contain sufficient information to determine the identity of individual patients. Access to such sensitive information, however, can occasionally be negotiated depending on the nature of the specific research study.

The most commonly used uniform patient identification number is the SSN, but this concerns many privacy experts. When Social Security was enacted in 1935, recipients received an SSAN—the number of a person's Social Security "account"—which was not intended as a personal identifier. In 1943, President Roosevelt signed an executive order stipulating that all federal agencies implementing new record systems (such as the Internal Revenue Service) use the SSN to identify individuals. The Privacy Act of 1974 prohibited states from using the SSN, but the Tax Reform Act of 1976 undermined that restriction. States with unique patient identifiers attached to hospital discharge abstracts (e.g., California, Massachusetts) typically use the SSN or some derivative. Outsiders cannot obtain actual SSNs. California, for example, carefully encrypts SSNs for public-use data files (Meux 1994).

In most instances, the SSN is unique and specific—a single individual has one and only one number. This is not the case in certain scenarios. Some states assign temporary numbers to persons without SSNs who require immediate Medicaid benefits; permanent and different numbers are given later (Bright, Avorn, and Everitt 1989). Family members may be assigned a relative's SSN. For instance, a wife may use her husband's SSN or an unborn child its mother's SSN. (Today, however, parents of 92 percent of newborns apply for their infant's SSN at the hospital after delivery.) Instances of single persons with multiple SSNs and multiple persons with a single SSN complicate record linkage. Nonetheless, these occurrences are rare and ways exist to disentangle data involving multiple persons with a single SSN (e.g., by tracking other identification information on individual records, such as sex, birth date, mother's name).

HIPAA Subtitle F, Sec. 1173(b)(1) stipulates that "The Secretary [of DHHS] shall adopt standards providing for a standard unique health identifier for each individual, employer, health plan, and health care provider for use in the health care system." Various options under consideration include an enhanced SSN, a new identification number based on bank card methods, and biometric markers. However, HIPAA also requires the secretary to protect individual privacy (see Chapter 6). It remains unclear how these two potentially competing goals will be reconciled and achieved.

Even without unique, patient-level numbers, analysts can often link records with some degree of certainty if adequate demographic and administrative information is available. Various computerized algorithms can match records showing exact agreement on specified characteristics (deterministic linkage). Algorithms automatically calculate a probability that given pairs of records refer to the same individual when they agree on only certain characteristics (Roos et al. 1996).

Having patient-level, linked data over time can solve some limitations of hospital discharge abstract information. As noted earlier, using linked data, analysts can identify conditions treated prior to hospitalization. Analysts can also look at patterns of diagnoses over previous hospitalizations or health care encounters to draw inferences about the course of illness. Linking Medicare Part A and B records provides an opportunity for "internal validation" of the quality of Medicare data—seeing whether hospital and physician claims agree on listed diagnoses and procedures. Risk adjusters like ACGs, DCGs, and CDPS use linked data to predict resource consumption for current or future years.

Longitudinal administrative data files offer a powerful tool to examine service consumption. These data may even be more accurate than directly asking patients about their experiences (Roos, Nicol, and Cageorge 1987, 43):

> Primary data collection must deal with both inability to locate individuals and refusal to participate; even well-run surveys employing multiple call-backs usually have 10–15% nonresponse. A database designed to capture utilization by an entire population "solves" the problem by registering ("locating") individuals and ensuring that utilization ("participation") results in a claim.

Tracking patients through longitudinal administrative databases minimizes concerns about nonrespondent bias that plague primary-data-based studies.

Medicare and VA files link readily with eligibility records indicating patients' vital status. Other data sets generally do not have a mechanism to track dates of death. In certain situations, one option for tracking patients' vital status involves tapping into the National Death Index (NDI). The NDI, maintained by NCHS since 1979, is a computerized record derived from states' vital statistics reports (Edlavitch, Feinleib, and Anello 1985). Matching criteria for the NDI include SSN, patient's first and last names, patient's father's surname, and patient's birth date. The NDI is updated approximately annually upon receipt of reports from states. Using the NDI requires data that are often protected for confidentiality reasons.

Another crucial structural question is whether the data are population based: Can analysts determine denominators? As described above, Medicare keeps updated enrollment files; once individuals join Medicare, their participation is generally "permanent" (i.e., patients do not often relinquish Medicare membership). Thus, calculating population denominators is fairly easy for Medicare patients. In contrast, eligibility for Medicaid waxes and wanes for many individuals as their financial and employment status changes. Determining the population covered by private insurers is challenging (Garnick et al. 1996). Many plans update their enrollment files annually, when groups renew coverage. In addition, most carriers only retain files on groups that are actively covered by their plans. Therefore, information disappears for those persons whose companies drop the health plan.

State databases pose problems with border crossing for services and residential migration across states, which are more likely in some states than others. Patients living in small states next to states with large, renowned, tertiary medical centers often cross state borders to obtain sophisticated services. Out-of-state services are not included in the database of the state where the patient resides. Thus, the numerator for calculating procedure rates, for example, in the small state would be biased downward by border crossing. Determining population denominators is particularly problematic for states with many illegal immigrants or migrant workers.

Finally, the size of administrative databases carries logistical and conceptual implications. Analysts must have computer hardware that can handle large volumes and other technical requirements (e.g., drives to download data). Huge sample sizes mean that even small differences appear statistically significant. Thus, *a priori* hypotheses about expected findings and associations are essential, as is a conceptual sense about what magnitude of differences is clinically meaningful.

Merging Administrative Data with Other Data Sources

Merging administrative data with other data sources can efficiently enrich administrative files (Lillard and Farmer 1997; U.S. GAO 2001). Using aggregate information collected by the decennial census, for example, researchers have linked person-level information with data on population characteristics (e.g., poverty level, racial distribution) within small geographical areas (Hofer 2001); sophisticated geographical information systems increasingly complement census-tract-based analyses (Rogers 1999). These studies must, however, recognize potential flaws in the data (e.g., errors in patient-reported zip codes, shifting geographic boundaries; Krieger et al. 2002). Linking information from the AHA annual survey allows insight (e.g., teaching status, bed size) into the institutions providing services. These examples involve merging information about individuals with aggregate, contextual information (e.g., about census tracts, neighborhoods, hospitals).

Linking two or more data sources containing information on individuals offers considerable additional insight. Most such merges include Medicare data because of their huge size and nationwide scope. One example merges two different sources from within Medicare itself—the Medicare Current Beneficiary Survey (MCBS) and the NCH file. The MCBS is an ongoing longitudinal survey of a representative panel of roughly 12,000 Medicare beneficiaries, with an oversampling of persons under age 65 and those 85 years of age and older (Adler 1994, 1995). Respondents typically remain empaneled in the MCBS for four years, with in-person interviews three times annually. Two types of surveys (based on residence within communities or institutions) solicit information about physical and sensory functioning, satisfaction with and access to care, out-of-pocket payments, and numerous other topics. Merging MCBS responses with Medicare claims facilitates varied analyses, such as examining screening and preventive services (Chan et al. 1999), satisfaction with care (Adler 1995; Rosenbach 1995; Hermann, Ettner, and Dorwart 1998), access to care (Rosenbach 1995; Foote and Hogan 2001), and out-of-pocket expenditures by ability to perform ADLs (Foote and Hogan 2001).

Surveys derived from national sampling have been merged with Medicare data, notably the Longitudinal Survey of Aging and the National Long-Term Care Survey, both of which contain extensive functional status information. Prior to linking these files, survey respondents must consent; 80 percent typically do, but consent rates vary across surveys (Lillard and Farmer 1997, 694). Analysts have used these linked files extensively to study patterns of service use, especially among elderly persons with functional deficits (Manton, Corder, and Stallard 1993; Mor et al. 1994; Culler, Callahan, and Wolinsky 1995; Stearns et al. 1996). Planning is underway to merge National Health Interview Survey (NHIS) responses with Medicare claims files, allowing wide-ranging analyses of service utilization associated with personal attributes and health-related attributes captured by the NHIS. To protect confidentiality, the content of these files and access to these data are carefully regulated.

A prominent interagency linkage involves merging Medicare claims files with the National Cancer Institute's (NCI) Surveillance, Epidemiology, and End Results (SEER) program data (Potosky et al. 1993; Warren et al. 2002a). The SEER program gathers information from 11 population-based cancer registries and three supplemental registries covering about 14 percent of the U.S. population (NCI 2002a). Started in 1973, the SEER database contains information on more than 2.5 million cancer cases, with about 160,000 new cases added annually. SEER routinely collects data on patients' demographics, primary tumor site, morphology, stage at diagnosis, first course of treatment (followed for up to four months), and vital status.

Data elements from the SEER program (SSN, name, sex, dates of birth and death) facilitate linkage with Medicare claims files. Using a deterministic matching algorithm, the first merge (for patients diagnosed from 1973 to 1989) matched 93.8 percent of persons diagnosed at 65 years of age or older (Potosky et al. 1993). NCI and CMS plan to update the merge every three years, adding Medicare claims during intervening years (NCI 2002b). To allow comparisons, the database also contains a 5 percent random sample of Medicare beneficiaries not in the SEER registry but residing in SEER areas (so-called "noncancer cases").

Researchers use the clinical detail of the SEER database to enrich analyses of cancer care conducted with Medicare claims (Warren et al. 2002a, 2002b). Riley and colleagues (1995) examined Medicare costs between diagnosis and death using merged files from 1984 through 1990, finding unexpectedly low costs for lung cancer, presumably because of short life spans. Studies have employed merged SEER-Medicare data to compare early detection of cancer for fee-for-service versus MCO insurance (Riley et al. 1994, 1999), outcomes of care by insurance type (Potosky et al. 1997, 1999), and mammogram experience by race (McCarthy et al. 1998) and age (McCarthy et al. 2000b). Analysts at the NCI have specified a method to identify comorbidities using administrative data within the SEER-Medicare file (Klabunde, Warren, and Legler 2002) and for measuring complications of cancer care (Potosky et al. 2002).

Some researchers leverage the broad reach of Medicare to enhance SEER analyses. For instance, using Medicare claims to identify incident cases, McBean, Babish, and Warren (1993) found that 1986–90 age-adjusted lung cancer incidence rates among Medicare beneficiaries residing outside nine SEER areas was 8 percent to 13 percent higher than rates for residents of the SEER regions. The researchers urged complementing SEER cancer incidence data with Medicare claims-derived rates, as Medicare covers the entire country and SEER sites may not be nationally representative.

Since the Social Security Administration (SSA) determines Medicare eligibility, particularly for persons with disabilities, one useful interdepartmental data merge links SSA and Medicare records. To examine Medicare costs for newly entitled disabled persons, for example, analysts at SSA and HCFA merged SSA's Master Beneficiary Record (records of entitlement and cash payments for all persons who ever received Social Security benefits), the Continuous Disability History Sample (a 20 percent sample of SSA disability determinations), and Medicare claims files. With this merged file, they examined long-term Medicare costs for disabled beneficiaries (Bye, Riley, and Lubitz 1987) and the potential costs to Medicare of eliminating the two-year waiting period between SSA disability determination and Medicare eligibility (Bye and Riley 1989; Bye et al. 1991).

Merging SSA disability and Medicare files required careful interdepartmental negotiations, primarily to ensure strict privacy and security of the data. With detailed information on SSA's disability determinations linked with

Medicare claims, even files stripped of specific identifiers (name, SSN) could pose potential privacy risks. Merged SSA and Medicare databases are not generally released to outside investigators.

Examples of Administrative Data from Other Countries

To a large extent, the fragmented nature of administrative data systems in the United States reflects the country's fragmented health care delivery system. In nations and regions where central authorities deliver health care to well-defined populations, comprehensive administrative data systems could facilitate monitoring of health and health care delivery (Nerenz 1996). The POPULIS data system in Manitoba, Canada, offers a good example (Roos and Shapiro 1995a; Roos et al. 1995; Currie 2002). POPULIS interconnects various data sets, tying factors affecting a population's need for health care to its use of health care services, to the supply of health care resources within defined geographical areas, and to the health status of the population.

At POPULIS's core is a population registry (e.g., births, deaths, geographical mobility) for defined geographical areas. Linked to this core are data sets containing indicators of socioeconomic status (derived from census-tract-level information on household income, employment, education, and cultural diversity), indicators of health (e.g., all-cause and cause-specific mortality rates, various indicators derived from hospital discharge abstracts and physicians' claims), and utilization of health care (e.g., payments to hospitals, nursing homes, physicians) (Roos et al. 1995). POPULIS also includes data on immunizations, prescription drugs, and home health care and other community-based services (Black, Roos, and Roos 1999). Researchers have used POPULIS to investigate "premature" mortality (Cohen and MacWilliam 1995), the association of socioeconomic factors with health status and service use (Mustard and Frolich 1995), and the effect of hospital bed closures (Roos and Shapiro 1995b). POPULIS is evolving into "a true system of population health information, of which health care services are only a part" (Evans and Mustard 1995, DS5).

Several other developed nations are building data systems similar to POPULIS (Zelmer, Virani, and Alvarez 1999). Examples of current trends include the following:

- Collection of data beyond acute, short-term hospitalizations and physicians' services (e.g., Australia, Canada, and New Zealand have started gathering mental health and home care information).
- Increased linkage and sharing of data definitions across information systems. For example, Australia is exploring linking person-level census data with health care data. In Canada, respondents to the National Population Health Survey are asked for consent to link their responses with data from administrative data sets, and most agree. Denmark uses

civil registration numbers to link information on various health care services for individuals.
- Efforts to protect individual confidentiality and privacy in linked data sets using consistent strategies across countries.
- Making health information more accessible, including reports on overall health and health system performance and international comparisons. Six of 18 European countries track progress against health targets, and another 8 are expanding their systems to permit such tracking. Many countries are developing user-friendly, web-based systems to share health statistics.

In Great Britain, the National Health Service has committed by 2005 to create lifelong electronic health records; offer 24-hour online access to patient records and information about best clinical practices; share information across delivery sites, including community-based services; and provide information for planners and managers (National Health Service Information Authority 1998). The National Health Service views administrative data as flowing from information required for clinical practice rather than being produced primarily for administrative purposes.

Future Issues

When we completed the manuscript for the second edition of this book in December 1996, the Internet remained a distant vision. E-mail was novel but clunky and often unreliable. At the close of that administrative data chapter, my speculation about the future failed to envision today's web-based transfers of massive quantities of health information. Today, my conjectures about the future begin by assuming that information technology shall make quantum leaps over the next years. Importantly, patients shall become involved, just as customers now go online for banking and other financial transactions. Clinical information will link increasingly with administrative information, as is happening today in the VA (see Chapter 8). Therefore, my comments here focus instead on factors that move more slowly (e.g., implementation of new code sets) or will require important political or policy decisions.

Privacy

Merging databases and constructing person-level files highlights concerns about individual privacy, an issue that could significantly affect creation and use of administrative databases in the future. In its report *Record Linkage and Privacy*, the GAO (2001, 70) found that "reidentification risks may be higher for data sets with person-by-person linkages than for their component parts," largely because of the greater depth of information on individuals. They describe strategies for protecting the privacy and security of linked data files, but some observers raise privacy concerns about even stand-alone administrative databases (U.S. GAO 1999a).

HIPAA required the administration to establish health information privacy regulations if Congress did not. Therefore, as President Clinton left office, his DHHS promulgated privacy rules, which the incoming Bush administration put on hold. On 9 August 2002, the Bush administration announced its final health data privacy rules (Pear 2002, A1):

> The administration decided to abandon the core of the Clinton rules, a requirement that doctors, hospitals and other health care providers obtain written consent from patients before using or disclosing personal medical information for treatment or paying claims. Instead, providers will have to notify patients of their remaining rights and have to make "a good-faith effort to obtain a written acknowledgment of receipt of the notice."

The new rules place important federal limits on outsiders' access to personal health information, making unauthorized disclosure for marketing or other nonroutine uses subject to civil and criminal penalties. The new regulations took effect 14 April 2003.

Patient privacy advocates decried the Bush administration's new policies, especially the abolishment of the informed consent requirements, and some Democrats vowed to pass legislation reinstating consent provisions (Pear 2002). Nevertheless, requiring individual informed consent before releasing administrative health information would largely stop research using these data. Unlike clinical trials, where informed consent theoretically protects the safety and rights of research subjects, studies using administrative databases have generally been absolved from requiring consent. This exemption recognizes that obtaining consent is burdensome and infeasible given the size and composition of administrative databases; requiring consent would yield biased subsamples of participants (Gostin and Hadley 1998).

Organizations may release private health information in administrative databases without individuals' permission, but only if recipients obtain a waiver from their institutional review board or privacy board (Gostin 2001, 3018–19).

> The waiver criteria include findings that (1) the use or disclosure involves no more than minimal risk; (2) the research could not practicably be conducted without the waiver; (3) the privacy risks are reasonable in relation to the anticipated benefits, if any, to individuals and the importance of the research; (4) a plan to destroy the identifiers exists unless there is a health or research justification for retaining them; and (5) there are written assurances that the data will not be reused or disclosed to others, except for research oversight or additional research that would qualify for a waiver.

Organizations like CMS, which releases administrative data for so-called "public use," routinely remove personal identifiers and require researchers to satisfy privacy and security standards. These public use files therefore meet the waiver criterion of posing minimal if any risk of breaching privacy.

The merging of detailed clinical data (e.g., laboratory, radiology, and other diagnostic test results) with administrative claims files will increase in coming years. Access to detailed clinical information overcomes many reservations about the limited clinical content of administrative data and would facilitate quality measurement, practice profiling, and health system monitoring. Research on large populations could potentially account for clinical factors that only painstaking chart reviews allow today. Yet, as with other merged data sets, the potential for identifying individuals will increase with more detailed clinical data. Fortunately, methods exist to address most privacy concerns, but these strategies must be applied systematically throughout the health care system, from the ground up (U.S. GAO 2001).

Setting Standards for Data Content and Electronic Transmission

Subtitle F, Sec. 261 of HIPAA touts standards as the means for administrative simplification:

> It is the purpose of this subtitle to improve the Medicare program under title XVIII of the Social Security Act, the Medicaid program under title XIX of such Act, and the efficiency and effectiveness of the health care system, by encouraging the development of a health information system through the establishment of standards and requirements for the electronic transmission of certain health information.

To share data electronically, it must be technically produced and transmitted in a standard fashion. For example, such standards throughout the banking industry now allow travelers to obtain cash from automatic teller machines worldwide. In health care, messaging standards will permit data exchanges across entire health systems, drawing from such sources as billing systems, bedside computers, physiologic monitors, and clinical laboratories. Committees representing various stakeholders (e.g., technology vendors, government, medical representatives, labor unions) are actively developing consensus standards for health care in the United States and internationally. Standards committees receive accreditation from organizations like ASTM International (formerly the American Society for Testing and Materials; http://www.astm.org) and the American National Standards Institute (ANSI; http://www.ansi.org). ANSI alone has more than 1,000 corporate, governmental, institutional, and international members. Committees seeking consensus typically meet over several years, obtaining external review and comment on draft standards before submitting them to a vote.

The resultant standards, represented by a baffling assortment of acronyms, are often interrelated. For example, the ANSI X12 standard directs communication of financial data to insurers and other outside health care organizations. HL7 standards, written by the Health Level Seven committee, govern sharing of clinical data. E1467 standards, developed by the ASTM E31.16 subcommittee, guide exchange of neurophysiological data from physiological monitors; these messages use identical syntax and most of the same segments as HL7 messages, but they incorporate data structures for continuous waveforms, such as electroencephalogram tracings. Various transaction standards typically are numbered (e.g., 837, health claims and equivalent encounter information; 834, health plan enrollment; 835, health care payment and remittance advice; 275, health claims attachment).

HIPAA requires all entities within the U.S. health care system to comply with standards stipulated by the DHHS.[18] Transaction standards for billing and related administrative functions must be adopted by 16 October 2003 by all payers and by all providers who bill electronically. The government has taken these standards from the ANSI Accredited Standards Committee X12N. So, for example, the 837 and 834 transaction standards will replace current formats, which are often idiosyncratic for each payer or health plan. HIPAA also mandates uniform code sets: ICD-9-CM, CPT, and HCPCS will become standard for coding diagnoses and procedures. These standardization efforts should not only improve efficiency throughout the U.S. health care system but also should make the resulting administrative databases more useful to researchers.

ICD-10 and Other New Code Sets

Starting in the 1980s, the WHO pursued its mandated responsibility to revise periodically the ICD nomenclature (Weigel and Lewis 1991). WHO and its various advisory bodies reviewed proposals for revisions from around the world from 1984 through 1987 and then drafted ICD-10. Delegates from 43 countries gathered in Geneva in 1989 to review the draft ICD-10, and the World Health Assembly approved the final version in May 1990. ICD-10 looks quite different from ICD-9, with its alphanumeric ordering scheme and new chapter titles; V and E codes, formerly supplementary listings, are now integrated into the main classification (WHO 2002). Volume I, the Tabular List, contains the classification at the three- and four-character level and runs to more than 1,000 pages. To underscore the statistical purpose of the nomenclature and its expanded scope, ICD-10's official title is the *International Statistical Classification of Diseases and Related Health Problems.* Numerous nations implemented ICD-10 for mortality reporting starting in 1994, and many countries (e.g., Australia, Brazil, Canada, England, France, Japan, Kuwait, Scotland, Thailand) now use ICD-10 to code both mortality and morbidity.

International treaty required the United States to report mortality statistics using ICD-10 by 1999. However, ICD-9 and ICD-10 differ. Whereas ICD-9 contained about 5,000 categories, ICD-10 has roughly 8,000. Chapters have been added and rearranged. "The shifting of deaths away from some cause-of-death categories and into others resulting from these changes creates discontinuities in cause-of-death trends from 1998, the last year of ICD-9, and 1999, the first year of ICD-10" (Anderson et al. 2001, 5). Whenever it implements a new ICD, NCHS therefore examines the effect of the new classification system on longitudinal trends of death rates by diseases.[19] Using more than 1.8 million death certificates from 1996 for all 50 states and the District of Columbia, analysts recoded cause of death using ICD-10. Preliminary results suggested that the change from ICD-9 to ICD-10 will result in discontinuities in cause-of-death reporting for certain conditions, including septicemia, influenza and pneumonia, Alzheimer's disease, and nephritis, nephrotic syndrome, and nephrosis.

In September 1994, NCHS and its consultants began reviewing ICD-10 to determine whether a clinical modification was necessary for morbidity reporting in the United States, as had been done with ICD-9-CM (see above). Although the review found that ICD-10 represented a substantial improvement over ICD-9, it nonetheless advised a clinical modification for American use. NCHS worked closely with a technical advisory panel, physician groups, clinical coders, and others to develop ICD-10-CM. They added many new codes to capture information about ambulatory encounters, injuries, and combinations of diagnoses and symptoms. A sixth digit was added to common four- and five-digit subclassifications. NCHS posted the draft ICD-10-CM on its web site for public comment from December 1997 to February 1998; a new draft ICD-10-CM was completed in May 2002. The NCHS web site contains information about this process and examples from ICD-10-CM.

Although ICD-9-CM contained procedure codes, ICD-10-CM does not. Instead, in 1995 HCFA (now CMS) hired 3M Health Information Systems (which updates the DRGs) to create an entirely new procedure nomenclature, ICD-10-PCS (Averill et al. 1998). This classification differs substantially from the procedure categories offered by ICD-9-CM, CPT, and HCPCS (see CMS web site, http://cms.hhs.gov/providers/pufdownload/icd10.asp). ICD-10-PCS codes are alphanumeric with seven characters. The second through seventh characters represent body system, root operation, body part, approach, device, and qualifier (the first digit is assigned 0).

No date has yet been set for the United States to implement ICD-10-CM for morbidity reporting or ICD-10-PCS for hospital procedure reporting. Once the final notice to implement them is published in the *Federal Register*, a two-year time window will be allowed for the switch. The mechanics of a full-scale transition from ICD-9-CM to ICD-10-CM will be costly and logistically complicated, requiring reprogramming of computers and retraining of thousands of coders from private doctors' offices to health clinics to hospitals. CMS will need to ensure that this shift will not significantly increase DRG-based hospital payment simply as a coding artifact. Although ICD-10-CM is superior to ICD-9-CM, by the time the United States implements it, the WHO may have moved on to ICD-11.

Notes

1. The HCUP database also contains information about ambulatory surgeries, and the Kids' Inpatient Database (KID) includes hospitalizations of persons 18 years of age and younger. Statewide hospitalization data are the one administrative source of information about uninsured persons; all admissions are captured, regardless of payer source. Questions and comments about the HCUP database can be e-mailed to hcup@ahrq.gov.

2. Some databases may assign the mother's identification number to her newborn infant; disentangling health care claims attributable to the mother and infant can become complicated.

3. In the *Federal Register* of 31 May 2002 (Vol. 67, No. 105, pp. 38044–51), the DHHS proposed that NDCs no longer be required on pharmacy-related transactions. For some health care providers (e.g., hospitals), using NDCs would have introduced complications for electronic transmission of claims.

4. The CMS Internet web site contains a listing called "CMS Files for Purchase Directory" (http://cms.hhs.gov/data/purchase/directory.asp, accessed 17 July 2002). According to this site, persons may purchase certain files if they qualify "under the terms of the Routine Use Act as outlined in the December 24, 1984, *Federal Register* and amended by the July 2, 1985, Notice."

5. The following example demonstrates the distinction between principal and primary diagnoses. Suppose a man is admitted routinely for a transurethral prostatectomy (TURP) to treat benign prostatic hypertrophy (BPH). On the day following an uncomplicated TURP, he falls and fractures his hip. He is stabilized and undergoes an open reduction and internal fixation (ORIF) to repair the fracture; postoperatively, he begins rehabilitation. Under UHDDS guidelines, BPH is the principal diagnosis because the patient entered the hospital for BPH treatment. The TURP surgery involved only one or two days, whereas the ORIF required an additional week in hospital. Thus, hip fracture is the primary diagnosis.

6. Changes to UHDDS proposed in June 1992 suggested that additional spaces be provided specifically for E codes, as well as allow the ability to designate whether an injury or poisoning was the cause of the hospitalization (the principal diagnosis).

7. We created the CSP, a computerized method using standard discharge abstracts, to screen for in-hospital complications and areas where care could be improved. The CSP identifies potential complications of adult medical and surgical hospitalizations using patients' age, sex, ICD-9-CM diagnosis and procedure codes, and number of days from admission to principal major surgeries or procedures. The structure of each of 28 CSP screens is similar. ICD-9-CM diagnosis or procedure codes called

"trigger codes" indicate that individual cases may have had a particular problem (e.g., postoperative pneumonia). The computer algorithm then looks for whether specified qualifying conditions are met. For example, pneumonia, other infectious diseases, pulmonary malignancy, or immunocompromise must not be the principal diagnosis, and the principal surgery must have occurred on the day of admission or the second hospital day. These qualifying statements aim to be brief and eliminate cases where the complication was caused by underlying disease, not substandard quality. If all qualifying conditions are met, the CSP flags cases as potential complications.

8. We were surprised to find many cases without any explicit clinical criteria or physician notes supporting the ICD-9-CM codes. One potential explanation is the "rule-out rule," described later in Chapter 5: We instructed nurse reviewers only to record confirmed clinical criteria and physician diagnoses, rather than potential, probable, or rule-out diagnoses.

9. AMI was especially susceptible to the rule-out rule and other coding guidelines, notably the statement that AMI could be coded up to eight weeks following the acute event. These coding instructions produced unintended consequences, as we found when studying patients admitted in 1984–85 to 15 hospitals in greater Boston (Iezzoni et al. 1988). Of 1,003 cases, 260 did not meet the clinical criteria for AMI. At tertiary teaching hospitals, 41.7 percent of cases failed to qualify, compared with 9.1 percent at nonteaching institutions. In a large fraction of cases, although an AMI was explicitly ruled out, the code was nonetheless assigned. An additional 66 teaching hospital cases did not qualify because the patient was admitted only for coronary angiography after an uneventful, post–myocardial infarction course, with almost one-third of these infarctions occurring five to eight weeks previously. On 1 October 1989, coding guidelines added a fifth digit indicating whether the diagnosis involved initial or subsequent treatment of the AMI.

10. Coding accuracy varied by condition, with the following diagnoses coded with the indicated accuracy: hypertrophy of tonsils and adenoids, 97.0 percent; cataract, 94.3 percent; hernia without obstruction, 89.1 percent; hernia with obstruction, 81.0 percent; low back pain, 56.3 percent; and chronic ischemic heart disease, 30.2 percent (Institute of Medicine 1977a). For most diagnoses with low accuracy rates, the chief cause of discrepancy involved erroneous sequencing—listing as principal diagnoses a condition that was actually secondary.

11. Investigators at RAND tried to "decompose" CMI increases into "true" changes and coding changes, using data from the organization that assesses the performance of peer review organizations (PROs, recently renamed QIOs), the SuperPRO (Carter, Newhouse, and Relles 1990, 1991). In the mid-1980s, each of approximately 50 PROs across the

country had been required to validate ICD-9-CM diagnosis coding for Medicare inpatients. SuperPRO medical record technicians, assisted by physicians, reabstracted a random sample of cases reviewed by each PRO. The RAND studies compared the ICD-9-CM codes assigned by the SuperPRO and the hospitals to determine the extent of DRG creep.

12. Major changes in the DRG algorithm itself contributed to some new coding approaches. The 1988 DRG grouper eliminated splits of DRGs based on age above and below 69 years. From that version forward, DRG pairs were split by the presence of complications or comorbidities only, not age (with the exception of DRGs pertaining expressly to pediatric populations and a handful split for other reasons, such as patient death). The 1988 DRG grouper also introduced special DRGs for patients receiving ventilator support. Not surprisingly, a considerable portion of the CMI changes between 1987 and 1988 were traceable to increased listing of secondary diagnoses representing complications or comorbidities and ventilator support codes (Carter, Newhouse, and Relles 1991).

13. The Office of Audit Services, OIG, U.S. DHHS continuously audits various public and private health care organizations paid by Medicare and Medicaid. Listings of the audit reports are posted at http://oig.hhs.gov/oas/oas/cms.html (accessed 29 July 2002).

14. Coding quality was "very good" for CHF, chronic renal disease, prior coronary bypass surgery, history of pacemaker, complete atrioventricular block, and shock; it was "intermediate" for epilepsy, other cerebrovascular disease, primary or secondary malignancy, and hypertension. This study of AMI patients admitted in 1990–91 also found that 7.6 percent failed clinical criteria for AMI and 23.7 percent had a "possible" AMI (most of the possible cases had either chest pain with borderline cardiac enzymes or positive enzymes without chest pain) (Wilson, Smoley, and Werdegar 1996, 14–23).

15. One hypothesis conjectured that the apparent "protective" effect of essential hypertension resulted from patients taking medications, such as beta-blockers, that improve survival among patients following AMI. Another hypothesis suggested that hypertensive patients have higher blood pressure than others even when experiencing an AMI and that these higher pressures produce better survival outcomes (Blumberg and Binns 1989). A further hypothesis held that the protective effect of coronary atherosclerosis in AMI results from increased formation of collateral vessels in patients with this chronic condition (Epstein, Quyymi, and Bonow 1989). Another hypothesis suggested that patients with chronic conditions (e.g., diabetes mellitus, hypertension) have more regular contacts with doctors and thus have their acute illnesses identified at earlier stages or lower severity.

16. Romano and Mark (1994) analyzed data from the California reabstraction study described previously. When only the first five codes were examined, persons who died had missing comorbidities significantly more often than those who lived (27 percent versus 12 percent; $p < 0.001$). However, when all 25 diagnoses were considered, decedents and survivors had equal rates of missing comorbidities.

17. Using the 1994 California data, our methods and case identification were identical (persons 65 years of age and older in four diseases; we used the fifth digit of the ICD-9-CM codes to select patients undergoing initial AMI treatment). This time, however, we used multivariable logistic regression to adjust for age and sex in calculating the odds of in-hospital death given the presence of specified secondary diagnoses.

18. In the past, even established data transmission standards left room for considerable diversity. For example, to encourage electronic claims transmission, in 1992 HCFA offered direct electronic payment for providers submitting at least 90 percent of their claims this way. However, each state added its own data elements to the electronic form. Some payers and software vendors therefore needed to support almost 50 versions of UB-92.

19. Using cause of death coded by ICD-9 and ICD-10 for the same sample of death certificates, NCHS analysts calculate comparability ratios (C) for cause of death i as follows:

$$C_i = (D_{ICD\text{-}10})/(D_{ICD\text{-}9})$$

where $D_{ICD\text{-}10}$ is the number of deaths due to cause i classified by ICD-10, and $D_{ICD\text{-}9}$ is the number of deaths due to cause i classified by ICD-9 (Anderson et al. 2001, 5).

CLINICAL DATA FROM MEDICAL RECORDS OR PROVIDERS

Lisa I. Iezzoni

When my hospital recently purchased a large piece of x-ray equipment, deciding where to put it was surprisingly easy. Because all radiographic images have been digital and stored electronically for several years, the old record room was empty; its shelves, formerly crammed with oversize envelopes of shadowy gray-black films, were bare. The sophisticated new machinery went there, into the old record room.

Hospitals and other practice settings nationwide are emptying their record rooms, one of many tangible manifestations of the new clinical information technologies insinuating throughout the health care delivery system. With electronic information should, theoretically, come efficiencies and improved patient care, as well as opportunities for clinically detailed, logistically feasible risk adjustment with potentially greater validity for detecting quality shortfalls and determining treatment effectiveness. As described in Chapter 8, the transition to exclusively electronic information is well underway at VHA hospitals, greatly facilitating risk adjustment of postoperative outcome measures. Some health care settings, notably ICUs, routinely obtain and record volumes of clinical information electronically from various monitoring and other devices during routine patient care.

Elsewhere, however, prior estimates of when the electronic information revolution would arrive in health care have proven overly optimistic. High costs have posed a huge barrier, as has changing the culture and mindset within clinical practice settings. Furthermore, although the mode of delivery is new, the content of electronic medical records remains remarkably similar to the handwritten tomes from decades ago. Therefore, risk adjustment using clinical information still often proceeds the old-fashioned way, relying on painstaking manual reviews of paper records, often documented with scrawled, illegible script and frequently missing data about critical risk factors.

Despite these difficulties, as described in this chapter, medical records and other clinical sources indisputably offer richer information about patients and their care than do administrative databases. Especially in teaching hospitals, records from a single admission can consume hundreds of pages and multiple volumes, with notations from dozens of clinicians and reports from numerous tests and procedures. Today's medical records nevertheless remain "second hand" in the sense that clinicians filter all observations (i.e., clinicians ask the questions and record the answers). Medical records thus reflect the realities of human discourse—forces involving both patients and clinicians—such as faulty memories, communication failures, subjective judgments, and conscious and unconscious distortions. Medical records do not always yield a straightforward, complete, and objective accounting of patients' risks, especially their preferences for care (see Chapter 3). This may change in years ahead, as patients begin annotating their own medical records.

History of Medical Records

Until recently, information about individual patients was not aggregated in one place. In the early nineteenth century, American hospitals kept records in bound volumes organized chronologically by admissions, not by patients. In conducting rounds, physicians walked from bed to bed, writing brief assessments of patients consecutively by order of encounter. Notations emphasized descriptions of patients and their symptoms, with scant information on physical findings, diagnoses, or treatment. A typical note is the following from Massachusetts General Hospital on 18 August 1824: "Skin nearly natural, tongue rather dry, with moist red edges. Countenance good. Took hasty pudding at 10 a.m." Other notes contained lengthier descriptions of patients' symptoms and physical findings, yet without diagnoses. This note, about a woman of unspecified age, also was written at Massachusetts General Hospital on 18 August 1824:

> Sense of fullness and oppression in the Chest. Dyspnea increased by exercise and by recumbent position. Sense of tightness across thorax. Pains in left side, not constant, but often darting to the epigastric region and to left shoulder. Inability of lying on left side, which brought on great distress and sense of suffocation. Tongue has thin pale coat. . . . Skin now cool and moist, says she has sweat much at times. Thinks she has not lost much flesh, being much swelled.

The colorful description of symptoms is revealing and suggests CHF with episodes of angina pectoris.

Even in the late nineteenth century, medical record notes remained primarily descriptive. The Mayo brothers in Rochester, Minnesota, generally did not record physical examinations, diagnoses, or treatments. Most of their medical records contained only the date, the patient's age and residence, and descriptions of symptoms, such as "gas on the stomach and poor sleep" and "night terrors—wetting bed" (Clapesattle 1941, 385). The so-called "unit" medical record, which accumulates all information on individual patients within a single record, was not fully implemented until 1916, at Presbyterian Hospital in New York City (Kurtz 1943).

Concerns about the quality of medical records soon arose. Throughout the early 1900s, the American College of Surgeons extensively discussed shoddy medical record keeping, and in 1917, its Conference on Hospital Standardization proclaimed, "If good records are kept, it is almost certain that good work will be done" (Hornsby 1917, 7). The conference asserted that 75 percent of hospitals kept "valueless" medical records because of missing information on histories, physical examinations, and diagnoses. Furthermore, the conference called the paucity of diagnostic information "premeditated" and "intended to cover up and hide carelessness or incapacity on the part of the surgeon to diagnose the disease" (Hornsby 1917, 7).

Ernest Amory Codman (1917), a founder of the College (see Chapter 1), envisioned a heretical new use for medical records: "Our record system should enable us to fix responsibility . . . for the success or failure of each case treated," noting the need for "clear, honest records, no matter how brief, if they fearlessly face the facts." One proposal stipulated that progress notes be written at least once every three days (Ramsey and Kingswood 1923). Raymond Pearl, the statistician to The Johns Hopkins Hospital, advocated standardized printed forms, bemoaning the diverse medical record formats used by physicians. As Pearl (1921, 187) observed, "The general scheme or outline which a history is to follow resides, far too often, in the head of the history writer, and there only. And heads, especially of human beings, do vary so!" In 1918, the American College of Surgeons (1918, 2) adopted Codman's vision for medical records:

> Consistent and fearless review of case records by the hospital staff, as here suggested, is a just and effective means to deal with incompetent medical and surgical work in a hospital. Facts are not debatable. . . .
> If the facts establish evidence that a physician or surgeon is unsafe in judgment, unworthy in character, untrained, lax, lazy, or careless, in all honor and decency that individual should either overcome his deficiencies or withdraw from practice. . . . A wise use of honest case records points the way to great advance in the medical profession.

Despite these exhortations, the medical record did not change significantly for more than four decades. The self-proclaimed independence of physicians, who railed against any hint of standardization or uniformity, underlay this inertia. Changes in charting came only in the 1960s with new clinical practices and burgeoning medical knowledge, which threatened to overwhelm physicians and their record keeping. In the visionary view of Lawrence Weed (1968, 593), it would "be necessary to develop a more organized approach to the medical record, a more rational acceptance and use of paramedical personnel and a more positive attitude about the computer in medicine." He proposed organizing documentation around a "problem list," a dynamic inventory of major clinical issues requiring attention. Weed (1971) developed the "SOAP" approach for documenting clinical problem lists, organizing information under the following four major headings:

- *Subjective*: symptoms and subjective feelings reported by patients, capturing patients' views about their health status and health care
- *Objective*: clinical findings, such as physical examination, laboratory test, and diagnostic procedure results
- *Assessment*: physicians' conclusions about the status of the problem based on the subjective and objective evidence
- *Plan*: diagnostic, therapeutic, monitoring, and other activities to address the problem

Weed's problem-oriented medical record and SOAP approach were widely adopted and taught to generations of medical students.

Despite the explosion of information technology, the structure and content of written medical records has changed little in the ensuing decades. Weed's early pleas for computerization were largely ignored for many years, except perhaps in laboratories (e.g., reporting blood test results, albeit on paper printouts). Some patients' medical records still spill into multiple volumes, containing hundreds of poorly fastened pages.

Several years after Weed's proposal, Lyons and Payne (1974, 714) reported "questions about how validly medical record information reflects the actual medical practice of the physician rather than only his record-keeping performance." They underscored the central role of medical records in communication among clinicians caring for patients, quoting Avedis Donabedian as saying that "the conditions that bring about good care are also responsible for bringing about good recording" (Lyons and Payne 1974, 714). A contrary view held that "classic casebook recording may be a defense for inferior practice and . . . the very best clinician may not use up the ink in one ballpoint pen in his entire career" (Lyons and Payne 1974, 715). Their research results, however, favored Donabedian's presumption: Better documentation and better quality were generally significantly correlated. Even the dramatic changes in medical practice over the last 30 years have probably not altered this fundamental relationship.

Reliability of Clinical Information

Risk adjustment is only as good as its underlying data. As described in Chapter 5, many structural factors raise concerns about the quality of administrative data, such as limitations of the coding scheme and financial incentives. The quality of clinical data, however, also prompts questions. For example, within several years of publication of New York state's CABG mortality reports, critics charged that some cardiothoracic surgeons exaggerated their patients' risks, such as the extent of lung and heart disease (see below). In clinical settings, the subjectivity of many medical findings hampers efforts to detect outright efforts at gaming and manipulation.

In the new millennium, debate persists about the boundaries between medical art and science. Interobserver variation in critical clinical findings can significantly and negatively affect patient care (Elmore and Feinstein 1992, 567).

> For the many phenomena in clinical medicine that are not easily measured and that lack a convenient or definitive "gold standard," the consequences of observer variability may be dramatic. A radiologist's interpretation of a mass lesion may lead to an expensive and invasive diagnostic work-up; a pathologist's reading of a tissue slide may determine whether a woman keeps her breast or loses it; a research technician's decision about primary clinical data may affect the final results of a research project.

The medical literature amply documents physicians disagreeing among themselves about the presence of a physical finding and the interpretation of common tests (e.g., chest radiographs, mammograms, ECGs) and sophisticated studies (e.g., endoscopy, angiography, radionuclide imaging). Research has also found tremendous intraphysician variability—physicians disagreeing with themselves on rereview of a physical examination or a test (Eddy 1984; Elmore and Feinstein 1992). Recently, physicians have mobilized to understand better the implications of and solutions for unreliable or questionable physical examination findings. The Society for General Internal Medicine sponsors a Clinical Examination Research Interest Group devoted to this concern. For the last several years, the *Journal of the American Medical Association* has published a feature called "The Rational Clinical Exam," where authors evaluate the quality of the evidence documenting various clinical conditions.[1] Based on extensive literature reviews, authors examine the precision of pertinent clinical findings, defining precision as the degree of interobserver and intraobserver variation, and the accuracy of diagnoses based on various findings and tests. In one such article entitled "Is this Patient Having a Myocardial Infarction?" Panju and colleagues (1998) found high precision of physical examinations for dyspnea and displaced cardiac apex beat but low precision for pulmonary rales and hepatomegaly. Precision of ECG interpretation may depend on physicians' level of experience. One study among residents found 70 percent disagreement about whether ECGs demonstrated an AMI; a study among cardiologists found 10 percent to 23 percent disagreement.

A group of Canadian investigators launched a nonprofit international collaborative of medical researchers to conduct studies on the Clinical Assessment of the Reliability of the Examination (CARE). As they note with asperity, "the all-too-common study of the accuracy and precision of the clinical examination comprises 4 experts examining 40 patients, the latter selected to confirm the biases and reputations of the former" (CARE 2002). The CARE team endeavors to enroll practicing clinicians from around the world to examine the accuracy and precision of specific elements of the history and physical examination.[2] One criterion for participation is a "well-developed sense of humour." CARE has published studies on chronic obstructive airways disease, and projects are underway concerning other conditions.

Questions about interrater reliability and the relative value of different clinical findings should therefore guide identification of candidate risk factors. Especially in observational studies, analysts generally cannot confirm independently whether clinical risk factor information is accurate or reliable. Even if analysts could rereview or reinterpret critical tests or findings (e.g., radiographs, ECGs), this could prove challenging. Without explicit review criteria, researchers are themselves susceptible to bias or interobserver variation. When possible, analysts conducting rereviews should be blinded to patients' outcomes or other critical factors that might bias their interpretations. This strategy pertains only to those clinical findings where "hard" data exist that can be retrieved and reviewed retrospectively (e.g., radiographic images, pathology tissue slides, ECG tracings). Rereviews are typically infeasible for risk factors where findings are ephemeral, are transitory, or require patients to be available for reexamination (e.g., physical findings).

The CSI relies heavily on detailed clinical information. Roughly half of the CSI's clinical factors represent numerical values, like vital signs or laboratory findings, whereas others are largely descriptive and qualitative (Iezzoni and Daley 1992). Many factors represent findings that are often measured unreliably, such as jugular venous distention, Kussmaul respiration, rales, and pulsus paradoxus. Other items require patients' reports and thus depend on recall or patient thresholds for pain and complaint, acuity of self-observation, and willingness to reveal personal facts. Examples include nausea, anorexia, numbness, tingling, and severe headache. Most differences in patients' reports of these factors probably vary randomly across providers. Nevertheless, systematic differences could occur across patient populations in the detail and nature of such self-reports relating to language, culture, education, and socioeconomic status.

The CSI's situation illustrates the dilemma surrounding use of potentially unreliable clinical findings for risk adjustment. First, regardless of whether such findings are unreliable, they are what clinicians use to make therapeutic and prognostic judgments about patients. Therefore, disregarding these types of findings in judging risk is problematic, especially if the purpose of the risk-adjusted information is to motivate clinicians' behaviors. Second, when using such findings, analysts must remember their inherent subjectivity. Given these two considerations, the major question becomes whether a potential for bias exists: Could any systematic factors bias assessments of these clinical findings by affecting the subjective interpretations of clinicians? The answer to this question depends on the purpose: For example, the public reporting of risk-adjusted death rates might motivate cardiothoracic surgeons in New York state—at least theoretically—to modulate reporting of risk factors requiring subjective interpretation.[3]

Quality of Medical Records and Other Risk Factor Documentation

According to Bradbury (1990, 25),

> The clarity and logic of medical recording is a direct reflection of the clarity and logic (or lack thereof) of the medical practitioner's thoughts. An ambiguous, illegible chart with a confusion of orders and counter-orders, incomplete physical examinations, and absence of clear impressions or plans most likely reflects the same confusion in that patient's physician.

As noted earlier, the completeness, accuracy, and validity of medical records have raised questions for decades. Physicians' indecipherable handwriting, a long-standing joke, has serious consequences. Photocopied records, for abstraction outside hospitals or physicians' offices, are even less legible than the originals. In studying the reliability of various severity measures, Thomas and Ashcraft (1989, 487) could not abstract 40 percent of their 431 charts using MedisGroups, which requires detailed information from physicians' notes. Photocopying made key elements in the clinical record unreadable.

Although computerized medical records solve critical problems of legibility, questions about the content and organization of clinical information remain. Errors or incomplete documentation impede identification of risk factors. Measuring the magnitude of this problem is complicated. A flawless investigation requires an omniscient observer continually monitoring clinicians who are unaware of being observed, with the observer simultaneously performing independent and objective evaluations of patients. Clearly, this is impossible.

Not surprisingly, therefore, relatively little has been published on the completeness and accuracy of medical records. This limited literature suggests that medical records suffice for certain purposes but that records often fail to completely or accurately represent certain risk factors and the care patients receive (Romm and Putnam 1981; Zuckerman et al. 1975). Data from outpatient settings are missing more often than is inpatient information (Feigl et al. 1988).[4] A comparison of medical records with patients' reports found that 83 percent of cases demonstrated at least one error in medication documentation (Beers, Munekata, and Storrie 1990).[5]

One study observed hundreds of patient visits to a primary care pediatric clinic, evaluating whether the doctors (interns and residents) chose a free-text medical record versus a structured encounter form (Duggan, Starfield, and DeAngelis 1990). When physicians used the structured form, they recorded significantly more information (overall care, history, physical examination, developmental assessment, guidance, and follow-up) than with free-text records. However, these physicians also documented a more comprehensive physical examination than was actually observed. Therefore, at least for examinations, "use of the structured form exerted a greater impact on recording than on performance" (Duggan, Starfield, and DeAngelis 1990, 111).

...tial Biases in Quality of Medical Records

...factors could bias the extent of medical record documentation. In our ...udy to validate the CSP (see Chapter 5), we designed abstraction instruments for trained nurse researchers to search medical records for explicit indicators of quality of care. They reviewed more than 1,000 records of elderly Medicare beneficiaries, failing to validate the CSP as a quality measure (Iezzoni et al. 1999). However, patterns of findings led us to speculate about potential biases in medical record documentation: When complications do arise, clinicians may more carefully document all activities and findings in the medical record than in the absence of complications. Therefore, even routine monitoring would be documented more thoroughly in the charts of patients with complications than for those without.

Completeness of documentation may vary by hospital type, especially between teaching and nonteaching hospitals. We found that physicians' notes at nonteaching hospitals generally focused exclusively on the acute presenting illness (Iezzoni et al. 1989, 1990). We hypothesized that nonteaching hospital physicians did not document chronic coexisting diseases because these physicians generally were the patients' primary providers, with detailed knowledge of their histories from prior encounters. Furthermore, these physicians generally supervised all inpatient decisions, making it unnecessary for them to inform other physicians about the patient's history through extensive notations.

In contrast, at teaching hospitals, physicians' notes contained copious information on both acute and chronic conditions. These documentation differences likely reflected differences in roles between teaching and nonteaching physicians. At teaching hospitals, interns or residents unfamiliar with the patient generally wrote the admission note, which therefore contained information extracted during a comprehensive review of the patients' clinical situations. Furthermore, as interns and residents extensively cross-cover each other during weekends and evenings, the medical record serves as the vehicle for transmitting critical information to covering physicians.

Records at both teaching and nonteaching hospitals contained scant information on functional status and social history. Most functional and social information, when it was recorded, appeared in nurses' notes. We had initially intended to create a measure of patients' living situations (e.g., whether they lived alone or with others) but could not do so because of missing documentation. Other investigators confirm the absence of social history information in medical records (McDiarmid, Bonanni, and Finocchiaro 1991; Mansfield 1986). A recent study of inpatient records found inadequate documentation of elderly patients' functional deficits not only in physicians' notes but also in medical record entries by nurses and physical and occupational therapists (Bogardus et al. 2001; see Chapter 15).

At teaching hospitals, trainees often write copious individual notes. Furthermore, multiple levels of trainees document records (from interns to subspecialty fellows), as do various attending physicians (e.g., patients' primary physicians, specialist consultants), nurses, therapists, pharmacists, social workers, and others. This frequently produces inconsistencies in information about specific risk factors. Data collection guidelines can therefore affect risk factor information. MedisGroups, for instance, required that reviewers abstract most information from physician notes, except for vital signs. While this strategy speeds chart reviews, it could affect comparisons across hospitals with different levels of physician coverage. Patients at tertiary teaching hospitals, with round-the-clock teams of physicians, could have multiple physician notes, whereas identical patients at a small community hospital could receive only one daily physician note. Documentation differences are particularly relevant to clinical findings that wax and wane, such as wheezing, pericardial friction rubs, or S3 gallop heart sounds.

The downside of having multiple physician notes is dealing with frequent discrepancies. We encountered this situation when we hired research nurses to review medical records using MedisGroups (Iezzoni et al. 1992b). The medical records came from complicated patients at tertiary teaching hospitals. The sheer volume of many medical records, especially at tertiary teaching hospitals, undermined the reliability of data abstraction. Patients with complicated conditions underwent numerous procedures and thus had voluminous records, and one reviewer or another frequently missed a particular notation or laboratory report. Furthermore, the MedisGroups vendor instructed reviewers to take clinical information from the notes of the most senior physician (i.e., attending physicians' notes took precedence over those of interns). Not unexpectedly, the reviewers encountered instances where senior specialists from different disciplines disagreed about their clinical observations. These occurrences compromised our ability to meet the designated MedisGroups data collection target of 95 percent accuracy.

When physicians' notes do not contain complete information about important risk factors, a reasonable option involves reviewing notes of nurses or other clinicians. The CSI uses all documentation in the medical record, including countersigned notes of trainees (Iezzoni and Daley 1992). This approach can prolong reviews and raises questions about interdisciplinary variability in assessing clinical findings. Nonetheless, this strategy broadens the range of candidate risk factors.

Biases in the extent of documentation of risk factors across hospitals could result directly from critical differences in practice patterns, including variations in use of diagnostic tests. Nonrandom variations in practice patterns could compromise analysts' abilities to produce unbiased assessments of patients' risks across providers. When physiological values are not measured, they cannot contribute to assessing risks.

The story recounted in Chapter 3 about the Pennsylvania hospital with high death rates among apparently mildly ill cancer patients exemplifies this situation. All Pennsylvania hospitals must report MedisGroups information to risk adjust their mortality rates; MedisGroups relies on extensive KCFs abstracted from medical records. When oncologists at this hospital investigated the worrisome deaths, they found that they involved patients, often with widely metastatic disease, who desired comfort measures only—eschewing even routine blood draws for serum chemistry (e.g., sodium, potassium) and hematology testing (e.g., hematocrit, white blood cell counts). No physiological KCFs were available to capture the patients' true risks of imminent death.

In some situations (e.g., risk adjusting CABG mortality rates), relying on technologically sophisticated tests for specifying risk factors is reasonable: With few exceptions, all CABG patients undergo extensive evaluations before surgery. As practice patterns shift, documentation of preoperative test results may extend across outpatient and inpatient records, complicating retrieval of the information. In other contexts, using test results could potentially bias estimates of risks across patients and providers. For example, early versions of MedisGroups tried to minimize reliance on inherently unreliable findings by seeking information from supposedly "objective" sources, such as technologically advanced diagnostic tests (Iezzoni and Moskowitz 1988). Later versions of MedisGroups rely instead on more routine tests (Steen et al. 1993).

Effects of Published Performance Reports on Data Quality

Biases arising from external forces also raise questions about clinical risk factor data. In locales that publish outcome information using clinically detailed risk adjusters, some observers have speculated that providers increased testing to identify more risk factors. Although this possibility remains unproven, it nevertheless heightens concerns about inappropriate services and paradoxically increasing costs, especially in competitive health care marketplaces. A related question is whether documentation of risk factors changes even without adding tests. Especially when performance reports identify physicians individually by name, incentives to color (or manipulate, distort, or game) documentation of risk factors may prove irresistible.

Manipulating clinical information is certainly possible. Even physiological parameters can be "normalized" or modulated in gravely ill patients: " 'Aggressive' treatment may mask extreme changes in physiology that would be identified in another ICU that waits and reacts to changes in patients' physiology" (Teres and Lemeshow 1994, 95). Some manipulation will be subliminal or reflect honest uncertainty characteristic throughout clinical practice. For instance, if during a manual blood pressure reading the Korotkoff sounds disappear around 104 to 106 mm Hg, the decision about which value to record could be subconsciously affected by knowing that a diastolic pressure of 105 mm Hg or greater results in a higher risk rating. Therefore, the incentives imposed by public or private data-collection mandates can significantly affect data quality.

Whether such documentation shifts occur—and whether they reflect fact or fiction—is difficult to assess (Shahian et al. 2001). The best-studied example involves report cards on CABG mortality rates, like those in New York state (see Chapter 1). Clinicians consulting with New York's Department of Health had specified the CABG risk factors, including low cardiac ejection fraction, stenosis of the left main coronary artery, unstable angina, New York Heart Association functional class, and various chronic illnesses (Hannan et al. 1990). Therefore, physician leaders felt assured of the clinical credibility of the risk-adjustment models. In 1991, however, *New York Newsday* published information on CABG volumes and mortality by individual cardiothoracic surgeon after winning a Freedom of Information Act lawsuit, and a public furor ensued.

Green and Wintfeld (1995, 1230–31) analyzed the prevalence of risk factors reported quarterly around the public releases of New York's CABG mortality reports, finding that "the reported prevalence of chronic obstructive pulmonary disease, unstable angina, and low ejection fraction increased sharply in the first quarter of 1990, just after the first mortality report had been distributed to hospitals." In the years 1989, 1990, and 1991, reported prevalence of chronic obstructive pulmonary disease was 6.9 percent, 12.4 percent, and 17.4 percent, respectively; corresponding prevalence of unstable angina was 14.9 percent, 21.1 percent, and 21.8 percent (Green and Wintfeld 1995, 1231). Some increased reporting resulted from changes in how risk factors were defined, but (Green and Wintfeld 1995, 1231):

> Patterns in the data suggested that some institutions outpaced the overall trend toward an increased reporting of risk factors. For example, at one hospital, the reported prevalence of chronic obstructive pulmonary disease increased from 1.8 to 52.9 percent; at another hospital, the reported prevalence of unstable angina increased from 1.9 to 20.8 percent. Variation in the reporting of some risk factors was far greater each year than could reasonably be attributed to differences in case mix. For example, in 1991 the prevalence of chronic obstructive pulmonary disease reported by surgeons ranged from 1.4 to 60.6 percent, and for unstable angina, the range was 0.7 to 61.4 percent.

New York state officials were also concerned about shifts in reporting of risk factors, and they instituted mechanisms to monitor this practice by independent audits and requests that hospitals revise problematic documentation. Nevertheless, "there will always be some room for judgment . . . in determining whether a patient has certain risk factors" (Chassin, Hannan, and DeBuono 1996, 396). Some risk factors are inherently subjective (e.g., New York Heart Association functional class). Completely evaluating the accuracy of such factors would require independent examinations of patients; rereview of medical records does not suffice. Mark R. Chassin, M.D. (2002, 47–48), who oversaw the initial years of New York's CABG report cards, remains convinced:

> Of course, the acid test for whether the risk factor data are accurate or not is how well the logistic regression model that is used for risk adjustment works to predict mortality. On this score, the model has proved extremely robust over the years, with C-statistics averaging just over 0.8 and tests of calibration demonstrating accuracy of predictions over all levels of predicted mortality.

Missing Records

Finally, a separate but important issue involves records that are altogether missing. In any study using medical records, some records inevitably are unavailable for various reasons. The obvious question is whether missing records represent significantly different patients and experiences. One hospital's study of obstetrical outcomes could not locate 25 percent of medical records (Westgren et al. 1986). Missing records involved a larger fraction of newborns with low birthweight and low gestational age than records that were found; the researchers believed that missing records significantly biased their findings.

A recent and ambitious study examining quality of care attempted to retrieve inpatient and outpatient records from physicians' offices for enrollees of six major health insurers nationwide (DiSalvo et al. 2001, 298). The researchers failed to receive complete sets of records for 20 percent of cases sampled for AMI and CHF; only 3 percent of records were unavailable for hypertension cases. However, the researchers eliminated an additional 9 percent of AMI and 19 percent of CHF cases because the medical records failed to confirm the principal diagnosis from the administrative data used to sample the case.

Privacy and Obtaining Clinical Records for Research

The study with the six insurers described above confronted another dilemma (DiSalvo et al. 2001, 298, 299, 302):

> Enrollment at one site was significantly lower because a confidentiality law in that state prevented access to records without a patient's explicit consent, and only 7% of the patients invited to participate at that site agreed to do so. . . . Failure to obtain patient or provider permission, despite repeated attempts, was the primary reason we could not obtain medical records. . . . Obtaining consent added a delay of 2 weeks to 2 months. . . .

Although DiSalvo and colleagues do not name the health plan requiring patient consent, one of their study sites was Minneapolis, Minnesota, home to a far-reaching state law to protect privacy of medical records (Melton 1997). As of 1 January 1997, the law required providers in Minnesota to do the following:

1. inform all patients in writing that their medical records may be released for research and that the patient could object;
2. obtain from patients a general authorization, which could be revoked, to release records for research; and
3. on request, inform subjects whose records were released and provide information on how to contact the researchers.

Melton (1997, 1467), at the Mayo Clinic, argued that this requirement would disrupt almost a century of observational research within Rochester, Minnesota, exploring the health and health care of the local population: "Any potential social benefits of epidemiologic research were discounted in favor of privacy."

Over the last few decades, the medical record has increasingly assumed roles beyond supporting actual clinical care or research, such as utilization review, quality assurance, cost containment, medicolegal activities, and other administrative purposes. Members of a patient focus group convened by the Mayo Clinic in 1996 voiced their strongest concerns about potential abuses of data from genetic testing, the fear that insurers or employers could discriminate in coverage, insurance premiums, or hiring (Melton 1997).

History of Privacy Concerns

Access to medical records beyond immediate caregivers seems antithetical to the common presumption that medical information is private. Nonetheless, the U.S. Constitution does not guarantee an explicit right to privacy. An 1890 legal opinion from Supreme Court Justice Louis D. Brandeis, as well as various amendments to the Bill of Rights, found a presumed right to privacy as the basis for a civil action (Donaldson and Lohr 1994). In a 1977 case, *Whalen v. Roe*, the Supreme Court accepted privacy within a general "right to be left alone" (Institute of Medicine 1997, 43). Nevertheless, the court let stand a New York state program that kept computerized lists of patients receiving prescriptions for dangerous medications, balancing the patients' privacy rights against society's interest in monitoring these drugs.

Patients were frequently unaware that they had authorized broad access to their medical records (Donaldson and Lohr 1994, 150).

> A patient may be asked to accede to disclosure by signing a blanket consent form when applying for insurance or employment. In such cases, however, consent cannot be truly voluntary or informed. Such authorizations are often not *voluntary* because the patient feels compelled to sign the authorization or forgo the benefit sought, and they are not *informed* because the patient cannot know in advance what information will be in the record, who will subsequently have access to it, or how it will be used.

Confidentiality of medical records was theoretically guaranteed by the Uniform Health Care Information Act, which stipulates that providers cannot give any information about patients or their health care to a third party without the patient's consent (McCabe 1988). The act identified exceptions to the patient consent requirement, through which providers could release medical records or health information without specific consent. The guiding principle for such exceptions was to meet patients' best interests, like sharing records among physicians in health care emergencies. Nonetheless (Donaldson and Lohr 1994, 17):

> As a practical matter, policing redisclosure of one's personal health information is difficult and may be impossible. At a minimum, such policing requires substantial resources and commitment. With the use of computer and telecommunications networks, an individual may never discover that a particular disclosure has occurred, even though he or she suffers significant harm—such as inability to obtain employment, credit, housing, or insurance—as a result of such disclosure. Pursuing legal remedies may result in additional disclosure of the individual's private health information.

Despite this legislation, many more persons not directly involved in patients' care obtained access to their records. This situation may have changed the content and character of medical record documentation in ways that alter risk factor information (Burnum 1989, 483):

> The loss of confidentiality of medical records has caused physicians and patients alike to withhold clinically important, but sensitive, personal information from medical records that might harm the patient if brought to public view. Furthermore, physicians are being forced to censor essential chart information patients might find objectionable now that patients have the right to read their own records.

Certain areas are especially affected, such as documentation of mental health disorders and symptoms, cognitive dysfunctions (such as dementia), substance abuse, sexual practices, and HIV status—important risk factors for many outcomes. Word choices and terminology are modulated to meet the expectations of various persons who now have access to medical records (e.g., HIPAA compliance officers, utilization reviewers, quality assessors, billing offices, lawyers, patients). To justify a patient's continued hospital stay, "chart notes have become increasingly gloomy" (Burnum 1989, 483). Documentation for HIPAA compliance with coding requirements, with the risk of civil penalties for nonadherence (see Chapter 5), has further affected the content of inpatient and outpatient medical records.

Patients' access to their own records generates ambivalence among some clinicians. Society undoubtedly advocates the rights of health care consumers, but the awareness that patients might read their records constrains what some physicians record. Physicians choose their words carefully or censor altogether their written assessments of patients' clinical status or prognoses. Concerns over malpractice litigation also affect medical record documentation. To protect themselves, many physicians extensively document not only treatments provided and patients' clinical responses but also instances where patients' explicitly decline tests or interventions.

HIPAA and Privacy

Given this environment, creating federal standards for privacy protection became a key provision of HIPAA (see Chapter 5). If Congress failed to enact federal privacy legislation by August 1999, the Secretary of the DHHS was to promulgate federal regulations. Since Congress did not act, DHHS did. The Clinton administration issued a proposed privacy rule in the *Federal Register* in November 1999 soliciting public comment and received more than 52,000 responses (Gostin 2001, 3016). The incoming Bush administration put Clinton's final rules on hold, reopening the comment period. This time, more than 24,000 additional comments were received. The Bush DHHS announced its final privacy rule on 9 August 2002, and the new regulations took effect 14 April 2003.

Two points deserve comment. First, HIPAA does not permit DHHS to preempt state laws conferring more stringent privacy protections than the federal regulations. DHHS therefore explicitly "sets a national 'floor' of privacy safeguards, but permits states to provide additional protections" (Gostin 2001, 3020). Minnesota's statute would therefore trump federal privacy regulations. This can complicate matters for national health care organizations, which must comply with both federal protections and the laws within jurisdictions where they operate.

Second, researchers seeking access to medical records and clinical information must still meet Federal Policy for the Protection of Human Subjects requirements—regulations known as the "Common Rule" (Gostin 2001, 3018). Investigators must seek approval from institutional review boards or privacy boards and meet their stipulations about minimal privacy risk and protection of identifiable data. Institutional review boards may require researchers to obtain consent from study subjects before gaining access to their medical information.

Circling back to the study by DiSalvo and colleagues (2001) that opened this section, the organizational, logistical, and fundamental data challenges to conducting medical record studies have become increasingly daunting in the last few years. This is ironic given the greater availability of electronic information and the technical ease of access to huge volumes of clinical information. The study's final paragraph conveyed a sobering message (DiSalvo et al. 2001, 303):

> Our results indicate that the feasibility of routinely implementing this or other sets of measures in managed care settings is affected

adversely by data system deficiencies, diagnostic disagreement between medical records and principal discharge diagnoses, inadequate annotation of clinical care rendered, low rates of eligibility for key performance measures, small sample sizes, and low survey response rates. Given these limitations, measuring quality of care in a way that is convincing to providers is problematic, and benchmarking providers will be difficult, if not impossible.

The problems encountered in this ambitious, six-site study certainly do not apply to smaller, targeted projects, but they nonetheless present a cautionary tale for researchers conducting medical record studies.

How Much Clinical Information Is Enough?

Studies using clinically based risk adjusters must answer the basic questions posed in Chapter 2; different studies will certainly vary in the extent and nature of the required risk factors. Clearly, in many settings, clinical information is superior to administrative data—or offers different answers. Ghali and colleagues (2002) found that discrepancies between men and women in coronary revascularization rates following cardiac catheterization disappeared after accounting for clinical risk factors. Initial adjustment using only administrative data variables failed to erase disparities by sex. A study from 22 St. Louis hospitals found that predictions of in-hospital mortality improved substantially when clinical laboratory values were added to diagnosis codes from administrative data (Pine, Jones, and Lou 1998). A study of almost 5,000 dialysis patients found significantly better predictions using detailed clinical data compared to administrative information (Mesler et al. 1999). Most sobering, survival predictions among the sickest patients were one-third shorter using the clinical versus administrative risk adjusters.

Hannan and colleagues (1992; the academic team that oversaw New York's CABG modeling effort) compared the ability to predict in-hospital CABG deaths using an administrative file derived from the New York Statewide Planning and Research Cooperative Systems, and the clinical database compiled through the Cardiac Surgery Reporting System. The latter contained detailed CABG risk factors, whereas the former included standard administrative information. The cardiac surgery model was significantly better able to discriminate between persons who lived and died, although adding only three of the Cardiac Surgery Reporting System's risk factors (reoperation, ejection fraction, and > 90 percent narrowing of the left main trunk) significantly improved the predictive ability of the other model. Both models chose somewhat different facilities as high and low outliers in terms of risk-adjusted mortality (Hannan et al. 1992, 903).

Thus, . . . the importance of using a clinical data base rather than an administrative data base for CABG surgery is dependent on the purposes of the data base. If the information is used for internal quality assurance purposes or to target hospitals for state or federal site visits, the administrative data base may suffice. However, if the information is used to inform consumers of relative quality of hospital care, the differences in hospital ratings between the two systems as well as the potential damage to a hospital's reputation are probably too great to risk using an administrative data base.

We found that predictive performance differed little between Medis-Groups (derived from dozens of clinical variables) and physiology scores (based on 12 and 17 physiologic variables) (Iezzoni et al. 1995a, 1996a, 1996e; Landon et al. 1996) (Table 6.1). In other words, a handful of clinical variables can be equally as useful as dozens of variables abstracted from medical records.

We explored the ability of six different models to predict in-hospital death of patients 65 years of age (Iezzoni et al. 1992c). One model used only administrative information, including age, sex, and comorbid illnesses defined by ICD-9-CM diagnosis codes (Table 6.2). The other five models used the values of KCFs abstracted during the first few hospital days using the MedisGroups chart review protocol. From more than 500 potential KCFs, we identified, for each condition, KCFs present in at least 1 percent of the cases or those clinically judged as important (e.g., ventricular fibrillation); this process produced 40 to 65 KCFs per condition. The administrative model performed least well. Despite being based on numerous KCFs, MedisGroups did better than the pseudo–APACHE II APS models for only AMI. The "ALLKCFs" model never had better cross-validated performance than the "10KCFs" model.[6]

Starting in the late 1980s, HCFA spent several years experimenting with a massive computerized tool to abstract clinical information from hospital records of Medicare beneficiaries, the Uniform Clinical Data Set System (UCDSS). Medicare PROs in six states conducted a pilot test, finding that individual UCDSS chart abstractions sometimes required hours. The UCDSS data-entry software contained 1,800 data elements: The PRO pilot found that pneumonia patients averaged 365 items and stroke patients 371 items (Hartz et al. 1994, 883). For these two conditions, Hartz and colleagues (1994) found that small numbers of these variables significantly predicted adverse events and LOS.[7]

The UCDSS experiment offered several important lessons. First, even data-abstraction tools containing almost 2,000 data elements may exclude important factors, such as functional status information. Second, predictive models sometimes distill hundreds of data elements down to a handful. Third, data gathering initiatives can die under their own weight. In test sites, UCDSS abstraction times averaged from 67 to 115 minutes per discharge (Jencks and Wilensky 1992, 901), and HCFA finally abandoned the UCDSS partially

TABLE 6.1

c-Statistics for
Predicting
In-Hospital
Death

Severity Measure	Condition			
	AMI	CABG	Pneumonia	Stroke
Many Clinical Variables				
Original MedisGroups	0.80	0.73	0.81	0.80
Empirical MedisGroups	0.83	0.74	0.85	0.87
Relatively Few Clinical Variables				
Physiology score 1	0.82	0.73	0.78	0.80
Physiology score 2	0.83	0.73	0.82	0.84

SOURCES: Iezzoni et al. 1995a, 1996a, 1996c; Landon et al. 1996.

because of its expense. In many instances, hospitals must absorb costs of government-mandated collection of risk-adjustment information. Given that expenses can rise into hundreds of thousands of dollars, some government initiatives to produce performance reports have switched from medical-record to administrative-data-based risk adjusters.

Today's electronic information could perhaps map directly into some future generation of UCDSS. Nevertheless, fundamental relationships—between predictor variables and their outcomes—are unlikely to change. Even if analysts electronically obtain huge numbers of clinical variables, perhaps only a dozen will do most of the work predicting specific outcomes.

Information Technologies and the Future

Futurists within health informatics have long anticipated the move toward paperless medical records, and some health care providers have largely "gone digital." Computerized medical records offer significant advantages (Raymond and Dold 2002), such as improved organization of massive quantities of data, easy access to individual data elements, the potential to prompt collection of specific data elements (e.g., complete physical examination findings), the inclusion of pictorial representations (e.g., radiographs, ECGs, even video footage from endoscopic procedures), legibility, and decreased space for storage and processing. Because computers are inherently interactive, they can also function as important partners in actual clinical care. For example, computers can transmit reminders about screening tests or preventive services for specific patients; computerized physician order entry programs can check medication prescriptions for potential errors (e.g., dosage, drug interactions); programmed alerts can warn clinicians when patients are at risk (e.g., triggered by specific laboratory values for patients taking particular medications); and

Model	Cross-Validated $R^2 \times 100$					
	Stroke	Lung Cancer	Pneu-monia	AMI	CHF
Administrative: age; age squared; sex; principal diagnosis; and comorbidities defined by ICD-9-CM codes (diabetes, chronic pulmonary disease, cancer, chronic liver disease, chronic renal disease, cerebrovascular degeneration or chronic psychosis, hypertensive disease, and chronic cardiovascular disease)	2.3	2.4	6.1	6.5	2.3
Original MedisGroups Score: 0, 1, 2, 3, and 4	9.6	5.8	15.4	19.5	7.5
P-APS: pseudo version of APACHE II APS constructed from MedisGroups KCF values for 12 physiologic variables	22.4	14.9	16.4	15.0	13.7
APSKCFs: values of the 12 APS variables plus age and sex in a regression analysis predicting in-hospital death within each condition	23.5	20.7	22.1	17.4	18.3
10KCFs: first ten KCFs to enter forward step-wise regression following age and sex within each condition	23.3	24.2	24.3	18.0	19.6
ALLKCFs: all 40 to 65 KCFs plus age and sex in a regression analysis predicting in-hospital death within each condition	20.8	5.4	24.0	15.7	19.6

SOURCE: Adapted from Iezzoni et al. (1992c).

TABLE 6.2
Performance for Predicting In-Hospital Mortality for Six Models within Five Conditions

computerized practice guidelines can assist in "real-time" therapeutic decision making.

Computerized information collected during routine patient care can be funneled into expert systems or downloaded into other databases to compute risk scores for predicting various outcomes (Hornbrook et al. 1998b). Health Evaluation through Logical Processing (HELP) at LDS Hospital in Salt Lake City was one of the earliest advanced, computerized hospital information systems (Kuperman, Gardner, and Pryor 1991). HELP obtains electronic data from numerous sources, including laboratories, pharmacy, computerized nursing charting, and computerized respiratory care charting (for persons on ventilators). For ICU patients undergoing hemodynamic monitoring, HELP captures information directly from physiologic probes on cardiac output, blood pressure, and pulmonary pressures and from pumps administering intravenous medications. ICU rounds often start with reviews of computer printouts to examine trends in physiologic parameters and drug infusions. HELP algorithms automatically calculate APACHE scores.

Algorithms for electronically computing ICU risk scores are increasingly sophisticated. A recent German study examined completely automated calculation of a risk score developed by the European Society of Intensive Care Medicine (SOFA; Junger et al. 2002). The computerized SOFA algorithm relatively easily captured laboratory values. However, although level of consciousness (e.g., Glasgow Coma Score) is critically important in assessing ICU risk, information for computing Glasgow Coma Scores is often embedded in free-text physical examination notes. Junger and colleagues (2002) designed structured query language (SQL) scripts to retrieve relevant information from physicians' clinical examination texts to compute surrogate Glasgow Coma Scores. The SQL scripts also helped identify artifacts from the automated vital signs monitor. For instance, during routine flushing of arterial lines, the automated monitor falsely records zero values for blood pressures, which would seriously distort SOFA scores.

HIPAA requires that DHHS examine standards (e.g., code sets, vocabularies) for computerized medical records, and the National Committee on Vital and Health Statistics has held many hearings on this topic. An important decision involves choice of a standard vocabulary to uniquely represent clinical concepts, terms, and relationships (Campbell et al. 1997). Standardized vocabularies would support collecting, comparing, and indexing information across disparate health care sites: "The terms enable computer systems firstly to capture and then retrieve on demand patient information in a natural clinical language" (National Health Service 2002).

A leading candidate is the Systematized Nomenclature of Human and Veterinary Medicine–Reference Terminology (SNOMED-RT). The College of American Pathologists developed the original SNOMED more than 20 years ago; SNOMED-RT indicates relationships among clinical codes and terms, thus facilitating linkages among clinical settings that use different words to describe identical concepts. SNOMED-RT is merging with Clinical Terms Version 3 from the National Health Service in Great Britain to further expand its coverage of clinical concepts. The new vocabulary, SNOMED-CT (clinical terminology), could become the accepted health care vocabulary worldwide.[8]

An important goal involves using algorithms based on SNOMED-CT or other vocabularies for automated coding of diagnoses from free texts or clinicians' notations. Natural language processing techniques use vocabularies or other word-based algorithms to extract various clinical concepts from clinicians' textual notes (Friedman and Hripcsak 1999). Natural language processing methods like the Medical Language Extraction and Encoding System show promise for extracting clinical concepts from texts, such as radiology reports (Hripcsak, Kuperman, and Friedman 1998).[9]

Nonetheless, many technical, conceptual, and cultural challenges remain before computer-based patient records will be widely used in daily clinical care. Technical challenges range from establishing electronic transmission standards to finalizing standardized vocabularies to ensuring data security, while practical challenges include expense and changing physician behavior (Institute of Medicine 1997; Dick, Steen, and Detmer 1997; McDonald 1997).

> . . . Few details have been worked out and agreed upon. For example, there is no common model for the CPR [computer-based patient record], no common set of data elements, no common vocabulary, and no common set of scenarios that are supported. These requirements are fundamental if developers are to create a person-centered CPR that links care across different sites, specialties, and circumstances.
>
> Many systems still follow the traditional organization and characteristics of the paper-based system and have simply automated that system. Narrative documentation, for example, is far more prevalent than structured text. Even though most new CPRs support a multimedia record, new data forms have not been smoothly integrated into the record, and little has been done to evaluate their true worth. Finally, the concept of incorporating patient-derived information (e.g., health status) as part of the patient record has not been implemented to any significant degree. (Dick, Steen, and Detmer 1997, 11)

Although hospitals are increasingly moving toward electronic data systems, private physicians' offices and small group practices lag far behind. Transforming raw clinical data into electronic information may require extra time for physicians (e.g., entering notes into the computer, reviewing computerized transcripts of dictations) and is sometimes less flexible than personal, customized, paper-based record keeping. Redesigning work processes and training clinicians is costly and time consuming. Clinicians' contributions to computerized records remain primarily unstructured free texts, which are problematic to analyze and interpret. SNOMED-CT or other vocabularies or natural language processing might ameliorate this problem.

Patients can also directly enter information into their medical records. Wald and colleagues (1995) designed a "health history interview" that queried patients about physical and psychiatric symptoms, health-related behaviors, and various risk factors. New patients were asked to come early for scheduled appointments, and prior to their physician visits, they entered responses to interview questions at terminals in the waiting room. Patients' answers were downloaded directly into their computerized medical records, and paper copies were printed for the patient and physician. The computerized interview took an average of 27 minutes. Although 42 percent of the older patients had no prior keyboard experience, patients rated the computerized interview as positive; 65 percent preferred the computer-administered survey, whereas 15 percent preferred face-to-face interviews (Wald et al. 1995, 149). Patients conveyed fairly sensitive information: 13 percent reported serious domestic violence in the prior 12 months, and 16 percent reported suicidal ideation.

Even if medical records are completely computerized, their general content and problem orientation will probably not change dramatically in the near future. They will continue to report providers' impressions, assessments, and plans for patients and their treatments. Regardless of the medium (paper or computer), questions will likely remain about the reliability, objectivity, and completeness of medical record information.

Notes

1. The web site of the Clinical Examination Research Interest Group of the Society of General Internal Medicine is http://www.sgim.org/clinexam.cfm (accessed 11 November 2002). This web site contains links to other organizations worldwide interested in evidence-based medicine and understanding reliability of the physical examination. It also lists complete citations from the rational clinical examination feature in the *Journal of the American Medical Association*.

2. CARE studies aim to enroll clinicians at any stage of training or experience (http://www.carestudy.com/CareStudy/Default.asp, accessed 12 November 2002). For each project, the goal is to involve at least 100 clinicians seeing more than 1,000 total patients. The examination under review should take fewer than two minutes per patient, along with data entry via the Internet; the studies last only two weeks. At this time, more than 160 physicians have joined CARE. Leaders of CARE began their efforts in collaboration with the prestigious Centre for Evidence-Based Medicine located at the John Radcliffe Hospital in Oxford, United Kingdom (http://minerva.minervation.com/cebm/docs/adminpage.html, accessed 12 November 2002). To address the innumerable questions about etiology, diagnosis, prognosis, and treatment raised in every patient encounter, the Centre is producing systematic evidence-based reviews called "Critically Appraised Topics." Designed for ready accessibility in various computer formats, the reviews aim to be useful for clinicians in routine patient care and may therefore also prove useful in identifying risk factors for specific conditions.

3. A potentially subjective risk factor is the New York Heart Association functional classification for cardiovascular disease patients, which reflects how cardiac symptoms impede usual activities and is based both on observation and patients' reports.

4. Feigl and colleagues (1988) compared inpatient and radiation therapy records for patients diagnosed with certain cancers. While inpatient records amply documented laboratory and other diagnostic test

results, consultations, and specific inpatient treatments, important information from outpatient settings about the extent of the cancer (e.g., mammography results) was poorly documented.

5. This study examined the accuracy of the medication histories documented in the medical records of 122 elderly persons admitted to two teaching hospitals in Los Angeles (Beers, Munekata, and Storrie 1990). Within 48 hours of admission, the investigators independently interviewed all subjects and abstracted the medication history recorded by the admitting intern or attending physician. Errors represented failures to record a medication the patient reported taking, not differences in dosages or administration schedules. When all medications were included in the analyses, at least one error occurred for 83 percent of subjects; 46 percent had more than two errors. Considering only "important" medications, 60 percent of subjects had at least one error, whereas 18 percent had more than two.

6. In lung cancer, the R^2 for the ALLKCFs model produced on the fitting data set (0.34) was much higher than that following cross-validation (0.05) (see Chapter 9). Although some ALLKCFs models, with 40 or more explanatory variables each, achieved high R^2 values, these models were initially overspecified: In the cross-validation analyses, they performed no better, and in lung cancer did far worse, than models based on the ten most important clinical variables (10KCFs).

7. Despite its 1,800 data elements, the UCDSS did not collect functional status indicators, such as the need for assistance with basic ADLs. One study empirically derived predictive models for hospital LOS and occurrence of adverse events for pneumonia and stroke patients (Hartz et al. 1994). Only a handful of data elements were statistically significant and retained in the final models. For example, just four factors appeared in the model predicting adverse events for stroke: lethargy, stupor, or coma; labored or abnormal breathing; increase in pulse rate of 20 beats per minute; and ischemic heart disease (Hartz et al. 1994, 890). When available, functional status items (need for bathing assistance, restrictions on out-of-bed movement) were among the items retained for two of the four models.

8. Many organizations are involved with defining and refining clinical vocabularies for applications to computerized medical records and electronic collating of clinical information. In the United States, the National Library of Medicine plays a leading role. SNOMED is proprietary, owned and copyrighted by the College of American Pathologists (http://www.snomed.org, accessed 7 August 2002). Giving SNOMED a prominent, government-sanctioned role therefore requires negotiation. Information about the clinical terminology version, SNOMED-CT, a collaboration with Great Britain, is available

at http://www.nhsia.nhs.uk/terms/pages/snomedct/sno_faqp1.asp (accessed 7 August 2002).

9. The web site for the Medical Language Extraction and Encoding System not only describes the methodology but also offers an interesting demonstration: http://cat.cpmc.columbia.edu/medleexml/demo/medlee.html (accessed 25 July 2002).

DATA FROM SURVEYS OR ASKING PATIENTS

Lisa I. Iezzoni

In proposing fundamental redesign of the U.S. health care system, the Institute of Medicine (2001a) anointed patients' perspectives as the "true north" to guide radical health care change (Berwick 2002). Among six suggested aims for health system reform is patient centeredness: "providing care that is respectful of and responsive to individual patient preferences, needs, and values and ensuring that patient values guide all clinical decisions" (Institute of Medicine 2001a, 6). The only way to evaluate patient-centered care is by asking patients.

Patients are being asked many things these days by providers, health plans, employers, researchers, and state and federal governments. Potential respondents are selected randomly (e.g., through random-digit dialing of telephone numbers) or targeted by specific events, such as hospitalizations, or group membership, such as health plan enrollment. Some worry that the flurry of surveys is overwhelming a public weary of intrusive telemarketing and "spam," its Internet equivalent. In certain settings, response rates are dropping, perhaps further biasing the findings: Neutral or contented persons may not answer, leaving only disgruntled respondents. In 2002, one Massachusetts health plan abandoned its annual survey of enrollees' satisfaction with their physicians when the response rate fell to 10 percent (Safran and Rogers 2002, 9).

Nonetheless, the complexities of conducting clinically credible outcomes studies can make obtaining information directly from patients seem relatively simple. In 1995, the Massachusetts Health Quality Partnership debated about which quality measures to adopt for comparing hospital performance, up front dismissing administrative-data-based approaches as insufficient. Initial ideas involved targeting mortality rates during selected hospital admissions (e.g., for heart surgery), but deliberations stalled around the conceptual and logistical challenges of risk adjustment. The group decided that starting with comparing patients' experiences and satisfaction with care was easier and selected the Picker Institute survey of patients' experiences (Cleary et al. 1991, 1993), which used patient-reported health status as its major risk adjuster (Hargraves et al. 2001).[1] The partnership examined Picker surveys of more than 24,000 persons to produce performance reports for 50 Massachusetts hospitals (Rogers and Smith 1999).

Chapter 7 explores issues raised by using data from patient surveys. Here, I do not review technical attributes of survey methodologies, sampling procedures, sample-size issues, or analytic approaches but instead focus on aspects pertinent to risk adjustment. I draw examples primarily from efforts to risk adjust capitation payments using functional status information and the Consumer Assessment of Health Plans Study (CAHPS). Numerous nationally representative, health-related surveys are conducted by the federal government, such as the NHIS from the NCHS and the Medical Expenditure Panel Survey from AHRQ. Medicare's Health Outcomes Survey examines the functional outcomes of beneficiaries enrolled in managed care organizations (CMS 2002d; Cooper 1998; Cooper et al. 2001; Golden 2001; Safran 2001). The Behavioral Risk Factor Surveillance System survey is jointly sponsored by states and the federal CDC. These surveys and other federal health surveys are used frequently and productively for outcomes research, with results risk adjusted by data elements from them. Information about these surveys is available elsewhere, such as at the NCHS, AHRQ, CMS, and CDC Internet web sites.

Risk Factors and Patient-Reported Outcomes

With certain exceptions (e.g., research exploring capitation payment levels; see below), projects using survey data typically target outcomes reflecting patients' viewpoints, such as satisfaction with care or self-perceived overall health. Thus, patients generally define the "what" in the "risk of what" question (see Chapter 2). Survey-based projects can study more diverse outcomes than administrative-data-based projects, where outcomes measures must derive from items within fixed data sets, such as mortality, costs, and service use. In contrast, the major constraints facing survey-based projects are people's willingness to answer specific questions and logistical feasibility.

Numerous tools are now available to solicit patient-reported outcomes, such as overall health status, quality of life, symptoms, satisfaction with care, and adherence to therapy. The field of patient-reported measures has grown tremendously over the last two decades. In 1980, a MEDLINE bibliographical search found 389 articles under the "quality-of-life" key word, whereas a 2000 MEDLINE search found 4,133 published citations (Mapi Research Institute 2002). The Quality of Life Instrument Database, compiled by a European collaborative, lists 1,000 patient-reported outcome questionnaires and provides detailed information on more than 300 instruments on its Internet web site (Mapi Research Institute 2002). Some instruments are "generic" (i.e., relevant to all persons regardless of health conditions), whereas others are condition or situation specific. When doing a project on patient-reported outcomes, the first step therefore involves selecting the outcome of interest, then identifying an appropriate instrument. The third step is considering risk adjusting the outcomes.

The need to risk adjust patient-reported outcomes depends on the context. Risk adjusting results in comparing outcomes across groups of patients can mask differences by important patient characteristics; however, failure to risk adjust could bias these comparisons. Research suggests that patients' opinions about their health and health care are affected by many factors, including their age, sex, race and ethnicity, education, burden of illness, extent of functional impairments, cultural and religious beliefs and practices, and expectations and preferences—potentially most of the risk factors described in Chapter 3. One study using a large nationwide survey found that low education, unemployment, old age, poverty, and minority race and ethnicity significantly predicted self-reported fair or poor health (Shi and Starfield 2000, 546). Self-reported functional deficits are also strongly associated with the burden of chronic disease (Au et al. 2001). Nonetheless, Safran and Rogers (2002, 24) argue, "The research literature shows that measured patient characteristics explain little of the variation in patients' assessments of care—most often 5 percent or less."

Race and ethnicity have attracted special interest because of well-documented disparities in care (Institute of Medicine 2002b). Studies typically show that nonwhite patients are less satisfied with their care and experience worse health outcomes than do white patients, although the extent and direction of these differences varies by racial and ethnic subgroup as well as the specific outcome of interest. Black persons generally report the worst experiences, with Hispanic and Asian patients often also noting poorer outcomes than white respondents.

Efforts to characterize the role of black race in patient-reported outcomes have produced provocative findings. LaVeist, Nickerson, and Bowie (2000) oversaw telephone interviews of 1,003 white and 781 black persons with cardiac disease, asking for their perceptions of racism within the health care system, mistrust of medical providers, and satisfaction with care. Black patients were significantly less satisfied with their care than were white patients, but once perceptions of racism and mistrust of medical providers were added to multivariable regression models, black race no longer significantly predicted dissatisfaction. Such negative perceptions are perhaps mitigated when black patients see black physicians (Cooper-Patrick et al. 1999).

Other research provides different insight. A study of 854 black and white ischemic heart disease patients at five VA medical centers examined eight scales summarizing health-related beliefs, attitudes, and experiences (Kressin et al. 2002).[2] The scales included questions about such concerns as feeling respected by physicians, being treated with dignity, whether doctors knew patients' personal situations, and feeling that the treatment was proper and decisions were correct. Only one scale, attitudes toward religion, yielded statistically significant differences between black and white respondents: Black patients "placed stronger importance on God and religion in general, as well as in coping with their heart problems and in making decisions about their heart disease" (Kressin et al. 2002, 179).

Self-perceived health and functional status are often critical risk factors for predicting patient-reported outcomes. For example, age and self-perceived health status strongly predict patients' reports about hospitalization experiences: Younger patients and those in poor health report significantly more problems than do older and healthier patients (Hargraves et al. 2001, 637). The Picker measure of hospitalization experiences used by the Massachusetts Health Quality Partnership (see above) therefore adjusted for age and self-reported health. People who are sick (Schlesinger, Druss, and Thomas 1999; Druss et al. 2000) and those with disabilities (Jha et al. 2002; Iezzoni et al. 2002) are generally less satisfied with their medical care. One potential explanation is that people with greater needs for services have more interactions with the health care system and therefore more opportunities to be disappointed. Certainly, people with significant health problems are more likely than others to need timely care involving a range of services and to want information about their conditions, prognoses, and therapeutic options. With more treatment decisions and interventions comes more chance of mishap involving technical and interpersonal quality of care.

The role of functional status may vary by dimension of functioning and outcome of interest. A study of satisfaction with six domains of outpatient care among more than 2,600 veterans used the mental and physical subscales of the SF-12 Health Survey, an abbreviated version of the SF-36.[3] Both mental and physical functioning were associated with selected quality dimensions, but with differing directions (Harada, Villa, and Andersen 2002, 162). For example, compared to others, veterans with better mental functioning were more satisfied with telephone access, providers' technical skills, and sensitivity to race but less satisfied with the physical environment and courtesy of the office staffs. Veterans with better physical functioning were less satisfied with some but not all aspects of care.

Within subpopulations, important risk factors can become very specific. The study of satisfaction with outpatient care among veterans found that such factors as membership in veterans' organizations, use of non-VA services, and military combat exposure were significantly associated with satisfaction, in addition to sociodemographic characteristics like race and ethnicity (Harada, Villa, and Andersen 2002).

As noted in Chapter 3, patient preferences and expectations for health care are potentially important predictors of such outcomes as satisfaction with care. Strongly expressed patient preferences sometimes have little effect on the care they receive, perhaps for compelling reasons but sometimes not. For example, one multicenter study found that patients' desires did not determine their place of death: Even patients who strongly preferred to die out of hospital had a similar likelihood of dying in hospital as did others (Pritchard et al. 1998). Desires for or expectations of specific elements of care, such as labora-

tory tests, physical examinations, or referrals to specialists, may be unr
sociodemographic characteristics (Zemencuk et al. 1999). Neverthe
concordance between such desires and expectations and what patient:
receive may strongly influence satisfaction with care.

Finally, regardless of the statistical association between patient-
outcomes and risk factors, the choice of appropriate risk factors—
depends on the context. Commenting in the context of surveys to assess physician performance, Safran and Rogers (2002, 24) raise fundamental questions
about risk adjusting physician-level results:

> A dilemma that we face in adjusting survey-based performance data
> for patient characteristics is that, in some ways, it runs counter to
> efforts to promote patient-centered care. That is, by leveling the
> playing field with adjustment, we negate the differing needs of pa-
> tients served by different physicians, rather than holding physicians
> accountable for how well they serve their particular patient mix.
> Nevertheless, it is almost certainly imperative that we risk-adjust
> physician-level performance data. Without this, the data will be
> readily disregarded by those who feel that their results are biased
> downwards by the particular characteristics of their patient panel.

Accuracy of Patient-Reported Risk Factor Data

Patients can supply some information about almost all potential risk factors,
except perhaps physiological values and technical clinical findings. Surveys
gathering patient-reported outcomes therefore generally include questions
about potential risk factors. Sometimes such surveys are linked to other data
sources (e.g., health insurance enrollment or claims files) that generate the
sampling frame and contain information about basic demographic risk factors and coded diagnoses. In other circumstances, confidentiality concerns
demand that surveys be completely anonymous (i.e., precluding linkage to
other sources). In these instances, survey responses provide the only insight
into risk factors.

Risk factors taken from patient survey responses fall along a continuum
from those putatively objective or measurable attributes, such as the presence
of diseases or health behaviors, like smoking, to those that are intrinsically subjective, such as self-perceived health status. For subjective measures, assessing
accuracy is moot—their very subjectivity, a synthesis of individual views and
preferences, is their value. Despite the subjectivity of measures like global
self-perceived health, however, this single item can significantly predict important outcomes ranging from mortality to annual expenditures (Bierman et
al. 1999). Nevertheless (Cleary 1997, 4):

> Some researchers are uncomfortable with subjective variables because
> they are perceived as unreliable. Such people often think of data

from medical records as "hard" data, whereas they think of survey responses as "soft" data. Thus, rather than judging the relative theoretical value of objective and subjective measures, some researchers' selection of variables is unduly influenced by their negative opinions about the value of survey data relative to other types of information. However, medical records contain many types of data, including information about subjective states collected using unstandardized methods.

Efforts to examine the accuracy of patient-reported risk factors have generally focused on more "objective" items, typically comparing patients' reports to a medical record "gold standard." Comparisons find that patients are most accurate when asked about well-defined medical conditions (e.g., AMI, diabetes) and least accurate for less specific conditions like arthritis (Silliman and Lash 1999, 348). In general, older patients and those with lower educational levels provide less accurate reports than do younger, well-educated patients. Especially when older patients have multiple coexisting conditions, their reports may be incomplete (Gross et al. 1996). Although most studies have examined underreporting of chronic conditions by patients, overreporting also can occur. One study from the Netherlands found that persons with mobility limitations were especially prone to report conditions, such as chronic lung and cardiac disease, atherosclerosis, cancer, stroke, and arthritis, that were not noted by their primary care physicians (Kriegsman et al. 1996, 1411).

One study compared patients' reports of cardiovascular disease risk factors obtained through a telephone interview with findings during a subsequent clinic visit with trained physicians and nurses (Bowlin et al. 1996). Reported risk factors were compared to objective test results (e.g., exhaled carbon monoxide levels to identify smokers, blood pressure measured three times using an American Heart Association protocol, serum total cholesterol on fasting venous blood). Compared with these clinical gold standards, approximately half of the patients with hypertension and hypercholesterolemia misclassified themselves as not having the risk factor. Patients' reports of smoking were generally accurate. In the Medical Outcomes Study, physicians' reports of "tracer" diagnoses (e.g., diabetes mellitus) agreed better with confirmatory laboratory data (e.g., glycosylated hemoglobin) than did patients' reports on self-administered questionnaires or face-to-face interviews (Kravitz et al. 1993). A study of VA clinic patients compared self-reported chronic diseases with diagnoses documented in medical records. Patients accurately reported 97 percent of chronic obstructive pulmonary disease and 95 percent of coronary artery disease (Fan et al. 2002).

Some studies have compared numerical risk-adjustment scale results derived from patient reports with those based on medical record reviews. Katz and colleagues (1996) developed a questionnaire containing the Charlson comorbidity factors (see Table 3.4) to be either self-administered or answered during an interview. Kappa statistics (see Chapter 9) indicating agreement between patients' reports of individual comorbidities and medical record evidence of comorbidities ranged from 0.35 to 0.85. Charlson scores from patient-generated data produced a Spearman correlation coefficient of 0.63 when compared with medical-record-derived scores (Katz et al. 1996, 77). In a study of 303 women with stage I or II breast cancer, Silliman and Lash (1999) found high correlations (roughly 0.6; $p \leq 0.001$) between comorbidity scores derived from telephone interviews. Nevertheless, scores based on patient interviews were generally slightly higher than those from medical record review, suggesting that the interviews identified more comorbid conditions than did chart abstraction.

Other researchers have examined the accuracy of patients' reports of processes of care or events. For example, drug use may potentially indicate the severity or complexity of diseases such as diabetes. One study examined self-reports of care among persons with diabetes, comparing these reports with medical record and claims information (Fowles et al. 1999). In a subanalysis of drug use, the investigators found that self-reported insulin administration was virtually 100 percent accurate; about 10 percent of respondents overreported and 10 percent underreported use of oral hypoglycemic agents. In contrast, although hospitalization seems a memorable event, comparisons of patients' reports with administrative records show that patients systematically underreport hospital admissions (Clark, Ricketts, and McHugo 1996; Roberts et al. 1996). Not surprisingly, patients' memories are especially faulty if considerable time has elapsed. Other studies, however, have found that patients accurately recall cancer screening services such as mammography (Degnan et al. 1992; Gordon, Hiatt, and Lampert 1993; Zapka et al. 1996).

Assessments of some risk factors may vary depending on who is asked. A good example is the discordance between perceptions of patients and clinicians about functional status (see Chapters 3 and 15). One study of agreement between outpatients and their physicians found kappa values ranging from 0.14 to 0.37, reflecting substantial disagreement between patients and physicians in perceptions of patient functioning (Calkins et al. 1991, 453). Agreement between patients and doctors was generally highest for measures of physical functioning and lowest for indicators of social functioning. The majority of disagreements involved physicians' underestimation of patients' disabilities.

Sometimes patients cannot answer surveys, and proxies respond. Explanations vary: Subjects may be too sick or cognitively compromised to respond; they may be healthy and out working or socializing when the telephone rings; they may be illiterate and rely completely on others to complete written materials; or they may be too young to respond themselves. With longer surveys, self-respondents may tire midway and rely on proxies to complete interviews or questionnaires, unless they drop out altogether. Therefore, the direction and nature of potential "respondent" bias varies depending on the context. Studies comparing self-reports to proxy reports generate varied results. Some suggest that proxies rate both physical functional status and overall health as more impaired than do patients, whereas other studies reach the opposite conclusion. An analysis using the federal NHIS found that proxies underreported disabling conditions among persons under age 65 but overreported disability for older persons (Todorov and Kirchner 2000).

In summary, despite concerns about accuracy, asking patients may be both better and easier than obtaining information from clinicians or medical records. Surveys are especially valuable to capture global concepts like functional status (Cleary 1997, 3–4):

> Patients can be asked whether they have difficulty going up and down stairs, or an observer can visit their homes to observe whether they can or cannot climb stairs. This is a situation in which objective measures are available and can be more reliable and valid, if properly administered, than patient self-reports, but such methods are often prohibitively expensive. . . . Medical records frequently contain functional assessments that were obtained by health care professionals with no training in standardized measurement and that are largely subjective measures. Such variables may be measured more efficiently, reliably and validly with standardized subjective measures.

Patient self-reports using well-validated functional status measures are now widely accepted. In a critical sense, patient-generated data are the only authentic data about patients' perceptions, functioning, health status, and quality of life. Nevertheless, these reports inevitably reflect the complexities and constant contradictions of life. For example, persons viewed by others as being in "poor" health often place relatively high values on their health, having adjusted their lifestyles and expectations to their capabilities (Dolan 1996). Conversely, young, apparently healthy people may devalue their health, given high and possibly unrealistic expectations about what optimal health should be. Neither perception is "inaccurate" when viewed as the patients' perspective, but appreciating nuances of these reports is important.

Logistics and Feasibility

Researchers argue that medical record reviews are particularly costly and inefficient in outpatient settings and that administrative data are insufficient to predict clinical outcomes (Silliman and Lash 1999; Fan et al. 2002). They therefore turn directly to patients. To develop a comorbidity index predicting two-year mortality and hospitalization, Fan and colleagues (2002) mailed VA medical clinic patients questionnaires inquiring about 24 chronic medical conditions. Their final comorbidity model included only seven chronic conditions plus age and smoking status.[4] Although the researchers did not report the costs of gathering the survey data, they propose that "a simple 9-item questionnaire could be sent to subjects" to calculate a statistically valid comorbidity score (Fan et al. 2002, 378).

Similarly, Katz and colleagues (1996) were concerned about the logistics and expense of paying trained nurse abstractors to gather medical record information for the Charlson comorbidity index. As described above, they therefore developed a questionnaire to obtain information directly from patients, either by mailed questionnaire or during an interview. Relative costs of obtaining comorbidity information by patient report versus chart review were estimated as follows: $0.93 for mailed, self-report questionnaires; $1.67 for patient interviews; and $3.50 for chart abstraction (Katz et al. 1996, 79). In studying type II diabetes, researchers turned to patients because of concerns about irregular laboratory testing and missing chart data (Greenfield et al. 1995). They created a composite, global measure by aggregating 15 individual severity scales using data from a patient questionnaire containing 130 items and taking about 15 minutes to complete.

Perhaps the greatest threat to the validity of information from surveys is low response rates, refusals to answer specific questions, and respondent bias. One can safely assume that persons who refuse to answer surveys or specific questions within surveys differ in potentially important ways from persons who do provide answers. Respondents and nonrespondents may diverge in characteristics considered key risk factors, such as age, gender, race and ethnicity, and health status. To reduce respondent burden and bolster response rates, most survey designers therefore aim for efficiency. For example, the SF-36, containing 36 questions, derived from a much longer questionnaire (Stewart and Ware 1992); a streamlined version, the SF-12, aims to achieve even higher response rates. People may refuse to answer questions covering sensitive topics, notably income.

The Partners in Health Survey was created to assess the health of communities. Using a broad conceptual framework, the survey captures multiple domains of health and well-being, contains 118 questions, and requires 22 minutes to administer by telephone (Bazos et al. 2001). A pilot test randomly telephoned households in central Pennsylvania, yielding a 66 percent overall response rate. Given the sampling scheme, the researchers could not determine the characteristics of nonresponders. However, respondents willingly answered even sensitive questions: For example, the percentage of missing values for various queries was 0.9 percent for smoking, 1.0 percent for having had at least one alcoholic drink in the last month, and 2.3 percent for keeping a loaded and unlocked firearm. However, 21.6 percent of income data were missing.

Obtaining information directly from patients raises numerous logistical considerations. As noted above, some patients may be physically or cognitively unable to respond. The use of proxies can improve the efficiency of surveys: Surveyors can get information from whomever is available within a household, for example, rather than waiting for a specific respondent. However, the decision to use proxy respondents must consider the ultimate audience for the information derived from the survey. The debate about whether to query proxies "polarizes survey methodologists and disability advocates more than any other" survey-related topic (Parsons, Baum, and Johnson 2000, 5). Disability advocates, for example, feel strongly that proxies cannot adequately represent the experiences of people with disabilities.

Many studies limit themselves to respondents who speak English, given the costs and linguistic challenges of translating questionnaires (i.e., ensuring that the translation has the same meaning as the English version). Rigorous techniques for translating questionnaires require multiple translations from English to other languages and back again. Cross-cultural differences in attitudes toward health, symptoms, and disease are crucial considerations in translating surveys for use across nations or across linguistic groups within populations (Ware et al. 1995; Mathias, Fifer, and Patrick 1994).

Linguistic differences can affect scoring metrics, such as the words used to weight either extreme of a Likert-type scale. For instance, the global, self-perceived health status question is typically phrased: "How would you rate your health? Excellent, very good, good, fair, or poor?" During a study of Chinese immigrants who spoke either Mandarin or Cantonese, Ngo-Metzger and colleagues (2003) found that respondents perceived "excellent" as an almost superhuman quality virtually unattainable by average persons. They changed the word weighting the upper end of the scale to one meaning roughly "very very very good."

Cultural differences are especially important in cross-cultural or international studies. One project looked at self-reports by cataract patients in the United States, Manitoba (Canada), Barcelona (Spain), and Denmark of global visual functioning (i.e., overall trouble with vision, rated as "a great deal," "moderate," "a little," and "none") (Alonso et al. 1998, 870); visual acuity was measured using standard Snellen-type charts. Among respondents with 20/40 or better visual acuity, 34.5 percent of U.S. respondents reported "a great deal" of trouble with vision, as did 32.1 percent of those from Denmark, but only 22.2 percent and 14.8 percent of persons from Barcelona and Manitoba, respectively, responded this way (Alonso et al. 1998, 873). Across all respondents, comorbidity significantly increased risk of reporting trouble with vision.

Designing survey methodologies for persons with disabling conditions requires special thought. Beyond concerns about sampling persons with disabilities and considering the appropriateness of proxy respondents (see above), significant logistical questions arise (Parsons, Baum, and Johnson 2000). Interview and telephone surveys with persons who are deaf or hard of hearing are especially challenging. Telephone surveys could potentially employ teletypewriter (TTY) or Telecommunications Device for the Deaf (TDD) equipment, but these technologies pose serious impediments to conducting surveys.[5] For instance, sometimes the length of typed text allowed is too short to accommodate entire questions. In addition, persons whose primary language is American Sign Language may not have complete facility communicating in English, similarly to other linguistic minorities. Designing written materials for persons who are blind or have low vision must consider alternative modalities like Braille, large print, or audiotape. Persons with speech impairments who use communication technologies also require special accommodations.

The mode of survey administration can affect responses. Self-reported health status scores are generally more positive when respondents are interviewed; perhaps people hesitate to admit health status problems to interviewers that they would report on impersonal mailed surveys. The 7 percent of Americans without telephones differ in important ways (e.g., socioeconomic status, psychosocial factors) from those with phones (Gfroerer and Hughes 1991). Health plans and providers are increasingly distributing surveys via e-mail and the Internet. Electronic responses are readily accessible to the analytic database, maximizing the timeliness of results. Nevertheless, only 41.5 percent of households in mid-2000 had Internet connections (Institute of Medicine 2001a, 177); persons without access are disproportionately poor and disadvantaged. Anecdotal reports suggest that younger, well-educated persons are the primary respondents to e-mail queries.

While mail or e-mail questionnaires are indisputably cheaper than in-person or telephone interviews, concerns about respondent literacy arise. Many adult Americans are functionally illiterate. The type II diabetes study developed an 11-question "questionnaire literacy screen" to judge whether study subjects could complete self-administered questionnaires about their diabetes and other characteristics (Sullivan et al. 1995). Based on the screening results, subjects were assigned an appropriate modality of survey administration, being interviewed only when necessary. In this urban, midwestern teaching-hospital population, 35 percent of respondents failed the questionnaire literacy screen (Sullivan et al. 1995, AS187).

Using Survey Data for Risk Adjustment

As noted earlier, publications about patient-reported outcomes are growing. Most such studies either look at associations between the outcome and potential risk factors or risk adjust the outcomes in making comparisons across subgroups of patients. Survey studies generally involve relatively few institutions and target well-defined patient populations. However, survey-based risk adjustment has also assumed center stage in larger policy-relevant contexts—determining appropriate capitation payments and evaluating plan performance. Surveys seem especially suited to the managed care environment, where respondent populations are relatively well circumscribed and contact information (e.g., names, addresses, telephone numbers) is typically available. Below, I briefly review two such initiatives.

Using Functional Status to Set Capitation Payments

Interest in using survey-based data to risk adjust capitation payments to MCOs stems from fundamental concerns about the limited clinical content of the administrative data typically used for this purpose. Survey data could presumably provide essential information missing from administrative data.

As noted in Chapter 1, to pay more fairly for sick and disabled enrollees, the 1997 Balanced Budget Act required Medicare to link MCOs' capitation payments to health status—to risk adjust reimbursement. Risk-adjustment methods for setting capitation payment levels typically rely on demographic characteristics and diagnosis codes.[6] However, ICD-9-CM offers scant insight into functional deficits, such as those experienced by frail elderly persons and disabled Medicare beneficiaries. Without considering all aspects of patients' clinical presentations, payments may not reflect true costs of caring for particularly vulnerable persons (Iezzoni et al. 1998). MCOs may avoid these needy patients.

Medicare already uses functional-status information to pay certain providers (see Chapters 15 and 16). Medicare's prospective payment systems for nursing homes, home care agencies, and inpatient rehabilitation facilities use functional-status information provided by clinicians rather than obtained directly from patients. In these care settings, clinicians routinely record patients' functional status. Therefore, gathering these data for payment purposes—although administratively potentially burdensome—does not demand entirely new documentation practices.

Researchers have examined whether functional status and other patient-reported information, alone or combined with data on diagnoses, improves predictions of costs for persons enrolled in MCOs. Results have been mixed. Some studies have found that self-reported functional-status information, gathered using SF-36 questionnaires (Hornbrook and Goodman 1995, 1996) or through the Medicare Current Beneficiary Survey (Gruenberg, Kaganova, and Hornbrook 1996), substantially improves predictions over models using only demographic or diagnostic information. Others, however, have found that self-reported health status performs less well than risk adjustment using diagnoses, specifically ACGs (Fowles et al. 1996) and DCG/HCC models (Pope et al. 1998). Patient-reported health behaviors, such as smoking, do not appear to predict annual costs of care (Hornbrook et al. 1991; Fowles et al. 1996). Perhaps the negative health effects of smoking do not declare themselves within one year, the time frame of these analyses.

Most researchers agree that adding patient-reported functional-status information significantly enhances predictions of annual health care costs but is insufficient alone. Instead, self-reported functional status and overall health complements more standard predictors—sociodemographic characteristics and chronic conditions (Gruenberg, Kaganova, and Hornbrook 1996; Hornbrook 1999). The focus then turns to strategies for gathering this information accurately and efficiently. Widespread patient surveys would add significantly to MCOs' administrative costs and risk the potential for gaming or manipulation. Hornbrook (1999, 1747) proposed using self-reported functional status information not only to set payments but also to measure plan performance and identify persons with unmet health needs:

> The importance of having dual-purpose payment and performance assessment is that it provides countervailing incentives for gaming. Risk adjustment [for payment] provides an incentive for providers [and plans] to encourage their members to deflate their health status scores to make the members appear sicker in order to obtain higher revenues. On the other hand, outcomes assessment provides an incentive for plans . . . to inflate health status scores so that they appear to have healthier enrollees and better outcomes than their competitors.

CMS's Health Outcomes Survey could offer that counterweight of measuring plan performance.

CAHPS

Medicare, Medicaid in many states, and hundreds of health plans have implemented the CAHPS survey, generating a database representing at least 400,000 persons (Westat 2001). Investigators can apply to obtain the CAHPS national database for agreed-upon analyses. Details about CAHPS are available on the CAHPS Survey Users Network Internet web site (http://www.cahps-sun.org).

CAHPS aims to measure important aspects of health plans' performance from the consumer's viewpoint. Data are gathered either through mail or telephone surveys from random samples of health plan enrollees. Applicable to public and private managed care and fee-for-service health plans, CAHPS contains a core set of questions for adults and for parents concerning their children's experiences. Additional modules of CAHPS apply to persons with chronic conditions and special health care needs. Most CAHPS questions are sorted into five major groups: getting needed care, getting care without long waits, how well physicians communicate, courtesy and helpfulness of office staff, and customer service of the health plan. Several years ago, CAHPS interviews cost $20 to $40 per completed survey (Zaslavsky et al. 2000, 173).

An ultimate goal of CAHPS is to provide consumers useful information to choose among health plans. Risk adjusting CAHPS results is therefore key to producing valid comparisons across plans. As noted throughout this chapter, the types of measures contained within CAHPS could be strongly associated with respondents' characteristics. However, CAHPS collects relatively limited information that can serve as risk factors. For its early version, "The general CAHPS recommendation, based on a literature review and analyses from CAHPS demonstration sites, is to adjust for age and health status" (Zaslavsky et al. 2000, 166). CAHPS asks respondents to rate their health status on a five-point scale from excellent (5) to poor (1). The CAHPS risk-adjustment recommendation drew from studies showing that younger persons and those in worse health provide more negative evaluations of their care than do older and healthier persons. Medicare MCOs differ significantly in the overall health status of their enrollees (Zaslavsky and Beeuwkes Buntin 2002). Nevertheless, early work showed that adjusting for respondents' risk factors (in some models including educational status and proxy respondent) had little effect on comparative CAHPS performance across health plans (Zaslavsky, Zaborski, and Cleary 2000). Another study controlled for age, health status, education, and interactions with specific health plans; it found that risk adjustment decreased variability in ratings across plans but did not dramatically alter perceptions of plan performance (Elliott et al. 2001).

CAHPS risk-adjustment models appropriately do not control for race and ethnicity, as those attributes might be linked to plan performance, the very quantity being studied. At least among adults, experiences with care vary little by racial and ethnic group (Morales et al. 2001). However, compared to white parents, racial and ethnic minority parents were less happy with their children's experiences in getting needed care, timeliness of care, provider communication, staff helpfulness, and plan service (Weech-Maldonado et al. 2001). Language barriers explain a large portion of these negative experiences, with Hispanic and Asian parents who do not speak English noting the most difficulties.

In examining CAHPS results, respondent bias could skew the findings. CAHPS surveys in Medicare populations find overall response rates of 75 percent to 80 percent, much higher than for many other such surveys (Zaslavsky, Zaborski, and Cleary 2002). However, older beneficiaries, persons with disabilities, women, racial and ethnic minorities, and persons living in geographical areas with relatively high numbers of poorly educated and impoverished persons had lower response rates to mailed surveys. Inaccurate contact information explained some of these differences. Conducting telephone interviews of persons who did not return mailed surveys improved the representativeness of respondents. For-profit health plans, however, were significantly more likely than nonprofit plans to have inaccurate contact information and lower response rates. Most worrisome, "Plans with lower ratings on the CAHPS survey also had more bad contact information" and consequently lower response rates. "If experiences with health care affect propensity to respond, nonresponse might bias plan comparisons. The fact that CAHPS scores from respondents are related to plan response rates suggests that this might be happening" (Zaslavsky, Zaborski, and Cleary 2002, 497).

Notes

1. The Picker Institute disbanded in 2001. Picker instruments are now marketed by National Research Corp., Lincoln, NE (http://www.nationalresearch.com).

2. The eight scales addressed self-perceived disease severity, patient evaluation of physician, evaluation of VA care, attitudes toward religion, satisfaction with decision making, perceived urgency of catheterization, vulnerability to catheterization, and bodily impact of catheterization.

3. Satisfaction with outpatient care was assessed in six domains: accessibility, physical environment, costs, interpersonal aspects of care, technical experience or skill, and overall satisfaction.

4. The Seattle Index of Co-morbidity contains the following items (weights are listed within parentheses): age in five-year intervals (1); prior myocardial infarction (1); lung disease (1); pneumonia (1); stroke (2); diabetes (2); cancer (2); CHF (2); past smoker (2); and current smoker (4) (Fan et al. 2002). The two outcomes of interest were all-cause, two-year mortality and hospitalization.

5. All states offer TTY services. The deaf or hard-of-hearing teletype user types a message to an operator who reads it aloud to the hearing caller; the operator then types the hearing caller's response, transmitting the written message back to the deaf or hard-of-hearing caller.

6. For many years, Medicare had adjusted capitated payments using the adjusted average per capita cost formula, accounting for residence county and age, sex, Medicaid status, and institutional and employment status—information readily available in Medicare's administrative databases (Greenwald et al. 1998). After the Balanced Budget Act, risk adjustment started first by using diagnosis codes from hospitalizations (i.e., PIP-DCGs; see Pope et al. 2002a). Eventually, diagnoses treated in all care settings will determine Medicare's risk-adjusted capitation payments.

CONCEPTUAL AND PRACTICAL ISSUES IN DEVELOPING RISK-ADJUSTMENT METHODS

Jennifer Daley, Lisa I. Iezzoni, and Michael Shwartz

Developing credible risk-adjustment methods is challenging, costly, and time consuming. We therefore typically recommend taking an existing method "off the shelf" if it suits the purpose. Even if existing measures do not perfectly match a project's context and goals, the trade-off may be worth it. The convenience of an existing risk-adjustment method may outweigh the many costs of developing and validating a new approach. When a method does not precisely fit a project's setting and purpose, results obviously must be interpreted cautiously, recognizing the conceptual mismatches. Nonetheless, the ready availability of existing methods—even when imperfect—is powerfully attractive, especially for projects seeking timely results.

Sometimes, however, existing methods are inadequate. As noted in Chapter 1, most widely used risk-adjustment methods aim to meet broad policy objectives, such as setting payment levels or comparing hospital-level mortality rates. Often, the target audiences for the risk-adjusted results are willing to tolerate certain limitations, such as minimal clinical detail. When the target audience is clinicians, however, clinical credibility becomes vitally important. Using clinically valid and transparent risk-adjustment methods is especially crucial when trying to motivate clinicians' behavior (e.g., in a quality-improvement project) or convince them about the merit of particular therapies (e.g., from observational studies). Furthermore, within very narrow or specific clinical settings, "generic" risk-adjustment methods intended for broad clinical use might fail to capture critical complexities. In these instances, developing a new risk-adjustment method may be necessary.

This chapter describes important considerations in developing risk-adjustment methods. Again, before starting, we emphasize the complexity of this undertaking. We urge potential users to consider existing methods or even modifying an existing method, such as recalibrating it to fit a particular database (see Chapter 10). For example, when applying the pneumonia severity index developed by Fine and colleagues (1993, 1995) to their own patient population, Flanders et al. (1999) discovered that the index predicted about 2.4 times more deaths than were actually observed. This finding was not surprising. When transporting statistically derived measures, such as the pneumonia severity index, to another data set, users should expect such discrepancies.

Fortunately, relatively straightforward analytical methods, such as imperfect calibration, exist to identify and fix problems (Justice, Covinsky, and Berlin 1999).[1]

We intend this chapter not only for persons developing risk-adjustment methods, but also for those seeking to understand the development process and the consequent strengths and limitations of a risk-adjustment method. The chapter addresses diverse issues, including specifying predictor variables, the role of clinical judgment, and empirical modeling techniques. We do not replicate detailed technical discussions (e.g., on multivariable modeling) available in statistical sources. Instead, we focus on issues particularly pertinent to creating risk adjusters.

To make this discussion real, we draw examples from existing severity measures, as well as the experiences of one author with developing two risk-adjustment methods. (For convenience throughout this chapter, we describe the activities of Dr. Daley and her colleagues using the first-person plural pronoun, but the other two coauthors of this chapter claim no credit for this extensive work!) The first was a medical-record-based method for risk adjusting Medicare beneficiaries' hospital mortality rates within four conditions (AMI, CHF, pneumonia, and stroke)—the Medicare Mortality Predictor System (MMPS; Daley et al. 1988). The second, larger study developed risk adjusters to identify adverse surgical outcomes for patients within VA hospitals. This project began as the National Veterans Affairs Surgical Risk Study within 44 VA medical centers (Khuri et al. 1995, 1997; Daley et al. 1997a, 1997b). Between 1 October 1991 and 31 December 1993, the study encompassed 87,078 major noncardiac operations.[2] The investigators used multivariable logistic regression to empirically derive risk adjusters predicting all-cause mortality and specific morbidities (complications) within 30 days after the index procedure for all operations and eight surgical subspecialties.

In 1994, the risk-adjustment techniques derived in the Surgical Risk Study became part of ongoing quality assessment activities within the VA—the NSQIP (Khuri et al. 1998; Daley, Henderson, and Khuri 2001). The NSQIP tracks all major operations within the 123 VA hospitals with surgical programs nationwide. Between 1991 and 2000, NSQIP accumulated data on more than 700,000 cases within nine surgical specialties (Daley, Henderson, and Khuri 2001, 282).[3] The data include more than 60 preoperative risk factors, 17 intraoperative characteristics, and 33 outcome variables. When the VA initiative began in 1991, trained nurses gathered the data by hand. Now, about one-third of the preoperative and most of the intraoperative variables are captured electronically by the VA's medical record system. Nurses continue to track or validate some preoperative variables, and they validate the intraoperative CPT-4 codes. Nurses also still do concurrent review and surveillance for the postoperative adverse events because they are consistently underreported or inaccurately classified in the records.

Getting Started

The first step in considering risk-adjustment involves answering four questions (see Chapter 2): Risk of what outcome? Over what time period? For what population? For what purpose (i.e., what is the goal of comparing risk-adjusted outcomes or producing risk-adjusted results)?

A reality of research is that projects can only study outcomes for which data are available. Studies have therefore generally concentrated on mortality, costs (or charges), use of specific procedures or services, complications or adverse events, and patient-reported satisfaction with care—a modest subset of the range of potentially important outcomes (see Chapter 2). Little is systematically recorded about patients' symptoms, functional status, quality of life, or whether care met patients' stated or implicit goals. This situation may change with the advent of electronic medical records, especially as patients themselves begin entering information into these files (see Chapter 6). As noted above, data collection for some NSQIP variables is largely electronic (e.g., laboratory data are automatically transmitted from each hospital's electronic laboratory system to the central NSQIP database).

Outcomes must be clearly and reliably defined. According to the NSQIP investigators, "Reliability is the most important prerequisite for the use of outcome data in the comparative assessment of the quality of care" (Khuri, Daley, and Henderson 1999, 123). In addition to tracking postoperative mortality, the NSQIP examines multiple morbidity outcomes, including superficial and deep wound infections, postoperative pneumonia, unplanned intubation, pulmonary embolism, acute renal failure, stroke, myocardial infarction, sepsis, coma, and bleeding more than four units of blood. Considerable efforts were expended on initially defining each of these outcomes so that data would be gathered reliably and consistently across institutions. Early on, some outcomes eluded clear, consistent definition and were therefore jettisoned (e.g., postoperative ileus, peripheral neurological injury). From a clinical perspective, each of the NSQIP morbidity outcomes could be expected to generate its own set of risk factors. For instance, even two similar outcomes—postoperative respiratory failure and postoperative pneumonia—yielded slightly different sets of risk adjusters from empirical modeling with NSQIP data. Important risk factors for respiratory failure included type of surgery, age, whether surgery was performed emergently, low albumin, high BUN, dependent functional status, and history of chronic obstructive pulmonary disease (Arozullah et al. 2000, 250). Pneumonia generated similar risk factors, but with notable variations (e.g., different ranges for BUN, surgical types) and some additional items, such as alcohol intake and blood transfusions (Arozullah et al. 2001).

The outcome must also be frequent enough for statistical modeling (see below). Even within a massive database such as the NSQIP file, some outcomes can be too rare to support separate risk-adjustment modeling. A good example is modeling postoperative mortality for transurethral prostatectomy and other urological procedures. Although NSQIP data contain more than 200,000 of these procedures, mortality is so low that stable models are impossible. Numbers plummet further when looking at individual hospitals' performance, the primary goal of NSQIP. Researchers often try various approaches for aggregating different outcomes into a single superoutcome measure. For instance, the NSQIP investigators considered several ways to combine 21 morbidity indicators, including the total number of morbidities reported, weights derived from regressing postoperative LOS on the 21 morbidities, and mean ratings by 44 chiefs of surgery, on a scale of 1 to 5, of the likelihood that the morbidity could cause death, disability, prolonged hospitalization, or patient dissatisfaction (Daley et al. 1997b; Gibbs et al. 1999). A simple summary measure—the presence or absence of one or more of the 21 morbidities—performed just as well in predicting postoperative LOS as the more complicated metrics.

Optimal assessment of the effectiveness of care requires investigation of various outcomes, positive and negative. Positive outcomes include amelioration of symptoms, improvement in functional status, prevention of death, and lower costs. Adverse outcomes include mortality, complications, lack of improvement or worsening functional status after surgery, dissatisfaction with care, and higher costs. Trade-offs among these outcomes may arise, especially when balancing clinical benefits and resource use. In some scenarios, better clinical outcomes (e.g., survival, functional ability) are possible but at a high price, such as lengthy stays in NICUs for low-birthweight newborns.

Because gathering data on risk factors can become expensive, an important question is whether a "minimum," or "core," set of risk factors can be used to adjust for risks of different outcomes, such as mortality, complications, and costs. Considerable research has assessed this hypothesis. Although important risk factors are often similar across different outcomes, relationships between these factors and particular outcomes (i.e., the "weights," the empirical parameter estimates) vary by outcome. One study used forward stepwise regression techniques to select the ten most statistically important MedisGroups KCFs to predict hospitalization costs and in-hospital death among patients at least 65 years of age (Iezzoni, Moskowitz, and Ash 1988, 119–20, 128–29). Results from three conditions suggest that the ten most important risk factors vary widely for predicting cost versus death (Table 8.1).

Examining outcomes is inherently a comparative exercise. What groups or "units" are compared depends on one's purpose and varies by context. Options include individual patients, individual providers, groups of providers (e.g., clinicians with capitated versus fee-for-service reimbursement), hospitals, groups of hospitals (e.g., teaching versus nonteaching facilities), or geographical areas (Whiting-O'Keefe, Henke, and Simborg 1984). These units are not mutually exclusive: Smaller units are often nested within larger units. As described in Chapter 12, the interrelationships among units of observation may demand special statistical techniques, such as hierarchical modeling.

TABLE 8.1

Top Ten Key Clinical Findings Entering Stepwise Regression Models to Predict Costs and In-Hospital Death for Three Conditions

	Stroke		Pneumonia		AMI	
Step	Cost	Death	Cost	Death	Cost	Death
1	Oxygenation	Coma	Oxygenation	BUN	CHF	Cardiac arrest
2	Lethargy	Respiratory rate	Hematocrit	Cardiac arrest	BUN	BUN
3	Creatinine	Cardiac arrest	Calcium	Systolic blood pressure	Cardiac arrest	Oxygenation
4	Myocardial ischemia	Stupor	Carbon dioxide	Arterial pH	Creatinine phosphokinase	Systolic blood pressure
5	Edema	Glucose	Calcium squared	Stupor	Positive sputum culture	Coma
6	Potassium	Pulse	Cardiac arrest	Respiratory rate	Cardiomegaly	Bundle branch block on ECG
7	Wheezing	BUN	Lethargy	Coma	Calcium	AMI on ECG
8	PTT	High-density brain mass	Premature ventricular contractions	Alkaline phosphatase	Potassium	Stupor
9	Calcium	Systolic blood pressure	Sodium	Pleural effusion	Pulse	Atrial flutter
10	AMI on ECG	History of diabetes	Blood in stool	Arterial pH squared	AMI on ECG	Positive sputum culture

NOTES: For physiological parameters that can have both high and low abnormal values, the value of the parameter squared as well as the raw value were entered into the model.

Units of analysis may also be defined by different time windows (see Chapter 4). The characteristics of the database may inherently constrain these time windows. For example, in most states, hospital discharge abstract data still cannot be linked at the person level (see Chapter 5). In this situation, the only available unit of analysis is the individual hospitalization. In databases with linked longitudinal information, the unit can be an individual patient observed during an episode of illness or over a set time period, such as a year.

Different risk-adjustment strategies have been developed for different units of observation. For example, the clinical criteria version of DS assigns a severity stage to each disease experienced by a patient. Thus, patients with several coexisting conditions could have multiple severity ratings (Gonnella, Hornbrook, and Louis 1984). Conceptually based on the four-level staging system for cancer, these DS severity levels are not equivalent across all diseases. For instance, stage 3.2 prostate cancer does not carry the same risk of short-term mortality as stage 3.2 pneumonia. This version of DS does not compute an overall severity score for the patient—diseases, not patients, are scored. Other versions of DS combine disease-specific information to generate overall scores for patients (see Chapter 2 tables).

The characteristics of the study population have implications for the risk-adjustment strategy (see Chapter 3). Research targeting one particular disease (e.g., diabetes) will not need to adjust for the presence of the disease, although one may wish to adjust for disease-specific severity (e.g., extent of end-organ damage, such as retinopathy, peripheral vascular disease, and renal insufficiency). The VA Surgical Risk Study population was 96.7 percent male (Daley et al. 1997b, 331); because of the large sample size, retaining women in the analytical database did not cause analytical problems.[4] As study populations expand (e.g., comparisons across states or regions), it becomes less necessary to adjust for risk factors that are likely to be distributed evenly across large populations (Gatsonis et al. 1995). One should probably always assume that patients admitted to different hospitals vary in a nonrandom fashion: Individual hospital populations, even for large academic medical centers, are too small to eschew risk adjustment when comparing their outcomes.

Whether risk adjustment should be condition specific or generic (diagnosis independent) depends on the context. As noted above, within the NSQIP, risk-adjustment methods differed even for such closely related outcomes as postoperative respiratory failure and pneumonia. With increasing sophistication in risk-adjustment methods and improvement in data quality, the recent trend has been toward developing disease-specific risk models. The evolution of APACHE is illustrative. Developed to predict the probability of in-hospital death for ICU patients, the original APACHE computed a generic score combining information about age, chronic diseases, and acute physiological parameters (Knaus et al. 1981). Because data did not yet exist, this initial APACHE relied largely on clinical judgment. Ten years later, with a database containing thousands of cases, the empirically derived APACHE III calculated the same score for any patient admitted to an ICU; however, the algorithm for predicting probability of in-hospital death with this score considered 78 disease groups (Knaus et al. 1991).

The VA Surgical Risk Study investigators collected identical risk factors across all surgical cases. In deriving their empirical risk-adjustment models, however, the researchers first created a generic version encompassing all operations, then separate models within each of the eight surgical specialties (ninth models cut across specialties). The investigators faced considerable challenges in interacting with their clinical colleagues. In the beginning, many surgeons and peer reviewers demanded procedure-specific models. Because postoperative mortality is relatively rare, developing stable models for most surgical procedures was not possible until adequate numbers of cases accrued. Even now, procedure-specific models are infeasible except for very prevalent operations with a relatively high mortality rate (e.g., abdominal aortic aneurysm repairs, partial colectomies). Modeling complications is often easier because they are more prevalent.

Finally, often the ultimate aim of risk-adjusted outcome analyses is to evaluate quality of care and motivate improvement (Chassin, Hannan, and DeBuono 1996). This motivation has important implications for risk-adjustment and the overall analytic strategy. Designing clinically credible, statistically robust risk-adjustment methods must recognize that the participating hospitals may vary widely in size and patient mixes. To motivate behavior change, all clinicians, not just those in large academic institutions, must feel comfortable with the methodology. Sometimes, hospital staffs that view themselves as treating a special mix of patients can derail an entire quality-improvement undertaking, as in the CHQC program described in Chapter 1.

Identifying Risk Factors

Sometimes, choices of risk factors are limited. When using administrative data, few options exist. Gathering additional information is generally infeasible unless one links the database to another administrative source (see Chapter 5). Since many administrative-data-based risk-adjustment methods exist, however, taking one off the shelf may be more appropriate than developing an entirely new method. Even if an existing method does not exactly suit the purpose, using components of these methods could prove useful. For example, the ACGs, CDPS, and DCGs (see Chapter 2) rate patients depending on their patterns of diagnosis codes; each method (and its software) groups ICD-9-CM diagnosis codes into clinically related categories. Using their own administrative databases, researchers could use these ICD-9-CM groupings to predict the target outcome. This strategy spares researchers from creating their own ICD-9-CM groupings, an arduous task.

Even with administrative data, however, it is essential to develop *a priori* clinical hypotheses about how potential risk factors relate to the outcome(s) of interest. Otherwise, empirical modeling to develop a risk adjuster could lapse into "data dredging"—allowing the computer to identify key risk factors and specify their relationship to the outcome (i.e., the coefficients or weights). Although data dredging can yield models with compelling p-values and strong performance metrics (e.g., R^2 values, c-statistics) in the developmental data set, dangers exist. These models may not validate well in other data sets (see Chapters 9 and 10), and they may lack clinical credibility: They can suggest relationships between risk factors and outcomes that do not make clinical sense. If clinicians do not believe in the risk-adjustment method, they are unlikely to trust the results.

Researchers can use several strategies to identify candidate risk factors and develop hypotheses about how each relates to the outcome(s) of interest. Published reports from randomized trials and other clinical studies may help. The clinical literature, however, is richer in some fields than in others. In particular, randomized trials are relatively limited—an explicit motivation for observational studies. RCTs generally provide little information about risk factors for predicting costs, functional status, and quality of life.

Another strategy is to ask clinical experts or panels of practicing clinicians. Clinical knowledge derived from patient care experience, as well as experts' syntheses of the literature, is critical for informing model development, as well as its ultimate acceptance. Involving clinicians in developing risk adjusters helps achieve essential clinical credibility. Individual interviews with clinical experts can also generate hypotheses about important risk factors. In developing the MMPS, we convened subspecialty physician panels and provided them with complete literature reviews concerning patient risk factors for 30-day mortality. We identified panelists based on recommendations from subspecialty societies and other major research projects concerning the four target diseases. In the Surgical Risk Study, we convened expert panels to identify patient risk factors for postoperative mortality and morbidity and to group similar surgical procedures according to likelihood of adverse outcomes. Chiefs of surgery at the participating hospitals became deeply involved in overseeing all aspects of risk adjustment and other methodological decisions.

The "herding cats" metaphor is used frequently to describe work with panels of expert clinicians, many of whom hold strong opinions, forcefully articulated. Nonetheless, their advice is invaluable and generally worth the effort. To identify candidate risk factors, expert panels must remain focused on the specific outcomes and time frames of the intended analysis. Frequent reminders to discriminate among specific risk factors relevant to different conditions or outcomes are important. For example, to determine a parsimonious set of risk factors for a planned chart-review tool, we asked MMPS panelists to suggest small numbers of risk factors predictive of mortality across all four conditions and to propose several condition-specific variables.

Researchers should ask clinical experts to specify exactly how candidate risk factors relate to the outcome(s) of interest. For instance, risk factors like body temperature are abnormal at both high and low levels: How, therefore, should temperature be entered into a statistical model? Having clinicians draw pictures or graphs clarifies these relationships. With increasing body temperature on the x-axis and increasing risk of death on the y-axis, the relationship between temperature and mortality risk forms roughly a U-shaped curve. This strategy worked well in developing the MMPS. Clinicians noted the critical importance of low body temperatures as well as fever in predicting the likelihood of imminent death in pneumonia. In the Surgical Risk Study, panels of clinicians reviewed all the candidate risk factors and drew sketches or graphs depicting the relationship between the continuous risk factors (e.g., laboratory variables, age) and the outcomes. This allowed them to succinctly summarize complex thinking (e.g., U-shaped curves suggest elevated risk at both high and low abnormal values).

Translating clinically important concepts into variables that can be measured reliably and validly using available data sources presents a significant challenge. The Surgical Risk Study began in 1991 after analyses of VA discharge abstract data and retrospective medical record reviews failed to provide findings with clinical credibility acceptable to surgeons practicing in VA facilities. Inconsistent coding across the 123 hospitals performing major surgery and the inability of discharge abstracts to distinguish preoperative from postoperative diagnoses compromised the utility of the VA discharge abstract database, the PTF (see Chapter 5). Retrospective chart review of six major surgical operations in a sample of VA medical centers demonstrated poor interrater reliability; in addition, important risk factors were missing from the charts.

The VA and its surgeons decided that the only way to ensure reliability, validity, and clinical credibility was to have trained nurse reviewers concurrently gather data on major surgery patients during their hospital stays. Project staff places the definitions and variable names in the charts of each surgical patient, and staff orients all attending surgeons and surgical residents to the data-collection procedures at each institution. Data gathering is prospective, although every patient need not have all relevant risk factors measured. Although all preoperative and intraoperative risk factors could probably come from electronic sources, we learned that a human being must survey, identify, and correctly classify the adverse postoperative events in a reliable way across institutions. The VA deemed that the direct costs of prospective data collection, analysis, and reporting—then about $50 per case—were worthwhile to produce comparative information across hospitals that chiefs of surgery would believe.

The eventual implementation of a systemwide computerized information system, the Decentralized Hospital Computer Plan, to all VA hospitals facilitated electronic data collection and transmittal and fostered communication among sites nationwide. The NSQIP Surgical Package of the Decentralized Hospital Computer Plan (now called VISTA) captures required data elements and permits range checks, verification, and reporting of surgical volume, risk assessment, and operative information at each site. In 1998, NSQIP reportedly cost $38 for each major surgery assessed by the program, or $4 million across the VA system (Khuri et al. 1998, 499).

Researchers may not appreciate fully the challenges of gathering risk-factor data until they try it. For studies using retrospective record reviews, especially of paper or electronic narrative records, researchers should first examine five to ten charts to determine their level of detail and completeness. Prospective data collection, although generally more reliable and valid, also requires pretesting of data-collection procedures and protocols. In the Surgical Risk Study, pilot data collection of wound, blood, sputum, and urine culture bacteriology results revealed wide variations across hospitals in how they reported culture results. This variability precluded collecting these data even prospectively, although now these data can be downloaded electronically from VISTA. Thus, institutional differences in how standard tests are handled may compromise their use in multicenter projects.

Lack of standardization among common diagnostic procedures can become problematic. In developing the MMPS pneumonia models, clinical experts suggested that the number of lobes showing an infiltrate on a chest radiograph is a risk factor for imminent death. We were unable to collect this information routinely from the chest x-ray reports for two reasons. First, among this sick elderly population, many chest radiographs were portable anteroposterior films in which the number of lobes could not be assessed. Second, even among those patients with posteroanterior and lateral films, the radiologists' readings rarely noted the number of lobes involved with pneumonia. Although the patients' physicians may have known the number of lobes involved by physical examination or through their reviews of the radiographs, we could not obtain this information on retrospective chart review.

In the Surgical Risk Study, we restricted patient risk factors to those typically recorded in routine preoperative assessments and laboratory evaluations. As in developing MMPS, a six-hospital pilot study confirmed that ECG results were too time consuming to collect. Laboratory values were collected through software programs that automatically scan laboratory databases in each hospital and transmit the information for analysis. In such a large-scale observational study, we avoided using certain cardiac, pulmonary, or vascular test results as candidate risk factors for several reasons: high rates of missing values (i.e., a small fraction of patients have these tests), inconsistent interpretation of results across facilities, and unacceptable data-collection burden.

Finally, risk factors should reflect only patient attributes, not some component of processes of care, such as performance of a diagnostic test (see Chapter 6). This issue, however, highlights the complex trade-offs in designing operational risk-adjustment methods: Researchers may balance conceptual purity against practical results. For example, the VA chiefs of surgery believed strongly that surgical type and emergency status must be considered when assessing patients' risks for mortality or morbidity. The surgeons themselves invested considerable effort in quantifying surgical complexity (Khuri et al. 1997, 317):

> To account for differences in the complexity of operations performed between medical centers, groups of subspecialists were asked to rank the complexity of each index operation in their subspecialty *above and beyond the risk factors that patients would typically bring to the operation* [italics added], on a scale of 1 to 5. The average score for each index operation, identified by CPT-4 code, was used as a measure of the complexity of that operation.

Across the NSQIP database, the "operation complexity score" was the eleventh most important predictor of mortality and the third most important predictor of morbidity; "emergency operation" was the fourth most important predictor for both outcomes (Khuri et al. 1998, 499). Other NSQIP risk factors, such as steroid use, blood transfusion, and ventilator dependence, also carry treatment connotations. ASA class, which is a subjective decision by the anesthesiologist, is another example.

Using risk factors related to processes of care could particularly confound comparisons by hospital teaching status and size. Not surprisingly, VA teaching hospitals see patients with statistically significantly higher operation complexity scores than do VA nonteaching hospitals (Khuri et al. 2001, 373). Teaching-hospital patients generally had much higher rates of serious risk factors than did those at nonteaching hospitals. After risk adjustment, 30-day postoperative mortality rates did not vary across teaching and nonteaching hospitals. Risk-adjusted 30-day morbidity rates were significantly higher at teaching than nonteaching hospitals for patients undergoing general surgery, orthopedic, urology, and vascular surgery operations. In contrast, a study of eight common surgeries found no relationship between risk-adjusted 30-day mortality by hospital volume (Khuri et al. 1999, 418).

Timing of Risk Factors

The NSQIP primarily focuses on improving surgical outcomes within the VA. As noted above, to isolate that elusive quantity, quality of care, the NSQIP predictive models of 30-day postoperative mortality and morbidity control only for preoperative findings. If intraoperative or postoperative factors were incorporated, results would be confounded by processes of care, and thus, quality. However, when evaluating postoperative LOS, the NSQIP researchers considered a range of factors from the entire hospitalization. For major elective surgery, the following risk factors were generally important for predicting postoperative LOS: older age; nonwhite race; ASA class 3; partially dependent functional status; intraoperative blood transfusion; operative time of three or more hours; postoperative urinary tract infection, ileus, or pneumonia; return to the operating room; and complication counts of two or three or more (Collins et al. 1999, 254). The researchers concluded, "Although preoperative factors were independently associated with a prolonged LOS, the factors generating the highest risks for a prolonged LOS were the intraoperative processes of care and postoperative adverse events" (Collins et al. 1999, 251).

A related topic involves when to measure pertinent risk factors. For example, APACHE (Knaus et al. 1985, 1991) aims to predict in-hospital death. Because most physiological parameters are measured repeatedly in ICUs, numerous values for APACHE's risk factors are typically available. Which values of these physiological parameters should be used for risk adjustment? The first? The worst over some time period? What time period?

The answer to this question depends on the context (see Chapter 4). Nonetheless, the decision holds implications for data collection. Although APACHE's developers recommended using the most abnormal value in the first day of ICU treatment, studies of cases at their own institution showed that in 88 percent of the physiological measurements, the worst value was that observed on ICU admission (Knaus et al. 1985, 825). Depending on the time interval considered, worst values might reflect the results of therapeutic or diagnostic mishaps. For example, blood pressure may become further deranged from its admission value because of incorrect therapeutic decisions. In addition, during manual record reviews, identifying the first value is easier than finding the worst value: Reviewers require less training, and data abstraction reliability is thus probably higher. Extensive analyses by APACHE's developers showed no significant difference in APACHE risk models based on physiological parameters collected initially and those gathered within the first 24 hours. However, calculating APACHE prognostic estimates daily during an ICU stay usefully tracks patients' clinical trajectories, differentiating patients who are improving from those who are worsening (Wagner et al. 1994). Electronic availability of risk factor information should facilitate the use of values from different time periods.

In the Surgical Risk Study, we assessed risk using 65 factors measured prior to surgery. Preoperative risk variables were captured as closely as possible to when patients entered the operating room, but we used some information from up to 14 days prior to surgery. Longer preoperative windows are especially common for low-risk, elective surgeries. For example, while we wanted the most recent hematocrit and white blood cell count values, we needed to accommodate elective surgery; patients underwent ambulatory preoperative clearance sometimes up to two weeks prior to their operations.

The longer the period from which data are collected, the greater the possibility of confounding the quality of care with patient risk before treatment. If the time period is too short, however, levels of missing information may be unacceptably high. One study to predict in-hospital mortality at a tertiary teaching hospital used information from a computerized repository of all laboratory test results obtained on hospitalized patients (Davis et al. 1995). To avoid confounding quality with patients' risk factors, the researchers initially intended to include only laboratory values from the first 12 hours of the hospital stay: Certainly the house staff thoroughly worked up patients immediately upon admission at their facility! However, to their surprise, they needed to expand the time window to the first 48 hours of hospitalization. Otherwise, too many values were missing, even for routine laboratory tests. Shortening hospital LOS may change timing of testing and the availability of certain test results during the hospitalization.

Other Feasibility Considerations

Some variables are such important risk factors that one may reasonably devote considerable time and effort to collecting them. In contrast, marginally useful risk factors may not be worth expending energy to collect. In developing the MMPS, we conducted feasibility studies to determine the most reliable sources of risk information in the chart, which led to a hierarchy specifying where data abstractors should obtain particular pieces of information. Because we sought the first values of vital signs obtained in the hospital, for example, we focused on emergency room information first and then reviewed the initial admission history and physical. We then examined all progress notes in the first 24 hours.

In teaching hospitals, we abstracted information from the attending physician, resident, intern, and medical student—in that order.

We also collected variables that we considered important but difficult to abstract: functional status and DNR status. Functional status information was available in only two-thirds of the charts and was rarely noted by the physicians (even now, functional information is rarely available in acute care hospital records; see Chapter 6). The initial nursing admission note, however, often contained basic information about patients' capacity to ambulate and feed themselves. We therefore used nurses' notes as the source of functional status information. We collected DNR status only if present on admission. DNR status usually appeared on both the emergency room admitting sheet and in the admitting orders, but it was designated very differently across institutions (e.g., DNR, do not resuscitate, care and comfort only, no code 99, no code blue). Therefore, we specified synonyms that qualified as DNR orders.

As suggested above, prospective data collection can solve some problems relating to variable definition, standardization, reliability, and validity. Data-collection instruments and guidelines are written in advance, and data collectors are taught and tested during a training period. Pilot tests of data-collection procedures can determine the feasibility of collecting specific data elements.[5] Certain important risk factors involve sensitive information that is difficult to obtain reliably regardless of how data are gathered. For example, although sexual behaviors and use of illicit drugs are associated with selected outcomes, this type of sensitive information is often underreported in medical records (see Chapter 6). In prospective data gathering, respondents often refuse to answer, lie, or are so offended by being asked such personal information that they refuse to answer subsequent questions.

Building the Risk-Adjustment Model

For building risk-adjustment models, experience has convinced most researchers that combining clinical judgment and empirical modeling is better than either approach alone. Different risk-adjustment methods have emphasized different development approaches, generally depending on whether large data sets are available for empirical modeling. Especially in the late 1970s and early 1980s, few large data sets, even administrative files, were available. Methods dating from that era often relied primarily on the normative judgment of expert clinicians with limited empirical testing.[6] Nowadays, the widespread availability of large electronic files, even those containing extensive clinical information, offers new opportunities for deriving both clinically credible and statistically rigorous risk-adjustment methods. Nonetheless, as noted above, this abundance of data poses a strong temptation for data dredging—a poor strategy for developing valid risk adjusters.

Clinicians can help identify candidate risk factors and hypothesize about their relationships to the outcome(s) of interest. Without empirical input clinicians are generally unable to quantify precisely the effects of risk factors, but statistical methods alone can yield clinically suspect results. In the Surgical Risk Study, one clinical variable—smoking in the two weeks prior to major surgery—demonstrated an unexpected statistical relationship to mortality. Patients who reported not smoking in the two weeks prior to surgery had much higher mortality rates than those who did report smoking, a relationship opposite of the one predicted. We therefore examined other risk factors of nonsmokers compared to smokers and discovered that nonsmokers had much higher risk profiles (i.e., more diabetes mellitus, ischemic heart disease, chronic pulmonary disease) than those reporting smoking in the two weeks prior to surgery. Contrary to our initial hypothesis, nonsmokers appeared very sick, perhaps unable physically to smoke in the two weeks preoperative. We did not include this smoking variable in our final risk-adjustment models. We now determine smoking status by asking whether patients smoked in the year prior to surgery and how many pack-years they have smoked.

Assembling an Analytic Data Set

Unless it is based solely on clinical judgment, developing a model of risk requires a data set. Before beginning analyses, data often require "cleaning." Standard data cleaning involves range checks (e.g., looking for values that are not plausible, such as centigrade temperatures of 102°), identifying impossible occurrences (e.g., female patients admitted for prostate surgery), finding invalid data elements (e.g., ICD-9-CM codes that have no meaning in the current version of the coding system), and describing the frequencies of missing or poorly specified data elements (e.g., the frequency of missing values for liver function tests in patients undergoing cholecystectomy). Multivariate checks should also be analyzed: Is the systolic blood pressure always higher than the diastolic blood pressure? Is the most extreme or worst value during the first 24 hours of admission always higher or lower than the first recorded value of risk variable X? Analysts acquire a valuable in-depth knowledge of their data sets through this process.

How much a raw data file needs cleaning and editing depends on the source of the data. In general, more cleaning is needed when the data have not been used before for a similar purpose. Some analysts obtain administrative data files that have already gone through extensive data checks (e.g., by the state agency that compiled the data). For example, one study (Iezzoni et al. 1994a) used the 1988 statewide computerized hospital discharge abstract data set obtained from the California Office of Statewide Health Planning and Development and found that the following key data elements were missing or invalid less than 0.001 percent of the time: age, sex, discharge disposition (e.g., death), and principal diagnosis (no cases were missing principal diagnoses). The state had performed routine editing before releasing the data.

If the data were entered using computer software that includes internal range checks, implausible values may have been rejected as the data were gathered. In developing MMPS, we created data-entry computer software that has internal data consistency checks and ranges of permissible values, thus preventing the entry of illogical or invalid values for many parameters. Some data files from chart review or prospective data collection may require considerable data cleaning. When data are acquired from external sources, clarifying variable definitions, coding conventions, missing data, and organization of the data set is often necessary. Clinical consultants may especially assist this process. For example, clinicians can specify ranges for clinical variables that are physiologically impossible and therefore represent data errors.

Treatment of Missing Values

In most data sets, values of some variables are missing. This problem is encountered most frequently in data collected from retrospective medical record reviews, but it also occurs in administrative databases and even with information that is gathered prospectively (Marshall et al. 1995). This problem invariably raises questions about how to handle missing information. The literature on severity measures addresses missing data concerns most commonly in the context of acute physiological parameters (see Chapter 2). These variables are typically clinical guideposts for physicians caring for acutely ill patients, and most (e.g., vital signs, complete blood counts, serum chemistries) are measured routinely and with minimal technological intervention (e.g., venipuncture). One reason that certain variables were eliminated in creating APACHE II was that they were measured infrequently (e.g., serum osmolarity, lactic acid level, skin testing for anergy), whereas others reflected a treatment decision (e.g., right atrial pressure measured through a central venous pressure line). Fortunately, the remaining variables—albeit generally available and easily measured—yielded good ability to predict in-hospital death (Knaus et al. 1985).

Given that most of these physiological parameters are measured routinely, how should one interpret missing data? *A priori*, this question has no correct response; it must be answered in both the research and clinical contexts. For example, APACHE assumes that unmeasured parameters are likely to be normal. This assumption is reasonable, as APACHE pertains explicitly to ICU patients who are generally aggressively treated and monitored. The MMPS also substitutes normal values for missing values; our analyses suggested that this choice maximizes predictive accuracy and reliability (Daley et al. 1988).

The approach toward missing values, however, may differ in other clinical contexts. For instance, gravely ill patients, such as those with widely metastatic cancer, may explicitly refuse even routine monitoring by blood tests—accepting so-called "comfort measures only" (e.g., intravenous morphine for pain control). In this setting, absence of information about serum electrolytes or hematological indices reflects patient preferences, not physiological status. In still other clinical contexts, missing data result when patients die before tests can be performed, which may explain Blumberg's findings (1991) that AMI patients with missing laboratory values were more likely to die within 30 days of admission than were patients with complete information on routine tests.

Depending on the database used to assess acute physiological parameters, two further explanations for missing values require consideration. As discussed in Chapter 6, practice patterns vary even for collecting routine physiological information (Selker 1993). For example, in a study of 15 metropolitan Boston hospitals (Iezzoni et al. 1989), important differences were apparent in even routine testing across teaching and nonteaching hospitals. Another source of missing data can be the specific data-collection protocol, such as that used in an older version of MedisGroups: Reviewers were instructed not to record values of clinical findings if they were in a "normal" range. Although this strategy aimed to facilitate the abstraction of literally hundreds of data elements, it had potentially problematic results: (1) when KCFs were missing, analysts could not determine whether the test was not performed or whether its result was normal and (2) because the normal ranges were very broad (e.g., systolic blood pressures were recorded only if <90 mm Hg), many cases had missing values (Iezzoni et al. 1993). Later versions of MedisGroups gathered all values, not just those outside the defined normal ranges. Downloading these data directly from computerized laboratory information systems increases the feasibility—and decreases the costs—of gathering all laboratory values.

Some information is frequently missing but has important predictive value as a risk factor. For instance, in the MMPS data set, only two-thirds of the patients had a simple measure of functional status (ability to ambulate independently) recorded in their charts, usually in the nursing notes (Daley et al. 1988). Our analyses included this variable; it proved a significant predictor in some models. We assumed that the absence of functional-status information implied full ability to ambulate independently and substituted "fully independent" for the missing values.

In addition to the clinical and data-collection implications of missing values, the way missing values are handled may dictate how many cases will be available for analysis using some modeling techniques. For example, many computerized statistical routines drop cases with any missing value among any of the variables in the model. Even if each variable is missing for only a few cases, many cases will have at least one missing value if numerous variables are considered. Thus, many cases could be eliminated during statistical modeling in data sets with numerous missing values. This situation may bias the models toward characteristics of that subset of patients with complete data—patients who are unlikely to be a random sample. In addition, when examining two models—one with few explanatory variables and a second with many—the second model may actually be fit to a much smaller data set (i.e., the subset of patients without any missing values). This argues for using the same standard data set when comparing models built with different variables.

Given the potential confounding of patient risk with data quality, availability, and practice patterns, how one treats missing data assumes some significance. In some contexts, it is very reasonable to substitute normal values for missing values of clinical measurements under the assumption that abnormalities would be recorded in the medical record. We used this approach in devising the MMPS, justifying this decision by observing that "studies . . . on other data sets indicate that this rule maximizes predictive accuracy and replicability" (Daley et al. 1988, 3620). This is an example of a more general approach called "single imputation," that is, substituting a single replacement value for a missing value. For variables for which there is no natural normal value (e.g., education), the substituted value might be the mean of the observed values for all people or certain subsets of people with similar characteristics to those whose values are being imputed (which might be estimated using a regression model). A problem with single imputation is that, if standard analyses are performed on the data set without explicitly taking into account the increased uncertainty introduced by using imputed values, standard errors associated with estimates from the data set will be too small.

Multiple imputation deals with problems associated with single imputation (Rubin 1987; Little and Rubin 1987; Schafer 1997; Shafer [1999] and particularly Patrician [2002] provide less-technical descriptions). Multiple imputation replaces each missing value with a set of m > 1 plausible values drawn from a probability distribution of the missing value. The result is m complete data sets (usually three to five imputated data sets are sufficient), which are then analyzed in the standard way. The variation among the m data sets reflects the uncertainty with which missing values can be predicted from observed ones (Schafer and Olsen 1998). Rubin (1987) shows how to combine results from the m data sets to obtain overall estimates and standard errors.

Only recently has computer software become available for easily determining from observed values the probability distribution from which imputed values are selected. Two web sites discuss some of these programs (http://stat.psu,edu/~jls and http://www.herc.research.med.va.gov/FAQ_19.htm). SOLAS, developed in collaboration with Rubin (http://www.statsol.ie/solas/solas.htm), was one of the first programs to facilitate use of multiple imputation. Both SAS and SPSS now have procedures for performing multiple imputation, which are likely to significantly increase the use of this approach for dealing with missing data.

In the national VA Surgical Risk Study, all patient preoperative risk factors were more than 99 percent complete, except the preoperative laboratory values. Most of the preoperative laboratory variables (e.g., complete blood count, serum sodium, BUN) were more than 95 percent complete, but a handful of preoperative laboratory values (serum albumin, serum bilirubin, SGOT) were missing in a substantial minority of cases (e.g., serum albumin was missing for 39 percent of cases). Analyses demonstrated that patients with missing albumin and liver function tests were less sick (i.e., lower incidence of other risk factors) and had lower mortality and morbidity and shorter LOS than those patients with values for those laboratory tests. Extensive analyses compared incorporating imputed missing values using a regression procedure with substituting a normal value for each missing laboratory variable. These comparisons found similar results for the two approaches.

In certain contexts, especially regions with aggressive "report card" initiatives (see Chapter 11), how missing values are handled could have practical consequences. If missing values are assumed to be normal, clinicians will learn that, to have their patients classified as "sick," they must record the problems they find. This could affect testing practices, for example, increasing laboratory testing even when clinical suspicions of an abnormal result are low.

Structure of Continuous Independent Variables

Exploring the effect of the form of each risk factor—whether it is entered into the model as a categorical or continuous independent variable—is important. The most common continuous risk factor, age (see Chapter 2), is a case in point. The relationship of age to outcomes (e.g., in-hospital mortality, LOS, charges) is unlikely to follow a simple straight line, especially over a wide age range. Age can be treated as a continuously valued variable or categorized into two or more groups. For example, as described in Chapter 2, PRISM weights physiological values differently for two age levels, infants and children, thus incorporating an interaction between age and physiological status (Pollack, Ruttimann, and Getson 1988). APACHE III assigns points for patients in different age categories (Knaus et al. 1991). Different risk-adjustment measures use different ways of weighting age with regard to outcomes.

Other clinical variables, such as blood pressure and temperature, have complex relationships to various outcomes, including death. For instance, the very high and low extremes of blood pressure are associated with increased likelihood of imminent death as compared to the middle or normal ranges. However, although high blood pressure is a risk factor for long-term mortality, it may not be highly predictive of 30-day mortality; low blood pressure is associated with short-term mortality (see, e.g., Lemeshow et al. 1985). U-shaped relationships with mortality may not be symmetrical for high and low values of some variables. For instance, the likelihood of death may be much higher for incremental decreases in temperature and blood pressure than for similar incremental increases above normal values. In pneumonia, for example, we modified the APACHE II scoring system for the MMPS to account for the much increased likelihood of death in the Medicare elderly presenting with very low body temperatures (Daley et al. 1988).

Most clinical variables have a nonlinear relationship with the outcome. In general, clinical judgment combined with statistical analyses is used to determine ranges for continuous variables and relationships with the outcome within these ranges. Computer-based "smoothing techniques" can help delineate these relationships. For example, Le Gall, Lemeshow, and Saulnier (1993) used the LOWESS (locally weighted least squares) smoothing function (Cleveland 1979) to produce a smoothed plot of the relationship between outcomes and candidate independent variables. "Cutpoints" in the smoothed function (points where a large change in outcome occurs for small changes in independent variables) can be used to define categories of independent variables, which are then represented in the final model by dummy variables. Cubic splines (Harrell, Lee, and Pollock 1988) are also used to produce smoothed functions. For example, in developing APACHE III, Knaus et al. (1991, 1632) did the following:

> The physiologic variables were divided into clinically appropriate ranges based partly on cell size and partly on clinical judgment. They were then incorporated into the analysis as a series of separate predictor variables for each range. The initial results from these analyses were compared with basic clinical and physiologic relationships. Where discrepancies existed . . . we adjusted the ranges. Most of these variations were due to small sample sizes in the original designated ranges. In a few cases where the results of the analyses remained incompatible with established physiologic patterns, we adjusted the estimated weights using clinical judgment. Patterns of weights were also checked using restricted cubic splines functions. Cubic splines is a statistical smoothing technique that allows assignment of a continuous varying weight to a physiologic variable. . . . In this data base, however, the use of cubic splines did not substantially increase total explanatory power.

In the VA Surgical Risk Study, panels of clinicians were asked to sketch the relationship between the outcomes of interest and the continuous variables of age and preoperative laboratory tests. Age and serum albumin, empirically and by clinical judgment, demonstrated a linear relationship to the outcomes. Actually, albumin produces a flat relationship when greater than 3.5, but below 3.5 the relationship is an exponential function. Age is linear in all the models. Selected laboratory variables (e.g., serum sodium, serum potassium, white blood cell count) demonstrated a U-shaped relationship to the outcomes and were trichotomized for the final analyses (i.e., serum sodium < 136 mEq/mL, serum sodium > 148 mEq/mL, and a reference group of serum sodium > 136 mEq/mL and < 148 mEq/mL).

A continuous variable that often appears in many disease-specific mortality prediction models is the serum BUN. In healthy patients, BUN ranges from 2 to 20 mg/dL, but in patients with multiple cardiac, renal, and metabolic abnormalities, BUN may rise to 500 mg/dL. In the MMPS, BUN was transformed and standardized to values greater than 40 mg/dL, and a continuous function of BUN above 40 mg/dL was constructed. In the VA Surgical

Risk Study, a similar relationship was found, and BUN greater than 40 mg/dL was used in all of the risk models.

Need for Data Reduction

Despite the many data limitations described in Chapters 3 and 4, much useful information is nonetheless available for deriving risk-adjustment models. The quantity of information can be overwhelming, and researchers are likely to need to reduce the data set to a reasonable number of potential risk factors for modeling.

An example of the potential perils of incorporating too many predictors was demonstrated by a study that modeled in-hospital mortality for 16,855 patients 65 years of age or older discharged from 24 MedisGroups member hospitals (Iezzoni et al. 1992c). Several risk models were examined (Table 8.2). The first model was the five-level old admission MedisGroups score (a categorical variable with values from 0 through 4). The second and third models used KCFs specified within each condition to derive empirically a model for predicting in-hospital death. From the more than 500 potential KCFs contained in that early version of MedisGroups, the investigators identified, for each condition, those KCFs that were present in at least 1 percent of the cases or that were viewed clinically as important predictors of death (e.g., ventricular fibrillation). Between 40 and 65 KCFs were identified in each of the five conditions. The second model allowed the first ten KCFs to enter a stepwise regression following age and sex within each condition. The third model used all 40 to 65 KCFs plus age and sex within each condition.

The R^2 statistic from an ordinary least squares regression was used to compare the utility of different models in predicting death (see Chapter 10). R^2 values were first computed on half of the data used to derive the model, then validated on the remaining half. The two empirically derived models had the best fits (i.e., highest R^2 values). Although the model with all KCFs fit the development data somewhat better than the model using only ten KCFs, its cross-validated performance was never superior to that of the ten-KCFs model. In lung cancer (total $n = 1,244$; 23.9 percent in-hospital deaths), the drop for the all-KCF model from the fitting R^2 value (0.344) to the cross-validated value (0.054) was particularly striking. Thus, although the models with 40 or more explanatory variables each achieved the highest R^2 values, these models appeared to have been overspecified: In the cross-validation analyses, they performed no better, and in one instance did far worse, than the models based on the ten most important clinical variables (Iezzoni et al. 1992c).

A variety of approaches are available to trim the number of predictor variables prior to modeling. For example, as in the study described above, inspection of the frequency distributions of the variables may reveal items that appear too infrequently to be retained in the analysis. Removing variables that are of suspicious quality or poor reliability is prudent, apart from statistical concerns. Examining univariate associations between individual predictors and

Condition	Sample Used for Model Performance	Model Performance (R^2)		
		Admission MedisGroups Score	Top Ten KCFs	All KCFs
Stroke	Fitting	0.122	0.299	0.330
	Cross-validating	0.096	0.233	0.208
Lung cancer	Fitting	0.049	0.280	0.344
	Cross-validating	0.058	0.242	0.054
Pneumonia	Fitting	0.137	0.247	0.278
	Cross-validating	0.154	0.243	0.240
AMI	Fitting	0.204	0.243	0.276
	Cross-validating	0.195	0.180	0.157
CHF	Fitting	0.069	0.208	0.234
	Cross-validating	0.075	0.196	0.196
All cases	Fitting	0.134	0.260	0.293
	Cross-validating	0.133	0.225	0.195

SOURCE: Iezzoni et al. (1992c).

TABLE 8.2
Fitting and Cross-Validating Model Performance in Predicting In-Hospital Mortality (R^2)

the outcomes is a common approach. Model development then employs only those factors that are statistically significant at a prespecified level (e.g., $p \leq 0.10$).

Another example using MedisGroups, with its dozens of KCFs as potential explanatory variables, illustrates the approach of starting with univariate analyses. Van Ruiswyk and colleagues (1993) employed these MedisGroups KCF data to develop a model to predict 30-day mortality for AMI patients. Chi square tests were used to identify individual predictors of 30-day mortality. However, "When several univariate predictors represented the same physiologic abnormality, a composite variable was formed that indicated an abnormality in any of the findings" (Van Ruiswyk et al. 1993, 154). After eliminating variables that revealed abnormalities in fewer than 0.5 percent of the sample, the remaining univariate predictors were entered into a backward stepwise logistic regression to create an empirical model of risk (see below).

Two distinct concerns arise when using rare risk factors as predictors. One is that too few cases are present in the model development data set to assess accurately the association between the rare risk factor and the outcome. For example, with 3,000 cases for modeling, a risk factor present in fewer than 0.5 percent of the cases occurs fewer than 15 times. This problem is minimized by a sufficiently large data set for model fitting. The other problem is practical. If data are gathered through chart review, do we want to expend costly effort finding rare risk factors? The answer may be yes in three instances: First, the rare risk factor is strongly associated with the outcome; second, it independently predicts the outcome even after other variables are included in the model; and third, clinicians feel that failure to include it either substantially reduces the model's clinical credibility or penalizes certain providers who see a disproportionate number of rare cases.

As suggested earlier, statistically significant univariate associations between risk factors and outcomes that appear opposite to the clinically hypothesized relationships must be carefully reviewed. They may reveal problems with the original data sources, database itself, or coding of the independent variables. A variety of computer-intensive approaches are increasingly used to identify important variables to include in models. Normand and colleagues (1996) used such an approach to identify candidate variables for a logistic regression model predicting 30-day postadmission mortality of AMI patients. From an initial sample of 14,581 patients, three 25 percent subsamples of patients were selected. For each of the three subsamples, 20 "random starting models" were identified. In each of the 60 models (3 subsamples times 20 starting models), four clinical variables closely related to left ventricular ejection fraction were forced into the model. Using a stepwise procedure, other statistically significant independent variables were stepped into the model. For each of the three subsamples, the model with the best fit among the 20 random starting models (measured by the likelihood estimate) was selected. The set of variables from these three "best-fit" models then became candidate variables for further regression models.

Similarly, Hornbrook and Goodman (1996) used a computer-intensive approach to analyze the importance of self-reported illness, functional status, perceived health status, and demographic characteristics in predicting annual HMO expenses. They made 25 random splits of the overall database. For each split, they used half of the data for model development and the other half for model validation (see Chapter 6). Thus, they produced 25 multiple regression models. The sign and statistical significance of the coefficients, as well as variance across the 25 replications, were examined. Conclusions about the predictive role of specific variables were viewed as more reliable when their coefficients consistently had the same sign, consistent statistical significance, and low variance across the 25 replications.

There are formal analytical techniques for data reduction, such as cluster analysis and factor analysis. However, these have rarely been used in building risk-adjustment models in part because clinical interpretation of the composite measures is difficult. As discussed earlier, if clinicians do not feel comfortable with the resulting models, much of their value is lost.

Multivariable Modeling Techniques

Detailed descriptions of multivariable modeling techniques, their underlying assumptions, strengths and weaknesses, and appropriate diagnostic measures are beyond the scope of this volume. Readers are referred to standard texts of statistical methods for detailed discussion of approaches for building multivariable models. In large part, the availability of clinical knowledge about the relationship of independent variables to outcomes is the main factor that distinguishes risk-adjustment modeling from general multivariable modeling.

In Chapter 10, we discuss two main types of multivariable models used in risk adjustment: multiple regression models, when the outcome is continuous; and logistic regression models, when the outcome is dichotomous. In Chapter 11, we briefly discuss proportional hazard models, when the outcome is time to an event, such as death. Researchers have evaluated a variety of alternative modeling approaches, particularly for dichotomous outcomes. However, logistic regression models have been shown to perform well compared to these alternatives (Marshall et al. 1994; Selker et al. 1995; Hadorn et al. 1992).

For the three types of models, stepwise procedures are usually used to build the models. Briefly, forward stepwise regression procedures build the model by adding one variable at a time. At each stage, the variable added is the one that contributes the most to model fit at that step. The backward elimination approach begins with all variables in the model and then, one by one, eliminates those variables that contribute the least to model fit. Using each technique, options allow variables previously added to be dropped (forward elimination) or variables previously dropped to be added (backward selection). In addition, some "stopping rule" is necessary. Usually modeling is considered complete when the variables added to the model are statistically significant at a $p \leq 0.05$ or 0.10 level (or those dropped are insignificant at one of these levels).

Harrell and colleagues (1984) performed simulations demonstrating that, if logistic regression models are built on data sets with fewer than 1,000 observations, significant deterioration of the c-statistic (see Chapter 10) can occur on model validation for models developed using stepwise procedures. With a dichotomous outcome such as mortality, the number of cases in the smaller of the two groups (i.e., those with or without the outcome) is usually the limiting factor. The work of Harrell and colleagues (1984) suggests that first clustering the variables and then developing indices from each cluster (using all the variables, a subset of variables, or both) performs better than traditional stepwise procedures. Most severity models have been developed on large data sets with well over 2,000 cases, where stepwise procedures seem to validate as well as other approaches.

A major challenge in developing a model is to identify important interactions, or nonadditive effects, among predictor variables. Even when a moderate number of predictors are under consideration, there are generally far too many possible interactions to use unguided statistical exploration to detect the important interactions. For example, ten predictors generate 45 possible paired interactions and 120 three-way interactions. Knaus and colleagues (1991) used logistic regression results plus clinical judgment to study interactions among physiological variables in APACHE III, evaluating both individual and combined weighting of variables. An important example involved the variables reflecting clinical acid-base disturbances (i.e., serum pH, pCO_2, and bicarbonate). Using their database including more than 17,000 ICU admissions, Knaus and colleagues (1991, 1621) found empirical relationships incompatible with established physiological principles:

> The computer-derived weights for serum pCO_2 above 50 mm Hg were consistently estimated as having little or no significant relationship to risk of death. We hypothesized that this was because the appropriate weighting for pCO_2 is also dependent on the associated serum pH (i.e., whether there is a primary or secondary respiratory disorder). Therefore, we developed a combined variable, which included serum pH and pCO_2 to establish weights for common acid-base disorders.

They then derived the weight for this combined variable as they had for individual variables. Knaus and colleagues (1991, 1621) also found important statistical interactions between urine output and serum creatinine and among respiratory rate, $PaCO_2$, and ventilator use. Combined variables were created from each of these sets. The weights assigned to the combined and individual variables were compared for their clinical validity.

As suggested earlier, a major concern in model development is model "overfitting"—including variables that may be useful predictors in the development database but do not have the same relationship to the outcome in other databases. The lung cancer example in Table 8.2 exemplifies this problem (Iezzoni et al. 1992c): Using all MedisGroups KCFs in stepwise regression models resulted in models that did not validate as well as simpler models. Chapter 10 discusses these issues further. Briefly, two main tactics are used to guard against model overfitting: first, employing both clinical and statistical criteria in making decisions about which variables to include and second, limiting the number of candidate variables. For example, when predicting a continuous variable, the number of independent variables should never be more than one-tenth of the number of cases. A ratio of at least 30 cases to each predictor variable is preferable. When predicting a dichotomous variable, the number of candidate independent variables should be fewer than 10 percent of the number of cases who experienced the event of interest. Using no more than one predictor for every 20 positive cases is safer.

One must decide not only about the number of independent variables to include but also whether to transform them before adding them to the model. Again, a combination of clinical judgment and statistical criteria underlies this decision. For example, in developing MMPS, we used the first 600 cases to select variables and choose the form in which each variable was expressed (i.e., APACHE II points, logarithm of the variable, or some other transformation), using goodness of fit measured by chi square analysis (Daley et al. 1988). Using an additional 300 cases, we next tested a few models, examining the overall goodness of fit but not the coefficients of individual variables. Only after the final functional form for the model was produced did we determine coefficients from the entire sample.

After a model is fit, one often must turn its output into a scale or score (see Chapter 10). In some cases, the results of the logistic regression model (e.g., parameter estimates, intercept terms) are used directly as the risk score. An example is the empirical version of MedisGroups that produces a probability of in-hospital death directly from the output of validated logistic regression equations. In other cases, however, modifications are made. For example, to produce a score for predicting morbidity and mortality for CABG patients, Higgins and colleagues (1992) first ran logistic regression models. Then, each significant variable was assigned a score of 1 to 6 points based on the univariate odds ratio, level of significance in the logistic model, and clinical input. "Different weights were evaluated for each factor to optimize performance of the clinical model" (Higgins et al. 1992, 2345).

Conclusions

Work to date in developing risk adjusters supports the use of empirical techniques whenever appropriate data are available. No matter how sophisticated, however, empirical methods are generally not enough—clinical judgment is also required. Even state-of-the-art statistical approaches and very large databases may yield clinically implausible findings. A model that is not clinically sensible (i.e., that contradicts established physiological principles) is not valid regardless of the statistical rigor used in its derivation. Studies that use clinically credible risk-adjustment strategies are far more likely to yield findings that will be trusted, believed, and, most importantly, acted on. Because assessment of health care outcomes aims ultimately to affect clinical practice, believability of the risk-adjustment method is essential.

Validity is thus a crucial attribute that encompasses both clinical and statistical considerations. Chapter 9 focuses on validity measurement primarily from a clinical perspective, whereas Chapter 10 addresses statistical measures of predictive validity.

Notes

1. Justice, Covinsky, and Berlin (1999) suggest ways to address concerns about what they call the "external validity" of prognostic measures derived from statistical models. They emphasize two broad concepts: accuracy (whether predictions match outcomes), assessed by examining calibration and discrimination; and generalizability, the extent to which the model provides accurate predictions in different patient samples. Generalizability itself has multiple components: reproducibility in comparable patient populations and transportability across different dimensions, including

place and time. Justice, Covinsky, and Berlin (1999) offer a systematic approach for evaluating performance of prognostic models, but, as they note, the relative importance of different aspects of external validity depends on one's purpose.

2. Efforts to risk adjust cardiac surgery outcomes had been underway within the VA for a number of years (Grover, Shroyer, and Hammermeister 1996; Grover, Hammermeister, and Burchfiel 1990; Grover et al. 1994, 2001; Shroyer et al. 1994, 1995; Grover, Cleveland, and Shroyer 2002; Hammermeister et al. 1995).

3. The nine surgical specialties included in NSQIP are cardiothoracic, noncardiac thoracic, general surgery, vascular surgery, orthopedic surgery, urology, plastic surgery, otolaryngology, and neurosurgery.

4. For some types of analyses, such as the regression models used by the VA Surgical Risk Study, small numbers of cases within key predictor variables (such as sex) can cause analytical difficulties (e.g., models may not converge).

5. The pilot study of the Surgical Risk Study prospective data collection identified various logistical problems. At the time, most laboratory data were gathered through automated software that downloads required information directly from the hospitals' laboratory systems. ECG results, however, were not available in the automated system. In a feasibility study, data collectors spent unacceptably long periods retrieving ECG results from patient charts and the ECG laboratories, to the detriment of collecting other important data elements. In addition, despite clear definitions of what constituted a nosocomial infection (i.e., postoperative wound infection), ascertainment bias became evident across the sites because of different practices for obtaining wound cultures. Adoption of the CDC definitions for superficial and deep wound infections and pneumonia and urinary tract infections, which are also used as the infection control definitions systematically throughout the VA, permitted standard case finding (see above).

6. APACHE was originally based solely on clinical judgment, using clinical variables and weights assigned by clinicians (Knaus et al. 1981). APACHE II was also derived primarily using the clinical judgment of its developers and their consultants (Knaus et al. 1985). In contrast, APACHE III was developed mostly empirically using a large database (Knaus et al. 1991). This third version incorporated several new acute physiology risk indicators (e.g., blood glucose, BUN, total bilirubin, serum albumin, urine output), and the weights assigned to all variables were calculated using a database of 17,440 patients admitted to 40 ICUs across the country. In creating the comorbidity component of APACHE III, the developers considered "the magnitude and direction of the influence of each comorbid chronic disease variable on mortality (a coefficient of 0.05) and the overall statistical significance of the influence" (Knaus

et al. 1991, 1633). These considerations guided selection of the seven chronic conditions included in APACHE III from among 34 candidate conditions. Thus, as data became available, APACHE evolved from a solely clinically based system to one that relies heavily on empirical modeling techniques.

VALIDITY AND RELIABILITY OF RISK ADJUSTERS

Jennifer Daley, Arlene S. Ash, and Lisa I. Iezzoni

Most researchers believe they understand the phrase "valid and reliable." It has a "mom and apple pie" ring: Of course risk adjusters should be valid and reliable! However, it is less clear how to demonstrate validity and reliability in observational studies with sometimes messy databases representing limited populations. Concerns extend from the risk-adjustment method to the underlying database and population sample. The important question is not "Is this risk-adjustment method valid and reliable?" but "How believable and trustworthy are our findings when we use risk-adjustment method X in the following way to answer question Y?"

Validity and reliability are multidimensional concepts, with no clear boundary between them. According to Donabedian (1980, 101),

> The concept of validity is itself made up of many parts; and there is no precise way of saying what belongs to it, or what belongs more appropriately under another heading. . . . I would say that the question of validity covers two large domains. The first has to do with the accuracy of the data and the precision of the measures that are constructed with these data. The second has to do with the justifiability of the inferences that are drawn from the data and the measurements.

Donabedian's observation highlights the difficulties in distinguishing between attributes representing validity and those connoting reliability or some other concept. Data accuracy and measurement precision present good examples. For instance, as described in Chapter 6, clinicians use many physical examination findings (e.g., S3 gallop heart sounds, pericardial friction rubs, jugular venous distension, rales) to indicate patients' cardiac or pulmonary status, although these quantities are measured unreliably across physicians. Does this unreliability make them invalid as risk factors? Is this a problem with validity or with reliability? If the differences involve random errors, only accuracy is affected. If systematic differences occur among groups of policy relevance, validity is threatened. Reliability also may not be meaningful as a stand-alone concept; it requires context: "reliability for the purpose of X." For example, two temperatures read to the nearest 0.1°F are likely to differ, yet most repeated readings will yield the same conclusion about whether patients have fevers.

Most existing risk-adjustment methods are repeatedly revised or updated to reflect new data, accommodate new diagnosis or procedure codes, and address problems identified by new users addressing novel purposes. As risk adjusters change, or simply as time passes, their validity or reliability may change. For example, biomedical discoveries and new therapies may make old risk factors and weighting schemes obsolete. New models will address previous deficiencies more or less successfully. In the ensuing pages, drawing examples again from the VA NSQIP (see Chapter 8), we separate these concepts—first discussing validity, then reliability. Our overarching goal is to address comprehensively those issues raised by risk adjustment relating to validity and reliability, regardless of which ones fall under which heading.

Dimensions of Validity

Evaluating the validity of a risk adjuster involves answering the following question: How well does the adjustment method account for the true risk of a specified outcome within a particular time frame for a particular patient population for a specific purpose? As noted throughout this book, embedded within risk-adjustment methodologies are answers to four questions (see Chapters 2 and 8). Risk adjusters developed for specific outcomes, time frames, populations, and purposes are generally most valid when applied to projects with similar parameters. As an extreme example, a risk adjuster designed to predict newborn mortality within NICUs will have poor validity for predicting annual costs for elderly Medicare beneficiaries in managed care.

Evaluating the validity of scales or classification systems falls within the purview of psychometrics or clinimetrics (Feinstein 1987; Stewart, Hays, and Ware 1992; Streiner and Norman 1995). Methodologists distinguish numerous dimensions of validity; Table 9.1 summarizes eight. These different dimensions, however, often overlap. In assessing risk-adjustment methods, the most important are face validity, content validity, criterion or construct validity, predictive validity, and attributional validity. Here, we do not recreate detailed technical discussions available in psychometric or clinimetric texts. Instead, we discuss these five validity dimensions, highlighting those issues most crucial in risk adjustment.

Face Validity

Face validity indicates whether a method appears on its face to measure what it claims to measure. In other words, will the method's users accept it as "valid" in the everyday sense of the word? Face validity, while not a rigorous concept, is critically important. Poor face validity seriously impedes overall acceptance, especially by practicing clinicians with little knowledge of more technical issues in risk adjustment. Clinicians generally judge the acceptability of a risk adjuster against their own internal standards: How well do the ratings match my sense of how sick a patient is?

Validity Dimension	Definition	Example
Face validity	A measure contains the types of variables that will allow it to do what it aims to do	A method for adjusting for in-hospital mortality for AMI includes clinical variables that on face value are the types of variables clinicians consider important risk factors
Content validity	A measure contains all relevant concepts	A method for adjusting for in-hospital mortality from AMI includes all clinical variables that are important risk factors
Construct validity	A measure correlates with actual indicators of risk in the expected way	A method for adjusting for in-hospital mortality from AMI correlates with actual measures of cardiac function
Convergent validity	A measure has a positive correlation with other indicators of actual risk	When a method for adjusting for in-hospital mortality from AMI shows increasing risk, actual measures of cardiac functioning also show increasing risk
Discriminant validity	A measure has a stronger correlation with indicators specific to its purpose than to other indicators	A method for adjusting for in-hospital mortality from AMI correlates more strongly with actual measures of cardiac function than with measures of ambulation
Criterion validity	A measure correlates with the gold-standard measure	A method for adjusting for in-hospital mortality from AMI correlates with a clinical scale derived from intensive, continuous cardiac monitoring
Predictive validity	A measure explains variations in outcomes	A method for adjusting for in-hospital mortality from AMI predicts accurately which patients have died
Attributional validity	Findings using the measure permit one to make statements about the causes of what is observed	In-hospital mortality rates, adjusted using the measure, permit one to attribute differences to effectiveness or quality of care

TABLE 9.1

Different Dimensions of Validity

SOURCES: Donabedian (1980); Thomas, Ashcraft, and Zimmerman (1986); Stewart, Hays, and Ware (1992).

Clinicians are skeptical of risk-adjustment methods that diverge from their clinical expectations about a patient's prognosis. For example, physicians expect patients with chronic renal failure requiring dialysis to face higher risks of dying when hospitalized (e.g., for major surgery) than otherwise healthy patients. Risk-adjustment methods that rely solely on the serum BUN to capture the effect of renal failure may underestimate the likelihood of death for patients on hemodialysis; dialysis machines lower patients' BUN levels, which, without dialysis, would be grossly elevated. In populations including some renal dialysis patients, risk-adjustment methods need to consider clinical risk factors beyond BUN to have face validity (i.e., to predict poorer outcomes for dialysis patients than for others).

Examining face validity of a risk-adjustment method requires evaluating its inner workings. The logic of the method (including risk factors and weights) should be fully available for clinicians and methodologists to examine. Over the last two decades, the internal workings of many commercial risk adjusters have been hidden, viewed as trade secrets by their vendors. However, to assess face validity, clinicians need to consider whether the risk adjusters include all important risk factors and whether the direction and weight of each feels appropriate for the outcome. As suggested in Chapter 8, risk factors that behave differently than clinicians expect raise questions about face validity and may cause them to reject an entire risk-adjustment method.

A key step in assessing face validity is perhaps the most difficult—translating the analytic structure of a statistical risk-adjustment model into something accessible to clinicians so that they can test it against their clinical experience. This translation is especially difficult when empirical models include highly correlated factors and numerous interaction terms. Determining in what manner and how much weight is attributed to the effect of various independent or predictor variables becomes complicated. Graphical representations of the independent effects of various risk factors on the outcome can help here but may not fully resolve this problem.

Content Validity

Content validity refers to the extent to which the included risk factors represent the universe of risk factors that should be included. Models of risk can always include more factors (see Chapter 3). Examining content validity asks whether important risk factors are missing. Information to judge this dimension is typically drawn from the clinical literature and expert clinicians, as described in Chapter 8. Again, relevant risk factors will depend on the outcome, time window, and population of interest.

Assessing content validity is complicated when the independent variables are highly correlated, causing some clinically important variables to be excluded. For example, in the national VA Surgical Risk Study, general surgeons examining the final risk models for 30-day mortality and morbidity often commented on the absence of key laboratory values, such as bilirubin and liver function tests, for assessing the presence of acute and chronic hepatobiliary disease. Initially, the surgeons questioned the validity of these models. After discussion, however, they appreciated that serum albumin level (an included variable) was an excellent predictor of surgical outcome, representing risk from both hepatobiliary disease and poor nutritional status. Therefore, although important variables may not appear in a final prediction model, other closely related variables may capture essentially the same information.

Thus, an individual clinical parameter can capture a range of clinical concerns. Serum BUN is another such variable that appears in many acute care risk-adjustment models. It reflects multiple clinical causes: intravascular volume depletion, diminished cardiac output, renal insufficiency, significant gastrointestinal bleeding, or an increased catabolic state. In contrast, fully representing some clinical risk concepts may require several risk factors. For example, a highly valid representation of risk of death from sepsis or septic shock involves very low or very high body temperature, low blood pressure, very high or very low peripheral white blood cell count, and the presence of positive blood cultures. No one or two of these variables alone has full clinical validity for predicting the risk of death from sepsis.

Other risk variables may only weakly represent the risk concept. For example, in CHF and AMI, acute neurological damage or diminished levels of consciousness are important risk factors for imminent death. The Glasgow Coma Score, developed as a measure of severity of acute coma in patients admitted to neurological and neurosurgical ICUs, serves as a surrogate for acute neurological damage, as well as a measure of coma for some risk-adjustment methods (Knaus et al. 1985, 1991; Daley et al. 1988). Although the Glasgow Coma Score does identify patients with acutely diminished levels of consciousness, it poorly represents other aspects of neurological damage, such as paralysis, paresis, or chronic mental status changes.

Content validity is ultimately limited by the information in the data source. While administrative data in particular contain limited clinical insight (see Chapter 5), key risk factors may be unavailable from any practical source. For example, even medical charts contain little information regarding functional status. The absence of routinely collected data on psychosocial functioning and quality of life limits the utility of risk-adjustment methods for certain purposes.

Criterion and Construct Validity

Criterion validity represents the extent to which a given measure correlates with a gold standard or criterion. While no gold standard exists for an abstract, multidimensional concept like "risk," some validation procedures can be useful. Construct or correlation validity is verified by finding a strong, positive association with another credible measure, for example, determinations of risk by a panel of expert clinicians.[1]

In one project, physicians estimated 180-day survival for 4,028 patients; computers estimated the same outcome for the same patients using an empirically derived risk model (Knaus et al. 1995, 195). The c-statistic, the area under a receiver operating characteristic curve (see Chapter 10), was identical for the physicians' and model's predictions, 0.78; the physicians and the computer performed similarly in discriminating between those who lived and those who died.[2] However, the physicians were more pessimistic than the empirical model, judging more patients to be at high risk of dying (<0.15 likelihood of survival).

Comparing scores among risk-adjustment methods is another way to investigate construct validity. Different risk-adjusters have relatively rarely been compared, however, partially because of the proprietary ownership of commercial methods. Sometimes, major policy initiatives compel head-to-head comparisons. For example, when considering which risk adjuster should support capitated Medicare payments following the 1997 Balanced Budget Act, Medicare sponsored research comparing various risk-adjustment methods using identical data and methods. Nonetheless, few researchers have directly compared different risk adjusters using the same databases.

Comparing performance measures, such as R^2 or c-statistics, calculated on different data sets can be misleading (see Chapter 10), as some data are more difficult to model than others. Ideally, comparisons should use the same patient population, outcome measure, and statistical approaches for assessing predictive validity (see below). If this is impossible, careful attention to how the data sources differ with respect to distributions of the dependent and independent variables, as well as reviews of performance characteristics of other models in similar settings, can help in interpreting results. Sample sizes also must be adequate to accommodate random variation at the chosen level of analysis (e.g., patient, institution, groups of institutions). Finally, the goal of the analysis is important. Methods for validating risk-adjustment measures may differ when considering predictive accuracy for individual patients as opposed to accuracy for groups of patients (Chang 1989; Hornbrook and Goodman 1995; see Chapter 10).

Predictive Validity

Predictive validity refers to how well a risk adjuster predicts an outcome. Chapter 10 discusses predictive validity in detail, examining statistical measures of model performance. Here, we consider conceptual issues in assessing predictive validity.

When considering predictive validity for an empirically derived risk adjuster, it is important to distinguish between the model's performance on the data set used to develop or "fit" the model and its performance in "validation" data. An empirically derived risk adjuster typically performs better in development data than in other data.[3] However, the true test of a model's predictive validity is how well it works on new data.

Researchers typically work to create a specific, well-defined database (analytic file) for their studies. Administrative databases can contain hundreds of thousands, even millions, of observations; data from chart review or clinical studies are generally much smaller, typically only several hundred cases. Often, researchers split their cases into two or more subsets, using one to develop their predictive model and another (or others) to test (validate) this model. The more data used to develop the risk-adjustment model, the greater the ability to identify important risk factors (predictor variables) and accurately quantify risks. However, holding some data aside for independent validation is valuable.

Although split-sample cross-validation is appealing, it has its drawbacks. Because all the data are not used in initial model development, analysts should report both split-sample performance measures and final models derived on the entire database. Although results in the validation sample will not directly pertain to the model developed using the full sample, the full-sample model should perform even better than the validation measures suggest. To develop a model whose specific coefficients will be used repeatedly, examining whether the models developed on subsets of the data have the same coefficients and predictive validity increases understanding of the extent to which a full-sample model captures real and stable relationships. If subsample models display considerable variability, analysts may require additional data to establish fully credible models. In databases with hundreds of thousands of cases, reserving no more than 100,000 for validation should be sufficient. Analysts can also use bootstrapping (Efron 1979) to examine the stability of coefficients and measures of predictive validity in different data sets (see Chapter 10).

Deriving a risk-adjustment method requires multiple steps, guided by extensive examination of the development data. This includes deciding how to code risk factors, identifying which risk factors to include, and assigning weights to each factor for predicting the outcome of interest. At each step, the opportunity to "overfit" the data (i.e., to make a choice that is "optimal" for these particular data) arises, leading to a model that fits these data better than can be expected with any future database. This leads to inflated performance measures. The cleanest way to avoid being overly optimistic about how well a model will perform in the future is to look at the development data during the entire model-building process and use the validation data only at the end to see how well the model performs.

With limited data, analysts often circumvent the ideal approach, for example, using the entire database to identify the model's predictor variables and validating only the choice of coefficients that arise from fitting the model. However, methods to reduce the number of variables, such as stepwise selection, can produce unstable results. Repeating the entire modeling process on data subsets can help reveal the extent of that problem in a particular situation. Interpreting cross-validated performance measures requires understanding whether the entire model-building procedure, or only selected components, was validated.

When available, external validation with entirely independent data is best for testing predictive validity. However, especially when the mean of the outcome variable is substantially different in the new data, at least some recalibration of the development model should be considered. Chapter 10 discusses such issues more fully.

Attributional Validity

Finally, Donabedian (1980) described a critical concept that he called "attributional validity." In the context of risk adjustment for studying health care outcomes, attributional validity reflects the extent to which observers can identify the real causes of variations in outcomes across patients (e.g., the reason for differences in mortality rates) (Donabedian 1980, 103).

> When outcomes are used to make inferences about the quality of care, it is necessary first to establish that the outcomes can, in fact, be attributed to that care. We may call this the problem of "attribution," and its satisfactory solution may be said to confirm "attributional validity."

When using risk-adjusted outcome information to motivate practice changes or monitor providers, attributional validity is key. It is, however, difficult to measure. In the health policy arena, many now assume that if a risk adjuster meets other validation standards (e.g., face validity, a certain level of predictive validity or R^2), one can safely eliminate differences in patient risk factors as an explanation for difference in outcomes, such as mortality rates in performance profiles (see Chapter 12). However, attributing causes from risk-adjusted outcomes—even with the "best" measure for risk—should be pursued cautiously.

Several relevant examples come from the mid- to late-1980s, soon after Medicare implemented DRG-based prospective payment for hospitals. With the new case-based payment approach came concerns that hospitals would discharge patients "quicker and sicker." Observers also worried that hospitals would skimp on services, seeking profits by keeping costs below the DRG reimbursement. Quality of hospital care therefore became a high-priority issue, and researchers studied the relationship between risk-adjusted hospital mortality rates and more process-oriented measures of the quality of hospital care.

After adjusting for patients' risk of dying on admission using APACHE II, Dubois, Brook, and Rogers (1987) found that hospitals with higher death rates cared for sicker patients than did hospitals with lower mortality rates in three high-mortality conditions (pneumonia, stroke, and AMI). The researchers conducted explicit and implicit chart reviews on samples of cases in each disease category from high- and low-mortality outlier hospitals (Dubois and Brook 1988). Explicit reviews detected no differences in effectiveness of care. After adjusting for differences in patient risk, implicit reviews demonstrated that patients with stroke and pneumonia had a 5 percent incidence of preventable deaths in high-mortality outlier hospitals, compared with 1 percent preventable deaths in low-mortality outlier hospitals. High outlier hospitals may have both sicker patients and less-effective care.[4]

A larger study of hospital quality following DRG implementation looked at risk-adjusted 30-day mortality after admission for CHF, AMI, pneumonia, stroke, and hip fracture (Keeler et al. 1992). After adjusting for sickness on admission, researchers studied the process of care using both implicit and explicit criteria. For both individual patients and groups of hospitals, the investigators demonstrated a relationship between risk-adjusted mortality rates and measures of process of care by implicit and explicit review criteria—hospitals with lower risk-adjusted mortality rates had better processes of care. Using Medicare administrative data, Hartz and colleagues (1993) correlated risk-adjusted mortality rates among hospitals caring for Medicare beneficiaries in 1987 with rates of quality problems reported by 38 PROs for the same hospitals. They found a weak but statistically significant relationship between PRO ratings of hospitals and risk-adjusted mortality rates. Findings were more striking for hospitals with similar characteristics (e.g., teaching status, size, urban location).

These studies demonstrate an important challenge in assessing attributional validity—finding measures of the ultimate target (e.g., quality of care) that are themselves valid. Especially in observational and health-policy-related studies, the risk adjuster may be easier to validate than the outcome measure. More recent chart review studies of quality of care continue to explore the difficulty of determining "truth" (Weingart et al. 2001, 2002).

Examples of Validation Studies

Validity should be assessed within the context (outcome, timing, population, purpose) in which a risk adjuster will be used. Often, however, because researchers' access to data is restricted and options for evaluating validity are limited, creative approaches are needed. Below, we describe two efforts to validate risk-adjustment methods and risk-adjusted results. The former draws from work we conducted using hospital-based severity measures in the mid-1990s; the latter comes from the NSQIP. Neither example demonstrates the current validity of any methodology (in fact, several of the methods are now obsolete). Instead, we aim to suggest strategies for validation studies.

Examining Hospital-Based Severity Measures

An important test of face validity is the extent to which clinicians feel the ratings of the risk adjusters agree with their own perceptions. One helpful technique is to ask clinicians to review specific clinical cases, producing their own rating of the patient's level of risk. Then, clinicians can compare their risk ratings with the scores of the case by particular risk-adjustment methods. Do the clinicians' ratings agree with the ratings of the risk adjusters?

In our study of hospital-based severity measures (see Chapter 5), we abstracted medical records for hospitalized patients, capturing all discharge abstract information, clinical events day by day, and detailed laboratory reports; we then developed narrative case vignettes (see Tables 5.8 and 5.10) and had cases "scored" using each of several risk-adjustment methods (Hughes et al. 1996). Comparing scores for cases offers insight into the role of the underlying data (clinical versus code-based methods), differences by targeted outcome (mortality versus resource consumption), and problems relating to the inability to distinguish diagnosis codes representing conditions present on admission from conditions arising later during hospital stays. Some risk adjusters appear more valid for predicting resource consumption, whereas others seem better suited to assessing clinical outcomes. As expected, face validity generally reflected the underlying purpose of the risk adjuster (e.g., whether the approach focused on predicting clinical versus cost outcomes; see Table 2.2).

Construct or correlation validation assesses how well one method correlates with other measures of the same concept. Our database contained several severity measures for each patient, allowing for the rare opportunity to assess construct validity. We report here on four conditions with enough in-hospital deaths for meaningful statistical analysis: AMI, CABG, pneumonia, and stroke (Table 9.2).[5] For each severity measure, we used logistic regression within each condition to predict in-hospital death from patient age, sex, and severity score (Iezzoni et al. 1995c). Here, we compare two clinically based methods (MedisGroups and a "physiology score" patterned after APACHE III's APS) and three measures derived from administrative data (APR-DRGs, DS, and PMCs). Each model produced a predicted probability of death for each patient. At each hospital, we added these to determine the expected number of deaths. We ranked hospitals from lowest (fewer deaths than expected) to highest (more deaths than expected) based on z-scores, calculated for each hospital as:

$$z = \text{(observed number of deaths – expected number of deaths)} / \text{(square root of the variance in the number of deaths)}.$$

We first asked the following question: Do different severity measures predict different likelihoods of in-hospital death for the same patients? Patients can be "flagged" as having different predicted probabilities of death in various ways, but regardless of the approach the answer was yes—the five severity measures scored many patients very differently (Iezzoni et al. 1995c, 1996b, 1996d). For the numbers presented here, we compared the adjusted odds ratios of death calculated by each severity measure (e.g., the odds of dying predicted by MedisGroups divided by the odds predicted by DS). When this ratio was less than 0.5 or greater than 2.0, we viewed patients as having very different probabilities of death predicted by the two measures (Table 9.2). Many patients had dissimilar likelihoods of death.

Patterns varied across conditions. Agreement between MedisGroups and physiology scores was high for AMI, but predictions diverged for 30.2 percent of pneumonia patients. Not surprisingly, code-based measures disagreed frequently with clinically based measures, but code-based measures also differed among themselves. For instance, PMCs and APR-DRGs disagreed for 60.7 percent of CABG patients.

Given these differences, an obvious question is, Which severity measures make more clinical sense? Because we could not return to medical

Severity Measures		Conditions			
		AMI	CABG	Pneumonia	Stroke
MedisGroups	Physiology score	19.5	4.1	30.2	17.8
MedisGroups	DS	51.4	32.8	47.6	57.8
MedisGroups	PMC severity score	45.6	42.0	46.9	61.6
MedisGroups	APR-DRGs	46.1	65.8	47.9	48.4
Physiology score	DS	51.6	32.3	38.9	52.0
Physiology score	PMC severity score	44.2	40.9	30.4	44.0
Physiology score	APR-DRGs	44.9	68.5	32.0	31.0
DS	PMC severity score	51.8	40.2	31.0	32.9
DS	APR-DRGs	49.5	56.4	30.4	41.3
PMC severity score	APR-DRGs	27.5	60.7	21.2	20.1

TABLE 9.2
Percentage of Patients with Different Odds of Death Calculated by Pairs of Severity Measures[a]

SOURCES: Iezzoni et al. (1995a, 1995c, 1996b, 1996d).
NOTE: MedisGroups = empirical version; physiology score = version 2.
[a] Comparisons were based on the ratio = (odds of death predicted by first severity measure)/(odds of death predicted by second severity measure). If this ratio were <0.5 or >2.0, then the odds predicted by the two severity measures were viewed as very different.

records, we explored this question using MedisGroups admission KCFs. We reviewed the medical literature to identify clinical characteristics viewed as predictors of in-hospital death and found the MedisGroups KCF that best captured each. We then looked at patterns of these KCFs for patients with discordant predictions of dying by pairs of severity measures (Iezzoni et al. 1995b, 1996b). Not surprisingly, the clinically based measures generally had more clinical credibility than code-based measures, except for CABG, where clinical and code-based measures were comparable.

Finding differences across severity measures for individual patients prompted a second question: Would judgments about whether hospitals look particularly good or bad differ when using different severity measures to risk adjust mortality rates? The answer to this question was again yes, but the findings were subtler than for individual patients (Iezzoni et al. 1995a, 1996a, 1996e; Landon et al. 1996). As before, several approaches can address this question. Here, we used severity-adjusted death rates the way hospitals or health insurers may employ the information (see Chapter 12). The z-scores described above identified hospitals falling into two extremes:

1. The best 10 percent: hospitals with the lowest severity-adjusted death rates. These hospitals could be designated as exemplary facilities, serving as benchmarks for quality-improvement initiatives.
2. The worst 10 percent: hospitals with the highest severity-adjusted death rates. Insurers and purchasers may refuse to contract with these institutions.

Table 9.3 shows how often pairs of severity measures agreed about which hospitals fell into the best and worst 10 percent; it also includes hospital rankings based on z-scores associated with raw mortality rates (unadjusted for age, sex, or severity). The immediate impression is that severity measures and unadjusted mortality rates often flagged different hospitals, but different severity measures also frequently flagged different hospitals (Iezzoni et al. 1995a, 1996a, 1996e; Landon et al. 1996). No clear pattern emerged, and findings differed by condition (e.g., MedisGroups and PMCs agreed relatively well for pneumonia but poorly for stroke).

When disagreements occurred, hospitals ranked in the top or bottom 10 percent by one severity measure often appeared in the next 10 percent (11–20 percent or 81–90 percent) when ranked by the other measure. However, differences in rankings were sometimes larger. For example, MedisGroups and DS agreed on 5 of 11 hospitals ranked among the top 10 percent for pneumonia. The remaining six, ranked as 4, 7, 8, 9, 10, and 11, respectively, by MedisGroups (where 1 = best), had the following rankings by DS: 57, 66, 25, 27, 43, and 30. Hospitals with widely discrepant rankings were not low volume, where small numbers could yield volatile results. For instance, the hospital ranked 7th by MedisGroups but 66th by DS had 266 pneumonia patients with 20 deaths (Iezzoni 1997).

Agreement between severity-adjusted and unadjusted mortality was often better than agreement between pairs of severity measures. For example, MedisGroups and DS agreed on only three of the ten worst hospitals for AMI, whereas MedisGroups and unadjusted rankings agreed on six. One set of severity-adjusted findings was therefore not obviously better than another, nor was it obviously better than unadjusted rankings.

For each pair of severity measures, we calculated a kappa statistic based on whether individual hospitals were flagged as among the best or worst 10 percent by one, both, or neither measure. Kappa assesses whether the observed agreement is greater than expected by chance (see below). The kappa values showed fair to excellent agreement among severity measures in flagging hospitals (Iezzoni et al. 1995a, 1996a, 1996e). For example, MedisGroups and DS agreed on only 5 of the 11 worst hospitals for pneumonia patients (Table 9.3), for a kappa of 0.39, indicating fair agreement (Iezzoni et al. 1996a). In contrast, the physiology score and PMC severity score agreed on 9 of the 11 worst hospitals, for a kappa of 0.80, suggesting substantial agreement.

Overall, these analyses suggest that individual hospitals might care greatly about which mortality rates are examined—unadjusted versus severity-adjusted rates—and about which severity measure is used. While severity measures agreed about flagging hospitals more often than chance, rankings for some hospitals differed dramatically across severity measures. Thus, these construct analyses suggest that, at both the individual patient and hospital levels, agreement across severity measures was often modest. The central question remained unresolved: Which severity measure best isolates that residual quantity—quality-of-care differences—across hospitals?

TABLE 9.3

No. of Times Pairs of Severity Measures Agreed on the 10 Percent of Hospitals with the Best and Worst Mortality Performance

Severity Measures, Including Unadjusted Mortality Rates		Conditions and Number of Hospitals in Best and Worst 10%							
		AMI ($n = 10$)		CABG ($n = 4$)		Pneumonia ($n = 11$)		Stroke ($n = 9$)	
		Best	Worst	Best	Worst	Best	Worst	Best	Worst
		Number of Hospitals on which Severity Measures Agreed							
MedisGroups	Physiology score	9	10	4	4	6	8	7	6
MedisGroups	DS	6	3	2	3	5	5	5	3
MedisGroups	PMC severity score	7	5	2	2	6	8	4	3
MedisGroups	APR-DRGs	6	4	1	2	6	7	6	4
MedisGroups	Unadjusted rates	5	6	3	4	3	6	3	5
Physiology score	DS	5	3	2	3	4	7	5	3
Physiology score	PMC severity score	6	5	2	2	7	9	6	3
Physiology score	APR-DRGs	6	4	1	2	5	8	6	3
Physiology score	Unadjusted rates	6	6	3	4	3	9	5	5
DS	PMC severity score	7	5	3	2	4	7	6	3
DS	APR-DRGs	7	5	2	2	4	6	7	3
DS	Unadjusted rates	5	4	1	3	1	7	5	3
PMC severity score	APR-DRGs	8	9	2	2	7	10	7	7
PMC severity score	Unadjusted rates	4	6	1	2	5	7	7	6
APR-DRGs	Unadjusted rates	6	6	1	2	5	7	6	5

SOURCES: Iezzoni et al. (1995a, 1996a, 1996e); Landon (1996).
NOTE: MedisGroups = empirical version; physiology score = version 2.
n = No. of hospitals in best and worst 10 percent.

NSQIP and Attributional Validity

The VA surgical outcomes initiative was designed to improve quality of care by giving surgeons information with sufficient clinical credibility to motivate self-examination and change (see Chapter 8). Although the VA investigators initially developed their risk-adjustment models at the individual patient level, they aimed to generate their most important reports for each VA medical center performing surgery. VA surgeons participated actively in ensuring the face validity of the risk-adjustment models constructed for individual patients (Khuri et al. 1995, 1997; Daley et al. 1997a, 1997b). In 1994, these risk-adjustment methods became central to an ongoing quality-assessment activity, the NSQIP, which tracks operative outcomes at 123 VA hospitals nationwide (Khuri et al. 1998; Daley, Henderson, and Khuri 2001). Attributional validity was key: Did a valid causal link exist between poor risk-adjusted hospital performance and the quality of its operative care? Did hospitals with higher-than-expected operative mortality and morbidity rates provide worse-quality care than hospitals with better-than-expected outcomes?

The VA investigators studied attributional validity in two ways: chart reviews and site visits. The chart review study examined 739 general, peripheral vascular, and orthopedic surgery records from the 44 VA hospitals participating in the national VA Surgical Risk Study (Gibbs et al. 2001; see Chapter 8). The researchers sampled cases for two levels of analysis: hospital (facilities with higher- and lower-than-expected mortality and morbidity rates) and patient (individual patients with high and low predicted likelihood of mortality and morbidity who had died or developed complications). Twenty-one VA general surgeons and eight VA vascular surgeons reviewed the records using a structured implicit review instrument modeled after a well-accepted approach (Kahn et al. 1992). Kappa analyses found fair to good agreement across the surgeons' judgments about quality (Gibbs et al. 2001, 190).

The chart review study produced mixed findings (Gibbs et al. 2001). Patients from hospitals with higher- and lower-than-expected mortality and morbidity rates had similar overall quality of care. However, patient-level analyses found that patients with low predicted likelihoods of adverse outcomes who nonetheless experienced adverse outcomes had worse quality of care than did those with high predicted risks. The researchers speculated that chart reviews may be relatively insensitive to hospital-level quality problems; medical records may not contain clues about systemic quality difficulties within institutions. Thus, the investigators themselves questioned the validity of the tool (chart reviews) they used to test the validity of risk-adjusted hospital findings as quality indicators.

The second attributional validity study involved site visits (Daley et al. 1997b; Young et al. 1997). Because many attributes of surgical practices within institutions cannot be evaluated through chart reviews, the researchers visited 20 outlier institutions: ten surgical services with the highest risk-adjusted mortality or morbidity rates and ten surgical services with the lowest mortality or morbidity rates. The visitors were blinded as to whether institutions were high or low outliers. Site-visit teams consisted of a chief of surgery, a surgical ICU nurse specialist, and a study investigator; teams spent two days observing and interviewing staff at each surgical service. The site-visit teams examined the technology, equipment, and physical structure of the surgical service; technical competence of the surgeons, anesthesiologists, nurses, and house staff; relationship with the affiliated university teaching programs; relationships with all other patient care services in the hospital (e.g., internal medicine, radiology, laboratory); quality monitoring and improvement activities on the surgical service; communication and coordination among surgery, nursing, and anesthesia; and leadership in surgery and the institution.

The site visitors identified significant differences between the high and low outliers in several dimensions. Surgical services with better-than-expected outcomes were more likely to have better technology and equipment (e.g., more up-to-date anesthesia equipment and monitoring equipment in the surgical ICU). These low-outlier institutions were more likely to standardize their approaches to routine patient care, such as using practice guidelines or clinical pathways for routine operations. Thus, care was typically better coordinated at low-outlier hospitals. The site visitors, unaware of the outlier status of the surgical services when they visited, rated overall quality of care higher among the ten low-outlier surgical services than among the ten high-outlier services. Site visit results therefore support the attributional validity of hospital mortality and morbidity rates as an indicator of quality of surgical care.

Reliability

An important indicator of the quality of a scientific measure is its ability to yield consistent, reproducible results. Statisticians call this characteristic "precision," whereas social scientists, psychologists, and health services researchers know it as "reliability." Both terms address this basic question: If this process were repeated, possibly by someone else but following identical rules, would the same results occur? Measures can be reapplied by the same observer or rater (to test intrarater reliability) or by different raters (interrater reliability). Agreement among different raters is a more rigorous test. As Feinstein notes, reliability matters:

> The crucial quality of scientific data is not accuracy, but reproducibility. There is no such thing as absolute accuracy, any more than there is . . . absolute truth. (1967, 345)

> No matter how the observations are made and described, the data will have scientific quality if the results of the observational process can be consistently reproduced by the same or another observer. (1987, 170)

Below, we explore reliability as it pertains to risk adjustment, drawing heavily from Hughes and Ash (1997). We do not comprehensively review technical methods for assessing reliability.

Reliability and the Data Source

As anticipated by Donabedian's quote at the outset of this chapter, the accuracy or reliability of the underlying data carries immediate implications for risk-adjustment methods. Chapters 5, 6, and 7 discuss reliability issues relating to the three main data sources (administrative databases, medical records, and patients). Here, we underscore several points.

The issue of reliability for a code-based measure revolves around how accurately and completely the coded information from the medical record was gathered—how consistently diagnosis and procedure codes were assigned. In studies using administrative data, returning to medical records to see if reabstractions would yield identical results is often infeasible. The reliability of administrative-data-based risk adjusters is thus not tested directly, but only inferred from studies of coding reliability. Such reports rarely pertain to the specific database being used; most relate to Medicare data (Hsia et al. 1988;

Fisher et al. 1992; Fowles et al. 1995; Lawthers et al. 2000; McCarthy et al. 2000a). This imperfect approach to assessing reliability is a concession to the realities and costs of data collection.

For risk adjusters based on clinical data, reliability considerations are more complicated. When data are drawn automatically from an electronic source, such as a laboratory reporting system, one can assume this process is performed reliably (although questions might arise about how accurately a laboratory determines a clinical parameter.) With manual data abstraction, reliability relates to the number of data elements, complexity and subjectivity of judgments required to identify variables, quality of the records themselves (e.g., completeness, legibility, organization), and other factors (see Chapter 6). Studies using medical records should conduct reliability testing. Unreliable data may not present problems when variations are random, but systematic variations can affect risk-adjusted findings. Data should not be used until reliability reaches acceptable levels.

Risk adjusters based on patients' reports must accept some level of unreliability or subjectivity (e.g., in reporting medical conditions or functional status). Studies using patient reports often trade off data quality concerns against ease of administration. The question then becomes whether differences in data quality are nonrandomly distributed across the units of observation, such as hospitals or health plans. Data quality may well vary nonrandomly, as the accuracy of self-reports may relate to education, income, and language abilities—quantities perhaps distributed nonrandomly across hospitals, health plans, and other groupings of patients and providers. Determining the reliability of patient-reported data is logistically complicated and costly.

Sources of Variability

Variability may be inherent within the underlying data elements (e.g., laboratory tests, self-reported functional status); it may result from performing the risk adjustment itself; or it may arise from the persons applying the risk adjuster. Feinstein (1987) called these three sources of variation "input," "procedure," and "user" variability, respectively. We discuss aspects of each concept below, recognizing that they may overlap.

In evaluating a biological variable, such as serum cortisol, where levels may vary systematically throughout the day, taking samples at a specified time could reduce diurnal variation. Similarly, repeated assessments of mental function of persons with dementia may yield different scores day to day relating to mood, level of sedating medications, or sleep adequacy. These examples illustrate variation in the entity under evaluation, or "substrate."

For risk adjusters, an analogous situation may involve medical records. For example, input variability pertains largely to the reproducibility of clinical information in the medical record. Medical records, once created, should not change. Nonetheless, several sources contribute to variability during the creation of records, including the setting and type of organization generating the record (e.g., tertiary teaching hospital, individual physician office); organizational documentation or information management practices, including the interface of electronic and paper data sources (e.g., how many diagnoses are retained); structure and size of the medical record; and types of illness under study (see Chapter 6). In risk-adjustment studies, these factors often vary across the units of observation, such as hospitals, physician practices, or health plans.

Procedure variability arises in applying risk-adjustment methods to medical records—extracting information from charts and applying the formula or algorithm to generate the risk score. Whereas input variability relates to creating medical records, procedure variability concerns their use. Procedure variability encompasses several components. First, risk factor information may be inherently unreliable. Although training, diligence, and close supervision of data abstractors can lessen this unreliability, it cannot be eliminated without automated, electronic algorithms. Even automated extraction of risk factors from narrative electronic information (e.g., clinicians' text notations) is susceptible to the vagaries of coding schemes and variations in language use. Thus, even with electronic records, risk factors fall into a hierarchy of reproducibility. Numerical values are abstracted most reliably, whereas those derived from narrative texts are generally least reliable.

A second source of procedure variability involves the replicability of the rating scheme—whether users can follow abstraction and rating procedures as readily as the original developers. Again, computerized scoring algorithms largely eliminate this concern. For manual methods, vague, ambiguous, or incomplete scoring instructions compromise consistent scoring. The third concern involves fragility, the extent to which risk adjusters are susceptible to a few influential risk factor values. Fragile risk adjusters are strongly influenced by rare but idiosyncratic findings, particularly those that are unreliably detected. Evaluating the fragility of a code-based risk adjuster involves, for example, examining how ratings change following modifications in the choice and ordering of diagnosis codes. By reabstracting medical records, Thomas and Ashcraft (1989) applied this approach to examine the reliability of three code-based methods (DRGs, DS, and PMCs). DRGs appeared much more reliable than DS or PMCs, largely because these two methods often rated cases based on a single diagnosis code. Thus, a single inconsistency in diagnosis coding could significantly affect the risk rating. In contrast, DRGs were less susceptible to coding variation because solitary diagnosis codes rarely, if ever, directed assignments.

Clinically based methods face similar concerns about fragility, especially when they rely on numerous data elements. Concerned about fragility, the developers of the CSI required two or more clinical criteria at a particular severity level before assigning patients to that level (Horn et al. 1991; Iezzoni and Daley 1992). For example, the CSI requires two oral temperature readings of ≥104.0°F to assign a pneumonia patient to severity level 4.

With the possible exception of some laboratory and diagnostic test results, all risk factors—from diagnosis codes to ratings of self-perceived health—carry some human component. Persons using risk-adjustment methods are motivated not only by their personal characteristics but also by external attributes, such as who employs them, how they perceive their role, how they are trained and monitored, stress and time pressures, work environment (e.g., ventilation, lighting), nature of their working relationships, and organizational culture. Different hospitals, for example, clearly vary in coding practices (Iezzoni et al. 1992a; Romano et al. 1997). Hospitals may aggressively pursue comprehensive coding if they are paid for treating sicker patients or worry about external publication of risk-adjusted report cards. On the other hand, the threat of prosecution for overcoding is a disincentive to coding conditions that may be present but would not be easy to defend in an audit.

The training and professional background of the person reviewing the record are critically important. Diagnosis and procedure coding using ICD-9-CM requires extensive training in coding guidelines leading to registered record administrator or accredited record technician degrees. Although hospitals usually employ individuals with such degrees to code their discharge abstracts, coders in other settings often have less training. The background of the reviewers can compromise reliability in unexpected ways. We once hired our own research staff to abstract medical records with MedisGroups (Iezzoni et al. 1992b). The reviewers were registered nurses with additional master's- or doctoral-level training who were uncomfortable following strict data-collection protocols established by the developers of MedisGroups to achieve high reliability. Although the guidelines often specified the exact words needed to establish the presence of a KCF, the reviewers wanted to use their extensive knowledge to interpret findings or reflect their own clinical sense of a case. Here, independent judgment, so highly valued in clinical care, led to unreliable data collection.

Assessing Reliability

Reliability assessment aims to determine the amount of agreement resulting from repeated application of the risk adjuster. The simplest measure is the percentage agreement between reviewers or raters. MedisGroups used this strategy to rate accuracy (Brewster, Bradbury, and Jacobs 1985). During training, new MedisGroups chart reviewers compared their KCFs with those identified by expert instructors; 95 percent agreement was required before the trainee qualified as a MedisGroups reviewer.

However, high percentages of exact agreement can occur even without skilled reviewers or reliable review instruments. To illustrate, imagine that rater A examines 100 cases, classifying 90 as high risk and 10 as low risk. Suppose that rater B labels patients as high risk randomly, each with probability of 80 percent. The expected percentage agreement between raters A and B is 74 percent: Raters A and B are expected to agree on 80 percent of the 90 high-risk cases ($n = 72$) and 20 percent of the 10 low-risk cases ($n = 2$). From this perspective, when one rater finds 90 percent high-risk cases and a second one finds 80 percent, 75 percent exact agreement is hardly larger than chance agreement. Furthermore, if rater C simply called all cases high risk, A and C would have 90 percent agreement.

Cohen's Kappa

Kappa is the most common measure of the reliability of instruments with categorical and ordinal scales (Cohen 1960). Kappa can take several forms. The simplest measures how much the level of agreement between two observers exceeds the amount of agreement expected by chance alone, computed as:

$$K = \frac{P_o - P_c}{1 - P_c}$$

where P_o is the observed agreement and P_c is the agreement that would have occurred by chance. In the previous example of raters A and B using a two-level scale, if the overall agreement rate had been 75 percent, kappa would be:

$$\frac{0.75 - 0.74}{1.00 - 0.74} = 0.04$$

How good is a kappa score of 0.04? In their seminal article, Landis and Koch (1977) assessed kappa values as follows: kappa < 0.0, poor agreement; kappa 0.0–0.20, slight agreement; kappa 0.21–0.4, fair agreement; kappa 0.41–0.6, moderate agreement; kappa 0.61–0.8, substantial agreement; and kappa 0.81–1.0, almost perfect agreement.

Although kappa is superior to percentage agreement, it becomes particularly unstable when the prevalence of the target outcome is small. For example, suppose two raters each reviewed the same 100 cases and each found two problem cases. Three scenarios are possible (Table 9.4): They found the same two problem cases; they agreed on just one case; or each found two different cases. Percentages of exact agreement for these three scenarios are 100 percent, 98 percent, and 96 percent, respectively; kappas are 1.00, 0.49, and −0.01. A shift in one or two cases thus can cause kappa to vary over the entire range of possible values.

The simple form of kappa applies when assessing agreement between two raters. With more than two raters, kappa scores can be computed for each rater pair and then averaged.

Weighted Kappa

In the basic form of kappa, all disagreements among raters are rated the same regardless of the magnitude of disagreement. Difficulties arise when raters have three or more choices on an ordinal scale, such as an edema (or swelling) score

TABLE 9.4

Example of Two Raters when Prevalence of Problem Is Small (by number of cases)

| | Rater 1 | | | | | |
| | Scenario 1 | | Scenario 2 | | Scenario 3 | |
Rater 2	No	Yes	No	Yes	No	Yes
No	98	0	97	1	96	2
Yes	0	2	1	1	2	0

NOTE: Kappa is 1.00, 0.49, and –0.01 for scenarios 1, 2, and 3, respectively; percent agreement is 100, 98, and 96 percent, respectively.

that ranges from 1+ to 4+. The basic formulation of kappa can apply here but could obscure important differences in reliability. For example, suppose two ordinal scales each yield possible scores from 1 to 4; both produce 70 percent agreement between two raters. For one scale, all disagreements are within one point. For the other, disagreements are frequently two or three points apart. Using the basic form of kappa, both scales achieve the same kappa value, although the sizes of disagreements for the two scales differ widely.

Landis and Koch (1977) proposed ways to weight kappa to give partial credit for small discrepancies or increase the penalty as the magnitude of the discrepancy in ratings increases. For example, when exact agreement is given a value of 1, ratings for an individual case within one rank might be given a $\frac{1}{2}$; those within two ranks given a $\frac{1}{4}$; and those more than two ranks apart given a 0. Another approach is to base the score on the square of the amount of disagreement, causing the penalty for disagreement to increase geometrically as the discrepancy in ratings increases. Because this form of weighted kappa depends on the squared value of the difference in ratings, it is a form of analysis of variance (ANOVA) procedure, providing opportunities for other statistical manipulations.

Other Measures of Reliability

The intraclass correlation coefficient (ICC), or interrater reliability coefficient (R_I), is based on one-way ANOVA and can be used in one of several forms to assess the degree of agreement among two or more raters. Because it is a proportion, the ICC ranges from 0 (complete disagreement) to 1 (complete agreement). Shrout and Fleiss (1979) developed several types of calculations for ICC, each a ratio of variance estimates. In each, the variance of ratings for different cases—the between-mean square (BMS)—is divided by a sum of BMS plus other variance components depending on the purpose of the particular analysis.[6] Because the ICC is based on one-way ANOVA, it treats risk adjusters as interval scales. As many risk adjusters produce ordinal scales, reliability results using the ICC could be misleading. Shrout and Fleiss (1979) provide an excellent discussion of considerations in selecting the appropriate form of the ICC.

Kendall's tau (sometimes called gamma) is useful in evaluating ordinal scales because it measures the degree to which two different observers rank cases in similar order. Kendall's tau is calculated by taking all possible pairs of cases and noting how often the pairs have concordant and discordant rankings (i.e., are ranked in the same order versus the opposite order by both observers; ties are not counted). Specifically, tau equals the number of concordant rankings minus the number of discordant rankings divided by the total number of pairs. The score can range from –1.0 (implying total disagreement) to 1.0 (total agreement). Several variations of tau—tau_a, tau_b, and tau_c—are useful if ties in ranks are present. Gibbons (1993) provides further description of these measures and simple examples.

Other Issues in Assessing Reliability

Different risk adjusters quantify risk along ordinal or interval scales, a distinction with important implications for reliability measurement. An interval scale provides a continuum of values; it suggests that a given increase in the scale always has the same implication for increased risk. On an interval scale, for example, the difference between scores of 5 and 10 conveys the same increased risk as the difference between scores of 25 and 30. In contrast, an ordinal scale conveys only a ranking; a higher score simply indicates greater risk. For example, on an ordinal scale, patients with scores of 3 face higher risks than those with scores of 2, but the difference between scores of 2 and 3 is not necessarily equivalent to the difference between scores of 3 and 4.

The reliability of a measure is to some extent an artifact. For example, suppose that two raters each rate 100 persons on a three-point scale, with the results shown in Table 9.5. The kappa value is $(60 – 34)/(100 – 34) = 0.39$, which is fair by the standards of Landis and Koch (1977). However, one can boost kappa to 0.52 (moderate) by collapsing the observations to a two-point scale (Table 9.6). The perceived improvement is somewhat real, as many misclassifications relate to distinctions between the scores 1 and 2. While one can often improve reliability by collapsing scores, reducing the number of categories can also cause kappa to fall. This would happen in the above example by using a different two-point scale (Table 9.7); here, kappa drops to 0.38.

These examples highlight two lessons: Do not rely too heavily on precise values of kappa, and do not compare kappas for risk adjusters with very different distributions of cases into categories. For instance, one should not compare a simple kappa for APACHE II, which has 72 scores (from 0 to 71), with a simple kappa for a four-level risk adjuster, such as the CSI. APACHE scores differ by one or more points much more easily than CSI ratings differ by an entire level.[7] A more fair approach is as follows: If 35 percent of cases fall into the CSI's lowest category, group together the 35 percent of cases with the lowest APACHE scores; if CSI level 2 includes 25 percent of the cases,

TABLE 9.5

Example of Two Raters and a Three-Point Scale

Scores of Rater 2	Scores of Rater 1			
	1	2	3	All
1	25	10	5	40
2	10	15	5	30
3	5	5	20	30
All	40	30	30	100

NOTE: Kappa = 0.39; percent agreement = 60.

TABLE 9.6

Example of Two Raters and a Three-Point Scale Collapsed to a Two-Point Scale: Case 1

Scores of Rater 2	Scores of Rater 1		
	< 3	3	All
< 3	60	10	70
3	10	20	30
All	70	30	100

NOTE: Kappa = 0.52; percent agreement = 80.

TABLE 9.7

Example of Two Raters and a Three-Point Scale Collapsed to a Two-Point Scale: Case 2

Scores of Rater 2	Scores of Rater 1		
	1	> 1	All
1	25	15	40
> 1	15	45	60
All	40	60	100

NOTE: Kappa = 0.38; percent agreement = 70.

group together the 25 percent of cases with the next highest APACHE scores; and so on. Then, one could calculate kappa scores using these four levels, with APACHE and the CSI groupings containing similar percentages of patients.

Although a risk adjuster's reliability is important, measuring reliability presents considerable challenges. A single measure of interrater reliability is generally insufficient. Although Thomas and Ashcraft (1989) demonstrated strong correlations among different reliability methods, they urged that reliability analyses employ several techniques simultaneously. Nevertheless, the ultimate test of reliability for any risk adjuster is not how well it performs under laboratory conditions but rather its performance in the real world. Real-world dynamics, such as financial motivations and concerns about public disclosure, may be the most powerful forces to compromise reliability.

Notes

1. Researchers have compared clinicians' ratings and risk scores. Kruse, Thill-Baharozian, and Carlson (1988) compared the predictions of 57 physicians and 33 critical care nurses with the APACHE II scores on 366 patients admitted to an ICU; clinical judgments and APACHE II scores had comparable accuracy. However, when Brannen, Godfrey, and Goetter (1989) compared the predictions of critical care physicians in one medical ICU with APACHE II predictions, their physicians did significantly better than the APACHE II score in predicting mortality. Another study in a surgical ICU found that clinicians' predictions were slightly better than APACHE II predictions. However, both physicians and APACHE II predictions misclassified as likely to die 40 percent of patients who subsequently lived (Meyer et al. 1992).

2. The c-statistic measures model discrimination, that is, how well the model distinguishes those who live from those who die. Two models with the same ability to discriminate could differ in how well they calibrate, that is, how well their prediction about the overall death rate in the sample compares to the actual death rate (see Chapter 10).

3. In a development data set, recorded relationships between predictor variables and outcomes are used to teach the model how to make "predicted" and actual outcomes conform as well as possible. (As the outcomes must be known in advance, this can be thought of as "predicting the past.") When validating a model in new data, we make true predictions—in the sense that they are made while ignorant of the "answers"—by applying the previously developed model to the predictor variables alone.

4. Given the public availability of APACHE algorithms, much effort has focused on the validity of APACHE, developed for ICU patients in the United States, for other populations of patients, including ICU patients in different countries. Because ICU practices vary internationally, APACHE's generalizability and validity must be studied anew in different environments; research using APACHE II has come from several countries, including Canada (Wong et al. 1995), Singapore (Chen, Koh, and Goh 1993), Israel (Porath et al. 1994), Britain and Ireland (Rowan et al. 1993, 1994), and Switzerland (Berger et al. 1992). In general, APACHE II demonstrated validity in these international comparisons. Variable results have arisen from attempts to validate APACHE II in specific diagnosis- or procedure-based populations, such as breast cancer patients (Headley, Theriault, and Smith 1992), neurosurgical patients (Hartley et al. 1995), AMI patients (Ludwigs and Hulting 1995), and trauma patients (Vassar and Holcroft 1994; Vassar et al. 1992; Rutledge et al. 1993).

5. The sample sizes were as follows: medically treated AMI, 11,880 patients from 100 hospitals with 1,574 (13.2 percent) in-hospital deaths (Iezzoni et al. 1995b, 1996e); CABG surgery, 7,765 patients from 38 hospitals with 252 (3.2 percent) in-hospital deaths (Landon et al. 1996); pneumonia, 18,016 patients from 105 hospitals with 1,732 (9.6 percent) in-hospital deaths (Iezzoni et al. 1996a, 1996b); and medically treated stroke, 9,407 patients from 94 hospitals with 916 (9.7 percent) in-hospital deaths (Iezzoni et al. 1995a, 1996d).

6. In general, a mean square is calculated from a sum of squares by dividing the sum of squares by $(n - p)$, where n is the sample size and p is the number of estimated parameters. The most familiar example of this is in calculating the variance of a set of data. The sum of squares total, or SST, is $\Sigma_i(Y_i - \overline{Y})^2$. The mean square, which in this simple case is used as an estimate of the population variance, is $\text{SST}/(n - 1)$. Here, n is the sample size and 1 is subtracted because just one parameter, the population mean, has been estimated (using $\overline{Y}$) from the data.

7. In comparing the reliability of several severity measures, Thomas and Ashcraft (1989) dealt with these issues by stratifying APACHE II, PMC Normative Cost Weights, and the DS Q-Scale, as well as DRG weights, into five categories, as had MedisGroups at the time. They determined the cutpoints for the APACHE II score in two ways. First, they approximated the distribution of rankings among the five MedisGroups severity levels; second, they determined the optimal cutpoints using the Automated Interaction Detector computer program to minimize variance (Thomas, Ashcraft, and Zimmerman 1986). With the latter method of recoding, the 90 percent of patients with scores of 15 or less were divided among the lowest four categories, whereas the remaining patients with scores ranging from 16 to 71 made up the fifth category.

EVALUATING RISK-ADJUSTMENT MODELS EMPIRICALLY

Michael Shwartz and Arlene S. Ash

The first question often asked about a risk-adjustment method is, "How good is it?" Questioners generally want a quick, bottom-line response— a number that allows them to compare one risk adjuster's performance to another's. They want to know its "predictive validity"—how well the risk adjuster accounts for actual differences in patients' risks for particular outcomes. As noted throughout this book, no single summary indicator of statistical performance can fully reveal how valid a risk-adjustment method is for an intended purpose. Other important dimensions of validity, including clinical credibility and reliability of the underlying data sources (see Chapter 9), help determine whether persons reviewing risk-adjusted outcomes data will believe and act on the information. Nonetheless, the ability of a risk-adjustment method to account for differences in patients' risks is often a key attribute, determining how much faith observers will place in risk-adjusted results.

Evaluating statistical performance generally involves comparing how well risk-adjusted predictions of patient outcomes "fit" the actual outcomes. As most risk adjusters derive from multivariable models (see Chapter 8), evaluations of their statistical properties can proceed generically, as one might assess any model. Many excellent textbooks discuss the principles and practices of empirical modeling, including classic works by Draper and Smith (1981); Neter and Wasserman (1974); Neter, Wasserman, and Kutner (1990); Mosteller and Tukey (1977); and Box, Hunter, and Hunter (1978).

Here, we examine special concerns relating to the use of multivariable models for risk adjustment when assessing health care outcomes. We discuss quantitative measures of predictive validity for predicting either continuous outcomes (e.g., LOS, costs of care) or dichotomous ones (e.g., death, complications). Throughout, we draw examples from existing risk adjusters (see Chapter 2) and our own work. First, we consider how to convert risk scores into predicted outcomes—the so-called "*PREDs*."

Translating Risk Scores into Predicted Outcomes

Risk adjustment requires estimating expected outcomes for individuals based on their risk factors. If Y is an outcome and *PRED* estimates its expected value for each person, the sum of the *PREDs* for a population equals the expected value of the sum of the observed Ys and the mean of the $PRED$s equals the expected value of the mean of the observed Ys. If Y is a 0/1 outcome, such as death, each $PRED$ is the predicted probability that an individual will die, the sum of the $PRED$s for a group is the expected number of deaths in the group, and the mean of its $PRED$s is the group's expected death rate.

For certain risk adjusters, the risk score for an individual already is the expected value of a particular outcome (see Table 2.5). For example, Medis-Groups assigns a $PRED$—a predicted probability of in-hospital death—to each admission based on the patient's KCFs. Analysts can compare the actual death rate in a group with its MedisGroups-adjusted expected death rate, its average $PRED$. Another MedisGroups model was developed to predict hospital LOSs. Expected LOS for a group of patients is again computed as the average $PRED$, here, predicted LOS.

Even when risk scores are derived explicitly to predict the outcome of interest, analysts may want to adjust or recalibrate the scores before using them as $PRED$s depending on the purpose of the analysis and the target population. As an illustration, suppose that 13 percent of 10,000 AMI patients hospitalized in California in 1999 died, but that their expected death rate based on a risk-adjustment model was 15 percent. To the extent that model predictions provide an appropriate standard, California outcomes are better than expected, perhaps because the quality of care there is better than the standard. However, purely "technical" factors can also cause observed and predicted outcomes to diverge; identifying the principal cause(s) of a difference is difficult and controversial. For example, declines in CABG mortality in New York state following publication of risk-adjusted mortality rates by hospital and surgeon have been attributed both to improved performance (Hannan et al. 1995; Chassin, Hannan, and DeBuono 1996) and to various non-quality-related factors (Green and Wintfeld 1995). One specific reason for caution is that more intensive coding of comorbid illness makes the same population "look sicker," causing its risk-adjusted outcomes to "look better." To the extent that coding intensity has increased over time or differs across settings, comparisons can be problematic.

Even if models developed in one population and applied to another do not predict the average outcome well, the "relative risks" encoded in the predictions can generalize. Recalibration (or simply calibration) refers to fitting a model developed elsewhere to a new data set, typically forcing the average expected outcome to exactly equal the average actual outcome in the new data. Recalibration strategies include adding the same amount to each score (e.g., in our California example, –2 percent), multiplying each score by the same amount (e.g., 13/15), or using more sophisticated regression techniques. When predictions are calibrated to a new population, they no longer provide an external standard for that population. However, recalibrated models are still useful for examining risk-adjusted differences in outcomes for policy-relevant subgroups of patients (e.g., Medicaid and private-pay patients) or for comparing different providers.

A "dimensionless" risk score must be calibrated to predict outcomes in a new population. For example, the DCG prospective relative risk score (RRS) represents next year's expected total health care costs as a multiple of average cost. RRSs are calculated from demographic data and a vector of health status information. An RRS of 1.2 means expected resource consumption is 20 percent greater than average. The simplest way to convert RRSs to *PRED*s in a population involves multiplying each score by a "proportionality constant" calculated as C/S, where C is the average outcome and S is the average score in that population. This is appropriate with any score that was developed to be proportional to the outcome of interest. A more flexible method of recalibration is required when the risk scores are likely to be systematically associated with the outcome but not necessarily proportional to it. One such method is "risk score bucketing." Analysts rank cases in the order of their risk scores and then assign cutpoints to delineate a small number of categories, so-called "buckets" or "bins."[1] No single bucket should contain most of the cases, and each bucket should contain enough cases to obtain a stable average.[2] The prediction for each case is calculated as the average actual outcome for all cases in the same bucket.[3] Bucketing approaches accommodate situations where risk scores were calibrated to one outcome (e.g., cost) but are being used to predict a related outcome (e.g., mortality). Large data sets permit more refined recalibrations by regressing the outcome in the target population on the risk score (or indicator/dummy variables for score buckets) plus other factors (such as demographic characteristics).[4]

If a model is used to generate the *PRED*s, it consists of equations that specify coefficients for each explanatory variable. These equations are then applied to new data to calculate a new risk score for each case.[5] To develop the model, the values of both explanatory and outcome variables are needed for each case. However, the model needs only the explanatory variable values for each case to create *PRED*s. The question of how well these *PRED*s match the outcomes in either the original data or in new data remains.

Model Performance in Development and Validation Data Sets

Before discussing specific measures of model performance, it is important to distinguish how a model performs in the data on which it was developed (called "fitting" or "development" data) from how well it performs when applied to new data (called "validation" or "confirmatory" data; see Chapter 8).

The more variables a model includes, the greater the importance of computing measures of performance on validation data. Thus, for example, to translate a risk score (*RS*) from an existing risk-adjustment method into a predicted cost (or other continuous outcome), analysts could calculate *PRED*s as:

$$PRED_i = \hat{a} + \hat{b} * RS_i$$

or for dichotomous outcomes (discussed later) as:

$$\ln[(PRED_i)/(1 - PRED_i)] = \hat{a} + \hat{b} * RS_i.$$

With only two coefficients to fit to a large data set, overfitting is not a major concern (see below). When the fitting data set is large and representative of likely future data, overfitting is also unlikely. However, in many situations, analysts use the same moderately sized data set to both specify the model (i.e., to determine which of many risk factors to include and the form in which to include them) and estimate coefficients for each included variable. In this setting, overfitting can occur: Variables are identified and parameters estimated to fit the particular development data set (and its idiosyncrasies) too closely. When fitting complicated models with many risk factors, a model fit to one data set is unlikely to predict outcomes equally well in new data.

When outcomes are approximately normally distributed, 30 cases per predictor variable are generally considered enough to establish reliable coefficients; for highly skewed outcomes, hundreds of cases may be needed. For example, the total health care costs of a general population during a fixed time period typically contain many $0 figures (for people who use no services), a large majority of cases with low costs, and a small fraction (generally fewer than 20 percent) with high costs. Within this last group, a few have extremely high costs. For example, in a national research database of people with employer-sponsored health insurance, about 25 percent had no costs and 50 percent used less than $500 in 1998. The top 20 percent averaged $1,300 each, consuming nearly 90 percent of all health care dollars, whereas the top 1 percent averaged $24,000 each, accounting for more than 30 percent of dollars (Ash et al. 2001). Extreme differences in health status and cost have sample size implications and heighten the need for validation. Especially when models include indicators for rare, expensive events, generic guidelines for the numbers of cases needed to achieve stable models—such as "no more than one predictor for each 30 cases" when predicting continuous outcomes and "no more than one predictor per 18 events" when predicting dichotomous outcomes—may not be sufficiently conservative.[6] Models built with fewer data are almost certain to be unstable and likely to predict substantially less well in new data than in the development data. However, even models built on larger databases should be validated on other data.

A practical impediment is the lack of data for validation. As described later in this chapter, various techniques allow analysts to estimate what performance would be on a validation data set by creatively using the development data.

Measuring Model Performance when the Outcome Is Continuous

When asking how well a risk adjuster predicts a continuous outcome like costs, many questioners want to hear about the R^2—a number representing how much of the total variability in the outcome is explained by the risk adjuster or how well the predictions fit the outcomes (Ash and Byrne-Logan 1998). Although several definitions of R^2 exist, the most common is:

$$R^2 = 1 - [\Sigma_i(Y_i - PRED_i)^2 / \Sigma_i(Y_i - \overline{Y})^2]$$

where $\overline{Y}$ is the average of the Y_is. In the term above that is subtracted from 1, the numerator is called the sum of squared errors (SSE) and the denominator is called the sum of squares total (SST). SST is determined by the data alone and not by the model, and it measures the variability of the outcome Y in the data. SSE measures the variability in Y that is not captured by the predictive model.

An ordinary least squares (OLS) algorithm chooses parameter estimates that minimize SSE. $(Y_i - PRED_i)$ is called the ith "residual," "deviation," or "error," and

$$SSE = \Sigma_i(Y_i - PRED_i)^2$$

with

$$PRED_i = \hat{Y}_i = \hat{a} + \Sigma_j \hat{b}_j * X_{ij}. \tag{1}$$

When estimating model parameters (a and the b_js) with OLS, $\hat{a}$ and $\hat{b}$ are selected to minimize SSE and thus maximize R^2. Therefore, R^2 is a particularly appropriate measure of performance for models derived using OLS.

R^2 can still be computed and is a useful summary measure of performance even if predicted values are developed some other way, such as using the binary split algorithm CART (Salford Systems, San Diego, CA, based on techniques developed by Breiman et al. 1984; see www.salford-systems.com/products-cart.html). Examining the same performance measure is often desirable when comparing models constructed with different algorithms, although these other approaches do not choose coefficients to maximize R^2. To easily calculate the R^2 for a set of $\{(Y_i, PRED_i)\}$ pairs, first calculate r, the Pearson correlation of Y and $PRED$, and then square it.

R^2 is often described as the fraction of total variability in the outcome (dependent variable) explained by or attributed to differences in risk among cases included in the model. Sometimes, analysts multiply R^2 by 100 to represent the percentage of variation explained by the model. For example, Shwartz and colleagues (1996b) found that DRGs explained 42 percent of the variability in costs among hospital admissions. After adding 23 comorbidity variables to the model, R^2 increased to 50 percent; thus, comorbidities increased the variability explained by nearly 20 percent ($[(50 - 42)/42] * 100$) over that explained by DRGs alone.

Most investigators routinely report R^2 to indicate how well risk-adjustment models explain continuous outcomes like health care expenditure or LOS. The Society of Actuaries, for example, recently compared how well methods based on administrative data predict next year's medical costs within commercially insured populations (Cumming et al. 2002). They examined the following seven models:

1. ACGs, Version 4.5. ACGs do not produce standard risk weights. Users calibrate models to their own data.
2. DCGs, Version 5.1. This version includes 32 age/sex cells and 118 condition categories.
3. CDPS, Version 1.7. This model assigns individuals to 1 of 16 age/sex cells and 1 or more of 67 medical conditions.
4. Medicaid R_x. This pharmacy-based model, originally developed for a Medicaid population, assigns individuals to 1 of 11 age/sex cells and 1 or more of 45 medical conditions based on prescription drug use, as recorded in National Drug Codes (not all NDCs are classified).
5. RxGroups, Version 1.0. This pharmacy-based system assigns people to 1 of 32 age/sex cells and 1 or more of 127 drug therapy categories. All NDCs are classified, without tying the categories to specific medical conditions.
6. RxRisk. This pharmacy-based system assigns adults to 1 of 22 age/sex cells and 1 or more of 27 medical conditions. Not all NDCs are classified.
7. Episode Risk Groups (ERGs), Version 4.2. This method first uses diagnoses, procedures, and medications to assign individuals to Episode Treatment Groups (ETGs; see Chapter 4). Based on this assignment, ERGs indicate which of 119 medical conditions are present.

The Society of Actuaries database contained almost 750,000 members of commercial employer groups in either preferred provider organizations or HMOs who were continuously enrolled in 1998 and 1999. We consider R^2 values from analyses in which models fit to 1998 data were used to predict 1999 expenditures. Each model (with the exception of ACGs) was evaluated twice: once using the risk weight for each condition category as supplied by the vendor of the particular risk-adjustment method, and again using risk weights from fitting a model with dummy variables for each category and using the coefficients from this model as the weights.

Table 10.1 shows the R^2 values for predicting raw (untransformed) total costs and "topcoded" total costs (discussed later), where total costs exceeding \$100,000 were set to \$100,000. Not surprisingly, R^2 was always higher when costs were topcoded; predicting less-skewed outcomes is easier. However, topcoded models do not account for all the dollars (i.e., the mean

Model	Prospective (Predicting 1999)				Concurrent (Predicting 1998)		TABLE 10.1
	Original Weights		Recalibrated		Recalibrated		Percentage of Variation* when Predicting
	Topcoded at $100,000	Full Range	Topcoded at $100,000	Full Range	Topcoded at $100,000	Full Range	Payments from 1998 Diagnostic
ACG[a]	NA	NA	14	10	38	28	and/or
CDPS[a]	13	10	19	15	42	36	Pharmacy Data
DCG[a]	18	14	20	15	55	47	
Medicaid Rx[b]	10	7	17	12	33	24	
RxGroups[b]	18	13	19	13	38	28	
RxRisk[b]	15	11	15	11	29	21	
ERG[a,b]	19	15	20	15	43	35	

SOURCE: Adapted from Tables 3.1, 3.2, and 3.3, Cumming et al. (2002).
* $R^2 \times 100$.
[a] Requires diagnostic data (ICD-9-CM codes).
[b] Requires pharmacy data (NDC) codes.

prediction for topcoded models equals the mean of topcoded costs, which is smaller than mean actual costs). Thus, the size of the increase in R^2 associated with moving from models predicting raw versus topcoded costs is uninteresting. As always, what matters is how different models compare when predicting the same outcome.

In contrast to the topcoding situation, how much R^2 changes with recalibration is interesting because analysts must choose between using risk scores from the vendors' algorithm and producing their own recalibrated weights. In the Society of Actuaries study, CDPS and Medicaid R_x had much higher R^2 values from recalibrated weights (Cumming et al. 2002). As Medicaid R_x had used Medicaid data to produce their weights, this is not surprising. The other methods produced only modestly higher R^2 values with recalibrated weights. This should reassure researchers wishing to use methods "off the shelf" to predict similar outcomes in roughly comparable populations as used to develop the method. Often, a full-scale model recalibration is impractical.

In the Society of Actuaries study, three risk adjusters relied on diagnosis codes, three scored persons using pharmacy data, and one used diagnoses, procedures, and pharmacy data. Despite these different data sources, most methods produced fairly comparable R^2 values. Given this, choosing among them will rely on other factors beyond statistical performance, such as feasibility, cost, availability, and appropriateness to purpose.

The last two columns of Table 10.1 show the R^2 values from models fit to 1999 data and then used to predict expenditures in 1999 (concurrent modeling). Not surprisingly, concurrent models produced much higher R^2 values than did prospective models. People with specified diagnoses in year

1 incurred costs in that year, as diagnoses are recorded during medical encounters. However, whether they use any health care at all next year, and how much, is subject to chance. Higher R^2 values from concurrent models relate primarily to their ability to "predict the past." Concurrent models "predict" what already happened, whereas prospective models predict the future. R^2 values from concurrent and prospective models are therefore not comparable.

Although R^2 is a valuable summary measure of model performance, it provides little intuitive feel for the ability of a model to discriminate among cases with high and low values for the dependent variable. To provide such insight, we suggest examining actual and predicted outcomes within deciles of predicted outcomes. Table 10.2 illustrates such a table for pneumonia patients (trimmed data) from our study of hospital-based severity measures. It shows that for APR-DRGs, which had an R^2 of 0.147, the predicted mean LOS of patients in the lowest decile was 5.5 days; the predicted mean LOS of patients in the highest decile was 12.8 days, slightly more than twice as long. For R-DRGs, with an R^2 of 0.170, the comparable LOS values were 4.1 days and 13.2 days, greater than a threefold difference. Table 10.2 shows the mean actual LOS values in each decile. In general, predicted mean LOS values in the extreme deciles were closer together than actual mean LOS values in these deciles. These deciles-of-risk tables usefully portray the ability of models to discriminate among different types of cases. We illustrate this in more detail when considering dichotomous outcomes.

Grouped R²

In calculating the traditional R^2 (i.e., $1 - SSE/SST$), each difference between a person's actual and predicted costs contributes to the model's error and reduces the R^2. Predicting an individual's future health care costs is difficult precisely because so much of health care spending is totally unpredictable (e.g., accidents) or largely unpredictable (e.g., strokes). As a result, in populations containing healthy and sick people, achieving high R^2 values for predicting costs is generally infeasible. In many settings, however, the main purpose of risk adjustment is not to produce correct predictions for each person but to produce correct average predictions within policy-relevant subgroups, such as persons enrolled in different health plans. Grouped R^2 measures how well models can distinguish among groups of individuals with predictably different outcomes.

When building models to predict next year's Medicare costs, Ash and colleagues (1989) sought to demonstrate that increasing R^2 even by a modest amount—from around 1 percent for a model using only demographic characteristics to about 6 percent for one based on discharge diagnoses—was important. Grouped R^2 values helped show that the diagnosis-based models were extremely useful for identifying subgroups of patients with predictably higher future costs.

TABLE 10.2
Actual and
Predicted Mean
LOS within
Deciles of
Predicted LOS
and R^2:
Pneumonia
Cases and
Trimmed Data

Severity Adjustment Method	Decile of Predicted LOS				R^2
	1	2	9	10	
	Mean Actual LOS (mean predicted LOS)				
AIM[a]	5.1 (5.5)	6.6 (6.8)	11.1 (10.9)	13.2 (12.8)	14.0
APR-DRGs[a]	5.0 (5.5)	6.6 (6.7)	11.6 (10.9)	13.0 (12.8)	14.7
DS Relative Resource Scale	5.1 (5.3)	6.4 (6.6)	11.2 (11.2)	13.4 (13.6)	14.4
PMC Resource Intensity Scale	5.2 (5.2)	6.4 (6.8)	11.0 (11.2)	12.6 (12.9)	12.2
R-DRGs	4.0 (4.1)	6.2 (6.5)	11.4 (11.5)	13.2 (13.2)	17.0
DS mortality probablilty	5.2 (5.3)	6.6 (6.9)	10.8 (11.0)	12.5 (12.6)	10.7
PMC severity score	5.1 (5.3)	6.5 (6.6)	10.8 (11.0)	12.6 (12.8)	12.2
Body Systems Count	5.1 (5.1)	6.5 (6.7)	11.0 (11.3)	13.0 (13.1)	13.3
Comorbidity Index	5.2 (5.3)	6.7 (6.9)	10.9 (11.0)	12.2 (12.5)	10.3
MedisGroups	5.2 (5.2)	6.5 (6.9)	10.7 (11.1)	12.4 (12.6)	10.9
Physiology score	5.1 (5.3)	6.7 (7.0)	10.6 (11.0)	12.1 (12.4)	9.9
Age, sex, and DRG only	5.2 (5.3)	6.8 (7.0)	11.0 (11.0)	11.9 (12.4)	9.7

SOURCE: Iezzoni et al. (1996c).
[a] From model with severity score interacted with DRG.

Unlike the traditional R^2, a grouped R^2 is not an intrinsic property of a population but rather depends on how the population is partitioned into groups, or "bins," such that each case belongs to exactly one group. Specifically, the grouped R^2 for a particular partition is defined as:

$$\text{grouped } R^2 = 1 - \text{GSS(model)}/\text{GSS(total)}$$

where GSS(model) equals the sum over all bins, B, of

$$(\text{No. of people in bin B}) * (\text{average } Y \text{ in B} - \text{average } PRED \text{ in B})^2$$

and GSS(total) equals the sum over all bins, B, of

$$(\text{No. of people in bin B}) * (\text{average } Y \text{ in B} - \overline{Y})^2$$

where $\overline{Y}$ equals the average cost in the entire population.

Looking at group totals (or averages) reduces random errors and highlights systematic differences between groups. The grouped R^2, for example, gives no penalty for predicting $1,500 for each of two people in the same group when one costs nothing and the other costs $3,000. Within the same group, positive and negative individual errors of prediction cancel each other out.

Different binning rules yield different values of the grouped R^2 for the same model. Analysts should decide, preferably in advance, which binning approaches are of greatest interest. (The same issue applies to the Hosmer-Lemeshow tests, described later.) To see how well a model captures differences in next year's cost based on differences in this year's cost, for example, we could form the bins using use deciles of current costs. More than for other statistical performance measures, the grouped R^2 value depends heavily on the specific data set and binning approach. Grouped R^2 values are therefore principally useful for comparing models in the same data to identify which approach better captures how the grouped subpopulations differ.

Rosenkranz and Luft (1997) used the grouped R^2 to study the performance of four models to predict health care expenditures: a single-equation model with demographic predictor variables only (called 1S), a single-equation model with demographic plus personnel predictor variables (i.e., marital status, length of employment, salary, zip code; called 1F), a four-equation model with demographic variables (4S), and a four-equation model with demographic plus personnel variables (4F). From a population of 5,000 employees enrolled in a fee-for-service health plan, they formed 100 bins of 50 persons each in two ways: randomly and based on predicted cost from the expenditure model being considered. Random groups mimic small employers identified without any risk selection. The risk-sorted groups mimic small employers identified with the most extreme selection possible based on the available risk factors. Table 10.3 shows the R^2 values. Individual R^2 values were very low, as expected. Random bins produced higher grouped R^2 values because predicting group averages is easier than predicting outcomes for individuals. However, as shown in the last column, when risk differed systematically across the bins, all grouped R^2 values were much higher.

However, comparing numbers within the columns of Table 10.3 does not necessarily reveal which model is best. One reason is generic to all comparisons of models using any statistical performance measure. Because the observed values of each measure are themselves random variables, concluding that one model performs better than another requires evidence that the observed differences are greater than those resulting from chance. One way to do this is by creating "bootstrapped" confidence intervals on the statistical performance measure (discussed later).

A second concern is specific to the grouped R^2: Its values are extremely sensitive to how the groups are formed. If different risk adjusters are evaluated based on bins formed using their own predicted risk scores for sorting, the bins will vary across risk adjusters. This is acceptable when informally evaluating the ability of risk adjusters to predict outcomes within risk strata. However, more rigorous comparisons across risk adjusters require use of a standard binning method before computing a grouped R^2.

As an alternative to grouped R^2, the Society of Actuaries study examined "predictive ratios" (Cumming et al. 2002). A predictive ratio (PR) is the ratio of the average predicted expenditures for persons in a group to their actual expenditures (Ash et al. 1989). In other words, PRs compare expected to observed outcomes—they are E/O ratios. The Society of Actuaries examined PRs for persons with specific diseases (e.g., breast cancer, CHF, asthma, depression, HIV infection) and for bins defined by quintile of actual expenditures. The asthma group, for example, included all people with asthma

R^2-Type Grouping	Individual None	Grouped Random	Grouped Risk Based
Model		$R^2 \times 100$	
1S	2.8	10.5	58.4
1F	2.6	11.0	54.2
4S	3.6	11.2	62.6
4F	3.4	13.0	70.3

TABLE 10.3
Comparison of Individual and Grouped R^2 Values for Groups Formed Randomly and Based on Risk

SOURCE: Adapted from Rosenkranz and Luft (1997).
NOTE: 1 vs. 4 = one- versus four-equation model specification; S vs. F = S predicts from demographics only, whereas F also uses marital status, length of employment, salary, and zip code.

regardless of other medical problems and all health care costs. Because people often have multiple diagnoses (and some have none), diseases cannot create the full-population partition that a grouped R^2 requires.

Not surprisingly, groups defined by a particular risk adjuster's classification system or by quantiles of its predicted risk yield grouped R^2 or PR values that are most favorable to that risk adjuster. Even a seemingly neutral approach, such as forming groups based on quantiles of the average *PRED* across all risk adjusters being compared, can be unfair. To see this, imagine that models 1 and 2 produce nearly identical predictions; model 3's predictions are equally powerful but somewhat different. If deciles are based on the average of the three *PREDs*, the grouped R^2 will suggest that models 1 and 2 perform equally well and better than model 3 at capturing the differences in deciles of average predicted risk. More generally, to the extent that several of the models produce very similar predictions, they will have higher grouped R^2 values than models whose predictions are least like the others, quite separately from their intrinsic ability to predict group averages. For this reason, we strongly recommend that grouped R^2 and PR values be based on groups that differ on features intrinsic to the data, such as prior costs, rather than differences in *PREDs*.

Sometimes, analysts use models to identify high-cost cases (or "top groups") for targeting disease management or other interventions. In this context, using R^2 to measure model performance does not directly address the relevant question: If each of several models are used to identify the same-sized top group, which one finds the "best" group? Ash and colleagues (2001) and Zhao et al. (in press) illustrate some approaches for comparing the ability of models to produce useful top groups, for example, those that contain (1) few "bad picks," persons whose next year's costs would be quite low (less than $5,000); (2) many "good" or "great" picks, persons whose next year's costs are high (at least $10,000 or $25,000); and (3) many people with potentially manageable diseases (e.g., diabetes, asthma).

Handling Extreme Values of the Outcome Variable

OLS estimates model parameters to minimize squared errors. Therefore, extreme values of a continuous outcome can substantially affect estimates. For example, health insurers may not care whether $10,000 in excess costs occur because the observed cost of a single case exceeds the predicted by $10,000 or because the observed costs for ten patients each exceed predicted costs by $1,000. However, the squared term associated with one large error far exceeds the sum of squares associated with multiple smaller errors that add to the same amount: $1 * 10,000^2$ is ten times larger than $10 * 1,000^2$. When fitting models to predict continuous outcomes with a few very extreme values (i.e., distributions with so-called "heavy right tails"), these "outlier" values can substantially distort predictions for cases with low or moderate values.

Health services researchers have several strategies for handling extreme or outlier cases. The most straightforward is simply to trim or eliminate cases with excessive or aberrant values from the data set. The effect of trimming on R^2 is not obvious. Dropping outlier cases reduces both SSE and SST. Because R^2 reflects the ratio of these two values, the effect of eliminating outliers depends on the relative magnitude of changes in the two terms.

Choosing which data to trim can depend on the purpose of the study. In projects examining hospital resource use, a common strategy involves defining either cost or LOS outliers, similar to Medicare's policy under DRG-based prospective payment, and then performing separate analyses including and excluding outlier cases. In our study of hospital-based severity measures, we used two strategies to identify high LOS outliers: Medicare's approach, which flagged all cases more than three standard deviations from the mean on a log scale; and a robust approach (one less sensitive to the actual distribution of the data) proposed by Hoaglin and Iglewicz (1987). For hip fracture patients, the Medicare approach eliminated 57 outliers (from a sample of 5,721), reducing the average LOS from 11.9 to 11.5 days; the Hoaglin-Iglewicz approach eliminated 414 outliers, shortening average LOS to 10.3 days (Shwartz et al. 1996a). Using the Hoaglin-Iglewicz approach, R^2 was higher on trimmed cases for only one of the 14 severity methods considered; using the Medicare trim points, R^2 was almost 50 percent higher on trimmed cases for eight methods. Likewise, in the study of pneumonia cases, R^2 was higher using the HCFA trim points for all severity measures (Iezzoni et al. 1996c).

A second way to handle outlier cases is to reset extreme values to some less extreme value—so-called "topcoding," "winsorizing," or "truncation." (The nomenclature used to distinguish these approaches in the health services literature is inconsistent.) In topcoding, the actual values for all cases with values greater than some number M are replaced by M. Thus, topcoding retains all cases but reduces the influence of high outliers by drawing them toward the mean. Topcoding is especially suited to situations where cases with particularly high values might be treated differently, such as reinsuring persons whose costs exceed a specified threshold. In winsorizing, equal numbers of both high- and low-value cases are replaced by specified values: For example, the five lowest values are reset to their maximum value and the five highest to their minimum. Winsorizing aims to create more stable estimates of means for essentially symmetrically distributed distributions (Dixon and Tukey 1968; Dixon and Massey 1969). Some researchers use the terms winsorizing or truncation when referring to what we called topcoding.

Various studies involving risk adjustment have used topcoding. In deriving APACHE III models to predict ICU LOS, Knaus and colleagues (1993) capped all ICU LOSs at 40 days. The Society of Actuaries study of risk-adjustment models performed analyses three ways: including all costs at their original values; topcoding costs greater than $100,000 at $100,000; and topcoding costs greater than $50,000 at $50,000 (Cumming et al. 2002). R^2 values were higher on topcoded data (see Table 10.1). When the topcode threshold was $50,000, R^2 values were even larger than for analyses with topcoding at $100,000.

We prefer topcoding to trimming because the most expensive cases are often very important and should not be completely ignored. We note that predictions from an OLS model fit to topcoded data occasionally exceed the topcode threshold. Such "out-of-range" predictions rather reliably mark the very sickest people; there is nothing to be gained by trying to "fix" them.

The effect of trimming or topcoding outliers may vary depending on how the risk adjuster is constructed. Methods that generate only a few categories (e.g., that assign scores of 1 to 5) may have defined a highest-risk category with few cases that are likely to have the most extreme outcome values. Conceptually, such risk adjusters should perform relatively better when outliers are included in the analysis than when they are excluded. Risk-adjustment approaches employing a continuous scale may distinguish better among non-outlier cases but not perform as well when cases with extreme values are included.

How and whether to trim or topcode data are best decided within the context of specific studies. In a payment policy context, for example, topcoding cases greater than $100,000 is consistent with a payment system that covers all costs below this threshold but pays for more costly cases out of a separate pool. Trimming or topcoding always understates expected costs (i.e., produces systematically smaller predicted than actual outcomes). This can prove misleading in a payment system with no special mechanism for handling outlier costs.

Another common strategy for limiting the influence of high-value cases is to transform the dependent variable, generally using a logarithmic transformation; the value of the dependent variable is replaced by its natural logarithm, producing a distribution of outcome values that is closer to normal. Lognormal transformations fall within the Box-Cox family of transformations (Box, Hunter, and Hunter 1978; Atkinson 1985; Spitzer 1982). With their more normal distribution, transformed data more closely conform to the assumptions of OLS modeling. Transforming continuous outcome variables is most appropriate when the goal is to identify statistically significant predictors of the outcome (to better meet the assumptions underlying the statistical tests). However, when the goal is to predict the value of the dependent variable, such transformations are less useful.

Predictions based on a transformed outcome variable must be retransformed to the original scale before calculating statistical performance measures. In particular, comparing R^2 values from predicting logged versus actual outcomes is inappropriate. As discussed above, OLS maximizes R^2 for the data to which the model is fit—whether on an original or transformed scale. Regardless of which scale is used in model development, statistical measures of model performance should be computed in the original scale (e.g., dollars, days).

Duan's (1983) smearing estimator is a widely used, theoretically attractive approach for retransforming log-transformed data. This estimator is a number (the average of the retransformed residuals) by which each prediction is multiplied to correct for the known bias associated with the retransformation. However, retransformed predictions often fail to achieve as high an R^2 as a model fit directly to the untransformed data. This is no surprise, as the OLS algorithm specifically estimates parameters so that predictions minimize R^2 in the scale of interest. In our study of hospital-based severity measures, we evaluated R^2 both on untransformed LOS data and log-transformed data, using Duan's smearing estimator to retransform predictions before calculating R^2. For both pneumonia and hip fracture cases, R^2 values were as high or higher using models fit to LOS rather than log (LOS) (Iezzoni et al. 1996c; Shwartz et al. 1996a).

As an alternative to transforming the data, the generalized linear model (GLM) provides a comprehensive framework for developing multivariable models with nonnormally distributed data. GLM assumes that some function of the outcome, called a "link" function, can be modeled as a linear function of the predictors. GLM seeks parameters to predict outcomes in their natural scale directly rather than in a transformed scale. The GLM framework also allows for independent specification of how variances might vary as a function of the mean value of the outcome (e.g., costs for expensive cases typically vary more than costs for inexpensive ones). GLMs are described in a classic but sophisticated text by McCullagh and Nelder (1989), which assumes knowledge of mathematical likelihood. Several books describe GLMs, especially their implementation in various software or programming languages (Chambers and Hastie 1992; Ripley and Venable 1994).

Another alternative for limiting the influence of outliers is to seek models with the smallest mean absolute prediction error, also called the mean absolute deviation (MAD), rather than the smallest squared error. MAD is the average of the absolute value of $(Y - PRED)$. The "deviation" in MAD denotes the same quantity as "error" in the phrase "mean squared error" (MSE).

Although standard software packages do not produce models specifically to minimize MADs, analysts can nevertheless compare risk adjusters based on their MAD values. The Society of Actuaries took this approach in evaluating risk-adjustment models (Cumming et al. 2002). Table 10.4 shows R^2 values and MAD when the models were used prospectively with either no topcoding or with topcoding at $100,000. Values of MAD are smaller (demonstrating better average fit) with topcoded data than with actual costs. In general, models with higher R^2 values have lower MADs. However, relative model performance can differ depending on the statistical performance measures. For example, CDPS, DCGs, and ERGs all had the highest, and similar R^2 values. However, with MAD, ERGs appeared best and RxGroups second best.[7]

Although MAD may seem like a more natural measure of model fit than R^2, analysts are comfortable with standard deviation (SD) as a measure of the size of a typical error. In a given data set, the model whose residuals have the smallest SD is the model with the highest R^2.[8] Furthermore, models are most commonly used to predict group averages, making predictive validity hinge on minimizing the "average of n deviations." When predicting averages for moderately large groups, models that minimize MSE are preferable to those that minimize MAD.[9]

Finally, when considering variable transformations and nonlinear modeling, transparent modeling logic is very important. Developers likely need to convince nontechnical audiences about the merit of their approach (a kind of "face validity"). They also need to engage others who are particularly knowledgeable about the specific context of the work in critiquing the model (see Chapter 8). OLS modeling is relatively transparent. Lumley and collaborators (2002) used simulations to show that, with large data sets, OLS generally handles nonnormally distributed data well, despite its underlying assumptions about normality.

Interpreting R²

With experience, analysts learn what values of statistical performance can be expected for "good" predictive models in specific contexts. For example, when predicting next year's health care costs for a Medicare enrollee from this year's data, actuaries and policymakers have looked favorably on models with R^2 values of 0.06 (Ash et al. 1989; Epstein and Cumella 1988). Although such small R^2 values indicate that individual *PRED*s might differ from the observed outcome by almost as much as if *PRED* always equaled the population mean,[10] these *PRED*s can identify subgroups with very different future costs.

The Society of Actuaries study demonstrates that validated R^2 values are now roughly 15 percent for models to predict next year's actual costs from demographic characteristics and this year's diagnoses or pharmacy claims. However, with more clinical information in administrative data sets (see Chapter 5), prospective models are beginning to produce R^2 values closer to 20 percent. Many observers remain unimpressed by models that explain only

TABLE 10.4
R^2 and Mean
Absolute
Deviation when
Models to
Predict Total
Annual Cost
Are Used
Prospectively
with
Recalibrated
Weights

Model	$R^2 \times 100$		MAD	
	Topcoded at $100,000	Full Range	Topcoded at $100,000	Full Range
ACG	14	10	2,100	2,193
CDPS	19	15	2,070	2,164
DCG	20	15	2,032	2,133
Medicaid Rx	17	12	2,062	2,159
RxGroups	19	13	2,014	2,113
RxRisk	15	11	2,091	2,187
ERG	20	15	1,983	2,079

SOURCE: Adapted from Tables 3.2 and 3.3, Cumming et al. (2002).

15 percent to 20 percent of the variation in cost. However, context is all important. Models that predict next year's actual costs will never approach 50 percent explanatory power because they cannot anticipate which specific individuals will experience acute illnesses or incur catastrophic expenses next year. Nonetheless, prospective models can identify the chronic problems that lead to large systematic differences in the future costs of groups.

When choosing among risk adjusters, analysts often look for the statistical performance measures reported in research publications. An important question is how well results from these published reports generalize to other settings and purposes. For instance, although APACHE II was developed explicitly to predict ICU deaths, it also has been used for non-ICU populations (Daley et al. 1988; Iezzoni et al. 1990; Keeler et al. 1990). APACHE III yielded a cross-validated R^2 of 0.15 to predict ICU LOS (Knaus et al. 1993). This figure comes from data drawn from a stratified random sample of 26 hospitals, plus 14 other volunteer hospitals that were primarily tertiary teaching facilities. The predominance of tertiary teaching hospitals raises questions about generalizability of this R^2 value to other hospital settings.

R^2 values depend on the cases in the database as well as the risk factors available for modeling. The dispersion of the independent and dependent variables significantly affects statistical performance, particularly R^2. Figure 10.1 shows three schematic diagrams of models to predict Y from a single variable X, where larger values for X indicate greater risks for poor outcomes. Graph A shows the classic bivariable normal situation. R^2 is approximately equal to:

$$1 - \frac{\text{variance in } (Y - PRED)}{\text{variance in } (Y)}.$$

The other two graphs in Figure 10.1 show what happens when only some of the data are available for modeling. In graph B, cases with extreme values of X are eliminated, producing less variation in Y but no change in

FIGURE 10.1

How Differences in the Data Modeled Affect R^2

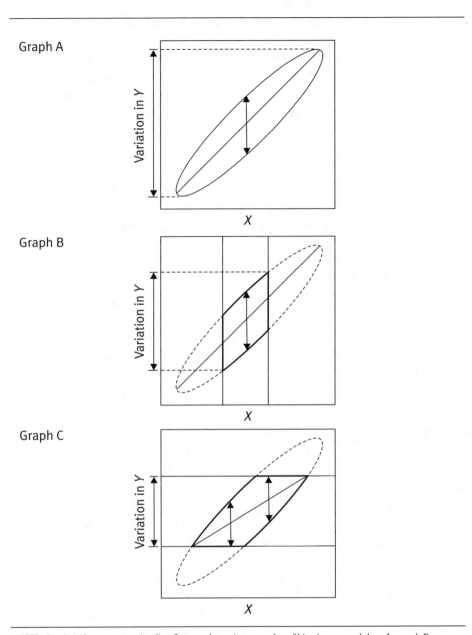

Graph A

Graph B

Graph C

NOTE: Graph A shows a regression line fit to a schematic scatterplot of bivariate normal data. In graph B, cases with extreme values of X have been removed; in graph C, cases with extreme values of Y have been removed. The shorter, vertical arrows in the body of each graph indicate variation in ($Y - PRED$). The smaller the ratio of variation in ($Y - PRED$) to variation in Y, the larger is R^2.

the variation in ($Y - PRED$) for the remaining cases. In this situation, R^2 should decrease. In graph C, cases with extreme values of Y are removed, which reduces both kinds of variation. The net effect on R^2 is unpredictable.

Another example illustrates how characteristics of the data affect statistical performance. Suppose two risk adjustment methods are applied to two different data sets and are equally accurate in predicting outcomes for cases across the range of independent variables (i.e., SSE/n is identical for each risk adjuster). The data set with more variability in the outcome variable generates a higher SST and, thus, a higher R^2 (Korn and Simon 1991). The difference in R^2 falsely suggests a difference in the power of the risk adjusters.

Certain data sets sample cases nonrandomly, oversampling particular types of cases (e.g., cost outliers, patients who died) to increase the amount of information available about them. Average outcomes for these oversampled cases often differ greatly from those in the general population. This artificially increases the variability of the dependent variable, usually leading to a higher R^2 than one for a general population. Such concerns lead some to conclude that R^2 is unsuitable for comparing models developed on different data sets (Cox and Wermuth 1992). More generally, comparing model performance on different data sets can be misleading, even with measures of model performance other than R^2.

Importance of the Form of the Risk Score for Interpreting R^2

As shown in Table 2.5, some risk-adjustment approaches rate cases by assigning categories of risk, whereas others yield scores with continuous values. To capture complex relationships between risk and outcome, analysts sometimes recode continuous scores as discrete categories. The approach used to create categories, including how outliers are handled, can affect the R^2.

To create categories, one approach involves distributing cases relatively evenly across groups (e.g., by defining five quintiles of increasing risk). In this instance, models generally perform better when outliers are excluded. In contrast, the top category may contain only a small percentage of cases, capturing those relatively rare cases with the highest values of the outcome of interest. These models typically perform better when outliers are included.

To some extent, the relative merit of different approaches for defining categories depends on the context and purpose. Suppose that two risk-adjustment methods each have risk categories 1, 2, 3, and 4. Within method A's four categories, respectively, 1 percent, 3 percent, 4 percent, and 8 percent of the cases have the outcome under study. Within method B's four categories, 0.5 percent, 3 percent, 4 percent, and 25 percent of cases have the outcome. At first glance, it seems obvious that method B discriminates better. Suppose, however, that 25 percent of cases fell into each of method A's four categories, whereas only 0.5 percent of cases were in each of method B's lowest and highest risk groups (categories 1 and 4). For many purposes, method A is more useful because it can meaningfully discriminate across relatively large numbers of people. If the goal is to find very small groups at particularly low or high risk, however, method B is better.

In comparing statistical performance measures across different approaches for creating discrete categories from continuous scales, it is important to know how the categories were defined and how cases distribute across the categories. If the categories were defined to maximize model performance in a development data set, the model's performance could deteriorate when applied to new data. A simple, informal way to examine how much discrimination categorical risk scores achieve is to tabulate the percentage of cases and average the values of the outcome in each risk category. Better models assign larger fractions of the population to risk categories with either very low or very high average outcomes.[11]

Measures of Model Performance for Dichotomous Outcomes

Suppose we compute a score measuring risk of in-hospital death and set a cutoff score such that we predict patients will die if their scores exceed this cutoff. We predict that patients with lower scores will live. We can array such data in a two-by-two table as shown in Table 10.5, leading to several useful quantities:

- True positive cases = A
- False positive cases = B
- True negative cases = D
- False negative cases = C
- Prevalence = $(A + C)/(A + B + C + D)$
- Sensitivity = $A/(A + C)$
- Specificity = $D/(B + D)$
- Predictive value positive (PV+) = $A/(A + B)$
- Predictive value negative (PV−) = $D/(C + D)$

The last four quantities measure the fraction of cases correctly classified taking different perspectives. Sensitivity is the fraction of deaths correctly classified by the prediction rule, whereas specificity is the fraction of live patients correctly classified. The PV+ is the fraction of patients predicted to die who are classified correctly, whereas PV− measures the fraction of those predicted to live who are classified correctly.

The cases used in denominators of PV+ and PV− depend on the classification rule. This complicates comparisons of different classification rules based on PV+ and PV−. In contrast, sensitivity (the true positive rate) and specificity (the true negative rate) use denominators defined by the death rate within the population under study. This makes sensitivity and specificity more suitable for comparing different classification rules involving the same population. The false negative rate is defined as 1 − sensitivity and the false positive rate as 1 − specificity.

Lemeshow and colleagues (1988) developed models to predict the probability of in-hospital death using data on 2,644 patients admitted to an ICU in a large tertiary teaching hospital. Three models were created, based on clinical findings at ICU admission, 24 hours into the ICU stay, or 48 hours into the ICU stay. The admission model, MPM_0 (Mortality Prediction

TABLE 10.5
Layout for
Comparing a
Dichotomous
Outcome with
a Dichotomized
Prediction

Risk Score Prediction	Patient Outcome		All Cases
	Dead	Alive	
Dead	A	B	A + B
Alive	C	D	C + D
All cases	A + C	B + D	A + B + C + D

Model with data from time zero), used data on 11 variables collected at ICU admission. Patients were predicted to die if the probability of death calculated from the MPM_0 model was greater than 0.50. In evaluating the performance of the MPM_0 model (using the 0.50 classification rule), they reported the following:

- Sensitivity = 0.448
- Specificity = 0.966
- Predictive value for dying = 0.762
- Predictive value for surviving = 0.879

Thus, this classification identified 44.8 percent of all cases who died, misclassifying only 3.4 percent of those who lived $(1 - 0.966)$. Of those predicted to die, 76.2 percent did die; of those predicted to live, 87.9 percent did live.

Evaluations of diagnostic rules in clinical practice often rely on two-by-two classification tables. In this context, the prevalence of a condition in a population affects the predictive values of a test (Ingelfinger et al. 1987). For example, the PV+ and PV– values for the above MPM_0 classification rule were computed in a population with just under 20 percent deaths. In a population with more deaths, a test with the same sensitivity and specificity would yield higher PV+ and lower PV– values. For instance, with 50 percent deaths, the PV+ and PV– are 0.929 and 0.636, respectively. Conversely, when the outcome is rare, PV+ falls while PV– rises. With a 1 percent death rate, for example, PV+ is 0.117, and PV– is 0.994. Not surprisingly, in a population where nearly everyone lives, predicting that a patient will live is very likely to be correct; accurately identifying those few who will die is much harder.

Sensitivity and specificity thus describe the properties of tests in the abstract, whereas PV+ and PV– address the consequences of using a test in a specific population. A major problem with using sensitivity and specificity determined from two-by-two tables to measure model performance is selecting a cutoff to dichotomize the risk score. For some purposes, defining the cutoff could closely mimic how the methodology will be used, such as using a score to identify a manageable number of high-risk patients to receive special follow-up. However, the "right" cutoff is situation specific, depending on such factors as the funds available to monitor the targeted patients. Typically, no single cutoff is clearly best.

The two-by-two table is poorly suited to comparing the performance of risk-adjustment methods. When different researchers describe performance of their risk adjusters, each using a different cutpoint, reported sensitivities can vary widely, impeding comparison of specificity values. When cutpoints are chosen to produce identical sensitivities, one can compare specificities. However, which model is judged better may depend on the value of the sensitivity used to establish the cutpoint. For example, one model may accurately identify a few cases for whom death is very likely while not discriminating well in the general population; another may identify a substantial fraction of cases where risk of death is much higher than average but still unlikely. In language defined later in this chapter, inconsistent judgments can occur whenever the receiver operating characteristic (ROC) curves for the different risk-adjustment models cross.

Models to Predict Dichotomous Outcomes

Logistic regression is typically used to model dichotomous dependent variables and performs well when compared to more complex modeling approaches (Feinstein, Wells, and Walter 1990; Hadorn et al. 1992; Selker et al. 1995). In logistic regression, the dependent variable is the (natural) logarithm of the odds of the event (written as ln O and called "log odds" or "logit"). If P is the probability that an event occurs and $Q = 1 - P$, then the odds of the event is P/Q. (For example, if the chance of an event is 3 in 4, $P = 3/4$, $Q = 1/4$, and the odds of the event is 3 to 1, or 3.00.) Letting O_i be the odds of the event for the ith case, the logistic regression model (analogous to Equation 1 above) is:

$$\widehat{\ln O_i} = \hat{a} + \Sigma_j \hat{b}_j * X_{ij} \qquad (2)$$

As with the multiple regression models for continuous outcomes, the X_{ij} terms may be dummy variables representing risk classes, covariates plus the risk classes, covariates plus a single risk score, or a subset of significant variables identified using a selection procedure, such as stepwise regression. With a continuous outcome variable, such as cost, the predicted value for the ith person represents an estimate of the expected value of cost, $E(Y_i)$. In logistic regression, the predicted value for the ith person also estimates the expected value of the outcome for the ith person—P_i, the probability of the event for the ith person. However, single observations can only be 0 or 1; thus, they never equal their expected value, P_i.

An estimate of ln O_i, as in Equation 2 above, leads to a predicted probability of the event for the ith case, as follows:

$$PRED_i = \hat{P}_i = \frac{e^{\widehat{\ln(O_i)}}}{1 + e^{\widehat{\ln(O_i)}}}$$

Methods other than logistic regression may be used to estimate the numbers $PRED_i$, such as binary splits algorithms (e.g., CART), probit models,

OLS models (Cleary and Angel 1984), determinations by panels of clinical experts, or Cox proportional hazards regression models (Knaus et al. 1995). Many measures of model performance, including the traditional R^2 and the c-statistic (see below), may be calculated from the set of pairs of numbers, one for each case, consisting of (1) the estimated probability of the event of interest for that case (its $PRED_i$) and (2) the actual outcome Y_i (coded as 0 or 1).

Another measure of model fit is also a function of these pairs—the "likelihood" (L) of the observed data as predicted by the model. If the outcome of interest is death, L for a particular model is computed by multiplying together the predicted probabilities of living ($1 - PRED$) for each case that lived and the predicted probabilities of dying ($PRED$) for each case that died. Better models have larger $1 - PRED$ values for cases who lived and larger $PRED$s for those who died—thus, they have larger likelihoods. The Akaike Information Criterion (AIC) uses the likelihood to measure the deviance between the actual data and the model, building in a penalty for model complexity (Akaike 1973). Neither the likelihood nor the AIC is standardized to an interpretable scale, such as the 0 to 1 interval containing the c-statistic (see below). One likelihood-based measure that is standardized is a generalization of R^2. Similar to the traditional R^2, it summarizes the improvement in model fit for the full model over an intercept-only model (Nagelkerke 1991). Likelihood-based measures of model performance are sometimes reported in the health services research literature, but much less often than the traditional R^2 and c.

As with OLS modeling for predicting continuous outcomes, logistic modeling relies on certain assumptions. Results from logistic models are valid when these assumptions hold true. Nevertheless, both logistic and OLS modeling are performed when these assumptions are clearly not met. Both techniques are generally "robust" (i.e., results are not much affected by many common departures from the assumptions). More importantly, the performance of a risk-adjustment model is typically judged by how closely its predictions match reality, rather than the extent to which the data conform to underlying assumptions. When employed carefully, these modeling procedures yield reasonable and useful predictions.

Model Calibration and Discrimination

As discussed earlier, models are calibrated to a data set when the average of their predicted values matches the average of the actual outcomes. Overall calibration error is measured as $[\text{AVE}(Y_i) - \text{AVE}(PRED_i)]$, where $PRED_i$ is the predicted value of Y_i. For a dichotomous outcome, Y_i records the presence of the outcome event: It is 1 if the outcome occurs and 0 if it does not. With this coding, the average Y is the actual outcome rate in the population, and the average $PRED$ is the average predicted outcome rate for the same group. When a model is derived by fitting the model to a particular data set, the model is calibrated to those data. If modeling used OLS regression, the resulting calibration error is zero. However, if some other fitting approach is used (e.g., the maximum likelihood method employed by logistic regression computer software packages), the actual and predicted outcome rates may differ, although usually by a small amount.

For a given outcome like death, model discrimination represents the extent to which a model predicts higher probabilities of death (higher *PRED*s) for patients who died than for those who lived. Discrimination can be portrayed graphically by drawing two histograms of the predicted probabilities on the same scale: one for patients who die and the other for those who live. The histogram of *PRED*s for patients who lived should lie to the left of the histogram for patients who died. Figure 10.2 illustrates two such histograms, scaled for a situation where four times as many cases lived as died (i.e., a 20 percent death rate). Such a picture is called a covariance graph (Yates 1982). With better discrimination, the two histograms overlap less.

While good model calibration is desirable, discrimination is usually more important. To see why, imagine a population with a 10 percent death rate. A model that assigns $PRED = 0.1$ to every person is perfectly calibrated, but it cannot distinguish patients who live from those who die. On the other hand, suppose that a second model assigns $PRED = 0.8$ to every patient who lives and $PRED = 0.9$ to the patients who die. Although the second model produces entirely wrong numerical predictions, the model can perfectly predict the outcome. While recalibration can fix the problem with the second model, no simple change can make the first model useful for identifying patients who die.

The c-Statistic to Measure Model Discrimination

The *c*-statistic is commonly used to measure the performance of models predicting dichotomous outcomes (Harrell et al. 1984). The *c*-statistic has several equivalent definitions. To illustrate one, consider all possible pairs that can be formed, such that one patient dies and the other lives. The *c*-statistic equals the proportion of pairs in which the predicted probability of death is higher for the patient who died than for the patient who lived. Each tied pair counts as one-half.

The *c*-statistic also equals the area under a receiver operating characteristic (ROC) curve. ROC curves result from converting the information in a covariance graph into multiple two-by-two tables, such as Table 10.5, and then plotting sensitivity versus (1 – specificity) from each table. The following example illustrates the ROC curve using covariance graphs. First, the two histograms are converted to distributions by rescaling each curve so that it has an area of 1.00. Given a predicted probability of death for each case ($PRED_i$) and a specified cutoff (t), we make a rule as follows: If $PRED_i$ is greater than t, patients are expected to die, and if $PRED_i$ is less than t, patients are expected to live. Figure 10.3 displays the consequences of this rule for a particular value of t. The true positive rate (i.e., sensitivity) is the area to the right of t and

FIGURE 10.2

Schematic
Drawing of a
Covariance
Graph:
Comparative
Histograms for
PRED by
Actual
Outcome

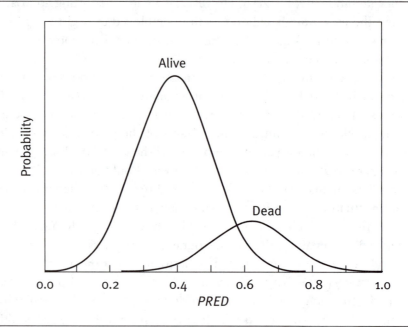

under the curve for the patients who die. The false positive rate (i.e., 1 –
specificity) is the area to the right of t and under the curve for the patients
who live. In this way, each t is associated with a pair of numbers: $P(t) = (x(t),$
$y(t)) = (1 - \text{specificity}(t), \text{sensitivity}(t))$. The ROC curve is the set of points
$P(t)$ that are traced on a unit square as t varies from its lowest to its highest
value (Figure 10.4). When t is lowest, all cases are declared positive and the
pair $(1,1)$ is generated. As the cutoff t increases, the vertical line in Figure
10.3 shifts to the right and fewer cases are called positive. Thus, both the true
and false positive rates decrease, and the new point lies to the left of and down
from the previous point. When t is highest, all cases are declared negative,
generating the pair $(0,0)$.

A model with good discrimination has a high true positive rate and a
low false positive rate. This generates a curve that passes close to the upper left
corner of the plot—the point $(0,1)$ in Figure 10.4. The area under this curve,
which is equivalent to the c-statistic associated with the model generating the
covariance graph, is close to 1. As marked on Figure 10.3, the cutpoint t
identifies a particular point $P(t)$ on this curve.

Most risk-adjustment models produce fairly continuous distributions
of predicted values. When that happens, drawing an ROC curve is relatively
straightforward. However, models with a small number of categorical independent variables generate only a few pairs of $(x(t), y(t))$. In these circumstances,
alternative approaches can estimate the presumably continuous underlying
ROC curve (Centor and Schwartz 1985).

Knowing the relationship between c and the rank sum statistic, S, gives
more insight into what the c-statistic measures. The rank sum statistic S tests

FIGURE 10.3
Distribution of
PRED by
Actual
Outcome with
Indications of
True and False
Positive Rates
as Determined
by a Cut Point *t*

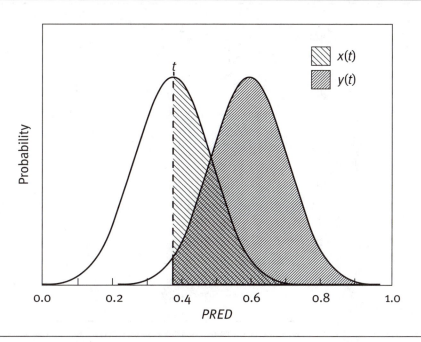

$x(t)$ = fraction of cases that live for which $PRED > t$
    = 1 − specificity
$y(t)$ = fraction of cases that die for which $PRED > t$
    = sensitivity
NOTE: The left-hand curve = alive; the right-hand curve = dead.

the following null hypothesis: The median value of *PRED* is identical for patients who live and those who die (which implies the model has no ability to discriminate). *S* is formed by combining the n_0 cases who live with the n_1 cases who die and assigning ranks according to the values of *PRED*. The case with the lowest value of *PRED* gets rank 1, the case with the second lowest value gets rank 2, and so on up to $n_0 + n_1$, the rank assigned to the case with the highest value of *PRED*. For cases with the same value of *PRED*, the ranks are averaged. For example, if four cases share the same lowest value of *PRED*, each is assigned 2.5 (which equals $[1 + 2 + 3 + 4]/4$).

The rank sum statistic *S* results from adding the ranks of all n_1 patients who die. The smallest possible value for *S* is achieved when all patients who die have a predicted probability of death (*PRED*) that is less than *PRED*s for cases who live. Then, $S_{min} = 1 + 2 + \ldots + n_1$. It can be shown that $S_{min} = n_1(n_1 + 1)/2$. This model has perfect discrimination, but it is wrong—persons who die have the lowest predicted probabilities of death and those who live have the highest. The largest possible value of *S* comes when the n_0 cases who live have ranks 1 to n_0, leading to $S_{max} = (n_0 + 1) + (n_0 + 2) + \ldots + (n_0 + n_1)$. The sum of these n_1 numbers is $S_{min} + n_0 n_1$. Such a model also has perfect discrimination, and it is right—the deaths have the highest predicted probabilities. Whatever the value of *S*, *c* is the following unique linear function of *S*:

FIGURE 10.4

ROC Curve
Associated with
Distributions
Shown in
Figure 10.3

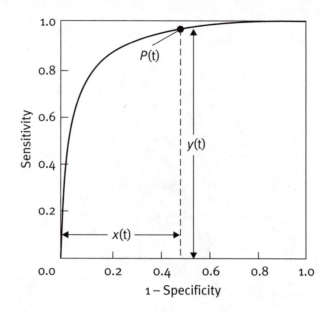

NOTE: $P(t) = (x(t), y(t))$ is determined using the particular cut point t shown on Figure 10.3. As t increases from 0 to 1, the ROC curve is traced out, starting in the northeast corner $(1,1)$ and finishing in the southwest $(0,0)$.

$$c = \frac{S - S_{min}}{S_{max} - S_{min}}$$

When $S = S_{min}$, $c = 0$; when $S = S_{max}$, $c = 1$. When the average rank of $PRED$ is identical for cases who lived and died (i.e., when S equals S_{mid}, a number halfway between its minimum and maximum), then $c = 0.5$. The c-statistic depends only on the ranks of predictions, not on their actual values. Thus, the value of c is unaffected by how close the average predicted values $[\text{AVE}(PRED_i)]$ come to the average actual values $[\text{AVE}(Y_i)]$ and, as a result, provides no information about model calibration.

In summary, the c-statistic measures model discrimination, achieving its maximum value of 1.0 when all $PRED$s for cases with the outcome are larger than any $PRED$s for cases without the outcome. When models have no ability to discriminate (e.g., probabilities are randomly assigned to cases with and without the outcome), the expected value of the c-statistic is 0.5. A c-statistic much less than 0.5 indicates model discrimination but with improper coding of the risk scores. This could be remedied by reassigning risk scores (e.g., each person's $PRED$ would become $1 - PRED$).

To suggest how various c values reflect different levels of discrimination, Figure 10.5 shows overlapping normal distribution curves when the distribution for the patients who die is shifted rightward from the distribution for patients who live by 0.5, 1.0, 1.5, and 2.0 SDs. Figure 10.6 shows the four ROC curves for the shifted distributions. The values of c associated with these shifts are 0.64, 0.76, 0.86, and 0.92, respectively.

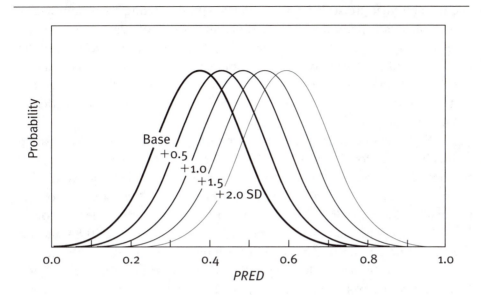

FIGURE 10.5
Overlapping Normal Distribution Curves Displaying Various Amounts of Shift

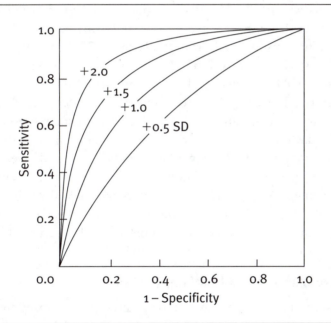

FIGURE 10.6
ROC Curves for Four Different Amounts of Shift between *PRED*s for Cases Who Live and *PRED*s for Cases Who Die

NOTE: The areas under the four curves are 0.64, 0.76, 0.86, and 0.92 for shifts of 0.5, 1.0, 1.5, and 2.0 SDs, respectively.

The c-statistic and ROC curve derive from measures of sensitivity and specificity. As noted earlier, these measures do not depend on the prevalence of the condition (e.g., the death rate in the population), a fact that has raised questions about c-statistics. Hilden (1991) argued that the value of a diagnostic test to clinicians depends on the prevalence of the targeted outcome in their patient population; hence, the insensitivity of c-statistics and ordinary ROC curves to prevalence represents a weakness. He proposed using ROC-like pictures that are scaled for prevalence (thus affecting total numbers of misclassified cases) and possibly for different "costs" of false positive versus false negative errors to the patient or society. Such graphs highlight the trade-offs associated with using different cutpoints for deciding when to call a case positive. Hilden (1991) also provides a disturbing example of two procedures that are logically equivalent yet lead to different ROC curves and different c-statistics.

Krakauer and colleagues (1992) reported c-statistics when comparing mortality models for almost 43,000 Medicare cases sampled from 84 hospitals throughout the country. They used logistic regression to develop two models to predict death: one from claims data submitted to Medicare for hospital payment and another from clinical data abstracted with the older version of MedisGroups. The c-statistic for the claims-based model was 0.84 and for the clinical model, 0.90. Knaus and colleagues (1991) reported a c-statistic of 0.90 for predicting death using APACHE III, based on the same 17,440 ICU patients from 40 hospitals used to develop the model. They also reported sensitivity, specificity, PV+, and PV– for three different cutpoints used to predict whether a patient would die: model-predicted probabilities greater than 0.1, greater than 0.5, and greater than 0.9. Moving from the lowest to highest cutpoint, sensitivity fell from 0.891 to 0.130 as specificity increased from 0.711 to 0.998. New York state's risk-adjustment model for predicting death following CABG surgery had a c-statistic of 0.79 (Hannan et al. 1994, 763). As described in Chapter 8, to examine quality of surgical care in VA hospitals, Khuri and colleagues (1997) developed logistic regression models to predict 30-day postoperative mortality using data from more than 87,000 noncardiac operations. Of 67 preoperative variables collected on each patient, 44 were statistically significant. However, the first ten variables entering the model contributed most of the explanatory power ($c = 0.87$ for the model with ten variables versus $c = 0.89$ for the model with 44 variables). Preoperative serum albumin level was the most important predictor; a model based on serum albumin alone achieved a c value of 0.79.

Methods for Measuring Model Calibration

The calibration curve graphically compares predicted probabilities of a dichotomous outcome with the actual outcomes (Yates 1982). To construct the curve, patients are divided into groups based on similar predicted probabilities of death. The averages of the predicted probabilities for patients in each group are plotted against the rate of actual outcomes in the group.

Lemeshow and Hosmer (1982) proposed a χ^2 (chi square) test derived from data organized similarly to the calibration curve. The Hosmer-Lemeshow χ^2 is often used in evaluations of risk adjusters to examine model calibration across the range of predicted probabilities. It does not check directly for overall calibration (i.e., whether the average of predicted outcomes is close to the actual outcome rate). Instead, it addresses whether average and predicted rates are similar within population subgroups. Although the Hosmer-Lemeshow method can be performed in several ways, the following four steps represent an increasingly standard application (using death as the target outcome):

1. Data are divided into ten subgroups based on deciles of predicted risk of death ($PRED$).
2. Within each subgroup, deviations between observed and expected numbers of deaths (O_{die} and E_{die}) and observed and expected numbers of live cases (O_{live} and E_{live}) are measured as is familiar from a standard χ^2 calculation:

$$\frac{(O_{die} - E_{die})^2}{E_{die}} + \frac{(O_{live} - E_{live})^2}{E_{live}} = \frac{(O_{die} - E_{die})^2}{n\hat{P}\hat{Q}}$$

where n equals the number of cases in the subgroup, $\hat{P}$ equals the predicted death rate for these n cases, and $\hat{Q}$ equals $1 - \hat{P}$. The expected numbers are average $PRED$s.

3. To assess whether deviations are larger than expected (under the hypothesis that each prediction is correct), these deviations are summed over the ten subgroups. The result is compared to a χ^2 distribution with 8 degrees of freedom.
4. The model is accepted if the p-value for this test is reasonably large (i.e., the observed deviations from the model predictions are fully consistent with the size of chance deviations that would occur if the model were correct).

As for any χ^2 test, a serious concern when using this or any version of the Hosmer-Lemeshow approach is that the decision about the adequacy of model fit depends heavily on the number of observations available. When the sample size is large, even small discrepancies between the model's predictions and observed counts (which may have little practical significance) can produce low p-values, causing rejection of the model. In contrast, when few cases are available, the null hypothesis (that the model is correct) may be accepted despite large differences between the expected and observed values.

Other applications of this test use different rules for assigning cases to subgroups or strata. With fewer cases, for example, analysts could split the data into five quintiles of predicted risk rather than ten deciles. When large fractions of the cases have very similar predicted probabilities, grouping cases requires a different strategy altogether. For example, if the $PRED$s for the healthiest half of the population are all similarly low, the lowest subgroup might contain the 50 percent of cases with the lowest $PRED$ values.

Strata do not need equal numbers of cases, but analysts should have a reasonably straightforward rationale for how they group. They should also show the distribution of cases among the subgroups. With k strata, the χ^2 with $k - 2$ degrees of freedom is the test statistic. The outcome of the test (i.e., the decision about whether the model is calibrated) can depend on the rule for grouping patients into strata.

Another concern with the Hosmer-Lemeshow χ^2 test is that $n\hat{P}\hat{Q}$ overestimates the variance of the deviations under the null hypothesis. If subgroups are formed using deciles of predicted risk, $n\hat{P}\hat{Q}$ and the sum of the $\hat{P}_i\hat{Q}_i$ are generally similar, causing little difficulty. However, when the subgroups contain cases with widely dispersed probabilities of death, the Hosmer-Lemeshow statistic is noticeably smaller than it should be—leading to the inappropriate acceptance of models with predictions that deviate greatly from actual outcomes.[12]

For the New York state CABG model, the p-value for the Hosmer-Lemeshow χ^2 statistic was 0.16, indicating good fit, particularly in light of having more than 57,000 cases in the database (Hannan et al. 1994, 763). The VHA models to predict 30-day mortality for noncardiac surgery cases were developed on more than 87,000 cases. Khuri et al. (1997, 320) reported, "The only goodness-of-fit statistics that were statistically significant at the 0.05 level were for all operations combined and for general surgery, primarily because there were a large number of cases in these categories." In contrast to most settings where statistical tests are performed, analysts here seek a p-value that is *not* statistically significant to provide reassurance of reasonable model fit.

In summary, the Hosmer-Lemeshow test has drawbacks, especially its sensitivity to the number of cases studied and the rule for assigning cases to subgroups. We therefore suggest that analysts treat Hosmer-Lemeshow test results as exploratory. In fact, differences in actual outcomes across the strata may be far more informative about the value of a model (how well it discriminates) than comparisons of actual and observed outcomes within strata (how well it is calibrated).

Model Performance Within Subgroups

The Hosmer-Lemeshow statistic forms a single summary measure of the match between predicted and actual death rates within subgroups of the data. Nevertheless, even with poor summary fit, analysts can look individually at each pair of observed and predicted outcome rates to see which deciles contribute most to the poor fit and to provide additional insight into model performance. Ash and colleagues (1990) used a deciles-of-risk calibration table to illustrate the ability of a model developed using administrative data available at the time of hospital admission to predict whether utilization reviews would deem the admission inappropriate. Based on a model fit to the whole data set (after examining models fit to two halves of a split sample), they examined calibration in deciles by comparing figures within rows, as in Table 10.6. Except for deciles 5, 9, and possibly 7, the observed and predicted problem rates are similar. The final column, which records each decile's contribution to the Hosmer-Lemeshow statistic, confirms that the other rows are not widely discordant. For the Hosmer-Lemeshow statistic not to reject the model fit, the sum of

TABLE 10.6
A Deciles-of-
Risk Calibration
Table

Decile	Predicted % Problems	Observed % Problems	Contribution to the Hosmer-Lemeshow Statistic
1	0.3	0.1	1.3
2	1.4	1.6	0.2
3	2.7	2.3	0.6
4	4.0	4.1	0.0
5	6.1	7.5	3.6
6	6.9	6.5	0.3
7	7.8	9.0	2.3
8	8.7	8.1	0.5
9	11.4	9.7	3.0
10	34.1	34.5	0.1

NOTE: The contribution to the Hosmer-Lemeshow statistic for decile i is $(O_i - E_i)^2/n_i\,p_i\,q_i$, where O_i is the observed number of problem cases in decile i, E_i is the expected number of problem cases in decile i, n_i is the number of cases in decile i, p_i is aver $(PRED)$ in decile i, and q_i is $1 -$ aver $(PRED)$ in decile i. The number of cases in decile i (n_i) is always within one of 1,030.5, since $N = 10,305$ is the full population size. The Hosmer-Lemeshow statistic is 12.0, the sum of the numbers in the last column. The probability that a χ^2 statistic with 8 degrees of freedom is greater than 12.0 exceeds 10 percent. Thus, the model is not rejected, $p > 0.10$. Observed problem rate = 8.334 percent. Predicted problem rate = 8.336 percent.

the numbers in the last column must be less than 15.5, which is the 95th percentile for a χ^2 distribution with 8 degrees of freedom. For a model to pass this test, only a few of the ten summands can be as large as 2. Here, the numbers add to 12.0, and the model passes this test of calibration.

Examining the observed percentage problems column of Table 10.6 provides further insight into model discrimination. If the model had no explanatory power, approximately 8.3 percent of the cases in each decile would have the outcome. Obviously, the outcome rate was dramatically higher for cases in the top decile than for other cases, and very few problem cases occurred in the lowest four deciles. Cases in deciles 5 through 9 had outcome rates relatively close to the outcome rate of 8.3 percent for the whole sample. Ash and Byrne-Logan (1998) use an analogous method to assess model performance when predicting a continuous outcome, next year's cost.

We can compute the fraction of all outcomes that occur in a decile or a group of deciles by adding the observed percentage of outcomes for these deciles and dividing by the sum of all the percentages (83.34 percent for Table 10.6). This computation addresses useful practical questions such as, "What percentage of all complications was found by looking at the 10 percent of the cases thought to be at greatest risk of complications?" Using the data from Table 10.6, the answer is more than 40 percent: $34.5/83.34 = 0.41$. In contrast, fewer than 10 percent of the outcomes occurred in the bottom four risk deciles.

Hannan and colleagues (1994, 765) used the Hosmer-Lemeshow statistic computed in deciles of predicted risk to examine the performance of New York state's CABG risk-adjustment model, concluding, "There was a reasonably good correspondence between actual deaths and expected deaths in each of the individual intervals." They noted that in the highest decile, predicted mortality was 36 percent and actual mortality was 32 percent; thus, the model appears to adjust sufficiently for the most severe cases.

The same kind of table may be constructed for other divisions of the data into subgroups (e.g., by age or payer class) to identify types of cases whose rate of death is not predicted well by the model. Analysts must then take the next step of understanding why predictions are poor for these cases.

Lemeshow and Hosmer (1982) argued that if models do not calibrate well, examining discrimination has little value. Harrell and colleagues (1984, 144) voiced another view: "The reason we argue for first priority to discrimination in judging a model's relative performance is that if discrimination deteriorates, no adjustment or calibration can correct the model. On the other hand with good discrimination, one can calibrate the predictor to attain reliability without sacrificing discrimination."

If the model is used to distinguish those with and without the outcome, actual values of the $PRED$s are not important. However, when a model is used to determine an expected outcome rate for comparisons with an actual outcome rate (e.g., as in profiling hospitals or physicians based on their risk-adjusted mortality rates; see Chapter 12), calibration is at least as important as discrimination. Both calibration and discrimination should be addressed when evaluating model performance.

R^2 and Dichotomous Outcomes

As for continuous outcome variables, R^2 for models predicting dichotomous outcomes can be defined in several ways. We use the same definition as for continuous outcomes:

$$R^2 = 1 - \left[\frac{\Sigma_i (Y_i - PRED_i)^2}{\Sigma_i (Y_i - \overline{Y})^2} \right].$$

The predicted probabilities ($PRED_i$) can come from any method of modeling, including OLS, logistic regression, or a binary splits algorithm. If a model targeting mortality is fit to data using OLS, R^2 exactly equals the amount by which the average predicted probability of death among those who died (AVE_1) exceeds the average predicted probability of death among those who lived (AVE_0). When predictions are derived using a logistic regression model, R^2 still closely approximates this difference.

The same issues associated with using R^2 to measure performance for modeling continuous outcomes discussed above arise when modeling dichotomous outcomes. Also, the same warnings about difficulties interpreting summary measures of model performance apply whether an R^2, a c-statistic, or another measure is reported. In particular, performance measures calculated on different data sets may not be comparable, especially if the populations vary markedly in the amount of total variability that the model attempts to explain. Many researchers fail to appreciate that this limitation pertains to the c-statistic as well as to R^2 and other measures.

Hadorn and colleagues (1992) explored the effect of the "hardness" of the data set on performance measures when modeling a dichotomous outcome. Based on predictions from a logistic regression model developed to predict mortality within 30 days of admission for patients with AMI, the overall data were divided into subsets that differed in the dispersion of the predicted probabilities. They ran both good and poor models on the harder and easier subsets of the data. Measures of performance for poor models on easy data often exceeded measures for good models on difficult data, nicely demonstrating the importance of comparing models on the same data (Hadorn et al. 1992). The problem of noncomparability can be partially addressed with a weighted analysis, but this is possible only if discrepancies between data sets result from well-documented and objectively quantified reasons (e.g., differences in the way in which cases were sampled within strata). While dissimilarity in the outcomes of two data sets clearly suggests noncomparability, similarity does not guarantee that the two data sets are equally easy to model (Hadorn et al. 1992).

Cross-validated (see next section) R^2 values for dichotomous outcomes have ranged generally from 0.10 to 0.30 in various studies of risk-adjusted death rates (Daley et al. 1988; Keeler et al. 1990; Iezzoni et al. 1995a, 1996a, 1996e). Wagner and colleagues (1994) modeled deaths for ICU patients using current APACHE III score and score change from the previous day, ICU admission diagnosis, age, chronic health status, and treatment before ICU admissions. These models achieved R^2 values of 0.34 (for predictions made on day 6 of the ICU stay) and 0.40 (for predictions made on day 1), and c-statistics ranged from 0.84 to 0.90 (Wagner et al. 1994, 1365). These are among the highest measures of performance reported for such models.

Typically, models with higher c-statistics have higher R^2 values, although exceptions do occur. However, when two models are applied to a single data set, R^2 values often differ even though the c-statistics are similar, illustrating that R^2 can convey information about relative model performance more strongly than the c-statistic (Ash and Shwartz 1999).

A public debate about R^2 and c-statistics involving New York state's CABG mortality model (see Chapter 1) arose in the *New England Journal of Medicine*, illustrating issues associated with these two measures (Green and Wintfeld 1995, 1230):

> The validity of risk-adjusted mortality as an indicator of the quality of care depends on the ability of a mathematical model to quantify baseline differences in case mix among providers accurately. Our analysis of predicted and observed outcomes revealed that the capacity of

[New York's] model to do this was limited. Predicted mortality rates assigned to surgeons by the model explained only a small portion of the variance in mortality ($R^2 = 7.3$ percent); the R^2 value for hospital was negligible (0.4 percent). The power of the model to predict outcomes for individual patients was also low ($R^2 = 8.0$ percent).

In their critique of New York's CABG model, Green and Wintfeld (1995, 1232) never mentioned c-statistics. Nevertheless, in their last sentence they warned, "To help ensure that report cards provide fair and informative comparisons, the data and methods used to generate them should regularly undergo a thorough, independent statistical evaluation." In 1996, New York officials responded, again in the *New England Journal of Medicine* (Chassin, Hannan, and DeBuono 1996, 396–397):

Statistically, the fit of a logistic-regression model is typically assessed on the basis of discrimination. . . . The R^2 statistic, or the square of the multiple correlation coefficient, is a measure typically used to assess linear regression models in which the dependent variable is continuous. In theory, values for R^2 range from 0 (representing no association between the predicted and observed values) to a 1 (representing a perfect association). In logistic-regression models in which the overall mortality rate ranges from 2 percent to 4 percent, however, R^2 is almost always less than 0.2. This limitation arises from the nature of logistic regression, in which the dependent variable must have one of only two values (in this case, survival or death). When the difference between actual and predicted mortality rates is calculated for each person (as part of the calculation of R^2), no matter how accurate the prediction is, the difference between the predicted value and the observed value for the mortality will be large, since the observed mortality must be either 0 or 1 and the prediction is a proportion between 0 and 1.

Discrimination in logistic regression, therefore, is usually measured by the c-statistic. . . . In analyses of the New York data, the c-statistic has typically been approximately 0.80; for 1992, it was 0.826. This value compares favorably with the c-statistics reported for other models of CABG-associated mortality, which range from 0.74 to 0.814.

It has been argued that the New York model does not accurately predict the future performance of hospitals or physicians and that therefore it functions poorly. Predicting performance is not a test of the model's validity, however, because it was not designed to foretell the future. Instead, the model was constructed to help hospitals and physicians improve their performance, precisely to avoid repeating problems encountered in the past.

The bottom line is that both c and R^2 are useful measures of the performance of models predicting dichotomous outcomes. With binary outcomes, however, many people do not appreciate how powerful models with small R^2 values can be. Thus, reporting only R^2 can expose a good model to criticism. In general, attempts to argue "policy value" require descriptions of model performance that are easier to grasp than either R^2 or c. A table of actual death rates within deciles of predicted risk (as described above) can be helpful in this context.

Model Validation

Models fit on specific data sets must undergo validation to determine how well they might perform in other settings. Analysts typically validate models using two approaches: cross-validation, in which part of the same data set used to develop the model is employed to validate the model, and independent validation, in which the model is applied to entirely new data.

Because analysts frequently do not have access to new databases, they commonly use a portion (e.g., one-half or two-thirds) of their data to develop the model, reserving the remaining data for validation. We used this approach to validate the contributions of comorbidities when predicting hospital costs, focusing on how R^2 increased when we added comorbidity variables to a model containing only DRGs (Shwartz et al. 1996b). On the first half of the data, the R^2 associated with DRGs only was 0.44; adding comorbidity variables increased it by 20 percent, to 0.53. When we reversed the roles of the development and validation data sets, R^2 in the validation set still rose 16 percent. When we fit the models to our entire data set, the nonvalidated R^2 increased roughly 20 percent (from 0.42 to 0.50). This validation analysis suggests that most, but not all, of the observed increase in R^2 is real; comorbidities add information about the cost of hospitalizations, even after accounting for DRGs. The cross-validation analysis confirmed that this increase did not simply result from overfitting.

In our study of hospital-based severity measures, we performed cross-validation as follows. First, we randomly split the data in half, into samples 1 and 2, and fit models to each sample. In sample 1, we computed SSE_1 and SST_1 as follows:

- $SSE_1 =$ the sum (within sample 1) of squared differences between each Y and the *PRED* predicted for it by the model that was fit to sample 2 and
- $SST_1 =$ the sum (within sample 1) of squared differences between the individual Ys and the average Y in sample 1.

From these, we computed cross-validated R^2, denoted CVR_1^2, as $1 - SSE_1/SST_1$. We repeated this process, reversing the roles of samples 1 and 2, to get CVR_1^2, a validated R^2 for the sample 2 data. We then averaged these two values to compute a summary CVR^2. This method provides insight into the variation associated with the resulting value. However, if a single number is desired, another approach is to calculate a single CVR^2 value on the whole database, using the following:

- $SSE = SSE_1 + SSE_2 =$ the sum (over all cases) of squared differences between each Y and the $PRED$ predicted for it by the model that was fit to the sample that did not contain it and
- $SST =$ the sum (over all cases) of squared differences between the individual Ys and the average Y in the whole population.

(Note that SST does not equal $SST_1 + SST_2$.)

     This approach offers the advantage of generalizing readily to settings where using half the data is viewed as inadequate for model development.[13] In this situation, a popular cross-validation approach involves dividing the data into a number of approximately equal parts (e.g., ten) and fitting models successively on all of the data except one part. Each model developed (e.g., on 90 percent of the data) is used to make predictions for the held-out part. Thus, the prediction for each case that goes into the SSE is based on a model that did not include that case in parameter estimation. Cross-validated R^2 values are then calculated from the actual and predicted values for all the cases.

     Knaus and colleagues (1993) held out successive tenths of cases in estimating the cross-validated R^2 for predictions of LOS using APACHE III. In creating the MMPS (see Chapter 8), Daley and colleagues (1988) used successive subsamples of 90 percent of the data to make predictions for the holdout 10 percent subsamples, then calculated R^2 values from the predictions and actual values in the ten holdout subsamples combined. To validate the VHA mortality prediction models, Khuri and collaborators (1997) developed their models on half the patients and tested the models on the other half. For the model for all types of surgeries, they repeated this process three times, comparing the c-statistics for the fitting and validation sample each time. On average, the c-statistic was 0.003 lower in the validation sample. For models developed for specific operations (which had much smaller sample sizes), the c-statistic in the validation sample generally fell within 0.05 of the c-statistic in the fitting sample. However, differences of that magnitude (0.05) in c are not trivial. Typically, models with c-statistics of 0.70 are noticeably more useful than those with c values of 0.65.

     In general, the smaller the holdout sample, the greater the concern about falsely assessing model performance. If each iteration holds out only small subsets of cases, the remaining main body of data is similar for each successive model fit (Picard and Berk 1990). Thus, the models are unlikely to differ much from a model fit to the entire database. Nevertheless, cross-validated R^2 values can sometimes differ substantially from R^2 values in the development data set even when only one case is held out. For example, Thomas and Ashcraft (1991) held out only one case during model development; nevertheless, they found much lower R^2 values on model validation, both for all cases and excluding outliers (with n approximately 1,700 and 1,400, respectively). Thus, even a single case can substantially affect model fit when samples are small.

Comparisons of R^2 values and c-statistics across different models must account for variability of the statistic. Bootstrapping allows analysts to estimate CIs for statistics whose distributional properties are not well characterized (see Chapter 8). To construct a bootstrap estimate of the CI for a model's R^2, for example, analysts sample with replacement from the original data set a large number (perhaps 1,000) of simulated data sets, each the same size as the original data set.[14] The model is fit to each simulated data set, and the R^2 is calculated. CIs for R^2 are constructed from the distribution of the 1,000 R^2 values. For example, if the 5th and 95th percentiles (i.e., the 50th from the lowest and 50th from the highest values of R^2) were 0.15 and 0.23, respectively, (0.15, 0.23) is a 90 percent CI for R^2.

In assessing the contributions of severity of illness to explaining cost differences between tertiary teaching and nonteaching hospitals, we estimated that severity plus other patient characteristics (e.g., admission source, discharge destination, transfer status, purpose of admission) explained 18 percent of the higher costs at teaching hospitals. We used bootstrapping to determine a 90 percent CI (from 4 percent to 33 percent) for this estimate (Iezzoni et al. 1990). Khuri and colleagues (1997) used bootstrapping to examine the stability of the important risk factors that entered stepwise logistic regression models to predict postoperative deaths. For each type of surgery, they drew 15 bootstrap samples and developed models. They measured the stability of each variable by the percentage of the models in which a given variable appeared. Serum albumin, the most important predictor, appeared in 92 percent of the replications, followed by age (84 percent), emergency status (84 percent), the American Society of Anesthesia classification (76 percent), and disseminated cancer (74 percent).

CIs for R^2 and the c-statitstic are usually estimated from bootstrap replications. However, Hanley and McNeil (1982, 1983) provide methods for analytically calculating CIs for c-statistics and for differences in c-statistics using either the same or different data.

Validating a model by applying it to a new data set is the strongest form of validation. However, if a model does not validate well, the model itself may not be the problem. As noted above, when model parameters are estimated in a development data set using OLS, the average predicted value from the model [AVE($PRED_i$)] equals the average actual value of the dependent variable [AVE(Y_i)]. When maximum likelihood methods are used to estimate parameters (e.g., in a logistic regression), the averages are usually close but not necessarily equal. However, when a previously developed model is applied to new data, AVE($PRED_i$) generally differs from AVE(Y_i). As discussed earlier, the significance of this difference depends on the purpose of the comparison.

If the goal is to assess model validity, the difference between AVE($PRED_i$) and AVE(Υ_i) measures model calibration. If the differences are large, it might suggest poor validation. Alternatively, "miscalibration" of the model may indicate that the two settings from which the independent databases come differ in important ways, such as in their quality or efficiency of care. There is no foolproof way to choose between these competing hypotheses—poor validation versus different setting. This is one reason that examining trends with a longitudinal data set can be so powerful (see Chapter 12). From year to year, data from the same setting are generally more comparable than data from completely independent sources.

As discussed, summary measures of model performance are likely to deteriorate when models are applied to independent data. The most complex models experience the greatest loss. However, such deterioration does not necessarily occur. For example, Ash and colleagues (in press) used data on more than 300,000 cases in 1995 to estimate parameters to predict one-year mortality following AMI using three models: a Charlson-like comorbidity model with 17 conditions, a DCG model with 118 conditions, and a model using 259 conditions defined by AHRQ's Clinical Classification software (http://www.ahcpr.gov/data/hcup/comorbid.htm). We then used these models to predict one-year mortality for AMI cases in 1999. The c-statistics from the models fit to 1995 data were 0.73, 0.80, and 0.81, respectively. Given the large numbers of cases involved, the validated c-statistics were also high. However, because of their many parameters, we expected some deterioration in the c-statistic for the DCG model and more for the model with 259 conditions. Surprisingly, in all cases, c-statistics increased by 0.01 in the 1999 validation data. The likely explanation is twofold: The 1995 data were sufficiently large to avoid overfitting, and the newer data were somehow easier to fit, perhaps because of better diagnosis coding.

In addition to evaluating validity with overall summary measures, assessing performance for subgroups of interest using both development and validation data sets is valuable. Suppose that a model developed to predict death is then applied to some subgroup of cases, either a subset of the model development data set or new cases that share a particular characteristic (as opposed to a randomly sampled validation data set). Suppose further that the observed death rate in the group being studied is significantly different from what the model predicts. If we believe that the model fairly captures and accounts for all important risk factors, we must then look for some other causal factor, such as lower- or higher-quality care. However, systematic mispredictions for subgroups of patients may reflect problems with the model.

Blumberg (1991) viewed poor model fit for specific patient subgroups as "biased estimation." To demonstrate the problem, he employed an old version of the admission MedisGroups severity score to adjust for 30-day mortality of AMI patients and found that estimates of expected mortality differed significantly from actual outcomes in subgroups defined by such attributes as patients' age, location of infarction in the myocardium, history of CHF, serum potassium level, BUN, pulse rate, and blood pressure. For instance, Blumberg reported a 38.4 percent death rate among 289 patients 85 years of age and older versus an expected rate of 27.2 percent. He concluded that this version of MedisGroups was biased by not accounting properly for the independent effect of age on mortality risk. Subsequent versions of MedisGroups specifically included age in the prediction models (Steen et al. 1993). Although age appears to be an independent risk factor for mortality (see Chapter 3), Blumberg's finding is also consistent with the possibility that very old persons receive worse quality of care, resulting in more deaths than expected.

When validating models on subgroups of the data, problems might arise because of intrinsic differences in the hardness of the data for modeling; performance measures for models applied to different subgroups are not comparable. Consider a situation where a data set contains patients representing three different diseases. If models are fit separately within each disease subgroup, the R^2 for making predictions in the whole data set is a sum of two quantities: the average of the three R^2 values for the three subsets and the R^2 for a model that assigns the average death rate for each disease to each patient with that disease. Thus, if the three diseases have very different death rates, the overall R^2 could be large simply because outcomes differ widely by disease, even if the ability to distinguish risk among patients with the same disease is negligible.

One should distinguish subgroups formed *a priori* (using variables similar to candidate risk factors) from subgroups formed based on observed outcomes (e.g., particularly high or low values of the outcome variable). Risk-adjustment methods may fail to calibrate well in extreme subgroups formed from observed outcomes, a problem sometimes called "compression." However, when groups are formed *post hoc*, based on extreme outcomes, the mean expected value of the group should be less extreme than the actual group value. This is especially evident when considering models to predict the total cost of next year's health services for a group of persons. For example, nearly 20 percent of Medicare beneficiaries generate no health care costs over one year. However, no Medicare recipient generates an expected cost of $0 during a year of enrollment. No matter how healthy a sizeable group of people was in a particular year, some expenditures will occur in the next year. Similarly, even if a group has high expected costs next year because of problems observed this year, their actual costs will likely be lower than the highest costs next year. Patients with the very highest or lowest costs in any one period are expected to have costs in the next period that are closer to the overall average in that period, a phenomenon called "regression to the mean" (Bailar and Mosteller 1986, 87).

Many subgroups of policy interest are defined by characteristics other than the targeted outcomes, such as urban versus rural hospitals, public versus private hospitals, Medicaid versus commercial insurers, and insured versus uninsured persons. For such groups, interpretation of discrepancies between observed and expected outcomes must be done carefully. For example, suppose that death rates in public hospitals are significantly higher than expected after risk adjustment using some particular set of variables to measure risk. Whether this difference indicates that care in such hospitals is poorer or that patients seen in public hospitals are sicker than patients in other hospitals in ways not measured by the model is critical to understanding this finding. Often, such findings flag the need for further research or, in its absence, give rise to pointed disputes about what the risk-adjusted findings mean.

Independent validation can extend beyond statistical assessment of the model to consider the purposes for considering risk-adjusted outcomes. As illustrated in the national VA Surgical Risk Study (see Chapter 9), researchers aimed to answer the question, "To what extent do model-based risk-adjusted measures of quality correspond to quality measured using different approaches?" Daley and colleagues (1997a) described site visits to 20 VA surgical services with either lower- or higher-than-expected risk-adjusted mortality or morbidity rates. Site visitors rated overall quality and technology and equipment much more favorably at hospitals with lower-than-expected mortality and morbidity rates compared to those with higher rates. Site visit teams blinded to the predicted outcomes of the hospital correctly determined the outlier status (i.e., higher or lower than expected) for 17 of the 20 surgical services visited. This is a powerful validation of the use of a risk-adjustment model to identify services with either high or low quality of care.

Given the strong public desire to compare risk-adjusted outcomes across providers (see Chapters 1 and 12), interest in the performance of risk-prediction models will increase. Of particular concern is the claim that worse-than-expected outcomes reflect the inadequacy of risk adjustment. The most rigorous way to test this claim is to collect data on the unmeasured risk factors believed responsible for the discrepancies and see how much of the difference is explained. Although theoretically attractive, this test is often impractical (see Chapter 3). Without further studies of the type conducted by the VA researchers, one must rely on judgments about the face and content validity of the risk-adjustment approach (see Chapter 8) and judgments about whether unmeasured risk factors might explain observed discrepancies. Thus, interpreting "objective" measures of performance must ultimately rely on more subjective assessments.

Conclusions

A variety of summary measures of model performance exist, including many not discussed here. However, regardless of what other measures are reported we believe that all publications and reports about risk-adjustment methods should present a core set of common measures. Our short list of important measures includes R^2 and deciles-of-risk tables for both dichotomous and continuous outcomes and, for dichotomous outcomes, additionally the *c*-statistic and the mean *PRED* for cases with and without the event.

Nevertheless, interpreting these quantitative measures of performance is not straightforward, and subjective judgments are often required. These judgments are influenced by such factors as the following:

- the specific context or origin of the sample under study (e.g., hospital types, whether certain groups were oversampled);
- the appropriateness of the outcome variable for this context;
- how well the independent variables represent baseline risks;
- the variability in the dependent and independent variables in the data set;
- whether and how outliers were identified and handled in the analysis;
- whether the risk adjuster is a continuous variable and, if so, whether and how discrete categories were formed for this analysis;
- whether data transformations were used and, if so, whether measures of model performance used the retransformed data; and
- whether performance measure estimates were validated or CIs reported.

Notes

1. The buckets could be chosen to contain equal numbers of cases (quintiles, deciles, or more generally, "quantiles"), to capture intuitive cutpoints (such as risks less than 1.0, between 1.0 and 2.0, between 2.0 and 5.0, and greater than 5.0), to distinguish a small but crucial high-risk subpopulation, or to match categories that have commonly been used before. There is no all-purpose best rule for creating buckets.
2. For cost outcomes, 500 or more cases per bucket are desirable.
3. With k buckets, this is equivalent to regressing Y on indicator variables for any $k - 1$ of them.
4. Unlike bucketing, multivariable regressions often produce negative cost predictions for some cases and negative coefficients for factors that logically should not subtract from expected costs. Eliminating such anomalies can require substantial work.
5. This broad statement is essentially true even when the prediction comes out of a "black box" methodology, such as a neural network.
6. Here, "number of predictors" is the number of model coefficients or parameters. For example, if $X = $ age is entered using X and X^2, it contributes two predictors.
7. One caveat is that it is not clear which, if any, of these distinctions is either statistically (or practically) significant (see discussion of bootstrapped confidence intervals later in the text).
8. This is because SST is a fixed characteristic of the data and does not vary for different models, and $R^2 = 1 - (n/\text{SST}) * (\text{SD})^2$.
9. The central limit theorem states that for large enough n and under

very general conditions, the average of a sum of n independent random variables is approximately normally distributed, with mean equal to the average mean of the Ys and variance equal to the average of the variances of the Ys divided by n. Thus, the larger n is, the more the distribution of average deviations will look like normal deviates, centered at zero, with variance = MSE/n, where MSE is approximately equal to SSE/n (assuming n is large). Because the shape of a normal deviate is fixed, the relationship between the mean squared error and the mean absolute deviation is also fixed: MAD $\sim 0.8 *$ MSE. (To make this exact, substitute $\sqrt{2/\pi}$ for 0.8.) Thus, in comparing two models, the one with the smaller individual MSE will have smaller MADs for its averages regardless of the relationship between the two models' individual MAD.

10. The SD for "an individual prediction error" equals $\sqrt{1 - R^2} *$ SD(Y).

11. Alternatives to creating categories are described in Harrell (2001). One option is to use computer-based approaches (e.g., "locally weighted scatter plot smooth," called LOWESS or LOESS—although technically distinct, in practice the acronyms are used interchangeably—or cubic splines) to produce a smooth plot of the relationship between an outcome and a candidate independent variable, such as a continuous risk measure. Change points in a smoothed function (places where the change in outcome is large for a small change in the independent variable) can be used to define "intelligent" cutpoints when creating risk score categories, which will then be represented in the final model by dummy variables.

12. Let n equal the number of cases in each decile, $\hat{P}$ equal the average predicted probability of death in the decile and $\hat{Q} = 1 - \hat{P}$. $\hat{P}_i$ and $\hat{Q}_i$ are the analogous probabilities for the ith person in the decile. In the Hosmer-Lemeshow statistic, variance in each cell is estimated as $n\hat{P}\hat{Q}$ rather than the sum of the $\hat{P}_i\hat{Q}_i$ terms, which is a better estimate of the variance. (If the P_is were known, rather than estimated, it would be exactly right.) Furthermore, $n\hat{P}\hat{Q}$ is generally larger than the sum of the $\hat{P}_i\hat{Q}_i$ terms. For example, if there are 50 cases with $\hat{P}_i = 0.90$ and 50 with $\hat{P}_i = 0.10$, the sum of the $\hat{P}_i\hat{Q}_i$ equals 9, whereas $n\hat{P}\hat{Q} = 25$. So, $(O_{die} - E_{die})/n\hat{P}\hat{Q}$ will be only 36 percent as large as would be correct (since $9/25 = 0.36$). On the other hand, if the $\hat{P}_i$ terms are split into two groups of 50 with more similar probabilities, say 0.40 and 0.60, the sum of the $\hat{P}_i\hat{Q}_i$ terms equals 24, which is 96 percent as large as $n\hat{P}\hat{Q}$. Using the sum of the $\hat{P}_i\hat{Q}_i$ terms instead of $n\hat{P}\hat{Q}$ in calculating the test statistic avoids this problem.

13. If using half the data is really inadequate for model development, all the data may still be too little. This is because doubling the size of the data only decreases the size of errors by a factor of $\sqrt{1/2} \sim 0.7$.

14. It may seem counterintuitive to sample N cases with replacement from the data set of N cases that we have. However, the data set we have is

our best estimate of the population from which the data arose. What we would really like to do is to repeatedly sample N cases from the population. Because we do not know the population, we sample from our best guess of what the population is—the data set of N cases that we have. In this sense, we are "pulling ourselves up by our bootstraps," the phrase giving rise to the name of the technique.

ESTIMATING THE EFFECT OF AN INTERVENTION FROM OBSERVATIONAL DATA

Michael Shwartz and Arlene S. Ash

Randomized controlled trials (RCTs) are the gold standard for evaluating the efficacy of clinical interventions (see Chapter 1). Because RCTs randomly assign patients to either an intervention or a control group, patients in each group will, on average, have similar measured and unmeasured baseline risk factors. Biases may arise in conducting clinical trials, for example, if outcomes are measured somewhat differently for study and control subjects. Nevertheless, presumed balance in baseline risk factors significantly strengthens confidence that an observed difference in outcome between the treatment and control groups is due to the intervention.

However, most clinical interventions are never subjected to RCTs because of practical, conceptual, and ethical concerns. RCTs basically depend on "coin flips" to assign subjects to the treatment or control group. To ethically justify such assignments, expectations about the benefit of the intervention must be sufficiently uncertain to withhold it from some patients and give it to others. In practice, many interventions become widely adopted before RCTs are performed, making it difficult to recruit subjects or their physicians because of strongly held beliefs about effectiveness. For example, there are too few data from RCTs for women over age 70 to know whether screening mammography is helpful in this population. While some believe that it is unethical to withhold this intervention with proven benefits in younger women, others are equally convinced that screening mammography is of little value for older women. However, "acknowledged uncertainty" rather than controversy is necessary to motivate clinical trials. Physicians and patients who already "know the truth" (whichever side they take) are likely to refuse random assignment.

To increase internal validity, RCTs often recruit relatively homogeneous subjects, for example, by excluding patients over age 70 or those with serious comorbidities. Furthermore, even among those eligible for inclusion, trial participants often differ from "refusers" in ways that affect study outcomes. Participants are typically healthier than the average eligible case, introducing a "healthy volunteer" effect. For example, perioperative mortality following carotid endarterectomy is higher in actual practice than reported in RCTs, even within institutions participating in the trials (Wennberg et al. 1998).

Thus, findings from RCTs may not generalize well to the patients seen in routine clinical practice. Clinicians' sense that study subjects are not like their patients slows the diffusion of RCT-validated interventions. Also, RCTs are expensive and often take years, during which time the targeted interventions may become obsolete.

Thus, most clinical interventions are not subjected to RCTs, and analysts must rely on quasi-experimental or nonexperimental observational studies.[1] In observational studies, some patients receive interventions while others do not, for reasons that are only partially captured by measurable factors. Analysts compare outcomes in the two groups, hoping to quantify the effectiveness of the intervention. However, directly comparing outcomes may be misleading; persons with and without the intervention often differ markedly in measured and unmeasured baseline risk factors and thus prognosis. The size and direction of these differences are generally unknown. Hence, it is difficult to determine whether differences in outcomes are caused by the intervention or largely by differences in baseline risk.

When assessing the value of an intervention from observational data, analysts typically use a multivariable model to adjust for baseline differences in risk. Standard multivariable models estimate treatment effectiveness without bias if every important risk factor is measured and if the relationship between the risk factors and outcome is correctly specified. However, this is a conceptual ideal. In this chapter, we first briefly discuss standard multivariable models used to make risk-adjusted assessments when the data and models approximate the ideal. Then, we describe two methods that are useful when the validity of these assumptions is in doubt: propensity score matching, which protects against biases caused by incorrect model specification, and instrumental variables, which address suspected differences in unmeasured risk factors.

Multivariable Models for Estimating the Effects of Interventions

Consider estimating the effect of an intervention, such as enrolling in a managed care organization (MCO). The data contain both people enrolled in MCOs and people who get their care through a fee-for-service arrangement. Historically, MCO enrollees have been healthier than those who remain in fee-for-service. If outcomes differ for those in the MCO, how much (if any) of that difference is due to managed care? The standard approach is to adjust for differences in baseline risk using multivariable models. The general approach is similar whether we are predicting a continuous (e.g., health care expenditures over a year), dichotomous (e.g., whether a person is admitted to the hospital over a year), or time-to-event (e.g., time to death following treatment) outcome.

First, consider a continuous outcome. Let Y_i be the actual value of the outcome variable for the ith person and X_{ij} be the value of the jth independent variable for the ith person, $j = 1, \ldots , J$. These J independent variables are the baseline risk factors. Let I be a variable that is coded 1 if the person is in an MCO and 0 if the person has remained in fee-for-service.

The standard multivariable linear regression model to assess treatment effectiveness is:

$$E(Y_i) = a + \Sigma_j \, b_j * X_{ij} + c * I$$

where $E(Y_i)$ is the expected value of the outcome variable for the ith person, a is a constant coefficient, the b_j terms are coefficients that measure the systematic effects of risk factors (the X_{ij} terms) on the outcome Y, and c is the coefficient that measures the effect of the intervention on Y. Imagine two people with the same values for all risk factors, one of whom is in managed care ($I = 1$) and the other in fee-for-service ($I = 0$). Under this model, the cost for a managed care patient is predicted to equal c + the cost for a fee-for-service person with the same risk factors. Managed care is demonstrated to influence cost if c is statistically significantly different from 0. The absolute value of c is called the size of the effect. For example, if $c = -500$, managed care is associated with a $500 reduction in yearly cost.

An interaction term allows the effect of a variable on the outcome to differ depending on the value of other variables. Interactions of risk factors with the intervention variable are often of particular interest. Consider a model with the following indicator variables: I for the intervention and F for female, coded as 1 for women and 0 for men. $I * F$ is an interaction between sex and treatment, which is 1 for a woman who receives the intervention and 0 for everyone else. The model might look like:

$$E(Y_i) = a + \text{effects from other risk factors} + b * F + c * I + d * (I * F).$$

This model form provides flexibility. Regardless of whether interventions occur, women are expected to cost some fixed amount b more than similar men.[2] Among men (for whom $F = 0$ and $I * F = 0$), the intervention adds c to their expected outcome; among women, the intervention increases expected outcome by $c + d$. Thus, the interaction term allows the model to assess the possibility that the intervention affects women and men differently. In general, to assess the effect of an intervention, we examine the CI and p-value associated with c, the coefficient of the intervention indicator I, and any other coefficients attached to the intervention, such as d in the model above.

When the outcome is dichotomous (e.g., being alive 30 days after hospital admission), logistic regression is the standard approach. The dependent variable is the log of the odds of an event of interest. If P_i is the probability of being alive for the ith person, O_i, the odds that person i is alive, is defined as $P_i/(1 - P_i)$.[3] A logistic regression model for assessing treatment effectiveness looks like:

$$\ln O_i = \ln[P_i/(1 - P_i)] = a + \Sigma_j \, b_j * X_{ij} + c * I$$

where ln represents the natural (base e) logarithm. This model allows the log odds of a person being alive to increase by a fixed amount c when the intervention is present. This equation can be rewritten as:

$$O_i = e^{a + \Sigma_{jbj} * X_{ij} + c*I} = [e^{a + \Sigma_{jbj} * X_{ij}}] * e^{c*I} = [\text{person-specific risk}_i] * e^{c*I}$$

showing that the effect of the intervention is to multiply a person's odds by e^c.[4] Under this model, if the odds of the event for a person with the intervention is divided by the same person's odds absent the intervention, the result is always e^c. Thus, e^c is called the odds ratio for the event, given the treatment. Treatments that make the event more likely have odds ratios greater than 1, and vice versa. This functional form assumes that the intervention has the same effect for all people regardless of their characteristics. Again, interaction terms could be added if this assumption is in doubt. As for OLS multiple regression, key interest is in the CI and p-value associated with c.

When time to an event (such as death) is the outcome, some cases may be lost to follow-up and others may be alive when the study ends. For these, we know that they were still alive at their last-seen date; thus, their date of death is partially known, or "censored." The proportional-hazards model is standard for modeling survival data with censoring (Cox 1972). Virnig and colleagues (2000) provide a more detailed yet introductory-level discussion of issues in survival modeling.

The dependent variable in the proportional-hazards model is the instantaneous hazard rate at time t, denoted by $h(t)$, which can be thought of as the probability that a person who has survived to time t dies (or experiences the event of interest) in some very small interval of time thereafter.[5] This is expressed as a function of a baseline hazard ($h_0(t)$, treated as a nuisance parameter) and other risk factors of interest. The model is:

$$h(t) = h_0(t) * e^{a + \Sigma_{jbj} * X_{ij} + c*I} = h_0(t) * e^{a + \Sigma_{jbj} * X_{ij}} * e^{c*I}$$
$$= [h_0(t) * e^a * e^{b_1 X_{i1}} * e^{b_2 X_{i2}} \dots] * e^{c*I}$$

Embedded in the structure of this model is the assumption that each independent variable affects the baseline hazard by a multiple that is the same for all patients regardless of other characteristics and at all times t. In particular, the effect of the intervention on the hazard rate is multiplication by e^c, called the hazard ratio (analogous to the odds ratio when the outcome is dichotomous). More complex, time-dependent models are appropriate if the effects of variables change over time (Kalbfleisch and Prentiss 1980).

As noted, the multivariable models described above will correctly adjust for differences in baseline risk between intervention and control groups if the important risk factors are measured and the relationships between risk factors and the outcome of interest are correctly specified. However, these two criteria are at best approximately satisfied. In the next sections, we discuss options for addressing situations where information about risk factors or their relationships with outcomes is seriously incomplete.

The first situation assumes that every important risk factor has been measured but we worry that relationships between risk factors and the outcome may not be correctly specified. If risk factors are both strongly associated with the outcome and distributed very differently in the intervention and control groups, model mis-specification can lead to biased estimates of the treatment effect. Propensity scores deal with this problem. In the second situation, there are important unmeasured risk factors that are distributed differently for persons with and without the intervention. We illustrate the use of an instrumental variable to assess treatment effectiveness in the presence of such factors. Winship and Morgan (1999) place both approaches in the more general framework of estimating causal effects from observational data. Volume 2, Number 3/4 of *Health Services and Outcomes Research Methodology* (2001) is entirely devoted to causal modeling.

Propensity Scores

Propensity scores are useful when

1. several measured risk factors have a strong relationship to an outcome,
2. persons who receive an intervention and those who do not have markedly different distributions of values for these risk factors, and
3. we are unsure about the true relationship between the risk factors and the outcome.

There are standard approaches for addressing this situation. First, with only a few important risk factors and many study cases, analysts can define risk strata and examine the effect of the intervention separately within strata. This eliminates the need to model the relationship between the risk factors and the outcome. For example, if age and gender are the only two risk factors considered important, one might compare the outcome of people with and without the intervention separately by gender within each ten-year age category. However, many risk factors would lead to too many strata with too few cases for meaningful analysis. While a correctly specified model solves the problem, it is not easy to verify that a model meets this rigorous test. Propensity score methods protect against the bias that an incorrect model can introduce when comparing outcomes in groups with notably different distributions of baseline characteristics (Rosenbaum and Rubin 1983, 1984, 1985; Rubin and Thomas 1996; Rubin 1997; D'Agostino 1998).

Here, we first provide a simple example illustrating how model misspecification can lead to incorrect estimates of the effect of an intervention. We then discuss how propensity scores can be used to reduce the effect of model mis-specification and finally briefly describe several applications in the published literature.

Hypothetical Example

Assume we have a summary risk score that varies from 0 (lowest risk) to 2, an outcome measure that varies from 0 (worst outcome) to 1 (best), and an S-shaped curve representing the unknown but true relationship between risk and outcome (Figure 11.1). At risk levels below 0.5, outcomes are good and worsen slowly with increasing risk; at risk levels between 0.5 and about 1.5, outcomes decline linearly and much more steeply than at lower risk levels; and at risk levels above 1.5, outcomes are poor but decline only gradually as risk increases further. The solid straight line in Figure 11.1 shows how we modeled the relationship between risk and outcomes—incorrectly specifying it as a straight line relationship. At lower risk levels, the model-predicted outcome is worse (lower) than the true outcome; at high risk levels, the model-predicted outcome is better (higher) than the true outcome.

Assume that persons at high risk differentially receive an intervention. Specifically, suppose that people receiving the intervention have an average risk of 1.5, whereas those in the control group have lower risks, averaging 0.4. Because of baseline risk alone, the average outcome in the control group would be 0.95 (see square a in Figure 11.1), while that for the group that undergoes treatment would be 0.05 (see square b in Figure 11.1). However, although the underlying difference in outcomes because of the different risk levels is 0.90, our model (illustrated by the straight line in Figure 11.1) underestimates that difference. Its predictions are overly pessimistic about the expected outcome for the lower risk levels, where control cases are more often found, and overly optimistic at the higher risk levels, where intervention cases are more often found. Specifically, our model expects outcomes for the control group to average 0.80 (see square c in Figure 11.1) and 0.25 for the intervention group (see square d in Figure 11.1), leading to an expected difference of 0.55.

Assume that the intervention improves outcomes for everybody who receives it by 0.30, bringing the average outcome in the intervention group up to 0.35. The intervention works: Without it, those in the intervention group would have had outcomes that were 0.90 worse than the others; with it, their outcomes are only 0.60 worse. The raw data suggest that the treatment harms people a lot (on average, by $0.95 - 0.35 = 0.60$). Because the intervention group was so much sicker at baseline, the model expected the treatment group's outcome to average 0.55 worse than the others. Given that they actually averaged 0.60 worse, it appears that the intervention harms people a little, on average, by 0.05. Thus, the model helps to "level the playing field" but still produces a biased finding about the effect. In summary, the observed difference is −0.60, the (improperly) risk-adjusted difference is −0.05, and the true difference is +0.30.

FIGURE 11.1

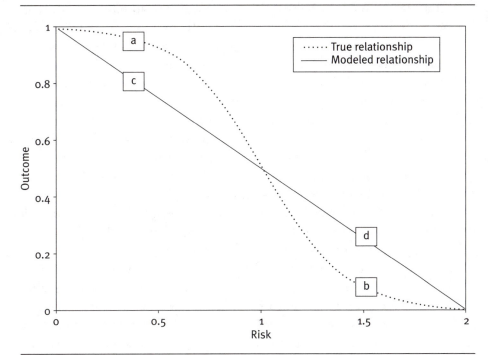

True and
Modeled
Relationships
between Risk
and Outcome

Propensity Score Approach

If we could compare outcomes within subgroups of study and control patients with similar risk profiles, the model's imperfections would matter less.
Propensity scores help identify such subgroups.

Consider a multivariable logistic regression model that uses risk factors
to predict receipt of the intervention as the outcome (by using an indicator,
or dummy variable of 1 when the intervention was received and 0 otherwise).
The propensity score for the ith case is the $PRED_i$ from this regression—the
predicted probability that the ith person receives the intervention. If subsets
of the intervention and control groups are chosen to have similar distributions
of the propensity score, these two groups will also have similar distributions
of the risk factors that comprise the propensity score model. Several standard
ways exist to identify subsets of study and control group members with similar
propensity scores. One simple way is by random subsampling within propensity
score category, as follows:

1. Develop a logistic regression model to calculate the propensity score
   (i.e., the probability of receiving the intervention as a function of the risk
   factors).
2. Rank the population from lowest to highest propensity score.
3. Divide the population into a few even-sized groups, such as quintiles,
   with similar propensity scores.

4. Within each propensity score quintile, divide people into the intervention and control groups (Table 11.1). Controls are most common in the lower quintiles (where the predicted probability of receiving the treatment is smallest) and least common in the higher quintiles.

5. Sample equal numbers of intervention and control cases from each quintile. As shown in Table 11.1, the smaller of either the number of intervention or control cases in each quintile limits the number that can be sampled. For example, with 12 intervention cases and 81 controls in the lowest quintile, we would select all 12 intervention cases and 12 of the 81 controls, for a total of 24 people. In the highest quintile, we would select all eight controls and eight of the 78 intervention cases, for a total of 16. The combined subsample of 206 cases, half from the control group and half from the intervention group, is identically distributed with respect to propensity score quintiles.[6]

6. Examine the distribution of risk factors between the intervention and control cases in the subsample to directly observe how their distributions of important risk factors compare. This illustrates one appealing feature of this approach. The purpose of the sampling is to achieve similar intervention and control groups, and the two groups can be examined to verify how similar their risk factors are.

7. Fit a new model to predict the effect of the intervention on the combined subsample. Because the intervention cases and controls in the subsample are similar with respect to baseline factors, raw and risk-adjusted estimates of the treatment effect should be similar. Although modeling can reduce the effect of residual differences between the subsampled groups, its main purpose at this stage is to produce a more accurate estimate (i.e., a narrower CI) of treatment effect.

Several points should be noted. First, if the database is large enough, it is useful to estimate the treatment effect separately within propensity score quintiles. If treatments are allocated rationally, patients with the highest propensity scores should experience the greatest benefits. Also, this could tell us how effective a treatment is for patients who ordinarily do not receive it. Second, dividing the propensity score into quintiles and then sampling within quintiles is generally adequate to produce balanced subsamples (i.e., little is gained from matching within narrower propensity score categories, such as deciles; Rosenbaum and Rubin 1984). Perfectly matched samples are unnecessary— only ones that have reasonably similar distributions of factors that importantly affect the outcome of interest—and this feature can be verified directly in the subsamples. Third, propensity score methods focus attention on how cases and controls in the full population differ on measured factors. This can help clarify reasons for differences in findings between standard and propensity score analyses.

Subsampling within quintile is relatively easy to do. Another relatively simple approach for achieving balanced subsets of cases and controls is "nearest

Quintiles of Propensity Score	No. of Cases		
	Intervention	Control	Analysis Sample
Lowest	12	81	24
Second lowest	30	67	60
Middle	44	38	76
Second highest	53	15	30
Highest	78	8	16
Total	217	209	206

TABLE 11.1
Example of Subsampling within Propensity Score Quintile

available matching on the estimated propensity score" (Rosenbaum and Rubin 1985, 35). Intervention group participants are randomly ordered. Then, in the first step, the first intervention group participant is matched with that control group participant whose propensity score is closest, and the pair is set aside. At each step, the next remaining study group participant is matched with the remaining control group participant whose propensity score is closest and set aside, until all study group participants are matched. This is an example of a "greedy algorithm," that is, a match once made is not reconsidered. Such an approach can be improved by setting a maximum acceptable distance between an intervention case and control case propensity score (called a "caliper"); when no control case within this distance is available for matching, the intervention case is discarded. This is done to avoid comparing outcomes between intervention cases and "extremely dissimilar" control cases. Note that both the greedy algorithm approach and subsampling within subgroups with similar propensity scores have a random component, so that somewhat different subsamples, and therefore potentially different "findings," can emerge when two analysts apply the same methodology to the same data. While this problem causes minimal practical difficulties, it is unsatisfying and can be avoided using more sophisticated approaches such as Mahalanobis metric matching either with or without calipers (Rosenbaum and Rubin 1985) or by using optimization models (Rosenbaum 1989).

Examples from the Literature Using Propensity Scores

We used propensity score matching to compare outcomes for two modalities for substance abuse detoxification within the publicly funded substance abuse treatment system in Boston: (1) acupuncture, which consisted of daily acupuncture sessions during the acute detoxification phase, followed by sessions two to three times per week for three to six months (in addition to acupuncture, patients received maintenance and motivational counseling, usually in groups), and (2) residential detoxification, which lasted approximately one week, with encouragement upon discharge to seek postdetox treatment. We were interested in whether clients were readmitted for detoxification within six months of an index detoxification admission (Shwartz et al. 1999).

Acupuncture clients were typically "better off" than those who received residential detox. For example, 13 percent of acupuncture patients were college graduates, compared to 4 percent of residential detox patients; 57 percent versus 13 percent were employed; 15 percent versus 3 percent had private insurance; 76 percent versus 55 percent lived with others; 3 percent versus 30 percent lived in a shelter; and 19 percent versus 43 percent had previous detox admissions in the year prior to the index admission. Among 1,104 acupuncture cases and 6,907 residential detox controls, we matched 740 cases and 740 controls on propensity score by subsampling within propensity score decile. The subsamples were quite similar. For example, 7 percent in both groups had college degrees; 42 percent of acupuncture versus 41 percent of residential detox patients were employed; 6 percent versus 9 percent had private insurance; 77 percent versus 72 percent lived with others; 4 percent versus 5 percent lived in a shelter; and 26 percent versus 27 percent had detox admissions in the previous year.

The estimated effectiveness of acupuncture in avoiding a detox readmission was relatively similar when the analysis was performed on either the full sample (odds ratio 0.71, 95 percent CI 0.53–0.95) or the propensity score matched subsamples (odds ratio 0.61, 95 percent CI 0.39–0.94). This similarity may relate to the extremely good predictive power (c-statistic $= 0.96$) of the original model fit to the full sample of cases, leaving little room for model mis-specification.

As noted, analysts can use propensity scores in several ways. In the acupuncture project, we used propensity scores to subsample patients, then estimated the intervention effect in the subsample. The approach is transparent: It highlights the similarities and differences between the people who did and did not receive the intervention. We had started with a standard multivariable analysis comparing the acupuncture and residential treatment program outcomes. Reviewers criticized these analyses, however, noting that users of the two treatment modalities were so different that their outcomes should not be compared. However, we found 740 residential detox patients who had very similar risk factors to a group of 740 acupuncture patients. Similarity of risk factors reduced concerns about the "black box" of multivariable adjustment. Ultimately, comparing outcomes in these subsets of similar residential detox and acupuncture cases was more convincing than relying on risk adjustment to compare outcomes in very different populations.

Analysts sometimes use propensity scores as a covariate in addition to other risk factors in a standard multivariable regression on the full sample of cases. Here, the goal is to adjust for a summary measure that reflects the likelihood of receiving the treatment in addition to other risk factors. However, this approach is unlikely to produce analyses that are robust to model mis-specification, as illustrated in the examples that follow.[7]

Propensity scores have been used in several studies of interventions for heart disease. We report results of some recent studies that compare estimates of effectiveness from standard and propensity score modeling approaches. First, we describe those that use propensity scores as an additional explanatory variable in a standard multivariable model. To illustrate, Stenestrand and Wallentin (2001) examined how early statin medications (drugs to lower cholesterol) affected one-year survival following AMI in almost 20,000 patients (of whom more than 5,500 received statins). Results were very similar using standard versus propensity score analyses. In a Cox regression analysis with 43 covariates, the relative risk associated with statins was 0.73 (95 percent CI 0.62–0.87); when propensity score was added to the model, relative risk was 0.75; and when propensity score was used alone, relative risk was 0.78. Other studies that used the propensity score as an additional independent variable in a multivariable model are those of Chan and colleagues (2002), Newby and colleagues (2002), Stenestrand and Wallentin (2002), and Osswald and colleagues (2001). In each of these studies, including the propensity score affected findings only minimally.

As noted, we support subsampling based on propensity score and advise against using the propensity score as an additional covariate. Connors and colleagues (1996) used propensity score subsampling to examine the value of right heart catheterization (RHC; also called pulmonary artery catheterization) during the first 24 hours in the ICU as a means to protect against serious perioperative cardiac complications. The 38 percent of patients who received RHC within 24 hours in the ICU differed substantially from those not receiving RHC. In a standard multivariable analysis, the odds ratio for a major cardiac event associated with RHC was 2.0 (95 percent CI 1.3–3.2). This ran counter to physicians' beliefs that RHC helps prevent major cardiac events. However, because the RHC group was sicker, the researchers also performed a propensity score analysis. Among 2,184 patients receiving RHC and 3,551 not receiving it, 1,008 RHC patients were matched on propensity score with 1,008 non-RHC patients, achieving similar risk factors in the two subsampled groups. Within the matched subsample, the odds ratio for a major cardiac event associated with RHC was 1.6 (95 percent CI 0.9–2.8). Although these findings are consistent with those from the standard multivariable analysis (the two CIs overlap substantially), the estimated size of the effect of RHC is somewhat smaller. Furthermore, the 95 percent CI of the odds ratio is wider (because of the smaller sample size) and now includes 1.0. Therefore, the evidence for increased risk with RHC is no longer statistically significant at the 0.05 level.

Gum and collaborators (2001) used propensity score matching to evaluate the effect of aspirin on all-cause mortality among more than 6,100 patients evaluated for coronary artery disease. Aspirin appeared to be even more effective in the matched subsamples than in the standard analysis. Elad and colleagues (2002) studied the effect of primary angioplasty on in-hospital mortality in more than 7,300 patients with AMI. In a standard multivariable analysis, angioplasty was associated with notably lower mortality (odds ratio

= 0.67, 95 percent CI 0.49–0.92). Almost 1,500 propensity score matched pairs were then analyzed, leading to an odds ratio for mortality associated with angioplasty of 0.73 (95 percent CI 0.53–1.01). Similar to the study of Connors and colleagues (1996) on RHC, the odds ratio from the matched sample was highly consistent with the odds ratio from the standard analysis. However, because the odds ratio from the subsample was both closer to 1 and its CI was wider, the finding was no longer statistically significant at the 0.05 level. Shavelle and coinvestigators (2002) studied the value of early angiography in more than 20,000 patients with ST-segment depression myocardial infarction. A standard analysis showed patients receiving early angiography had lower mortality compared to those receiving early conservative therapy (odds ratio = 0.76, 95 percent CI 0.60–0.95). However, among 1,405 matched cases and controls, the estimated intervention effect was somewhat weaker and no longer significant at the 0.05 level (odds ratio = 0.89, 95 percent CI 0.71–1.13). Clearly, healthier patients had received the intervention, and at least some of the apparent benefit indicated by the standard analysis may not be real.

The use of propensity scores is likely to grow and become a standard part of multivariable modeling used to assess treatment effectiveness, much as it has in the recent literature on heart disease interventions.

Instrumental Variables

Standard multivariable modeling and the propensity score are powerful tools for distinguishing the effect of an intervention from the effect of differences in baseline risk. However, these techniques can still mislead if additional risk factors that both strongly affect outcomes and are unevenly distributed between intervention and control cases have not been measured. Instrumental variables, used extensively in econometrics (Bowden and Turkington 1984), can be used to assess the effect of an intervention in the presence of unmeasured risk factors.

Accounting for the effect of unmeasured risk factors seems impossible. However, such analyses become possible if there is an additional observed variable (or set of observed variables) that meets two criteria: (1) the variable is associated with the likelihood of receiving the intervention and (2) the variable does not itself affect the likelihood of a good outcome. Such a variable is called an instrument (for studying the intervention). Angrist, Imbens, and Rubin (1996) state more formally the assumptions required for valid instrumental variables.

Here, we offer a simplified hypothetical example of the instrumental variable (IV) approach in the context of an RCT with incomplete compliance with the intervention (motivated by Greenland 2000a). The arm of the trial to which the person is randomized provides an excellent instrument. Persons randomized to the study group are much more likely to receive the intervention than those randomized to the control group. However, the value of the instrument (intervention versus nonintervention) is not directly associated with the likelihood of a good outcome, as those randomized to the study group are similar in terms of both measured and unmeasured risk factors to those randomized to the control group; in the absence of the intervention, their outcomes should be similar. Later, we discuss several examples in which IVs have been used in health services research.

Hypothetical Example

Consider 2,000 people, half randomized to a study group that receives an intervention and the other half randomized to a control group. Of the 1,000 people in the study group, only 600 comply with the intervention. None in the control group receive the intervention. The first section of Table 11.2 shows the numbers of people and deaths in each group.

The standard analysis of an RCT, an "intention to treat" analysis, compares outcomes among all people in the study group, whether they received the intervention or not, to outcomes among all those in the control group. In our example, the death rate is 5.2 percent in the study group (52/1,000) and 8.8 percent in the control group. An intention-to-treat analysis finds a 41 percent reduction in deaths because of the intervention.

An intention-to-treat analysis suggests that offering the intervention led to 41 percent fewer deaths than not offering it. It does not tell us what the effect of the intervention would have been if everyone in the study group had complied. As rates of noncompliance rise, intention-to-treat analyses increasingly underestimate the effect of the intervention on those who actually receive it.

One alternative to an intention-to-treat analysis is an "as treated" analysis, which compares the outcomes for people who actually received the intervention (the compliers) to those in the control group who did not. In our example, 12 of the 600 compliers died, for a 2 percent death rate. This represents a 77 percent reduction from the 8.8 percent death rate in the control group. The problem with as-treated analyses is that compliers are a nonrandom subset of the study group. They are usually better educated, of higher income, and more healthy, and they are expected to do better even without the intervention. As-treated analyses generally overstate treatment benefits because of this "healthy volunteer" bias. Because we do not know how study group "compliers" differ from the control group in terms of both measured and unmeasured risk factors, an as-treated analysis loses the credibility conferred by the original randomization. Thus, such analyses, once common, have fallen into disfavor.

A third approach builds on a "counterfactual" or "potential outcomes" framework, which can be used to estimate causal effects from observational data (Rubin 1974, 1977, 1978). The key idea is that individuals in a particular state (in our case, a control or study group) have potential outcomes in other

TABLE 11.2
An RCT
Example to
Illustrate
Instrumental
Variables

What we observe from the RCT

	Study Group			Control Group
	Compliers	Noncompliers	All	All
No. of patients	600	400	1,000	1,000
No. of deaths	12	40	52	88
Death rate (%)	2	10	5.2	8.8

Plausible underlying reality*

	Study Group		Control Group	
	Compliers	Noncompliers	Compliers	Noncompliers
No. of patients	600	400	600	400
No. of deaths	12	40	?	40
Death rate (%)	2	10	??	10

Data from the RCT

	Study Group	Control Group
No. of patients	1,000	1,000
No. of deaths	52	88
No. treated	600	0

* Because the total number of deaths in the control group was 88, one can reasonably assume that ? = 48 and ?? = 8.

states (here, the state to which they were not randomized). In our example, the counterfactual state for the control group is assignment to the study group. What are reasonable potential outcomes for the control group in their counterfactual state? Randomization gives us confidence that the control group is similar to the study group. Hence, it seems reasonable to assume that had the control group been offered the intervention, 600 people would have complied with the intervention and 400 would not have. Furthermore, it is reasonable to assume that the 400 noncompliers in the control group are similar to the 400 noncompliers in the study group. Hence, we would expect 40 deaths among these control group noncompliers in their counterfactual state (see the second section of Table 11.2). Because there were a total of 88 deaths in the control group, we would expect the rest of the deaths, 48, to occur among the 600 counterfactual control group compliers. Control group counterfactual compliers can be legitimately compared to study group "actual" compliers. There were only 12 deaths among the study group compliers. This suggests that the intervention reduced deaths by 75 percent in this group of 600 treated individuals.

The logic of IV analysis is similar to the analysis in the last paragraph, although the actual steps are somewhat different. The third section of Table 11.2 shows the data available from the RCT. The instrumental variable is group assignment. Note that as the value of the IV goes from control to study, two things happen: (1) the number of deaths declines from 88 to 52 and (2) the number of people receiving the intervention increases from 0 to 600. What could account for the decline in deaths? It is not differences in either measured or unmeasured risk factors, as the randomization makes these similar for each level of the instrumental variable. The lower death rate must be due to the increased number receiving the intervention in the study group.

The estimate of treatment effectiveness in an IV analysis is:

$$\frac{\text{(change in likelihood of dying, by level of the IV)}}{\text{(change in likelihood of receiving treatment, by level of the IV)}}$$

or:

$$(0.052 - 0.088)/(0.60 - 0.00) = -0.06.$$

To interpret the -0.06, note that the study saves 36 lives $(88 - 52)$ by providing the intervention to 600 compliers; for every 100 compliers, the intervention saves six lives; or for every complier, the intervention saves 0.06 lives. We know from the RCT results that 12 deaths occurred among the 600 compliers. As 36 lives were saved, we would have expected $12 + 36$, or 48, deaths among the 600 compliers if they had not been given the intervention. The intervention has reduced the number of deaths per 600 from 48 to 12, or 75 percent. Thus, this effectiveness estimate is consistent with the one that emerged from the counterfactual logic above.

The IV estimate of treatment effect does not apply to all people, only to the types of patients who would shift from not having the treatment to having treatment because of their IV level. Here, this means people similar to the 600 compliers who had been assigned to treatment. Whereas an intention-to-treat analysis estimates the effect of offering an intervention to a population, an IV analysis estimates the effect of an intervention in so-called "marginal patients"—those who would receive the treatment at one level of the IV variable but not at another (Harris and Remler 1998). An attractive feature of the IV analysis is that it estimates the effect of treatment on the people treated while avoiding the bias associated with an as-treated analysis.

The IV estimate of effectiveness illustrated above can also be calculated using a two-stage model. Unlike the simple calculation above, the two-stage approach generalizes to more complex situations. In stage I, we model the probability of treatment as:

$$PRED(T) = a + b * \text{IV}$$

where $\text{IV} = 1$ if the person is in the study group and 0 otherwise. In this example, $PRED(T) = 0.6$ when $\text{IV} = 1$ and 0 otherwise. Hence, $a = 0$ and $b = 0.6$.

In stage II, we model the outcome of interest, in this case the probability of death, $PRED(D)$, as a linear function of the value of $PRED(T)$ from the stage I model:

$$PRED(D) = c + d * PRED(T)$$

The coefficient d is the effect on $PRED(D)$ as $PRED(T)$ changes from 0 to 1. In our example, $c = 0.088$ and $d = -0.06$, as in the calculation above.[8] The two-stage approach allows important measured risk factors to be added as covariates at each stage.

Most standard statistical software packages accommodate two-stage modeling when outcomes are continuous, such as costs or hospital LOSs. If the outcome variable is dichotomous, the stage II model is usually formulated as a logistic regression. In this case, specialized software is needed to correctly estimate standard errors. Macros have been written, for example in SAS, for such analyses.

The assumption underlying IV analysis is that groups defined by different IV states are comparable in terms of unmeasured risk factors. In our example, the IV assumption allowed us to estimate that the 1,000 control cases would have produced 400 noncompliers and 40 deaths among these noncompliers had the control group members been assigned to treatment. If groups in different IV states are not comparable, results from an IV analysis can mislead. Unfortunately, there is no direct test of the IV assumption. In describing applications in the literature, we consider how respective authors have examined the validity of this assumption.

Examples of IV Analyses in the Literature

McClellan, McNeil, and Newhouse (1994) published a classic study using IVs in health services research. They examined the value of more intensive treatment of AMI (such as cardiac catheterization or coronary revascularization) in reducing mortality among elderly patients. The standard approach would compare the risk-adjusted mortality of those who do and those who do not receive intensive treatment. However, these two groups differed greatly in measured baseline risk, suggesting that differences in unmeasured risk factors might also be present. For example, 2.8 percent of the patients who received catheterization within 90 days had cerebrovascular disease, versus 5.4 percent of those who did not. One can easily imagine how differences in unmeasured risk might arise. Consider two people, one relatively hardy and the other frail, with the same measured risk factors. If only one is treated aggressively, it is likely to be the stronger individual, who would probably have fared better than the frailer patient even without treatment. Suspecting that such unmeasured risk factors had produced inappropriately optimistic estimates of treatment effect, McClellan, McNeil, and Newhouse (1994) used an IV analysis.

Their instrument was the extra distance (beyond the distance to the nearest hospital) a patient must travel to the nearest hospital that offers intensive treatment. The following assumptions led to selection of this variable as an instrument: (1) the shorter the extra distance, the more likely the patient is to receive intensive treatment and (2) unmeasured risk factors are likely to be similar for people with different amounts of "extra distance."

The data supported the first assumption. For example, 34 percent of patients whose extra distance was less than 2.5 miles received catheterization within seven days, versus 5 percent of those requiring longer travel. However, the second assumption—the key to the validity of an IV estimate—cannot be directly verified. Examining the plausibility of the IV assumption commonly involves comparing the distributions of measured characteristics in the IV-defined groups, which in this case were fairly similar. For example, in both groups 4.8 percent of the patients had cerebrovascular disease. If the groups have different patterns of measured characteristics, this casts doubt on the assumption that their unmeasured characteristics are similar. This does not mean that similarity on observed covariates implies similarity on unmeasured ones. However, comparable distributions of measured risk factors across IV states make the IV assumption more plausible.

A standard risk-adjusted analysis estimated a 28 percent reduction in four-year mortality associated with catheterization. The IV analysis estimated a 6 percent reduction. The reduction in estimated effect suggests that, as a group, patients who were catheterized were systematically healthier than those who did not receive it in ways that were not captured by the measured risk factors. However, IV estimates only pertain to "marginal" patients (i.e., patients who receive catheterization only when it is more readily available) (Harris and Remler 1998). In this example, place of residence did not affect receipt of intensive treatment for some AMI patients. The IV analysis reveals nothing about treatment effects for such cases. Nonetheless, finding 34 percent versus 5 percent seven-day catheterization rates for people with different IV states suggests that, for many cases, early intensive treatment is strongly influenced by whether the resources are immediately accessible. The IV estimate of effectiveness applies to such patients.

In contrast, estimates of effectiveness based on propensity score matching apply to intervention and control cases that are similar to each other on measured covariates. Thus, estimates of effects from IV and standard analyses could differ without either being incorrect. In particular, a plausible explanation exists for at least some of the 28 percent standard effect estimate versus the 6 percent IV estimate. Perhaps early aggressive surgical intervention is highly effective within a targeted set of people whose characteristics mean they almost always receive these therapies, whereas its benefit is minimal for people (marginal patients) with limited disease, for whom the chance of receiving aggressive therapy is more influenced by its ready accessibility.

The December 2000 (Part II) issue of *Health Services Research* is devoted to applications of instrumental variables in health services research. The next several examples come from this important publication (McClellan and Newhouse 2000).

Malkin, Broder, and Keeler (2000) used IV analysis to examine the effect of postpartum LOS on newborn readmission rates. A standard analysis would compare risk-adjusted readmission rates of short- and long-stay newborns. An IV analysis can account for the possibility that these two groups differ in ways not captured by the measured risk factors. In one analysis, they used hour of birth as an instrument: Babies born before noon had on average a longer LOS than babies born later. Thus, the IV related directly to the likelihood of the intervention, in this case a long hospital stay. There seems to be no reason why unmeasured risk factor should depend on whether birth was before or after noon. In terms of observable risk factors, babies born before and after noon were fairly similar. This increases our confidence in the key IV assumption that unobservable risk factors do not depend on the value of the instrument. The standard analysis suggested that increasing hospital stays by 12 hours reduced the newborn readmission rate by 0.3 percent. The IV analysis using time of birth as the instrument suggested that a 12-hour increase in LOS reduced the readmission rate by 0.6 percent, double the rate from the standard analysis. The standard approach may underestimate the benefit of a longer stay because babies with longer stays are sicker in ways not fully captured by measured risk factors.

Howard (2000) used IVs to analyze the effect of waiting time on liver transplant outcomes. A direct comparison of patients with short versus long waits would be misleading: Sicker patients have a higher priority for transplantation and hence shorter stays on the waiting lists. In this analysis, the patient's blood type was the IV. Type O blood is harder to match, and hence these patients wait an average of 52 days longer than patients with blood type A (thus demonstrating that the intervention, waiting time, differs by the IV state). However, blood type does not affect transplant failure rate, suggesting that both measured and unmeasured risk factors are similar across blood types. Graft failure was 15 percent for type O patients and only 12 percent for type A patients. In a standard analysis, waiting time did not significantly affect outcomes. In an IV analysis, longer waiting times were associated with a statistically significantly higher likelihood of graft failure.

Health services researchers are increasingly using IV analyses. Although much of the IV literature is highly technical, the report from McClellan, McNeil, and Newhouse (1994) is accessible, and we recommend it to researchers new to IVs. Other valuable descriptions of this technique include Newhouse and McClellan (1998) and Greenland (2000a). The challenge in an IV analysis is to identify a good instrument. Few instruments can match the benefits of randomized assignment, but plausible instruments can yield useful insights into the effects of interventions. Nevertheless, concerns remain about the inability to evaluate empirically the extent to which a particular variable satisfies the requirements of an instrument. IV assumptions are typically justified by examining distributions of measured covariates and discussing the magnitude and direction of plausible differences in unmeasured covariates. To the extent that an IV finding relies on untested assumptions, it is not definitive. However, a sizable difference between the effect estimates from a well-conducted IV analysis and a standard analysis raises important questions. The search for and testing of hypotheses to explain such differences is an important way that observational data can elucidate the true object of interest—the intervention's effect on outcomes.

Conclusions

Evidence from observational studies can be—and has been—misinterpreted, leading some to question their value (Sackett et al. 1997). However, several recent studies have challenged the hypothesis that observational studies contain systematic biases. Based on 136 reports from 19 treatments, Benson and Hartz (2000, 1878) "found little evidence that estimates of treatment effects in observational studies reported after 1984 are either consistently larger than or qualitatively different from those obtained in randomized, controlled trials." Likewise, based on 99 reports in five clinical areas, Concato, Shah, and Horwitz (2000, 1887) conclude: "The results of well-designed observational studies (with either a cohort or a case-control design) do not systematically overestimate the magnitude of the effects of treatment as compared with those in randomized, controlled trials on the same topic." Ioannidis and colleagues (2001) examined 45 topics in which both RCTs ($n = 240$) and nonrandomized studies ($n = 168$) had been performed. Across all types of studies, nonrandomized studies tended to show larger treatment effects; nonetheless, there were "few differences beyond chance when randomized trials were compared with prospective nonrandomized studies. . . . [In addition,] significant between-study variability was seen as frequently among the randomized trials as between the randomized and nonrandomized studies" (Ioannidis et al. 2001, 828).

However, recent reports questioning the safety of hormone-replacement therapy (HRT) present an important "cautionary tale" for analysts of observational data. Several previous analyses of large observational studies had led to the widespread belief that HRT decreases the risk of coronary heart disease (Stampfer and Colditz 1991; Grady et al. 1992). However, the Women's Health Initiative RCT found increased coronary heart disease, breast cancer, stroke, and pulmonary embolism risks for healthy postmenopausal women assigned to estrogen plus progestin (Writing Group for the Women's Health Initiative Investigators 2002). Commenting on an earlier RCT, Petitti (1998, 650) had described similar findings as "a sobering reminder of the limitations of observational research, the incompleteness of current understanding of the mechanisms of vascular disease, and the dangers of extrapolation."

The discrepancy between the RCT and observational findings probably resulted from inadequate risk adjustment for the many ways in which women taking hormone-replacement therapy outside research settings differed from those not taking such therapy. However, the observational data that produced misleading assessments of hormone-replacement therapy may nevertheless offer insight into the determinants of population-based health. For example, Berkman (2002, 2) suggests that researchers should now seek "to identify the types of women who took HRT to see what else it was about them that might be health promoting." Reexamining the earlier analyses and reanalyzing the same data could indicate whether current and better causal modeling techniques produce findings more consistent with the RCT results.

Volume 2, Number 3/4 of *Health Services and Outcomes Research Methodology* (2001) contains eight articles, both conceptual and applied, devoted to causal modeling. As these articles demonstrate, a solid foundation has been established for understanding the key components of well-designed studies to distinguish causes from associations in observational data. More empirical work is needed to better understand the magnitude of differences associated with different analytical methods and how these differences can help clarify "what is really going on."

Notes

1. In "quasi-experiments," patients who receive an intervention are distinguished from those who do not by a weaker mechanism than randomization. For example, an intervention might be implemented earlier in one part of a large geographical area than another as a way of learning about effect. In contrast, in a purely nonexperimental observational study, the intervention is offered throughout the geographical area, and those who receive the intervention are compared to those who do not. For our purposes, we note that data from a quasi-experimental observational study resemble those of a nonexperimental observational study in their need for risk adjustment.

2. If b were negative, women's expected costs would be lower. Notice that in the model the effect of sex is assumed to be the same amount b for all categories of patients—for example, between male and female 30 and 60 year olds. The way to escape this restriction is to include interactions between sex and other risk factors—for example, by using age-sex indicator categories, such as "30–34-year-old female."

3. "Odds" are familiar from gambling—as in, "the odds of winning are 5 to 2," or $5/2 = 2.5$. While probabilities must be between 0 and 1, odds can assume any positive value (and log odds can assume any value, negative, 0, or positive). This makes log odds more attractive for modeling than

raw probabilities. The relationship between the probability of an event and the odds is straightforward: $P_i = O_i/(1 + O_i)$. For example, odds of 1/2, 1, and 2 correspond, respectively, to log odds of -0.69, 0, and $+0.69$ and to probabilities of 1/3, 1/2, and 2/3.

4. For people who do not receive the intervention, $I = 0$ and $e^{c*I} = e^0 = 1$, whereas for those who did receive it, the multiplier is e^c.

5. To clarify the nature of the dependent variable in this model, note that the probability that an event (e.g., death) occurs in a small interval of time (from t to $t + \Delta t$) is the product of two probabilities: first, the probability that death does not occur prior to time t, and second, the conditional probability that a person who has survived until time t dies prior to $t + \Delta t$. This latter probability is called a hazard rate. For example, consider 100 patients alive at time 0. In the first six months, 40 patients die. In the next week after the six months, six more patients die. The probability of surviving six months is 0.6, and the hazard rate (for Δt equal to one week) is 0.10 (6/60), the probability of death among those 60 patients who lived to the start of the interval. The product of the two probabilities ($0.6 * 0.10 = 0.06$) is the observed probability of death in the interval from six months to six months plus one week.

6. In a data set with many more controls than cases, one may wish to retain two or even four times as many controls as cases in each propensity score quantile to improve the precision of the final estimate of treatment effect. Ratios larger than 4 to 1 do little to improve precision. In a data set in which there are very few cases or controls in the extreme quantiles, one may wish to eliminate those quantiles from the analysis to avoid any misleading extrapolation of estimates of treatment effectiveness to groups in which there are really very few people observed.

7. If both the propensity score model and the multivariable regression were linear (and if the propensity score model included the same risk factors as the regression to predict outcomes), it is a theorem that including propensity score as an additional covariate would have zero effect on model predictions. Thus, to the extent that the models with and without the propensity score covariate differ, it is a very small effect induced by the small differences in predicted probability caused by using a linear predictor of P versus a linear predictor of $\ln(P/1 - P)$.

8. We used linear models to predict probabilities here for ease of explanation. Logistic models are generally viewed as more appropriate for predicting dichotomous outcomes. Often, however, simple linear models applied to 0/1 outcomes produce similar findings to logistic models. In the case of the very simple models in this example, predictions from either type of model would be identical.

COMPARING OUTCOMES ACROSS PROVIDERS

Arlene S. Ash, Michael Shwartz, and Erol A. Peköz

Risk adjustment facilitates meaningful comparisons of outcomes across groups of patients by accounting for those differences in intrinsic patient characteristics that are related to outcomes. However, such comparisons are just a means to a larger end. Nightingale and Codman viewed comparing outcomes as a powerful way to motivate improvement of quality of care (see Chapter 1). As Nightingale wrote in 1863 (175–76):

> In attempting to arrive at the truth, I have applied everywhere for information, but in scarcely an instance have I been able to obtain hospital records fit for any purposes of comparison. . . . I am fain to sum up with an urgent appeal for adopting . . . some *uniform* system of publishing the statistical records of hospitals. There is a growing conviction that in all hospitals, even in those which are best conducted, there is a great and unnecessary waste of life . . .

Nightingale and Codman argued that simply comparing rates of events was insufficient. One must discover why differences in patient outcomes occurred and correct identified problems.

Jumping to the start of the twenty-first century, comparisons of outcomes are now central to scrutiny of the American health care delivery system and an important component of responses to competitive market forces. Patient outcomes are compared across individual physicians, group practices, clinics, hospitals and other institutional settings (e.g., nursing homes), and private and public health insurers. These comparisons are variously called performance or practice profiles, report cards, scorecards, and outcomes reports. As noted in Chapter 1, the growing interest in pay-for-performance schemes will likely put such profiles center stage, heightening the financial stakes of risk-adjusted outcome measures (Institute of Medicine 2002c).

Several types of questions motivate report card and profiling initiatives, such as:

- Do any particular providers stand out as either much better or worse than average?
- How strong is the evidence that provider A's performance has been (or, perhaps more importantly, will be) substandard?

Numerous decisions are required when designing a profiling approach and assembling the data to compare patient outcomes across providers and answer such questions (Table 12.1). In addition, interpreting results requires both good methodology and a thoughtful conceptual framework. This chapter discusses "principles of good design" as well as important practical considerations in performance profiling. We emphasize, however, that no all-purpose best way exists to compare patient outcomes across providers. Especially when using profiles to support decisions with serious patient care or financial implications, analysts must remain aware of how various methodological choices can shape their findings.

The Effect of Randomness on Comparing Patient Outcomes

Random fluctuations affect estimates of provider performance and thus limit the conclusions that can be drawn safely from performance profiles. To elucidate the role of randomness, we consider a contrived example targeting hospital costs as our outcome. We assume that the patients have identical clinical conditions and receive the same treatment across hospitals.

The simplest model views the costs of the n_A cases admitted to hospital A this year as a sample from a theoretically infinite population of cases that might be treated at hospital A. This year's observed average cost at hospital A, $\overline{Y}_A$, estimates the underlying average cost, μ_A, for all cases that might be treated there.

The distribution of observed costs for this year's patients provides information about the variability of costs among potential groups of patients at various hospitals. Examining this distribution is always advisable. For example, analysts should look at standard summary statistics: the mean, median, and standard deviation; minimum and maximum values; and values associated with different percentage points of the distribution (e.g., the value demarcating the upper 1 percent of cases). For facilities in hospital A's comparison group, side-by-side boxplots (sometimes called box-and-whiskers plots, discussed later; Figure 12.1) help to identify likely errors (e.g., hospital stays with negative costs) or values that are correct but extreme (Tukey 1977). For instance, a hospital with high average costs because all its cases were expensive differs from an institution where one very expensive case raised the average by nearly $10,000 (e.g., one "million-dollar baby" among 100 average-cost newborns).

The standard deviation (SD) is the most common summary measure of variation for a variable Y. It is estimated for a population from a sample Y_1, $Y_2, \ldots, Y_n$, by:

$$s = \sqrt{\Sigma_i (Y_i - \overline{Y})^2 / (n - 1)}$$

TABLE 12.1

Design
Considerations
for Provider
Profiling

What data will be used?
    Can information be linked at the person level?
    Can numerators and denominators be determined?
    What are the accuracy and reliability of the data?
    Which patient risk factors are captured in the data?
    What is the time frame encompassed by the data?
What outcomes can be measured from the data?
Which providers will be included?
    Are there reasons to exclude any providers?
        • Small sample sizes
        • Incomplete data
        • Known patient risks unable to measure with the data (e.g., public hospitals)
        • Policy considerations (e.g., small hospitals, rural hospitals)
Which patients will be included?
    What are the specific inclusion criteria (e.g., disease, surgery)?
    Are there reasons to exclude any patients?

FIGURE 12.1

Box Plots of
Expected LOS
at Six Hospitals

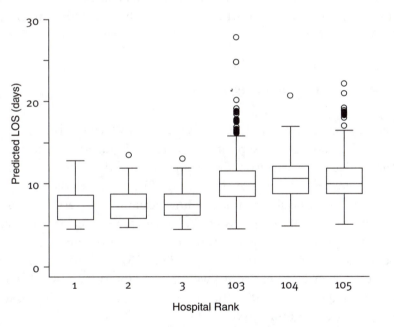

NOTE: Box plots from three hospitals with the lowest and three with the highest expected LOS using Disease Staging's Relative Resource Scale to determine expected values.

Just as $\overline{Y}_A$ is an estimate of an unobserved mean, μ_A, of a larger theoretical population, the SD in hospital A, s_A, is an estimate of σ_A, the SD of that larger population. SDs have the same units as Y (here, dollars). Regardless of the shape of the distribution of Y, most costs are likely to lie within two or three SDs of the average.

The usual model hypothesized when comparing hospitals (or any other provider unit) assumes that

- each case at hospital A has expected value μ_A, which may differ by facility; but
- the Y values at each facility are equally variable (i.e., there is a single, common value σ of the σ_As).

If all the SD$_A$s have the same value, σ, each s_A (computed by applying the above formula to the cases at hospital A) is an estimate of it. The "pooled" estimate of s is calculated from the s_As using weights that reflect differences in sample sizes, as:

$$s = \sqrt{\Sigma_A(w_A * s_A^2)}$$

where A indexes facilities and $w_A = (n_A - 1)/(N - K)$, with N being the total number of patients and K the number of facilities.

A common goal is both to estimate μ_A and measure the accuracy of these estimates based on what we observe, namely $\overline{Y}_A$, n_A, and s_A. For almost any distribution of Y, the observed average cost at hospital A, $\overline{Y}_A$, is very likely to fall within two standard errors (SEs) of the true average μ_A—that is, within the range $\mu_A \pm 2 * SE_A$, where SE_A, the (observed) SE of the mean at hospital A, is calculated as:

$$SE_A = s/\sqrt{n_A}$$

Thus, each interval $\overline{Y}_A \pm 2 * SE_A$ is likely to contain its true hospital mean value, μ_A.

For a given hospital A, μ_A (the value around which individual Y values are centered) and σ_A (a measure of how much the individual values are dispersed around μ_A) are properties of the population and do not depend on n_A, the number of cases at hospital A. In contrast, SE_A relates to the variability of an "estimator"; specifically, it measures how accurately $\overline{Y}_A$ estimates μ_A. As the number of observations at hospital A increases, SE_A decreases, reflecting the increased accuracy of $\overline{Y}_A$ as an estimate of μ_A. For example, suppose that we observe mean costs of \$5,000 with an SD of \$5,000.[1] With 100 observations, we are reasonably sure that μ_A will be in the interval \$5,000 $\pm$ 2 * 500, that is, from \$4,000 to \$6,000. With $n = 400$, we are reasonably confident that μ_A is between \$4,500 and \$5,500.

Even with the highly skewed distributions typical of health care cost data (see Chapter 10), unless n_A is small, the observed mean will be approximately normally distributed. This implies that an interval centered at $\overline{Y}_A$ and extending for two or three SE-sized units above and below will likely include μ_A. For many purposes, 30 cases is an adequate n_A. However, especially when the outcome variable is extremely skewed, producing a nearly normal distribution of $\overline{Y}_A$ may require hundreds of cases, as extreme values significantly affect the mean. When the underlying variable in the population from which the n_A cases were sampled is distributed normally, $\overline{Y}_A$ has about a 95 percent chance of falling in the so-called "prediction interval," $\mu_A \pm 2 * SE_A$. This is equivalent to saying that the interval $\overline{Y}_A \pm 2 * \mathrm{SE}_A$ has a 95 percent chance of containing the true value, μ_A. This latter interval is called the 95 percent confidence interval (CI). A CI specifies plausible boundaries for a parameter estimate (here, μ_A), whereas a prediction interval establishes boundaries within which an observed random variable (here, $\overline{Y}_A$) should lie. Although we know that cost distributions are not normal, cost averages, such as $\overline{Y}_A$, are more nearly so.[2]

Profiling is not a theoretical exercise in statistical science. Rather, these intervals provide a convenient "cutoff" for highlighting situations requiring further examination. A two-SE cutoff casts a broad net for identifying possible problems, many of which will be spurious. Three SE's might prove more appropriate for settings, such as public reporting, in which false flags have severe consequences.

The observed coefficient of variation (CV) is the ratio of the SD to the mean: $s/\overline{Y}_A$. Table 12.2 shows the half-widths of (approximate) 95 percent CIs:

$$2 * \mathrm{SE} = 2 * \overline{Y}_A * \mathrm{CV}/\sqrt{n_A}$$

for different values of CV and sample size. The figures in Table 12.2 demonstrate the combined effect of sample size and data variability on the range containing the average of a sample of size n. For example, with $\mathrm{CV} = 1$ and a sample size of 100, the approximate 95 percent CI for μ_A is:

$$(0.8 * \overline{Y}_A, 1.2 * \overline{Y}_A)$$

That is, we can estimate mean cost with about 20 percent error. Because accuracy is proportional to 1 over the $\sqrt{n}$, achieving estimates with 10 percent error requires 400 observations.

From a different perspective, assume that average costs are the same at each hospital. If μ_A equals μ, $\overline{Y}_A$ is likely to be within the interval $\mu \pm 2 * s/\sqrt{n_A}$.[3] Assuming a large number of patients across all hospitals, $\overline{Y}$ calculated from all patients is a good estimate of μ, the true mean cost for all patients. Hence, $\overline{Y}_A$ is likely to be within the interval $\overline{Y} \pm 2 * s/\sqrt{n_A}$. Suppose $\overline{Y}_A$ falls outside this interval. In the traditional hypothesis-testing framework, we conclude that hospital A's costs differ from average. Furthermore, suppose that we are judging 100 facilities and we flag any hospital as an outlier when $\overline{Y}_A$ is outside the interval $\overline{Y} \pm 2 * s/\sqrt{n_A}$. In this situation, hospitals designated as outliers have costs that are statistically significantly different than average at $p < 0.05$. Among 100 identical facilities (i.e., all $\mu_A = \mu$), this approach incorrectly flags about five outliers. This is an example of the "multiple comparisons" problem (Snedecor and Cochran 1980). Incorrectly flagging a typical hospital is called a type I error.

On the other hand, trying to avoid type I errors by being conservative about flagging outliers increases the chance that true outlier hospitals are missed—a type II error. To illustrate type II errors, assume that an inefficient

TABLE 12.2
Effect of Sample Size and Coefficient of Variation (CV) on the Half-Width of Approximate 95 Percent Confidence Intervals*

Sample Size (n)	CV (σ/μ)					
	0.5	1	1.5	2	2.5	3
10	0.32	0.63	0.95	1.26	1.58	1.90
25	0.20	0.40	0.60	0.80	1.00	1.20
50	0.14	0.28	0.42	0.57	0.71	0.85
100	0.10	0.20	0.30	0.40	0.50	0.60
150	0.08	0.16	0.24	0.33	0.41	0.49
200	0.07	0.14	0.21	0.28	0.35	0.42
300	0.06	0.12	0.17	0.23	0.29	0.35
400	0.05	0.10	0.15	0.20	0.25	0.30
500	0.04	0.09	0.13	0.18	0.22	0.27
1000	0.03	0.06	0.09	0.13	0.16	0.19

* Cells of the table are $2 * \mathrm{CV} / \sqrt{n}$. Half-width = $\overline{Y}_A *$ table cell.

hospital (hospital I) has costs 20 percent above an average of $1,000. This difference seems sufficiently large to be important. Suppose that we flag a hospital as an outlier only when its observed mean differs from $1,000 by at least 40 percent (roughly the cutoff for identifying a statistically significant difference at $p < 0.05$ when $n = 100$ and the CV $= 2$). Under this rule, hospital I will be flagged if its average cost exceeds $1,400 (i.e., the 95 percent CI for μ_I lies entirely above $1,000). However, with only 100 observations and a CV of 2, the chance that hospital I's observed mean will exceed this threshold is only 20 percent. Thus, hospital I has an 80 percent chance of avoiding an outlier flag.

The same considerations apply when examining a dichotomous outcome, such as death. Assume that P is the death rate in a large population of patients and $\hat{P}$ is the observed rate in a smaller population of size n (e.g., patients at hospital A). The estimated SE is then $\sqrt{\hat{P}(1 - \hat{P})/n}$. For different values of n and death rate P, Table 12.3 shows the half-width of an interval that is about 95 percent likely to contain P.[4] For example, if $\hat{P}$ were 10 percent in a sample of 100 patients, the interval from 4 percent to 16 percent is likely to contain P.[5] This interval is wide compared to reasonable differences between poor- and high-quality providers (Hofer and Hayward 1996; Ash 1996).

With any rule for flagging outliers, as the difference increases between a given hospital's underlying performance and typical performance, the likelihood of being flagged rises. Thus, depending on the (unknown) mix of normal and variously aberrant providers in a study population, roughly 5 percent of nonproblematic providers will erroneously receive outlier flags, whereas some (unknown fraction of) problematic providers will escape flags. Which flags are incorrect is generally not obvious. Using data on cardiac catheterization, Luft and Hunt (1986, 2780) illustrated that small numbers of patients and relatively low rates of poor outcomes make it difficult to "be confident in the

TABLE 12.3

Effect of
Sample Size
and Probability
of Death on the
Half-Width of
Approximate
95 Percent
Confidence
Intervals*

	Probability of Death (P)**							
Sample Size (n)	0.01	0.02	0.05	0.10	0.15	0.20	0.25	0.50
25	—	—	—	0.12	0.14	0.16	0.17	0.20
50	—	—	0.06	0.08	0.10	0.11	0.12	0.14
100	—	—	0.04	0.06	0.07	0.08	0.09	0.10
150	—	—	0.04	0.05	0.06	0.07	0.07	0.08
200	—	—	0.03	0.04	0.05	0.06	0.06	0.07
300	—	0.02	0.03	0.03	0.04	0.05	0.05	0.06
400	—	0.01	0.02	0.03	0.04	0.04	0.04	0.05
500	0.01	0.01	0.02	0.03	0.03	0.04	0.04	0.04
1,000	0.01	0.01	0.01	0.02	0.02	0.03	0.03	0.03

* Cells of the table (= half-width) are $2 * \sqrt{P * (1 - P)/n}$.
** When $n * P$ (the expected number of deaths) < 5, the normal approximation (the basis for calculations in this table) is unreliable (—).
NOTE: More precise CIs for proportions are described in Agresti and Coull (1998) and implemented in
http://www.graphpad.com/quickcalcs/ConfInterval2.cfm.

identification of individual performers." For example, suppose the death rate is 1 percent, but a hospital treating 200 patients experiences no deaths. Even using a lenient 0.10 significance level, determining whether that hospital had statistically significantly better outcomes is impossible. If the expected death rate is 15 percent and five deaths occurred out of 20 patients (an observed rate of 25 percent), the difference is insufficient to label the hospital as performing poorly. Thus, random chance plays a prominent role in determining outlier status when sample sizes are relatively small. In this situation, comparisons across providers must be interpreted cautiously.

Comparing Observed and Expected Outcomes

Calculating expected rates of outcomes is usually the first step in producing risk-adjusted performance profiles. The simple example above ignores the need for risk adjustment by targeting patients with identical clinical conditions. In most situations, different providers see different mixes of patients, so risk adjustment is essential.

Linear regression modeling is the most commonly used method for risk adjusting continuous outcomes (see Chapter 10). Thus, we might build a model as follows:

$$PRED_i = \hat{a} + \Sigma_j \hat{b}_j * X_{ij}$$

where $PRED_i$ is the expected outcome for patient i, who has characteristics $X_{ij}, j = 1, \ldots, J$ for the J predictors in the model. For patients treated by a specific provider, their expected outcome (E) equals the average of the $PRED_i$s.

In contrast, logistic regression, in which the log of the odds of the event is modeled as a linear function of the predictor variables, is generally used to predict dichotomous (yes/no) outcomes.[6] After fitting a logistic regression model, the predicted probability of death for the ith case ($PRED_i$) is calculated from the relationship:

$$\ln(\widehat{\text{odds}}_i) = \ln(PRED_i/(1 - PRED_i)) = \hat{a} + \Sigma_j \, \hat{b}_j X_{ij}$$

by solving for $PRED_i$:

$$PRED_i = e^{\ln(\widehat{\text{odds}}_i)}/1 + e^{\ln(\widehat{\text{odds}}_i)}$$

To determine the expected number of deaths in a group of n cases, we sum the $PRED_i$ terms; to determine the expected death rate, we divide this sum by n.

Comparing observed to expected outcomes is central to performance profiling (e.g., drawing inferences about the quality or efficiency of care). Various approaches have been used for comparing O and E. Neither ($O - E$) nor O/E is clearly superior. For example, suppose that hospital A treats cases expected to average \$5,000 (i.e., average $PRED_i$), but the actual cost is \$6,000. In contrast, hospital B treats cases that should cost \$10,000 but actually average \$11,500. Thus, both hospitals' costs are greater than expected, but how do they compare with each other? On an additive or difference scale ($O - E$), hospital B performs worse, as hospital A's excess is only \$1,000 per case, compared to B's excess of \$1,500. However, on a multiplicative or ratio scale (O/E), hospital A does worse, as its cases cost 20 percent more than expected, compared to only 15 percent more for B. Theory offers no insight into which hospital to prefer.

Consider another example. Which is worse: 2 percent complications when only 1 percent was expected (double the rate), or 50 percent complications when only 40 percent was expected (ten excess problems per 100 but only a 25 percent higher complication rate)? This question has no simple answer. Analysts can use their data to explore which model is more realistic— an additive model (where adding the same amount to each case represents the provider effect) or a multiplicative model (where provider-associated increases are proportionate to the expected outcome). Even when multiplicative models are chosen, observers typically still want to know how observed results compare additively to expected results, such as how many extra dollars a provider costs or how many extra complications have occurred.

Ratios, such as O/E, are centered at 1 but range from 0 to infinity. To put comparable distances between ratios below 1 and those above 1, analysts sometimes display $\log(O/E)$ values rather than O/E values (Roos, Wennberg, and McPherson 1988). On a graph where O values are on the x-axis and $\log(O/E)$ values are on the y-axis, a "broken" y-axis can be used to indicate the gap between the smallest $\log(O/E)$ associated with a positive observed

(O) and negative infinity (the value of the logarithm function at zero). On an untransformed scale, substantial differences among O/E values less than 1 are hard to see and thus may appear unimportant. In contrast, on a log scale, the distances between points representing O/E values of 0.25, 0.50, 1.00, 2.00, and 4.00 are equally spaced because each value doubles the one below it.

A drawback of the ratio O/E is that when E is small, its value changes dramatically with small changes in O. For example, if we observe 30 cases, each with a 1 percent risk of complications, the expected number of complications is 0.3. If 0, 1, or 2 complications are observed, O/E is 0, 3.3, or 6.7, respectively. A good guideline is to avoid examining such ratios when the expected number of events is less than 1.0. Some researchers advise against O-to-E comparisons unless E is at least 5.

Fortunately, when comparing O to E, findings as extreme as our examples above are unlikely. If expected costs at two hospitals are $5,000 versus $10,000, or if expected complications rates are 1 percent versus 40 percent, these hospitals should probably not be compared—their patient populations or other characteristics differ too much. When distributions of expected outcomes are roughly similar across hospitals, difference and ratio measures of performance will produce reasonably similar results. Examining expected outcomes across providers is therefore important to ensure that patients' risks do not differ radically across providers (see below). Reviewing common descriptive statistics (e.g., mean and median, SD, percentage cutoffs of the distribution, boxplots) is a useful first cut at comparing expected outcomes across providers.

In our prior work, we examined the extent to which severity explained differences in hospital LOS for pneumonia patients (Iezzoni et al. 1996c). To illustrate the relationship between the distribution of predicted LOS and severity, we examined these distributions for six hospitals (number of cases per hospital ranged from 73 to 316): the three hospitals with the highest and three with the lowest predicted average LOSs (which corresponds to the hospitals with the lowest and highest risk-adjusted severity). Figure 12.1 shows side-by-side boxplots of predicted LOS values at these six hospitals, using DS Relative Resource Scale as the severity measure. (We removed outliers using Medicare's definition: cases more than three SDs above the mean on a log scale; see Chapter 10.)

In Figure 12.1, the box shows the range encompassing the middle 50 percent of cases. Thus, 25 percent of cases have values below the bottom edge of the box, and 25 percent have values above the upper edge. The horizontal line within the box is the median. The length of the box is the interquartile range (IQR), sometimes called the "H-spread." The top of the box plus 1.5 ∗ IQR and the bottom of the box minus 1.5 ∗ IQR define the inner fences; the top of the box plus 3 ∗ IQR and the bottom of the box minus 3 ∗ IQR define the outer fences. The ends of the lines extending above and below the box indicate the highest and lowest values within the inner fences; circles indicate individual values between the inner and outer fences. (Different computerized statistical packages use different symbols, but the boxplot concept is similar.) The boxplots show that 75 percent of patients in the three hospitals with the least severely ill patients were expected to have an LOS below eight days, whereas 75 percent of cases at the hospitals with the most severely ill patients were expected to have an LOS above eight days.

Failure of O-to-E Comparisons to Adjust Fully for Risks

When examining death rates, epidemiologists often use standardized mortality ratios (SMRs). SMRs are *O/E* ratios, where the *E* values are calculated using indirect standardization. To illustrate the need for standardization (the epidemiologist's term for risk adjustment), consider a hypothetical situation involving two types of patients: low-risk, with a 1 percent mortality rate, and high-risk, with a 5 percent mortality rate (Table 12.4). Suppose further that half of all patients in a large population are low- and high-risk, yielding an overall mortality rate of 3 percent. Now consider hospital A, which treats 1,000 patients, 800 at low risk and 200 at high risk. Hospital A's experience with its low-risk patients is similar to the overall experience—a 1 percent mortality rate (8 deaths among the 800 patients). However, hospital A does poorly with high-risk patients; it has a 10 percent mortality rate, double the population average, leading to 20 deaths among the 200 high-risk patients. Despite this, because of its favorable case mix, hospital A's mortality rate is 2.8 percent (28/1,000), somewhat better than the 3 percent population average.

Indirect standardization determines a hospital's expected number of deaths by applying stratum-specific rates determined from all patients to the number of cases in each stratum in the hospital. In this case, a stratum is a risk category. Based on the overall data, we expect 8 deaths among the 800 low-risk patients (with a 1 percent mortality rate) and 10 deaths among the 200 high-risk patients (with a 5 percent mortality rate), for an expected rate of 1.8 percent.[7] The standardized mortality ratio for hospital A is 1.56 (28/18), since it has 56 percent more deaths than expected based on its patient mix.

One can report this discrepancy in other ways. Some prefer to express the hospital's performance on the same scale as the population average, giving a "risk-adjusted average." This is achieved by multiplying the SMR by the population average rate (e.g., $1.56 * 3 = 4.68$ percent). Another choice is to report the difference between the observed rate (2.8 percent) and the expected rate (1.8 percent); thus, hospital A has 1 percent more deaths than expected. All of these summary measures agree on the main point: After adjusting for its patient mix, hospital A has more deaths than expected.

Indirect standardization and its generalization via multivariable risk-adjustment modeling are powerful tools for making fairer comparisons among providers with different types of patients. Nevertheless, comparing outcomes across providers is complicated when patient mix both strongly affects the out-

TABLE 12.4

Hypothetical Hospitals with Different Patient Mixes and Death Rates

	All Patients in Population		Hospital A		Hospital B		Hospital C	
	Patient Mix (%)	Death (%)	n	Death (%)	n	Death (%)	n	Death (%)
Risk Category								
Low	50	1	800	1	200	1	800	1.25
High	50	5	200	10	800	10	200	12.50
Performance								
Observed death rate (*O*)		3	28/1,000 = 2.8%		82/1,000 = 8.2%		35/1,000 = 3.5%	
Standard mortality ratio (SMR) = *O*/*E*			28/18 = 1.56%		82/42 = 1.95%		35/18 = 1.94%	
Risk-adjusted mortality			3 * 1.56 = 4.68%		3 * 1.95 = 5.85%		3 * 1.94 = 5.82%	
Difference (*O* – *E*)			2.8 – 1.8 = 1%		8.2 – 4.2 = 4%		3.5 – 1.8 = 1.7%	

come and differs widely across providers. In the terminology of epidemiology, patient mix is a confounding factor when examining patient outcomes.

To illustrate, consider another institution, hospital B, with exactly the same mortality experience within each stratum as hospital A above, but with an unfavorable case mix. Hospital B treats 200 low-risk patients with 2 deaths and 800 high-risk patients with 80 deaths (see Table 12.4). Solely because of differences in patient mix, hospital B's unadjusted death rate is 8.2 percent, much higher than hospital A's 2.8 percent rate. When facilities differ widely in their patient mix, "raw" comparisons can mislead.

However, risk adjustment does not always do what we anticipate or hope that it does. For example, an indirect adjustment approach fails to make hospitals A and B look equally good. To perform indirect adjustment for hospital B, we first compute its expected number of deaths as 42 (0.01 * 200 + 0.05 * 800). Hospital B's SMR is thus 1.95, its risk-adjusted death rate is 5.85 percent, and its excess mortality rate is 4 percent (as opposed to 1.56 percent, 4.68 percent, and 1 percent, respectively, at hospital A). However reported, hospital B looks worse than A, although the same type of patient had the same outcome at either hospital. Results could be even more misleading. Imagine that hospital C is seriously deficient: It has the same favorable patient mix as hospital A but 25 percent higher death rates for both patient types (1.25 percent and 12.5 percent mortality, respectively, among low- and high-risk patients). Hospital C's SMR, risk-adjusted death rate, and excess mortality rate (1.94 percent, 5.82 percent, and 1.7 percent, respectively) look marginally better than hospital B's, although its performance is clearly worse.

Direct standardization, an alternative adjustment approach, produces results that feel more correct, but the method has conceptual and practical problems. In direct standardization, provider-specific rates are computed in each risk stratum and applied to a "standard" population case mix, producing an estimate of what might be expected if the provider were to treat this standard patient mix. For example, suppose that the standard population has 50 percent low- and 50 percent high-risk patients. Under this assumption, hospitals A and B have stratum-specific death rates that are estimated to yield 5.5 percent mortality in the standard population (0.5 ∗ 0.01 + 0.5 ∗ 0.10), as compared to hospital C's estimated 6.9 percent rate (0.5 ∗ 0.0125 + 0.5 ∗ 0.125).

In epidemiological studies, the strata are generally large, such as populations in different states broken into five-year age categories. Relatively reliable estimates of stratum-specific rates are possible using such large populations. However, in profiling individual providers for patients stratified by disease or other risk factors, stratum-specific rates are generally based on too few cases to provide reliable estimates. Furthermore, questions arise about whether a provider should be judged harshly for ostensibly doing poorly with types of patients that it rarely sees. For example, suppose hospital D treats 1 high-risk patient who dies and 999 low-risk patients, of whom only 5 die. Although its death rate is only half as large as the 1 percent expected rate for nearly all of its 1,000 patients, its projected death rate for the standard population is more than 50 percent (0.5 ∗ 0.005 + 0.5 ∗ 1.00). Thus, as this example demonstrates, which of several providers looks best can change depending on the patient mix of the standard population. Direct standardization is rarely used to profile physicians or hospitals.

Most performance profiles use more complex multivariable models to determine expected values. However, the fundamental approach is identical: Each provider's observed outcome is compared to expected outcomes based on the risk characteristics of its patients and the model-specified relationship between these characteristics and the outcome of interest. When providers treat very different populations, risk adjustment therefore cannot answer definitively "which is better." In reality, particular providers may do better with certain types of patients and worse with others. Thus, examining the data in multiple ways becomes particularly important, for example, examining provider performance within high- and low-risk strata of patients. In a rational world, providers would concentrate on their most successful types of cases, and performance profiles would help steer patients to providers who do well with similar kinds of patients.

Random Variation in Comparing O-to-E Outcomes

As discussed, standard errors capture the effect of random variation on the reliability of estimates from data. When each of n observations is an independent observation from a common distribution with mean μ and SD σ, we estimate μ by $\overline{Y}$ and σ by:

$$\hat{\sigma} = s = \sqrt{\Sigma_i\,(Y_i - \overline{Y})^2/(n-1)} \qquad (1)$$

The values of $\overline{Y}$ and s remain relatively constant as n increases, each becoming an increasingly accurate estimator of μ and σ, respectively. In contrast, the statistic that measures the accuracy of $\overline{Y}$ as an estimator of μ becomes smaller as n increases:

$$\mathrm{SE}(\overline{Y}) = s/\sqrt{n}$$

Properly estimating standard errors for predictions of providers' expected outcomes requires care. Consider predictions of a continuous outcome from a multivariable linear regression model. Most computerized statistical regression packages estimate the SE associated with an observed outcome. However, there are two SE values: the SE for the expected value of an observed outcome (i.e., for the mean of many patients similar to that one for whom the prediction is made), and the SE for that individual patient. For provider profiling, the latter SE is more relevant. It is larger than the first because it reflects not only uncertainty about estimates of parameters in the model but also uncertainty associated with the outcome of an individual observation given its expected value.

If s_i is the standard error for the ith observation, the SE for the average of a group of n cases is:

$$\frac{\sqrt{\Sigma_i s_i^2}}{n}.$$

An approximate 95 percent CI for the average outcome of n patients at hospital A is:

$$\overline{Y}_A \pm 2 * \frac{\sqrt{\Sigma_i s_i^2}}{n}.$$

The distributions of continuous outcomes like costs and LOSs usually have "long right tails," including some cases with extremely high values (see Chapter 10). Therefore, the logarithm (usually the natural logarithm) of these continuous values is often used in modeling because its distribution is more symmetrical than that of the untransformed data. In this situation, CIs can be computed on the log scale. However, achieving estimates on the original scale requires that the "point estimate" of the mean and the endpoints of the CI be retransformed by exponentiation (and adjusted for bias; see Chapter 10). Resulting CIs will not be centered at the estimated mean.

Consider a dichotomous outcome like death. The SD associated with an individual's predicted probability of death (corresponding to s_i for a continuous dependent variable) is:

$$\sqrt{\hat{P}_i (1 - \hat{P}_i)}$$

and the SD of the mean death rate of n persons, used to estimate the "real" death rate P that we cannot observe, is:

$$\frac{\sqrt{\Sigma_i \hat{P}_i (1 - \hat{P}_i)}}{n}.$$

When each provider's expected outcome (E) comes from a model fit to many cases, calculations of 95 percent CIs for O/E ratios can treat E as a constant. Then, one can calculate the CI around the observed number of deaths as:

$$O \pm 2 * \sqrt{\Sigma_i \hat{P}_i (1 - \hat{P}_i)}$$

and divide the resulting lower-, midpoint-, and upper-interval values by E. Multiplying each end of the CI by the area-wide rate yields a CI for risk-adjusted outcomes. Hosmer and Lemeshow (1995) found this approach was reasonable based on simulation studies, including a situation in which the observed cases were excluded from the data set used to build the model generating the expected findings.

Presenting Comparisons of O-to-E Outcomes

As noted throughout this book, risk-adjusted outcomes information—including performance profiles—is increasingly used by nontechnical audiences for a variety of purposes. Therefore, results must be presented in a clear-cut, easy-to-understand fashion. Because few users comprehend the methodological underpinnings of the computations, some performance profiles aim for the simplest presentation, even though it obscures important issues. For example, the 1996 profile of health plan performance produced by the Massachusetts Healthcare Purchaser Group initially arrayed ratings on a scale of one to five stars, establishing cutpoints to determine the numbers of stars. Apparently some health plans objected, noting that a single star, for the lowest-rated plan, sent a disproportionately negative message. The final version of the rating used only the center part of the five-star scale, with the lowest-rated plan having two stars and the highest having four. The *Boston Globe* published this rating on the front page of their business section, with the stars printed in bright red (Pham 1996a, C1). The numerical rankings appeared to the right of the stars, in small black print on a gray background. The lowest three-star plan had 89.8 percent overall satisfaction, while the sole two-star plan, Massachusetts Blue Cross and Blue Shield, had 87.3 percent, hardly a striking difference. Blue Cross withdrew from the voluntary rating program, noting that their low rating by the star method obscured the fact that their performance was numerically only slightly below their competitors' (Pham 1996b, C3).

However, the American public frequently sees results of opinion surveys presented alongside their "margin of error," especially around election time. People should therefore not have difficulty understanding that comparisons of observed-to-expected outcomes are also uncertain. How should this uncertainty be portrayed on the printed page? Producers of performance profiles use two common strategies to depict differences between O and E outcomes in a way that captures the effect of random variation: showing the observed value in relationship to a "prediction interval" of the form $\mu \pm 2 * \text{SE}$ or measuring the difference between observed and expected values in units of SE.

A report card on heart attack outcomes produced by the Pennsylvania Health Care Cost Containment Council (PHC4 1996) illustrates the first approach. PHC4 developed separate models for "direct admits" (patients receiving initial care for a heart attack) and for "transfer-ins." Figure 12.2, reproduced from the PHC4 report, illustrates a prediction interval generated from a multivariable model that adjusts for risk factors and a particular hospital's rate relative to the interval. Figure 12.3, also from the PHC4 report, shows an example of the results. The prediction intervals were wide, many spanning a range of 10 percent (e.g., from 5 percent to 15 percent). The interval for Aliquippa Hospital is typical; based on 87 cases, the interval ranged from about 3 percent to 13 percent. Butler Hospital, with 259 cases, had a narrower interval (from about 6 percent to 12 percent), whereas Corry Memorial Hospital's interval, based on only 46 cases, went from about 2 percent to 17 percent. Hospitals with higher or lower observed than expected rates are obvious, flagged by a small symbol to the left of the hospital.

For all hospitals depicted on the same page, readers can compare the relative widths of the prediction intervals, which are primarily a function of the number of cases treated. Hospitals with wider intervals treat fewer cases. Despite cluttering the presentation, showing the number of cases treated at each hospital would have been useful here, although detailed tables later in the report list the number of cases, percentage transferred out, and actual values with 95 percent CIs for mortality and LOS (PHC4 1996, 23–25).

In Figure 12.3, 4 of the 39 hospitals had rates outside the 95 percent prediction intervals, one with a higher rate than expected. The display invites the conclusion that the three below-interval hospitals had particularly high-quality care and the one above-interval hospital had low-quality care; however, 5 percent of ordinary hospitals fall outside the 95 percent prediction interval because of random chance alone. Thus, among 39 similar hospitals, about two would be spuriously flagged. Of the four that fell outside the interval, readers cannot know which, if any, are quality outliers. The traditional approach for adjusting for this "multiple comparisons" problem essentially expands the width of the prediction interval. This decreases the power of tests to identify hospitals that really do differ from expected and has been rarely used in performance profiling. As discussed later, hierarchical models handle the multiple comparisons problem better.

The PHC4 heart attack report showed the same findings for physician practices within hospitals, provided they treated more than 30 cases. As noted earlier, if a continuous variable does not have a widely skewed distribution, the mean of a sample of 30 cases is approximately normally distributed, probably the rationale for choosing a minimum sample size of 30. However, in this

FIGURE 12.2

Instructions for
Reading
PHC4's
Hospital
Performance
Reports

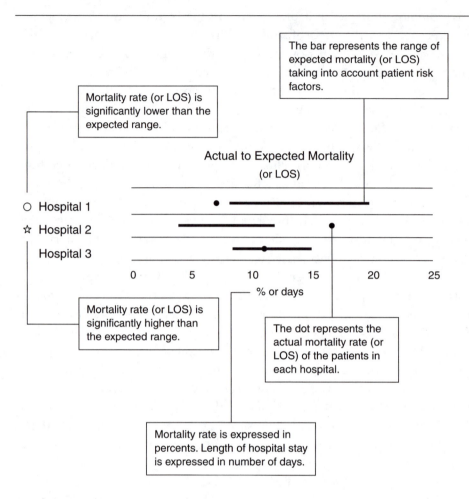

SOURCE: Pennsylvania Health Care Cost Containment Council (1996).

situation, PHC4 addressed a dichotomous outcome. With such an outcome, the normal approximation is generally reasonable when the event rate times the number of cases is at least five. Using this rule, 30 cases necessitate an event rate of more than 15 percent. This is higher than what occurred (Localio et al. 1997).

In both the mortality and LOS analyses, the PHC4 excluded patients from hospitals closing since 1993; who left against medical advice; under 30 and over 99 years of age; from hospitals treating fewer than 30 cases; involved in two or more transfers; and who were "clinically complex," with a preexisting or coexisting clinical condition not related to heart attack treatment and not included in the risk model. The LOS analyses also excluded patients who died, patients transferred out (who had "truncated" LOSs), and patients with "atypical" LOSs (more than 40 days or those discharged on the same day they were admitted). While PHC4 exempted hospitals with fewer than 30 cases from the mortality analysis, they included all hospitals in the LOS analysis.

FIGURE 12.3

Mortality Rates
and Prediction
Intervals for a
Sample of
Pennsylvania
Hospitals

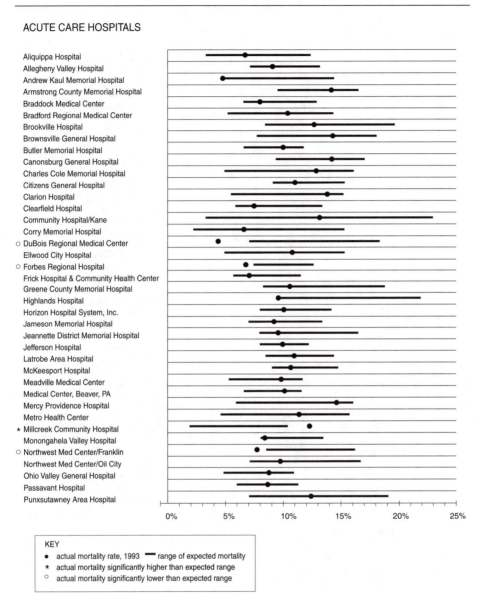

ACUTE CARE HOSPITALS

KEY
● actual mortality rate, 1993 ▬ range of expected mortality
★ actual mortality significantly higher than expected range
○ actual mortality significantly lower than expected range

SOURCE: Pennsylvania Health Care Cost Containment Council (1996).

The PHC4 LOS analyses used a log transform: ln(LOS) was the dependent variable. They calculated upper and lower endpoints for CIs in the log scale, then retransformed them by exponentiation. As illustrated in Figure 12.4, presentation of LOS data paralleled that for mortality. More hospitals fell outside the prediction intervals for LOS than for mortality.

Obviously, the number of cases treated is crucial in interpreting such data. For example, if a provider's expected death rate is 10 percent, an observed rate of 15 percent based on 400 cases is more worrisome than either an observed rate of 15 percent based on 100 cases or an observed rate of 20

FIGURE 12.4

Average LOS and Prediction Intervals for a Sample of Pennsylvania Hospitals

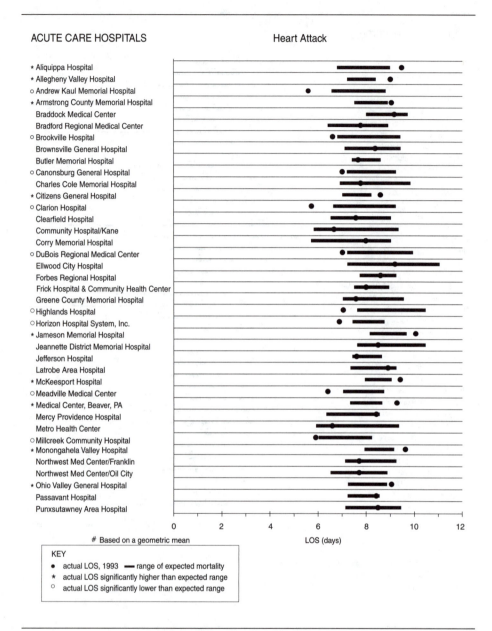

SOURCE: Pennsylvania Health Care Cost Containment Council (1996).

percent based on 10 cases. Figures 12.3 and 12.4 appropriately remind readers to pay less attention to deviations based on fewer cases.

Standardizing is a common statistical technique for converting a deviation (i.e., an $O - E$) into a measure that suggests whether the deviation is statistically meaningful. We consider:

$$z = (O - E)/\text{SE}$$

where SE is calculated as described above. If the observed rate pertains to a process whose expected value really is E, and if n is sufficiently large, this

quantity has approximately a standard normal distribution. This is called a "z-score," since z is used in statistics to denote the standard normal random variable. The standard normal is centered at 0; 68 percent of z-scores fall in the interval from −1 to +1; and slightly more than 95 percent are in the interval from −2 to +2. Widely available standard normal tables (or computer programs) are used to convert z-scores into p-values.

The p-value measures how likely it is for observed and expected rates to differ at least as much as they do, assuming that the observations reflect the hypothesized model. For example, a standard normal variate falls outside the interval −1 to +1 only 32 percent of the time. Thus, a z-score of either +1 or −1 (i.e., O and E differ by one SD) has $p = 0.32$. A z-score greater than 1.96 or less than −1.96 has a p-value smaller than 0.05. If a provider's O − E value leads to $z = 1.96$ ($p = 0.05$), its true rate may nonetheless be E. However, random deviations this large occur only one time in 20.

We used z-scores in study of hospital-based severity measures. Table 12.5 shows z-scores at five hospitals when we used different severity measures to determine expected rates of death for pneumonia patients (Iezzoni et al. 1996a). We selected these five hospitals for illustrative purposes from the 30 out of 105 hospitals in the study at which observed mortality rates differed significantly from expected ($p < 0.05$) when judged by one or more, but not all 14, severity methods analyzed. For example, at hospital B, observed mortality was significantly lower than expected when using DS's probability of mortality model ($z = -3.07$, $p < 0.01$), APR-DRG ($z = -2.30$, $p = 0.02$), or PMC-RIS ($z = -2.16$, $p = 0.03$). In contrast, observed rates were less than two SEs from expected, consistent with the null hypothesis of no difference, when using the original version of MedisGroups ($z = -1.33$, $p = 0.18$), physiology score 1 ($z = -1.53$, $p = 0.13$), or R-DRG ($z = -0.84$, $p = 0.40$), as well as other severity measures. Thus, whether hospital B was identified as a particularly high quality hospital, and perhaps used to benchmark performance at other institutions, depended on which severity measure was used for risk adjustment.

California's hospital report card initiative used a similar approach to portray outlier hospitals (Wilson, Smoley, and Werdegar 1996). However, rather than use the normal approximation to convert a z-score into a p-value, an "exact" p-value was calculated as described in Luft and Brown (1993). Figure 12.5, taken from the California report, shows how they reported their results.

Some critics complain that z-scores and p-values are not intuitive; many consumers of report cards would rather receive their information in such familiar terms as rates of excess problems or risk-adjusted problem rates. A deeper criticism is that any single-number summary (or point estimate) is likely to convey more precision than is justified, especially when ranking providers. Several strategies might combat this "tyranny of spurious precision." One involves using categorical reporting, as in Figure 12.5. This solves the problem of believing that one provider is better than another because 3.2 is bigger

TABLE 12.5

Examples of Relative Mortality Rate Performance from Five Hospitals: Pneumonia Patients

Hospital Performance Measure and Severity Method	A	B	C	D	E
No. of cases	200	317	88	267	132
No. (%) died	17 (8.5)	32 (10.1)	10 (11.4)	36 (13.5)	25 (18.9)
z-score (decile rank) from unadjusted model[a]	−0.53 (4)	0.29 (7)	0.56 (8)	2.14 (10)	3.63 (10)
z-score (decile rank) from severity-adjusted model[b]					
MedisGroups					
Original version	−2.30 (1)	−1.33 (2)	1.56 (9)	2.70 (10)	1.99 (10)
Empirical version	−2.73 (1)	−1.73 (1)	2.03 (10)	1.33 (9)	1.17 (9)
Physiology score 1	−2.25 (1)	−1.53 (1)	1.64 (9)	2.24 (10)	2.79 (10)
Physiology score 2	−3.12 (1)	−1.84 (1)	1.49 (9)	1.95 (10)	2.02 (10)
Body Systems Count	−1.74 (1)	−1.23 (3)	1.95 (9)	2.29 (10)	3.07 (10)
Comorbidity Index	−1.28 (2)	−1.13 (3)	1.32 (9)	2.11 (10)	3.16 (10)
DS					
Mortality probability	−2.51 (1)	−3.07 (1)	1.51 (9)	3.51 (10)	2.14 (9)
Stage	−2.05 (1)	−0.95 (3)	1.87 (9)	2.12 (10)	2.88 (10)
Comorbidities	−1.15 (2)	−1.66 (1)	1.45 (8)	2.05 (10)	2.57 (10)
PMCs: severity score	−1.99 (1)	−1.88 (1)	2.23 (10)	1.04 (9)	2.78 (10)
AIM	−1.54 (1)	−1.97 (1)	1.99 (9)	2.17 (10)	3.20 (10)
APR-DRGs	−2.25 (1)	−2.30 (1)	2.32 (10)	1.73 (9)	2.50 (10)
PMC-RIS	−2.05 (1)	−2.16 (1)	2.60 (10)	1.48 (9)	3.41 (10)
R-DRGs	−2.08 (1)	−0.84 (3)	0.60 (8)	3.04 (10)	1.79 (10)

SOURCE: Iezzoni et al. (1996a).
[a] Unadjusted model assumed 0.096 probability of death for all patients.
[b] Severity-adjusted model included age-sex, DRG, and severity score.

than 3.1, for example, at the cost of introducing harmful "edge effects" in which two nearly identical hospitals appear different because only one "made the cut" into a better category (as illustrated in the *Boston Globe* example at the start of the section). Another strategy is to report numerical performance measures using fewer decimal places (e.g., 3.1 rather than 3.14159). Displaying confidence (or acceptance) intervals is also helpful. Finally, performance reports should resist the urge to list providers in rank order from "best to worst."

Pictures often convey messages more powerfully than words or numerical tables. The graphical displays shown in Figures 12.3 and 12.4, for example, provide point estimates and prediction intervals for each hospital in a way that facilitates and encourages comparison. One important feature of such displays involves the order for listing data from different hospitals. The Pennsylvania report used alphabetical order, making it easier to locate

FIGURE 12.5

Portraying "Outlier Status" for a Sample of California Hospitals

FACILITY	Model A	Model B
Beverly Hills Medical Center	☐	☐
Beverly Hospital	☐	☐
Brotman Medical Center	☐	☐
California Hospital Medical Center ✉	☐	☐
Cedars-Sinai Medical Center	✪	✪
Centinela Hospital Medical Center	☐	☐
Century City Hospital ✉	☐	☐
Charter Community Hospital	☐	☐
Charter Suburban Hospital	☐	☐
Cigna Hospital of Los Angeles, Inc.	☐	☐
City of Hope National Medical Center	☑	☑
Coast Plaza Doctors Hospital	☐	☐
Comm & Mission Hospital–Huntington Park	☐	☐
Community Hospital of Gardena	☐	☐
Covina Valley Community Hospital	☐	☐
Daniel Freeman Marina Hospital ✉	☐	☐
Daniel Freeman Memorial Hospital ✉	☐	☐
Doctors Hospital of West Covina	☐	☐
Dominguez Medical Center	☐	☐
Downey Community Hospital	☐	☐
Encino/Tarzana Regional Medical Center	☐	☐
Foothill Presbyterian Hospital	☐	☐
Garfield Medical Center ✉	●	☐
Glendale Adventist Medical Center	☐	☐
Glendale Memorial Hospital & Health Center	☐	☐
Glendora Community Hospital	●	●
Good Samaritan Hospital ✉	●	☐
Granada Hills Community Hospital	☐	☐
Greater El Monte Community Hospital	☐	☐
Hawthorne Hospital	☑	☑
Henry Mayo Newhall Memorial Hospital ✉	☐	☐
Hollywood Community Hospital ✉	☐	☐
Holy Cross Medical Center	✪	✪
Huntington Memorial Hospital ✉	☐	☐
Inter-Community Medical Center	☐	☐
Kaiser Foundation Hospital–LA ✉	☐	☐
Kaiser Foundation Hospital–Bellflower ✉	✪	☐
Kaiser Foundation Hospital–Harbor City ✉	☐	☐
Kaiser Foundation Hospital–Panorama City ✉	✪	☐

✪ Significantly better than expected ● Significantly worse than expected
☑ Not significantly different than expected, no patients with adverse outcomes ✉ Comment letter received from hospital or hospital system
☐ Not significantly different than expected, one or more patients with adverse outcomes

SOURCE: Wilson, Smoley, and Werdegar (1996).

information for a particular hospital and harder to find the supposedly best and worst performers.

Displaying hospitals from highest to lowest performance draws attention to ranking, an unwise choice given the unreliability of rank determinations (Goldstein and Spiegelhalter 1996). Furthermore, when observed rates, *O/E* ratios, or risk-adjusted rates are used to establish a rank ordering, the most extreme rates are usually those based on few cases (such as 0 percent problems based on zero of ten cases). These extremes most likely reflect randomness and will likely change in subsequent periods. Reordering the same data may prompt new insights. For example, displaying hospitals by important characteristics (e.g., ownership, payer mix, teaching intensity) encourages comparisons among similar facilities. Such displays also highlight differences by type of hospital.

The art and science of good visual displays has advanced rapidly in recent years (Tufte 1983). Also, software for producing graphics is increasingly available, such as the many powerful display formats that have been implemented in the S or S+ computer language (Cleveland 1993).

Figure 12.6 shows how one might compare several providers (e.g., hospitals A, B, and C) on their performance with each of several kinds of patients (e.g., low, middle, and high risk) by portraying results separately within patient categories (Teres and Lemeshow 1993). Observing a multidimensional "signature" for a hospital might highlight areas that require explanation and reveal potential strategies for improvement (e.g., hospital A may do well with low-risk patients and poorly with others). Such an approach, however, requires enough patients to estimate rates reliably within each hospital or risk cell. Almond and colleagues (2000) suggest useful graphical displays for comparing a particular provider to other providers in the group.

Bayesian Models

Standard approaches for provider profiling present several problems. The first is how the "true" mean value of an outcome is estimated for each provider (e.g., μ_A for provider A). Traditionally, this is calculated separately for each provider as the average outcome of patients treated by that provider ($\overline{Y}_A$). However, the resulting set of provider estimates is often not as close as it could be to the true means and not the best predictor of what will happen in the future. Typically, $\overline{Y}_A$s are too extreme, the highest ones being higher than the associated true μ_As and the lowest $\overline{Y}_A$s being too low. When provider-specific averages are based on small numbers of patients, large over- and underestimates are especially likely.

In addition, traditional estimates of SE values (described above) may understate the amount of variability that is present, leading to CIs that are too narrow. Understating true variation causes more normal providers than expected to be flagged as outliers. One reason is that traditional methods recognize only one source of variation in the data—random variation of patients within a provider. However, variation across providers also exists. Standard errors are also often underestimated because patients treated by a particular provider may fall into groups such that patients in one group are more similar to each other (for whatever reason) than patients in another group. In other words, patients may not be independent observations but are "nested" or "clustered," often by some organizational hierarchy: For example, patients are clustered by their treating physicians; similarly, CABG surgeons are nested

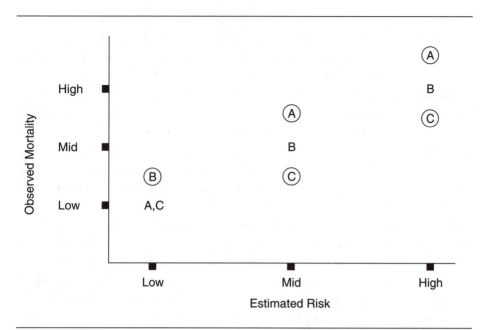

FIGURE 12.6
Portraying
Outcomes by
Risk Strata

SOURCE: Teres and Lemeshow (1993).

within hospitals. When analyzing units within which clustering occurs, effective sample sizes (in terms of the amount of information provided) are less than actual sample sizes. Approaches that do not adjust for clustering underestimate SEs (Greenfield et al. 2002). Bayesian hierarchical models (also called multilevel or random coefficient models) provide a comprehensive approach for dealing with such problems.[8]

The Bayesian Approach

Hierarchical models fit within a more general Bayesian perspective that views newly observed data within the context of prior knowledge. For example, suppose in ten coin tosses we observe one head. We know from our understanding of coin tosses that P (the true probability that a coin comes up heads) is quite close to 0.5. Therefore, our observed rate of 0.1 heads raises some question about whether the coin is truly fair.[9] However, if the coin looks normal, it still seems more reasonable to suppose that the P is more like 0.5 than 0.1. If we toss the coin more and continue to generate fewer than 50 percent heads, we grow more suspicious that P is less than 0.5. If the coin is biased, what is its true P? As the number of coin tosses increases, the observed proportion of heads increasingly becomes a more credible estimate of P.

Similar reasoning is useful for evaluating providers such as hospitals, where, without data, we assume that hospital A is ordinary and has outcomes like those at other hospitals. (Technically, this is called the exchangeability assumption.) If we receive a little evidence about hospital A's performance, we adjust this "prior" estimate slightly. As evidence accumulates, however, we place increasing weight on the new data and less weight on our prior belief.

At some point, the data may be enough to convince us that hospital A is of truly lower (or higher) quality or efficiency than other hospitals.

This is the sense in which Bayesian analyses interpret new data within the context of prior beliefs. To give another example, if we are uncertain about the safety of an operation but we observe one complication in ten operations, we may accept $\hat{P} = 0.1$ as our best guess for the true complication rate P. However, if we observed no complications in ten operations, we may feel uncomfortable with $\hat{P} = 0$, since we know that all surgery presents risks. Implicit in this is our belief that this operation is in some ways like other surgeries where complication rates around 10 percent are typically seen, but a complication rate of 0 percent is not.

Classical statistical methods capture the level of uncertainty in estimating P by putting confidence intervals on $\hat{P}$ (as described above). This approach has two major limitations: First, computations of $\hat{P}$ and a CI for P rely only on current observations; and second, the approach leads to "all-or-nothing" estimates. That is, if the difference between observed and expected values is statistically significant (e.g., because a 95 percent CI does not include the expected value or the p-value is < 0.05), we accept the observed mean as the best guess for the true mean. Otherwise, we continue to believe that the true mean equals the previously held expected value. Using traditional hypothesis testing, our ten coin tosses lead us to estimate P as 10 percent if we observe one head (i.e., after rejecting the null hypothesis that P is 0.5). However, if we observe two to eight heads, we would conclude that the coin is probably fair, and our best guess for P would be 0.5.

A Bayesian framework uses prior knowledge about a situation to produce estimates for the true mean that lie somewhere between the observed average and the expected mean based on prior knowledge. The resulting estimate is closer to the expected mean when the observed mean is based on few data and prior knowledge (e.g., about how fair coins behave) is strong. The estimate is closer to the observed mean to the extent that either outside knowledge is less certain (e.g., surgery with an unknown complication rate) or when more data are available (e.g., when the observed mean derives from 1,000 operations rather than just 10).

Historically, the Bayesian dependence on "prior knowledge" has generated considerable controversy. Two people examining identical data might reach different conclusions because of personal differences in their prior knowledge and assumptions. Nevertheless, Bayesian analysis has entered mainstream statistics, partially because powerful modern computers have overcome previously intractable computational problems associated with the approach. Furthermore, analysts can use a Bayesian framework without depending strongly on prior knowledge. One way is through an approach called "empirical Bayes"—using the data both as the basis for prior knowledge and to adjust this knowledge. Another strategy is to assume very vague prior knowledge, captured by placing noninformative prior probability distributions on unknown parameters (e.g., by conjecturing that complication rates associated with a new surgery are uniformly distributed between 0.1 percent and 80.0 percent). When prior knowledge is vague, the data primarily drive the Bayesian estimates.

Empirical Bayes Analysis

Casella (1985, 83) attributes the basis of "modern" empirical Bayes analysis to work by Efron and Morris (1972, 1973, 1975). As they discuss in an excellent nontechnical paper (Efron and Morris 1977), parametric empirical Bayes analysis derives from a theorem initially proven by Stein (1955) that challenged the fundamental assumption of traditional estimation theory, that the average of the observed data is usually the best estimate of the mean of the population from which the data were drawn. However, Stein proved that there are better ways to estimate jointly the (true) means of three or more normal populations than by using the three averages computed separately from samples from each population. The thinking inspired by Stein's theorem evolved into better ways to estimate means for several populations simultaneously. [10]

Empirical Bayes estimation extracts information from the current data set to function as the prior knowledge required for Bayesian estimates. For instance, in a particular database of 10,000 AMI patients treated at 100 hospitals, 13 percent die in hospital. This 13 percent serves as prior knowledge and provides a context for interpreting hospital A's experience—10 deaths out of 100 patients. The empirical Bayes estimate for the true death rate at hospital A will lie between 10 percent (the observed value) and 13 percent (our prior knowledge). Exactly where depends on the relative size of random variation in the observed death rate (10 percent) and the amount by which true hospital death rates differ from their mean of 13 percent.

To illustrate the empirical Bayes approach, consider comparing costs at four hospitals. A typical classical analysis considers two alternatives: (1) to accept the null hypothesis, in which case the true mean cost at each hospital is estimated as the common mean from the pooled sample of all patients, or (2) to reject the null hypothesis, in which case the mean of each hospital is estimated as the average of patients in that hospital. The empirical Bayes estimator represents a compromise, estimating each hospital's mean by giving weight to both the common mean and the mean at each hospital. Thus, the empirical Bayes estimate of the average cost in each hospital "shrinks" the hospital-specific cost toward the overall average.

Empirical Bayes estimates explicitly recognize two sources of variation in the data: (1) random variation within each unit examined (e.g., within each hospital, variation of individual patients' observed costs from the hospital's true average cost, measured by σ_A for hospital A) and (2) variation across hospitals in their true average costs (i.e., variation in the μ_i values for $i = 1$ to N, the number of hospitals). In making empirical Bayes estimates, the weight given to the observed mean in each unit is a function of these two sources of variation, measured by the variance (which equals the standard deviation squared):

$$\text{weight} = \text{variance across units}/(\text{variance across units} + \text{variance within units})$$

As variation within units (e.g., hospitals) increases, unit-specific averages receive less weight (i.e., estimates are shrunk closer to the overall average). As noted earlier, variation in the average is $s/\sqrt{n}$, making within-unit variation larger for smaller samples. Usually, the most extreme raw averages come from units with small sample sizes. Thus, their Bayes estimates are shrunk much closer to the overall mean, leaving units with less extreme raw averages based on larger samples with the most extreme Bayes estimates.

We used empirical Bayes techniques to profile small geographical areas based on hospitalization rates among people aged 65 and over in Massachusetts (Shwartz et al. 1994). Specifically, we examined so-called "relative hospitalization rates" (RHR) in each geographical area, defined as the observed number of hospitalizations minus the expected, expressed as a multiple of expected:

$$\text{RHR} = (O - E)/E$$

Thus, for example, RHRs of –0.5, 0.0, and +0.5 represent areas with 50 percent less than expected, as much as expected, and 50 percent more than expected hospitalizations, respectively. We determined expected numbers of hospitalizations using indirect standardization to adjust for differences in age and sex distributions of the population in each area. Consider the effect of empirical Bayes shrinkage on perceptions of hospitalizations for cardiac catheterization. The highest RHR for cardiac catheterization, 0.90, occurred in a very small area with only 4,955 residents over age 64. The second highest cardiac catheterization RHR, 0.84, came from a much larger area, with 40,390 residents over age 64. The empirical Bayes estimates for the two areas were 0.65 and 0.80, respectively. Because the first area had a small population, the empirical Bayes estimate gave less weight to its observed rate and more to the overall mean of 0. In other words, the rate estimated by empirical Bayes "shrank" much closer to the overall mean, from 0.90 to 0.65. Because the second area had a much larger population, far less shrinkage occurred. This illustrates how empirical Bayes techniques adjust point estimates to reflect the uncertainty associated with raw averages, helping to guard against drawing conclusions from extreme estimates based on a few cases.

Our study also found that the set of empirical Bayes estimates of hospitalization rates in small geographical areas generally matched the set of area-specific rates for the following year better than did the raw averages (Shwartz et al. 1994). For 62 of the 68 conditions studied, empirical Bayes estimates yielded smaller weighted average errors (weighting by the size of the areas) when used to predict next year's hospitalization rates.

It is important to note that a shrunken (Bayes) estimate may be worse than the average of the data for an individual unit. Across all units, however, shrunken estimates produce lower overall errors.

Hierarchical Bayesian Models

Hierarchical models generalize the idea of shrinkage and provide a comprehensive framework for explicitly incorporating variation at different levels of analysis (Bryk and Raudenbush 1992). The "hierarchy" derives from nesting, which arises when the data are not generated independently, but in groups. For example, patients are nested within provider (a group of patients treated by the same physician); in turn, providers may be nested within practice groups (e.g., physicians who work at the same hospital) and hospitals may be nested within types (e.g., teaching versus nonteaching). At each level of the hierarchy, the relevant independent variables and their influence may differ. Explicit modeling of the hierarchical structure recognizes that nested observations may be correlated and that different sources of variation can occur at each level.

Consider the cost for treating patients with a particular disease; to simplify, assume patients are clinically similar across providers. For profiling provider costs, we could use the following simple (although slightly unrealistic) hierarchical model:

- Y_{ij} has some distribution (e.g., normal truncated to be positive) with mean μ_j and variance σ^2 (stage I model)
- μ_j has some distribution (e.g., normal truncated to be positive) with mean λ and variance ν^2 (stage II model)

Y_{ij} is the observed outcome for person i treated by provider j. Provider j's true expected outcome is μ_j. This model assumes that random variation of outcomes is identical for each provider. It is measured by σ^2. Providers' true expected outcomes differ; in this example, they follow a normal distribution with mean λ and variance ν^2. Hence, we can generate a data point as follows: (1) by randomly selecting a μ_j from a positively truncated normal distribution with mean λ and some variance ν^2 and (2) by randomly selecting a Y_{ij} from a log normal distribution with mean μ_j and variance σ^2. Thus, the Y_{ij} values have two sources of variation, one due to variation within provider (the σ^2) and another due to variation across providers (the ν^2). In a Bayesian hierarchical framework, the stage II parameters λ and ν^2 are called hyperparameters. These parameters are usually given vague or noninformative prior distributions (which implies vague prior knowledge); for example, the distributions are uniformly (or nearly uniformly) distributed over some appropriately wide range that incorporates any feasible values. As a result, the data primarily determine the estimates. Analysts can easily enrich this simple model by incorporating individual-level risk factors or a risk score in the stage I model and provider-level covariates (e.g., physician specialty, practice site) in the stage II model.

Hierarchical models have several key features (Thomas, Longford, and Rolfe 1994). They

- explicitly model differences among providers (over and above what is explained by differences in patient mix);
- view provider effects as "random variation," with the measure of spread, v^2, estimated during model fitting;
- "shrink" the point estimate of a provider's outcome from the observed provider average toward a risk-adjusted expected value for the provider by an amount that depends on v^2, σ^2, and the provider's sample size;
- produce wider intervals around point estimates that appropriately reflect the uncertainty arising from both individual variation of patients within providers and variation of providers; and
- provide a framework for comprehensively addressing the problem of multiple comparisons.

Gatsonis and colleagues (1995) offer a good nontechnical illustration of hierarchical modeling in examining variations across states in the use of coronary angiography for more than 218,000 elderly AMI patients. Patients were nested within state; states were nested within region. Within each state, the probability that a patient received angiography was modeled using logistic regression as a function of patient age, sex, race, and comorbidities. The researchers coded independent variables so that the intercept in that state was the log odds that a baseline case (a 65-year-old nonblack man with no comorbidities) received angiography. These were the stage I (or level 1) models. In stage II, they modeled the intercepts from the stage I models as a function of region and a measure of the availability of angiography in the state. Stage II models were developed in the same way for each stage I model coefficient. Thus, for example, the log odds of angiography for black versus nonblack persons in each state were also modeled as a function of region and angiography availability.

This approach recognized several sources of variation: within the same region, for a given level of angiography availability, states vary; within state, for a given set of patient characteristics, patient outcomes vary; and finally, variation remains after accounting for both patient and state characteristics. Differences in observed rates across states reflect all three sources of variation. The approach is similar to the empirical Bayes method, which recognizes two sources of variation, within units and across units; thus, empirical Bayes represents a special case of hierarchical modeling and the same types of shrunken estimates result. For example, the log odds of angiography in a particular state is a weighted combination of the intercept from the model that only includes patients from that state (stage I model) and the predicted value from the stage II model based on the region and availability of angiography in the state. The coefficient associated with the effect of race on angiography is a weighted combination of the coefficient from the stage I model and the predicted value from the stage II model. As in empirical Bayes estimation, the degree of shrinkage is a function of the reliability of the within-unit estimate (here, within state) and the estimate of variation across states.

Interval estimates of parameter values from hierarchical models "quantify uncertainty," although they are not CIs.[11] Goldstein and Spiegelhalter (1996) illustrated this approach by reexamining the New York state CABG mortality data (see Chapter 1). They found very wide Bayesian intervals, which precluded definitive conclusions about most surgeons. For example, the analysis supported strong conclusions about whether rankings fell into the top or bottom half for only two of 17 surgeons. Green and Wintfield (1995, 1230) had criticized New York's CABG report because "in one year 46 percent of the surgeons had moved from one half of the ranked list to the other." Goldstein and Spiegelhalter (1996, 404) noted that "such variability in rankings appears to be an inevitable consequence of attempting to rank individuals with broadly similar performances." Furthermore (Goldstein and Spiegelhalter 1996),

> An over-interpretation of a set of rankings where there are large un-certainty intervals . . . can lead both to unfairness and to inefficiency and unwarranted conclusions about changes in ranks. In particular, apparent improvements for low ranking institutions may simply be a reflection of "regression to the mean."

Hierarchical models deal comprehensively and appropriately with the problem of multiple comparisons, as both point and interval estimates for each provider derive from all the data rather than just data for that particular provider. As Greenland (2000b, 920) notes:

> Giving the target parameters random components [as is done in hierarchical models] treats the problem [of multiple comparisons] with a global loss function quite different from that in classical adjustment: . . . modeling of the sort described here attempts to minimize estimation error by using additional background information, while classical methods only attempt to preserve global α-levels through purely arithmetic adjustment. It should come as no surprise, then, that critics of the latter find mixed [that is, hierarchical] modeling more acceptable.

In reanalyzing CABG mortality data from the Pennsylvania Health Care Cost Containment Council, Localio and colleagues (1997, 280) used simulations to demonstrate "the dramatic reduction in the number of false outliers with the use of hierarchical statistical models. The hierarchical models maintained adequate statistical power for detecting true departures from expected rates of mortality."

Hierarchical models rapidly become complex, requiring computer-intensive simulations to solve for parameter estimates, although computationally efficient approaches exist for conducting the simulations (Gelfand and

Smith 1990). New, easier-to-use software for personal computers is constantly evolving. The software package BUGS (Bayesian Inference Using Gibbs Sampling) is available free of charge from the United Kingdom's Medical Research Council Biostatistics Unit at the University of Cambridge Institute of Public Health (see http://www.mrc-bsu.cam.ac.uk/bugs/ for information on downloading and using the software). BUGS obtains solutions to the models using Markov Chain Monte Carlo simulation methods. This is a very powerful approach, although its use requires some statistical sophistication.

One advantage of simulation-based methods is that analysts can estimate more policy-relevant outcomes. Normand, Glickman, and Ryan (1996) did this in a study profiling hospitals for the HCFA Cooperative Cardiovascular Project in the early 1990s. Outcomes included the probability that hospital-specific mortality for average patients was at least 50 percent greater than median mortality, and the probability that the difference between risk-adjusted mortality (calculated for each hospital using a logistic regression model fit to the hospital's patients) and standardized mortality (predicted mortality based on a model developed from all patients) was large. Simulations enable relatively straightforward calculations of such statistics.

An Example Using Bayes Estimation

As an example of Bayesian methods, we simulated patient-level cost data and then used two approaches to estimate underlying parameters: shrunken estimates from a hierarchical model and averages calculated directly from the data. We illustrate two things: (1) Bayes estimates are more likely to "get it right" than traditional estimates and (2) how Bayes intervals and traditional CIs compare.

We assumed that the cost data were generated according to a slight enrichment of the simple hierarchical model described above. Specifically, each patient's cost was randomly sampled from a lognormal distribution with parameters that varied from provider to provider. For each provider, the parameters for the lognormal distribution were randomly sampled from a common normal distribution (truncated to be positive).[12]

We estimated parameters for the underlying distributions based on charge data for patients under age 65 admitted to Massachusetts hospitals in 1997 in DRGs 89/90 (simple pneumonia and pleurisy). Average costs per patient (more precisely, charges) were about $6,400, with an SD of roughly $4,000. We assumed hospitals' true mean costs varied from about 20 percent below to 20 percent above the average of $6,400.

For 25 hospitals, we generated data under two alternative assumptions about patient volume: first, assuming that each hospital treated 30 patients, often the minimum considered acceptable for producing profiles; and second, assuming that each hospital treated 100 patients, a relatively large number for a condition-specific profile. We generated five sets of simulated data under either scenario. From the simulated data, we estimated each hospital's mean two ways: (1) as the average of the data for the hospital and (2) using a hierarchical model with noninformative priors (corresponding to vague prior knowledge) on unknown parameters (i.e., the mean and SD of the normal distribution and one of the parameters of the lognormal distribution). We ranked hospitals from high to low cost based on their mean costs estimated each of the two ways. We then compared the rankings to rankings based on their actual mean costs, which we knew because we knew the distributions from which the data were simulated. We report two measures: (1) on average, how far hospitals' ranks were from their true ranks (calculated as the average of the absolute value of the difference in ranks) and (2) how often hospitals' ranks were five or more ranks away from their true ranks (which would put them in a different quintile).

With sample sizes of 30, ranks based on the mean cost of a hospital's patients were, on average, 4.8 positions away from true ranks; more than 40 percent of the ranks were five or more positions away from true ranks. Ranks derived from the hierarchical model were, on average, 2.1 away from the true ranks; fewer than 8 percent of ranks were five or more ranks away from the true ranks.

We found similar results with sample sizes of 100, a size usually thought sufficient to "get things right." The ranks based on the mean cost of a hospital's 100 cases were, on average, 3.6 away from the true ranks; more than 35 percent of the ranks were five or more positions away from the true ranks. Ranks derived from the hierarchical model were, on average, 1.6 away from true; fewer than 5 percent of the ranks were five or more positions away from true ranks. Simulation results, however, probably overstate the real value of Bayesian estimation because we used the correct underlying model to make the Bayesian estimates. In real life, the hypothesized model is only an approximation of the underlying reality.

Figure 12.7 shows, for sample sizes of 30, the raw averages and shrunken estimates for the 25 hospitals from one replication of the simulation. (To avoid cluttering the graph, we connect only some of the pairs of estimates.) The shrinkage is evident. Estimates for hospitals at the extreme are "pulled" toward the mean, suggesting by how much raw averages overestimate differences among hospitals compared to the estimates from hierarchical models. Because all sample sizes are equal, differences in the amount of shrinkage are caused by differences in the distribution of hospitals' cost data, especially the influence of outliers. Consider the two most expensive hospitals. The most expensive hospital's shrunken estimate was below that of the second most expensive hospital. The explanation is that two very expensive outliers caused the most expensive hospital's high average costs. In contrast, the second most expensive hospital had many cases with relatively high costs but no extreme outliers. The Bayesian estimates discount outliers and shrink the estimates more when outliers drive the raw averages.

Figure 12.7 also demonstrates that hierarchical models do not necessarily shrink all estimates toward the overall mean. In fact, the hierarchical model pulls the tenth most expensive hospital's cost away from the mean.

FIGURE 12.7

Average Cost (left) and Bayes-Estimated Mean Cost (right) by Provider*

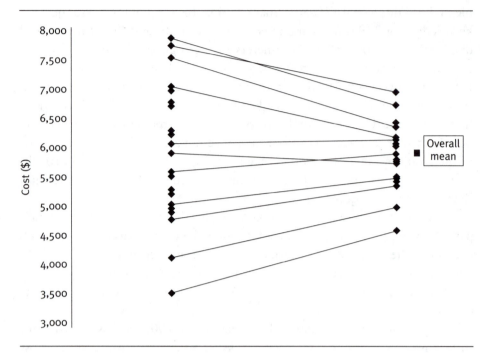

* Calculated from simulated data for 30 patients at 25 hospitals.

Examining the distribution of this hospital's costs is informative. This hospital had many inexpensive cases, but one very costly outlier pulled up the average. After reducing the effect of this outlier, average cost fell, and the shrunken estimate pulls this "average with outlier effect reduced" toward the mean.

For five hospitals, Figure 12.8 shows the estimated means as well as CIs and Bayesian probability intervals. Figure 12.8 makes two points. First, Bayes estimates pull extreme averages toward the overall sample mean, which is slightly under $6,000; second, Bayesian intervals are frequently wider than the CIs.

Hierarchical modeling provides an attractive framework for estimation when profiling providers. Shrunken estimates appropriately adjust for the influence of outliers and the increased unreliability associated with estimates from smaller samples. Furthermore, the Bayesian probability intervals better reflect the uncertainty associated with estimates than do traditional CIs. Nevertheless, hierarchical models have generally not been used to profile provider performance outside of research settings. One criticism is the extent to which results are based on the underlying probability models, although Greenland (2000c, 164) noted:

> Every inferential statistic (such as a p-value or confidence interval) is model based, in that some set of constraints (i.e., a model) on the data-generating process must be assumed in order to derive tests and estimates of quantities of interest. . . . Multilevel modeling is

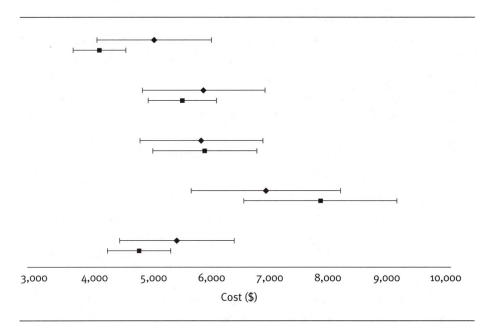

FIGURE 12.8
95 Percent
Bayesian
Probability
Interval* and
95 Percent
Confidence
Interval** for
Simulated Data
For Five
Providers

* Top interval of each pair, mean indicated by a diamond.
** Bottom interval of each pair, mean indicated by a square.

distinguished only by its unfamiliarity, which obliges one to make more effort to explain the model. But multilevel modeling need not involve stronger assumptions than ordinary modeling, and in fact provides an opportunity to use weaker assumptions.

A more serious problem is that hierarchical models "require substantial statistical sophistication to implement properly" (Shahian et al. 2001, 2162). Hierarchical models nonetheless offer substantial advantages, and ever-easier methods for implementing these models will likely continue to appear.

Comparing Outcomes over Time

Chapter 12 thus far has concentrated on cross-sectional comparisons—information relating to a single time period. However, a powerful profiling tool involves examining changes over time, so-called "longitudinal" analyses. As Donald M. Berwick, M.D. (1996, 4), a leading health care quality-improvement expert, observed, "Pick a measurement you care about, and begin to plot it regularly over time. Much good will follow."

Plotting measures over time highlights change. For simplicity, suppose that all patients have the same level of risk. Suppose that we examine the problem rate in two hospitals in year 1. Hospital A has a problem rate of 3 percent, with a 95 percent CI from 2 percent to 4 percent, whereas hospital B's rate is 5 percent, with a 95 percent CI from 4 percent to 6 percent. From the classical "hypothesis testing" perspective, we can reject the hypothesis that the underlying problem rates at the two hospitals (P_A and P_B) were identical in year

1 in favor of the alternative that hospital B's rate was higher. This conclusion does not mean that hospital B's problem rate will be higher than A's next year. Furthermore, even if in year 2 hospital A's problem rate is statistically significantly higher than B's, that does not mean that the assessment of which facility did better in year 1 was wrong. Hospital B could have improved.

However, provider profiles are useful chiefly to the extent that they reflect a persistent reality. As noted earlier, Green and Wintfeld (1995, 1230) criticized New York state's CABG mortality report. They said:

> The usefulness of the risk-adjusted data was also limited in that surgeons' rankings during two years of the study offered few clues about their position in the subsequent year ($R^2 = 4.9$ percent). . . . The fact that surgeons' performance ratings fluctuate so much from year to year means that by the time the data are published, users of the report can have little confidence that the ratings are still applicable.

Green and Wintfeld thus speculate that real differences in comparative performance are outdated by the time they become publicly available. However, Goldstein and Spiegelhalter (1996) provide a more fundamental critique, suggesting that such large changes in rank are likely when true differences in provider performance, even if real and stable over time, are small compared to random "noise."

For the NSQIP (see Chapter 8), Khuri and colleagues (1998) illustrated a way to portray *O/E* ratios over time. Such presentations suggest that providers' performance varies from year to year. From the numbers alone, however, we cannot know how much variability results from some providers improving more than others (i.e., last year's data are outdated) and how much from randomness (i.e., noise overwhelms the "signal"). In-depth study is required to disentangle these different possibilities. Nevertheless, longitudinal plots can reveal when providers' ranks change dramatically from one year to the next. When big yearly changes are common, both public reporting and decision making should be restrained. In particular, report cards should not list providers in rank order of their measured performance, as this reinforces the impression that the figures are reliable. Managers should think twice before disrupting provider-patient and network-provider relationships over findings that may be transitory, even if real.

Given the various methodological concerns and resulting questions about interpretation, profiles should be employed only where they are likely to be useful. For example, if last year's findings differ from this year's because relative quality can change rapidly among providers, profiling data will be most valuable for quality improvement and less useful to large purchasers and individual consumers of health care services aiming to select providers for the future. Even when longitudinal analyses show stability over time, legitimate concerns remain over whether consistently poor performers are the victims of inadequate risk adjustment. Future research must identify profiling information that is relatively stable over time and distinguish it from figures that fluctuate without obvious explanation. With most current profiling initiatives, random noise is a major consideration, as are unmeasured differences in patient risk. Small sample sizes for individual providers also raise concerns. These factors limit the inferences that can be drawn from practice profiles. Longitudinal plots often provide a sobering reality check to the evaluation process.

Despite methodological concerns, profiles are increasingly generated and used as important tools in ensuring health care "value"—a melding of cost and quality. Comparing patient outcomes across providers can be valuable, but much depends on how the profiles are used. Given the state of the art, however, relying on such profiles alone to make all-or-nothing business decisions (e.g., withdrawing business from outlier providers) is inappropriate. In this context, profiles are likely to generate (often well-founded) criticism and heighten adversarial relationships among providers, payers, and policymakers. Similarly, if such profiles are disseminated to a public unaware of the need for cautious interpretation, further controversy may erupt, impeding opportunities for useful dialog and improvements. If providers are given profiles without education about how to use them productively to identify areas for improvement, the information will likely be ignored.

Profiles comparing patient outcomes are most valuable in an environment of cooperation and collaboration, with incentives for learning and improvement. With increasing competitive pressures, however, this ideal environment may be more pipe dream than tangible reality.

Notes

1. The coefficient of variation, or CV, defined for a nonnegative variable as s/μ, is a useful summary measure. Hospital costs for a specified type of hospitalization often have a CV of around 1. In looking at total costs next year for a heterogeneous population (with many zeros and a few extreme outliers), the CV may be 4 or larger.

2. Recognizing that averages based on moderate sample sizes are only approximately normal, it makes sense to avoid the "appearance of precision" implied by using intervals with half-widths equal to $1.96 *$ SE. Thus, we use $2 * $ SE.

3. s is calculated as the weighted average of the SDs at each hospital, as described above. If the data were distributed normally, $\overline{Y}_A$ would be in this interval about 95 percent of the time. With highly skewed cost data and modest sample sizes, the probability is lower. As a result, under the hypothesis of no differences among providers, having more than 5 percent of "normative" providers fall outside these bounds is not surprising.

4. The calculations of Table 12.3 are only approximate. Especially when P is near zero, a reasonable 95 percent CI would not be centered

at $\hat{P}$. For example, after observing 5 deaths in 500 patients (1 percent), the modified Wald method that Agresti and Coull (1998) recommend yields the 95 percent CI 0.4 percent to 2.4 percent. Note, however, that the half-width of this interval is 1 percent, as suggested by the calculations in the table. For a clear discussion of these issues, see " 'Exact' Confidence Intervals Are Not Exactly Correct" at http://www.graphpad.com/articles/CIofProportion.htm.

5. A better CI—of approximately the same width—would be 5.4 percent to 17.6 percent.

6. Odds—the ratio of the probability of an event to the probability that it will not happen—are much used in the world of betting. For example, an event has 3-to-1 odds (i.e., odds = 3) when it has a $P = 0.75$ likelihood of happening and $P = 0.25$ chance of not occurring.

7. This expected rate is identical to that from a model that predicts probability of death from the whole population using the single predictor of high versus low risk.

8. Greenland (2000c) gives an excellent nontechnical description of the principles of multilevel modeling. McNeil, Pedersen, and Gatsonis (1992) also provide a nontechnical description of hierarchical models in the context of provider profiling. Shahian and colleagues (2001) discuss problems with traditional approaches and the advantages of hierarchical models as part of a review of cardiac surgery report cards. Normand, Glickman, and Gatsonis (1997) provide a technical discussion of statistical methods for profiling providers.

9. For ease of exposition, we ignore here the interesting observation that "you can load a die, but you can't bias a coin" (Gelman and Nolan 2002, 308).

10. Traditional thinking held that statistical estimators should be unbiased (i.e., the difference between the expectation of the estimator and the parameter being estimated equals zero). However, overall error, measured by the mean square error (MSE) has two components: bias in the estimated parameter and the spread of individual data points around the estimated parameter. Stein estimators minimize MSE but are biased. For profiling, it is probably fine to accept a small amount of bias if that leads to a smaller MSE.

11. A 95 percent CI is an interval that has a 95 percent chance of covering the parameter of interest; if data were resampled from the population 100 times and 95 percent CIs constructed, about 95 of these 100 intervals would include the underlying parameter. Note that in this interpretation, the intervals have a chance of covering a fixed parameter. Ninety-five percent CIs are often interpreted incorrectly as being the interval in which there is a 95 percent chance the parameter value falls. In this incorrect interpretation, the parameter is viewed as having a chance of falling into a fixed interval. The distinction is between the

chance the interval covers the parameter (which is what a CI is) and the chance that the parameter falls in the interval (the way in which a CI is incorrectly interpreted). A non-Bayesian framework assumes that the parameter value is fixed. Hence, considering the chance that the parameter value falls in an interval makes little sense. A Bayesian framework creates a probability distribution for parameters; therefore, considering the chance the parameter lies in some interval makes sense. This is the interval determined in a Bayesian analysis.

12. A lognormal distribution with parameters μ_j and σ^2 has mean $\exp(\mu_j + \sigma^2/2)$ and variance $\exp(2\mu_j + 2\sigma^2) - \exp(2\mu_j + \sigma^2)$. Here, we supposed σ^2 was fixed and that for each provider the parameter μ_j was generated according to a common normal distribution. Then, we generated patients' costs according to a lognormal distribution with parameters μ_j and σ^2 and took the true mean for a provider to be $\exp(\mu_j + \sigma^2/2)$.

RISK ADJUSTMENT IN PEDIATRIC POPULATIONS

Karen Kuhlthau and Timothy G. Ferris

C hildren are not merely small adults. Just as broader societal policies make provisions for factors specific to childhood, risk adjustment for pediatric populations must recognize unique issues pertaining to children. Several characteristics make children special: relatively low mortality and morbidity rates; the importance of developmental milestones; rapid growth, especially in the first years of life; and the early need for proxies, typically parents, to represent patients' views and experience. Children also require specialized pediatric services, such as neonatal intensive care; providers and institutions outside the traditional acute care delivery system, like school-based and public health clinics; and adult help and supportive environments (Forrest, Simpson, and Clancy 1997). Furthermore, important outcomes of interest differ in size (e.g., expenditures) or content (e.g., pharmacy use) between adults and children.

With some exceptions, risk adjustment for pediatric outcomes has received relatively little scrutiny. Perhaps this lack of attention reflects the historical impetus for risk-adjustment research. Most early studies of risk adjustment addressed Medicare concerns, such as designing prospective payment systems and examining Medicare hospital mortality rates. Today, however, interest in pediatric risk adjustment is growing as analysts increasingly grapple with designing pediatric quality measures and setting capitated payments for Medicaid programs, which cover many children nationwide. Some risk-adjustment methods have added children to approaches oriented initially toward adults, whereas others were developed specifically for pediatric populations. Here, we describe conceptual issues raised by risk adjusting outcomes for children and review the current state of pediatric risk adjustment.

What Is Special About Children?

Pediatricians generally define the pediatric population as starting at birth and continuing to "young adult years" (see the American Academy of Pediatrics web site, http://www.aap.org). Infancy includes children ages 0 to 11 months old, with the first 28 days comprising the neonatal period. Childhood is further broken down into early childhood (ages 1 to 4 years), middle childhood (ages 5 to 10 years), and adolescence (ages 11 to 21 years). The older adolescent period, over age 18, is also considered "adult" depending on the purposes for which distinctions are being made. This ambiguity over the "end" of the pediatric period is driven in part by adolescents themselves (switching to adult care systems), legal changes, and program eligibility. Disease epidemiology and care-seeking behavior of adolescents may be more similar to young adults (e.g., pregnancy, acute injury) than younger children (Schmidt and White 2002). For purposes of risk adjustment, arguments can be made for including adolescents and young adults with adults (e.g., measures related to pregnancy), as children (e.g., measures related to PICU outcomes), or as a self-contained category (e.g., measurements related to adolescent screening for sexually transmitted diseases). Several factors, discussed below, make risk adjustment for children different from approaches designed for adults.

Epidemiology

The first factor differentiating risk adjustment for children is the epidemiology of childhood disease and chronic conditions. Relatively low proportions of children have serious persisting illnesses or congenital conditions requiring medical attention. Unlike adults, children rarely have multiple coexisting diseases (van den Akker et al. 1998). Morbidity in childhood typically involves brief, acute viral or bacteria illnesses or accidental injuries. Children generally have much lower average health care expenditures than do adults (Thorpe and Machlin 2001). Because of these relatively lower costs, examining health care for children may appear less important than for adults (Richardson, Tarnow-Mordi, and Lee 1999).

Given this epidemiology, the number of children with any particular serious health condition is generally small, except in specialty clinics. Even for relatively common chronic conditions such as asthma, numbers of patients may be too small to produce rigorous risk-adjusted outcomes for children treated by individual physicians. Providers who treat persons of all ages, such as family physicians, rarely see enough children to assess outcomes for their pediatric patients. In addition, the relatively low use of hospital care by children (Krauss, Machlin, and Kass 1999) suggests that hospital-based outcome measures are less useful for pediatric than adult populations. Nonetheless, comparisons of outcomes across hospitals or hospital units treating many children (e.g., children's hospitals, neonatal intensive care units [NICUs]) are helpful. Such comparisons often require risk adjustment.

Risk Factors

Important risk factors for children and adults may differ. While diagnoses are often critical risk factors for older adults, developmental milestones, functional status, family supports, and social environment may be more important risk factors for children. ICD-9-CM, the diagnosis coding nomenclature in administrative databases (see Chapter 5), does not contain codes for many developmental, functional, or familial attributes, especially across different age ranges. Codes for symptoms and signs give little indication of their severity or chronicity. In addition, the clinical meaning of codes may differ for children and adults (e.g., heart murmur, urinary tract infection, chest pain, sleep disturbance, shortness of breath). Although codes do exist for some developmental conditions, they may not be coded because such conditions rarely motivate medical interventions. For example, although relevant codes exist,[1] using administrative databases to identify children with mental retardation is hampered by the absence of claims for mental retardation–specific services (Perrin et al. 1998a).

The quality of diagnosis coding in pediatric settings is unknown. Most studies of coding completeness and accuracy have targeted Medicare populations (e.g., Lamont et al. 2002; Cooper et al. 2000), as have most regulations, auditing, and oversight of coding and medical record documentation (see Chapter 5). Diagnosis coding and medical record documentation may therefore be even less accurate and clinically meaningful for children than for adults. Similarly to adults, some conditions, such as HIV infection and mental health conditions, are undercoded, perhaps because of fears of "labeling." Attaching socially disadvantageous diagnostic labels may have longer-lasting implications for children than for adults. On the other hand, parents may seek diagnostic labels to obtain services for their children, such as special education or other programs targeting dyslexia or attention deficit disorder.

Processes of Care

Processes of care often vary between adults and children, carrying consequences for some risk-adjustment approaches. For example, analysts generally avoid using processes of care, such as specific surgical interventions, as risk factors for adults, fearing that practice pattern variations could lead to manipulation or gameability of the risk adjuster (see Chapter 3). However, in designing their risk adjuster for congenital heart disease surgical mortality, Jenkins and colleagues (2002) argued that little if any discretion exists in the operations performed for various heart defects; they therefore built their risk-adjustment methodology around specific surgical procedures.

Some risk-adjustment tools rely on pharmacy claims (see Chapter 2 tables). For many conditions, patterns of medication use differ between adults and children (Ferris et al. 1998; Stafford et al. 1999). Among the ten most frequently used medications in children, only two would reliably indicate the presence of a chronic condition, whereas nine of the most common medications in adults are usually prescribed for chronic conditions. Moreover, drugs are often not tested in children; little evidence is therefore available to guide pediatric use. The Food and Drug Administration (FDA) only recently crafted regulations regarding the inclusion of children in clinical trials—the FDA Modernization Act, PL 105-115 (http://www.fda.gov/cder/guidance/105-115.htm) and the Best Pharmaceuticals for Children Act (http://www.fda.gov/opacom/laws/pharmkids/pharmkids.html#begin).

Care Settings

Most health care encounter databases include services covered by only one public or private insurer, but children often use services from diverse settings inside and outside the traditional acute health care delivery system. Use of school and public health clinics is generally not included in administrative databases; medical records in private doctors' offices generally do not contain information from school or public health settings. Thus, children who use early intervention, public health, and school-based clinics may appear healthier than they actually are simply because existing data sets do not include all health-related information. A related concern is that children use both the pediatric care system (including pediatric subspecialists, general pediatricians, and children's hospitals) and the adult care system. Since the pediatric care system likely serves children with more severe conditions (Kuhlthau et al. 2001), risk adjustment may be particularly important when comparing outcomes for children across pediatric and adult providers.

External Factors

Finally, parental, familial, and community factors strongly influence children's health and use of health care services. The local educational and health care environments affect access to important childhood health services. For example, some localities rely heavily on public health authorities to provide pediatric preventive care, whereas others favor physicians' offices; some cities and towns have access to children's hospitals, whereas others do not. These complex, interrelated psychosocial and environmental factors may be important risk factors for certain outcomes. For instance, timely delivery of childhood vaccinations is a common quality indicator for children. Although virtually all children require immunization, characteristics of families (e.g., living with mother and maternal grandmother, cash assistance eligibility, father living in the home with the child, presence of an additional preschool sibling, use of certain federal assistance programs) are associated with immunization rates (Alessandrini et al. 2001; Wood et al. 1995). Stratification of children by these factors may therefore be important for comparing immunization performance across health plans of providers. Few databases, however, contain information on these critical familial factors.[2]

The prominent role of the family and environment in which children live highlights concerns about medical care equity raised by the Institute of Medicine's (2001a) report *Crossing the Quality Chasm*. In producing performance profiles, ignoring these critical psychosocial, socioeconomic, and community factors could bias comparisons across health plans or providers. Unadjusted comparisons could appear fundamentally unfair to those seeing disproportionate numbers of vulnerable children. This could make plans or providers leery of enrolling or treating disadvantaged children, impeding their access to care.

Risk Adjusting Pediatric Costs

As noted earlier, pediatric populations have been incorporated in risk-adjustment methods oriented initially or primarily toward adults in addition to those developed explicitly for children. The first category of risk adjusters typically focuses on cost outcomes, whereas the second emphasizes quality indicators (e.g., NICU or congenital heart surgery mortality). This section introduces approaches toward risk adjusting cost outcomes for children.

As described in Chapter 2, various risk-adjustment methodologies using administrative data aim to predict future costs (typically total charges or payments) for a defined population, potentially to assist in setting capitated payment levels. Examples include the ACGs, DCGs, CDPS, and clinical risk groups (Muldoon, Neff, and Gay 1997). At some point, pediatricians helped create these methods, developing the clinical algorithms by grouping together clinically homogeneous ICD-9-CM diagnosis codes relevant to children. Some specifically tested their algorithms on child populations using Medicaid or private insurance databases (for a detailed tabulation of the characteristics of several of these systems, see Shenkman and Breiner 2001).

One strength of these methodologies for adults is their ability to quantify the combined effect of multiple coexisting conditions. However, children typically do not have extensive comorbid illnesses (van den Akker et al. 1998), so this advantage may not extend to predicting pediatric costs. Studies demonstrate that these risk-adjustment methodologies can predict pediatric costs, but systematic errors can occur for different subgroups of children. Fowler and Anderson (1996) tested DCGs, ACGs, ADGs (a component of the ACGs), and payment amounts for capitated systems using data representing Medicaid and privately insured children. Each risk adjuster improved the model fit as measured by R^2 statistics. However, some methods underpredicted expenditures for children with chronic conditions and overpredicted costs for children without chronic conditions. Using Medicaid data, researchers examined the predictive accuracy of risk-adjustment models (ACG, ADG, HCC, and DPS) for selected groups simulated to have different expenditure, hospital, and chronic health characteristics. In general, as expenditures, number of admissions, and burden of chronic conditions in simulated populations rose, the predictive accuracy fell below 1, indicating potential underpayment (Hwang, Ireys, and Anderson 2001). Using various risk adjusters (ACG, ADG, CDPS, and HCCs from the DCGs) and Medicaid data from several states, Kronick and colleagues (2000) found lower variance explained for child populations compared to adults.

The Chronic Disease Status (CDS) method, developed at Group Health Cooperative of Puget Sound, uses pharmacy claims to score individuals based on their chronic diseases, complexity of the medication regimen, whether the underlying condition is potentially life threatening, and whether the medications treat diseases and not symptoms (Von Korff, Wagner, and Saunders

1992). Controlling for health care utilization, the CDS is associated with physician-rated disease severity, patient-rated health, hospitalizations, and mortality. CDS excludes medications treating diseases of children. Fishman and Shay (1999) built on the CDS to create a pediatric-specific measure. The increasing availability of pharmacy information makes medication-based risk adjusters feasible for persons whose public or private health insurance plans provide prescription drug benefits.

Mental health problems (see Chapter 14) are among the most prevalent and morbid conditions in children, particularly adolescents. Mental health and substance abuse services are often "carved out" of existing health insurance contracts. In addition, insurers often place caps on the number of visits or services. Mental health and substance abuse services therefore require special attention in setting capitation rates. Using Michigan Medicaid data, one study predicted mental health and substance abuse expenditures with demographic characteristics, indicators of psychiatric disability,[3] and existing risk adjusters (ACGs, ADGs, or HCCs). The best model for children included a risk adjuster and the psychiatric indicators (Ettner et al. 2001). A privately insured population produced similar results (Ettner et al. 1998). The existing risk-adjustment systems performed better among children than among adults, although children had larger prediction errors (Ettner et al. 2001).

Risk Adjusting Pediatric Quality Outcomes

Researchers have used risk-adjustment methods to predict pediatric outcomes relating to processes of care, including subspecialist visits (Kuhlthau et al. 2001; Forrest and Reid 2001) and hospitalization and emergency department visits (Perrin et al. 2002). In each of these studies, risk adjustment substantially changed the results. Admittedly, these outcomes are closely correlated with expenditures. For investigations of quality for specific conditions, such as asthma care, risk adjusters designed to consider all diagnoses may not be as meaningful as those created for the specific condition (Shields et al. 2002). Several risk adjusters have been developed for specific pediatric care settings and particular conditions.

NICU Outcomes

Morbidity and mortality for newborns, particularly those treated in NICUs, are important child outcomes. Not surprisingly, therefore, risk adjustment for NICU populations has received considerable attention. Douglas K. Richardson and colleagues reviewed the literature on neonatal risk-scoring systems designed to predict neonatal mortality, LOS, and total costs (Richardson, Tarnow-Mordi, and Escobar 1998; Richardson et al. 1999). Table 13.1 shows the risk factors used to score NICU patients by three risk-adjustment methods. Richardson and coauthors (1999) concluded that neonatal risk measures

Risk Factor	CRIB	SNAP-II	SNAPPE-II	TABLE 13.1
pH		X	X	
Temperature		X	X	
Blood pressure		X	X	
Inspired oxygen	X			
PaO$_2$/FiO$_2$		X	X	
Urine output	X	X	X	
Seizures	X	X	X	
Congenital anomalies	X			
Worst base deficit	X			
Gestational age	X		X	
Birthweight	X		X	
Small for gestational age			X	
Apgar score			X	

TABLE 13.1
NICU
Risk-Scoring
Systems

NOTE: CRIB = Clinical Risk Index for Babies (the International Neonatal Network 1993); SNAP = Score for Neonatal Acute Physiology (Richardson et al. 2001); SNAPPE = Score for Neonatal Acute Physiology, Perinatal Extension (Richardson et al. 2001).

are an effective, important, and powerful tool for ensuring fair comparisons among NICUs.

Several risk-adjustment methods specifically target neonatal outcomes. Two have undergone rigorous independent evaluation (Pollack et al. 2000): the Clinical Risk Index for Babies (CRIB; International Neonatal Network 1993), and SNAP (Richardson et al. 1993a, 1993b) and its updates (Richardson et al. 2001). Other methods raise important questions. The Neonatal Therapeutic Intervention Scoring System (Gray et al. 1992) and the Berlin score include treatments when rating patients. A method created for the National Institute of Child Health and Human Development neonatal network (Horbar, Onstad, and Wright 1993) includes race. Including treatment and race variables may create unwanted biases in comparing NICU performance.

Despite publications documenting multiple uses for CRIB and SNAP in particular, neither has been extensively applied to comparing provider performance beyond research settings. Nonetheless, these studies suggest several important considerations when using them to compare NICU performance. These methods usefully risk adjust performance comparisons among NICUs (Horbar 1999; Roblin et al. 2000; Phibbs et al. 1996). However, the performance of these methods varies by the population of newborns and the time period represented. They rely on data from blood tests (e.g., arterial blood gas), and differences among institutions in testing procedures can affect their scores. Empirically derived risk adjusters like SNAP reflect NICU practices extant when the method was developed or recalibrated; with therapeutic advances, scoring algorithms require updating and additional recalibration.

Despite these caveats, NICU risk adjustment is sufficiently well developed and validated to use for comparing provider performance and profiling NICU outcomes. Considerable improvements in NICU care might result from widespread adoption (Richardson et al. 1999; Horbar 1999). As such improvements occur, the methods will require periodic review and updates.

PICU Outcomes

Methods for predicting mortality in PICUs have also undergone extensive study. The most commonly used tools include PRISM (Pollack, Ruttimann, and Getson 1988; Pollack, Patel, and Ruttimann 1996), the Dynamic Objective Risk Assessment (Heard, Fletcher, and Papo 1998), the Pediatric Logistic Organ Dysfunction approach (Leteurtre et al. 1999), and the Paediatric Index of Mortality (Pearson, Stickley, and Shann 2001). Dynamic Objective Risk Assessment permits daily updating of mortality risk as assessed by PRISM. The Société Française d'Anesthésie et de Réanimation (2002) maintains an Internet web site where risks of mortality from each of these instruments can be used to predict individual risks and compared (see Note 1, Chapter 1). Table 13.2 shows the risk factors used to score PICU patients by Pediatric Logistic Organ Dysfunction, Paediatric Index of Mortality, and PRISM III's APS.

PRISM and its revisions (PRISM III) have undergone the most extensive testing and use. PRISM scores, like the NICU scores, rely primarily on data from physiological measurements made within the first half or full day of admission to the PICU. Researchers have used PRISM to understand differences in PICU admissions between teaching and nonteaching hospitals and the effect of pediatric intensivists on mortality rates (Pollack et al. 1994) and to compare hospital LOS among institutions (Ruttimann, Pollack, and Fiser 1996). Although not currently used widely, PRISM could be employed across institutions to compare PICU outcomes.

Congenital Heart Disease and Other Pediatric Hospital Admissions

Surgery to correct congenital heart defects in children is relatively common at regional centers and, like adult cardiac procedures, is technically demanding. Also as in adults, in-hospital mortality following pediatric heart surgery varies widely, with high-volume institutions generally showing better outcomes (Jenkins et al. 1995). For these reasons, the outcomes of congenital heart surgery are logical targets for comparing hospital performance (Erickson et al. 2000).

Using various administrative and clinical databases, researchers have examined mortality following surgery for congenital heart defects. Risk of death appears to be closely linked to the type of procedure (Jenkins et al. 1995, 2000, 2002; Hannan et al. 1998), and use of procedure as the primary predictor of risk of mortality reduces the diversity among congenital heart conditions (Jenkins et al. 2002). Investigators have therefore felt comfortable designing risk adjusters around surgical type. Jenkins and colleagues (2002)

Risk Factor	PELOD	PIM	PRISM III-APS
Blood pressure	X	X	X
Heart rate	X		X
Respiratory rate			X
Temperature			X
pH			X
$PaCO_2$	X		X
PaO_2/FiO_2 ratio	X	X	
PaO_2			X
Absence of pupillary reflex	X	X	X
Base excess		X	X
Bilirubin	X		X
BUN			X
Creatinine	X		X
White blood cell count	X		X
Hemoglobin			X
Platelet count	X		X
PT	X		X
Sodium			X
Potassium			X
Calcium			X
Glucose			X
Albumin			X
PTT			X
Gutamic oxaloacetic transaminase	X		
Glasgow Coma Score	X		X
Mechanical ventilation	X	X	
Elective admission		X	
Specific diagnosis		X	

TABLE 13.2
PICU Risk-Scoring Systems

NOTE: PELOD = Pediatric Logistic Organ Dysfunction (Leteurtre et al. 1999); PIM = Pediatric Index of Mortality (Pearson, Stickley, and Shann 2001); PRISM III-APS = Pediatric Risk of Mortality–III Acute Physiology Score (Pollack, Patel, and Ruttimann 1997).

developed a method of risk adjusting in-hospital mortality for children under age 18 undergoing surgery for congenital heart disease. The RACHS-1 measure used expert consensus and empirical methods to determine relative risks of in-hospital death based on specific surgical procedure and other clinical characteristics. This method is new and requires further evaluation. Nevertheless, RACHS-1 or an analogous method could be used in initiatives to improve pediatric heart surgery outcomes (Mavroudis and Jacobs 2002), as has been done for adult cardiac surgery.

Pediatric cardiac surgery represents the technologically sophisticated end of the spectrum of acute care hospitalizations among children, which are generally relatively infrequent. Common reasons for hospitalization, such as asthma exacerbations, may be sensitive to the quality of outpatient care

(Perrin et al. 1989; Billings et al. 1993). In addition, significant numbers of pediatric hospitalizations involve supportive as opposed to curative care and may therefore be subject to wide variations in resource use. These two factors contribute to efforts to compare hospitalization rates and resource use for pediatric hospitalizations between populations or institutions. Risk adjustment is necessary to allow for these types of comparisons.

Among child hospitalizations, asthma hospitalizations and outcomes have received the greatest scrutiny. Asthma presents significant challenges to adequate risk adjustment. The most commonly used performance measures—emergency department utilization and anti-inflammatory medication use—are both indicators of severity as well as indicators of quality of care. Some researchers have used prior hospitalization in adjusting for risk on grounds that the higher threshold for admission to a hospital is more closely related to severity of illness than quality of care (Ferris et al. 2001). While hospitalizations for asthma are significantly related to asthma outcomes, they do not occur frequently enough among the total population of children with asthma to make them very useful as a risk adjuster. Risk adjusters derived from administrative data, such as ACGs, may have little value in adjusting asthma performance measures (Shields et al. 2002). On the other hand, clinical variables, such as oxygen saturation and respiratory rate, improve predictions of hospital admissions and subsequent short-term outcomes (Ferris et al. 2001; Finkelstein et al. 1995; Homer et al. 1996). These adjustment methods are limited insofar as they control only for severity of acute exacerbation of asthma (appropriate for short-term resource use and outcomes), not the severity of the underlying disease. Lieu and colleagues (2002) used parental reports of underlying (chronic) asthma severity as an effective adjustment for longer-term outcomes and comparing quality of care.

Table 13.3 shows two methods for assessing risk for child hospitalization from the emergency department. The Pediatric Comprehensive Severity Index (adapted from the CSI developed originally for adults) relies on physiological and other clinical measures to rate the risk of children, and it predicts individual outcomes and resource use (Willson et al. 2001; Horn et al. 2002). The index assigns a severity level to every child upon admission. Unlike Pediatric Risk of Admission, which uses a single set of risk factors regardless of diagnosis (Chamberlain et al. 1998), specific risk factors for the Pediatric Comprehensive Severity Index severity rating differ by each diagnosis. Willson and colleagues (2001) used this index effectively to show that practice variation accounted for large differences in institutional costs for infants admitted with bronchiolitis.

Conclusions

Risk-adjustment methods are much less developed for pediatric populations than for adults, with the possible exceptions of mortality adjusters for NICU

TABLE 13.3
Child Hospitalization Risk-Scoring Systems

Risk Factor	PRISA	PCSI*
Respiratory rate	X	X
Temperature	X	X
pH		X
PaO$_2$		X
PaCO$_2$		X
White blood cell count		X
Pulmonary findings on clinical exam		X
Radiology findings		X
Abnormal mental status	X	
Heart rate	X	
Blood pressure	X	
Glucose	X	
Platelet count	X	
Hemoglobin	X	
Arrival by ambulance or helicopter	X	
Referral by physician or other ED	X	
Age < 29 days	X	
Immunocompromised	X	
Dependence on medical device	X	
Asthma, taking medications in addition to bronchodilators	X	
Isotonic fluid bolus	X	
More than four nebulizations	X	

NOTE: PRISA = Pediatric Risk of Admission (Chamberlain et al. 1998); PCSI = Pediatric Comprehensive Severity Index (Willson et al. 2001); ED = emergency department.
* PCSI scores are diagnosis specific. The example used here is from the PCSI score for "lower respiratory tract illness."

and PICU. NICUs and PICUs, however, provide acute, high-technology care rarely needed by children. The vast majority of care for pediatric populations occurs outside such tertiary perspectives. For predicting costs, pediatric components have typically been added to methods covering adults, and statistical performance for pediatric subpopulations generally differs from that for adults (sometimes better, sometime worse).

Nevertheless, the distinctly nonrandom distribution of children across providers and health plans, some of which carry disproportionate numbers of disadvantaged children, drives the need for better pediatric risk adjustment. In addition, we must understand better the experiences of children with little or no health care and those who are "at risk" but not yet diagnosed with specific conditions. Children without longitudinal providers, who pop in and out of school and public health clinics, emergency rooms, outpatient departments, neighborhood health centers, and private practitioners' offices, present particular challenges to measuring risk.

Given current data limitations, capturing pertinent risk factors for children poses special challenges. Learning more about the role of families, communities, and local health care environments is essential to understand better their risks to the health of children (Halfon and Hochstein 2002). Linking information for parents with that of their children could offer crucial insight (Kahn et al. 2002; Minkovitz et al. 2002; Duncan, Brooks-Gunn, and Klebanov 1994; DiFranza and Lew 1996). Forging links among health data systems (if they exist) at public health departments, private practitioner offices, outpatient clinics, neighborhood health centers, and children's hospitals would require tremendous effort and expense. Nevertheless, sharing these data is important to obtaining population-based views of child health, various risk factors, and the unique and overlapping roles of different sources of pediatric care. This issue falls beyond the narrow topic of risk adjustment but suggests today's significant barriers to obtaining comprehensive information about child health, let alone the quality of pediatric care. As for adults, risk adjustment is inherently limited by inadequate or unavailable data.

A variety of technical issues need additional study. Improved methods for handling small sample sizes are essential for comparing risk-adjusted performance across providers seeing few pediatric patients. Changes in patterns of care (e.g., diagnostic testing, therapeutic interventions) and practice differences across settings could affect the data available for risk adjustment and relationships between risk factors and outcomes of interest. As elsewhere, empirically derived risk adjusters require periodic updating. Finally, as with adults, pediatric risk adjustment will never be perfect—including all pertinent risk factors is impossible. Understanding the effect of excluding potentially important risk factors on comparisons of outcomes across plans or providers is important. Given the ultimate goal of improving child health care, battles over measurement methods should not subvert resources, attention, motivation, and willpower, as has sometimes happened in adult settings.

Notes

1. ICD-9-CM codes are available for some developmental disabilities. Examples include mild mental retardation (317, IQ 50–70), moderate mental retardation (318.0, IQ 35–49), severe mental retardation (318.1, IQ 20–34), profound mental retardation (318.2, IQ < 20), and unspecified mental retardation (319). Mental retardation is in fact one of few conditions for which ICD-9-CM provides specific clinical definitions, as suggested by the indicated IQ levels.
2. As described in Chapter 5, one possible solution involves using data on socioeconomic status from the U.S. census to adjust measures such as physician performance profiles (Fiscella and Franks 2001).
3. Mental health and substance abuse indicators included any mention of an inpatient or outpatient ICD-9 diagnosis in the following categories: schizophrenia or other nonmood psychosis, bipolar

disorder, major depression, dysthymia or other depressive disorders, anxiety disorder, substance abuse disorders, adjustment disorder, personality disorder, disorders originating in childhood (including mental retardation/developmental disorders), and other mental health conditions (First 1994).

RISK ADJUSTMENT FOR MENTAL HEALTH CARE

Richard C. Hermann

Mental health and substance-use disorders are common and costly. Between 19 percent and 29 percent of Americans have a diagnosable disorder in a given year (Kessler et al. 1994, 11; Narrow et al. 2002, 119), and the nation spends $82 billion annually on treatment (Coffey et al. 2000, 13). The rationale for risk adjustment in mental health parallels that in other areas of health care. Dollars for care are constrained, and quality of mental health care varies widely (Dickey, Hermann, and Eisen 1998; Wang, Demler, and Kessler 2002). Coalitions of stakeholders—purchasers, public and private payers, MCOs, clinicians, and advocacy and oversight groups—are seeking ways to encourage evidence-based care and allocate resources more fairly. Comparing quality across delivery systems and aligning incentives to improve resource allocation require risk adjustment.

Unique features of mental health care also contribute to the context for risk adjustment (Mechanic 1998). State agencies, including mental health and substance abuse authorities and Medicaid, play large roles in financing or providing direct care, particularly for individuals with severe and persistent mental illness. These public entities have been in the forefront of quality-assessment and risk-adjustment initiatives. Mental health policymakers and advocacy groups increasingly view measurement and management of care as key steps to achieving parity in insurance coverage for mental health care. "Carve-out" arrangements, which manage mental health separately from other health care, have increased attention on resource use in mental health care but have also hindered efforts to integrate data sets for quality assessment and risk adjustment.

Although risk adjustment for mental health care has received more attention recently (Ettner and Frank 1998; Hendryx, Beigel, and Doucette 2001), it continues to lag behind the medical mainstream. Some prominent commercial risk-adjustment methods pay little attention to mental health. Many initiatives that compare quality of mental health care across facilities or plans are not risk adjusted. Mental health care lacks a frequent, meaningful, and consistently collected indicator of short-term outcome. No objective laboratory tests are available to quantify the severity of mental illness.

Nevertheless, mental health care offers unique advantages for risk adjustment. An extensive nosology exists with well-defined, criteria-based diagnoses of established reliability—the *Diagnostic and Statistical Manual of Mental Disorders, Fourth Edition* (DSM-IV) (American Psychiatric Association 1994). In addition, a long tradition of psychometric study has produced numerous instruments assessing symptoms and functioning in varied domains of mental health and illness. The sections that follow describe outcomes of mental health care, dimensions of risk, and examples of risk adjustment applied in mental health care.

Outcomes of Mental Health Care

Clinical outcomes of mental health care are primarily defined by changes in symptoms, functioning, and quality of life. Expectations for outcomes vary by condition and course of illness. In general, therapeutic goals for the treatment of chronic conditions, such as schizophrenia, include delaying or diminishing exacerbations of symptoms and improving functioning and well-being. For individuals with acute or episodic illnesses who function well between episodes, treatment seeks to achieve remission of symptoms, restore functioning and well-being, and prevent relapse or recurrence. Other desired outcomes are specific to individual disorders (e.g., abstinence in substance abuse) or societal goals (e.g., reduction in involvement with the criminal justice system).

Many mental health care outcomes mirror those in other clinical areas, including somatic symptoms; social, occupational, and other role functioning; health-related quality of life and well-being; and patient satisfaction. More unique to mental health are specific emotional and behavioral symptoms, such as depression, mania, psychosis, anxiety, trauma, and substance use. Cognitive functioning, self-care, and behavioral disturbances associated with dementia are important concerns in treating geriatric populations. For children and adolescents, additional areas for assessment include adaptation and adjustment, attention, school performance, and conduct-related problems. For persons with severe and persistent mental illness, socially mediated outcomes are particularly relevant and include issues surrounding poverty, exposure to risks for physical illness, adequacy of food and shelter, and safety from crime (Rosenblatt and Attkisson 1993).

Hundreds of instruments assess mental health symptoms and functioning; many are well-tested, covering nearly every mental health condition and outcome (IsHak, Burt, and Sederer 2002; Task Force for the Handbook of Psychiatric Measures 2000). Most were developed for clinical research but are applied increasingly to evaluating health care services. Sequential measurements permit construction of change scores, which are used to assess treatment outcomes. Thresholds established for some rating scales allow identification of remissions, relapses, and recurrence (Frank et al. 1991).

Symptom rating scales are designed to be completed by patients or their clinicians; they may be generic or condition specific. The Hamilton Rating

Scale for Depression, for example, requires a clinician to complete 24 items that rate depressive symptoms and severity (Hamilton 1967). In contrast, the Symptom Checklist (SCL-90R) is a 90-item, patient self-administered questionnaire covering nine symptom clusters (Derogatis 1994). Both instruments are widely used in clinical and health services research and have been extensively tested.

Instruments measuring mental health functioning and disability vary widely in their complexity and specificity. The Global Assessment of Functioning Scale illustrates one end of the spectrum. Clinicians evaluate a patient's symptoms and social and occupational functioning on a single scale with a range from 1 to 100 (Endicott et al. 1976). Strengths of this instrument include its brevity, widespread use, and moderately good reliability in formal testing. Weaknesses include the merging of symptoms and functioning into a single scale—because their severity may differ—and a paucity of data assessing reliability in routine use. The WHO Disability Assessment Schedule is more extensive but more burdensome to administer (Epping-Jordan and Ustun 2000). Clinicians assess 36 items in six functional domains, which are compatible with the ICF (WHO 2001; see Chapter 15).

Multidimensional instruments have been developed specifically for evaluating mental health outcomes in facilities and delivery systems. Researchers at the University of Arkansas have created modules for assessing schizophrenia, depression, alcohol use, and panic disorder, along with risk-adjustment approaches. For example, the Schizophrenia Assessment Module assesses symptoms and functional status over the course of treatment, along with selected patient characteristics for risk adjustment (Cuffel et al. 1997). The Behavior and Symptom Identification Scale (BASIS-32), a patient self-assessment, was designed for heterogeneous populations of psychiatric inpatients. Its 32 items yield scores in five domains: depression and anxiety, psychosis, impulsive and addictive behavior, relation to self and others, and daily living and role functioning (Eisen, Grob, and Klein 1986).

Other measures of health care quality evaluate processes of care. Process areas measured in mental health care include illness detection, access, assessment, treatment, continuity, coordination, and safety (Hermann et al. 2000; Hermann and Palmer 2002). Examples include performance measures developed by NCQA and the National Association of State Mental Health Program Directors Research Institute. Some process measures apply only to relatively homogeneous patient populations, obviating the need to risk adjust for patients' clinical characteristics. However, risk adjustment is particularly important for other measures in mental health care, where patients' actions and preferences often drive their care. Although clinicians fully control some clinical processes, patients influence other aspects of care. Persons with severe and persistent mental illness, for example, fail to attend up to half of scheduled visits (Smoller et al. 1998). While clinicians can influence adherence and service use, patient characteristics (e.g., illness severity, comorbid substance-use disorders) also play a role. Risk adjustment for these and other characteristics can be important to ensure fair comparisons across providers.

As elsewhere in health care, assessing resource consumption is critical in mental health care. Despite decades of deinstitutionalization, inpatient care continues to consume substantial portions of the mental health care dollar (Coffey et al. 2000). Efforts to align reimbursement incentives with patients' needs for inpatient care have motivated studies of risk adjustment for LOS (Jencks et al. 1987), costs (Fries et al. 1990), and staff hours (Essock-Vitale 1987; Hirdes 2002). Risk adjustment has been less frequently applied to outpatient care (Wood and Beardmore 1986) and setting capitation payments for clinical services for mental disorders (Ettner et al. 2001; Kapur, Young, and Murata 2000) or substance-use disorders (Rosen et al. 2002). In health plans that integrate medical and mental health care, risk adjustment of capitation rates reduces incentives to avoid individuals with mental health and substance-use disorders. In plans that carve out mental health services, risk adjustment helps diminish selection against sicker patients.

Risk Factors in Mental Illness

Diagnoses and Illness Severity

The American Psychiatric Association's DSM-IV criteria and codes are widely used for diagnosis and reimbursement throughout the U.S. mental health system. As illustrated in Table 14.1, DSM-IV assesses patients on multiple axes. Axes I and II focus on mental health and personality disorders, respectively, whereas Axis III lists associated medical conditions. Axis IV describes psychosocial problems, and Axis V assesses illness severity. Detailed diagnostic criteria for each disorder describe signs and symptoms, time course, and threshold levels of disability. For the most part, DSM-IV diagnostic codes are consistent with five-digit ICD-9-CM codes (see Chapter 5).[1]

Most risk-adjustment methods for mental health consider diagnoses because the information is clinically meaningful and readily available in administrative databases. Strategies for incorporating diagnoses vary but typically begin with a primary Axis I diagnosis, such as major depressive disorder (or affective disorders, if broader groupings are used). Next, risk-adjustment models often incorporate concurrent Axis I diagnoses, such as secondary mental disorders and substance-use disorders, based on expectations that comorbid conditions complicate treatment, increase costs, and worsen outcomes. Concurrent personality disorders (Axis II) and medical conditions (Axis III) may be added to these models as well.

DSM-IV criteria have enhanced the reliability of recorded mental health diagnoses. Nevertheless, reliability varies by clinicians' adherence to the criteria, information available at the time of diagnosis, consistency of patients' clinical presentation over time, and quality of documentation. In addition, diag-

TABLE 14.1
DSM-IV Axes
and Examples

DSM-IV Axis	Examples
Axis I	
Clinical disorders	Major depressive disorder, single episode, mild
Other conditions that may be a focus of clinical attention	Adverse effects of medication
Axis II	
Personality disorders	Avoidant personality disorder
Mental retardation	
Axis III	
General medical conditions relevant to mental disorder	Diabetes mellitus, type I
Axis IV	
Psychosocial and environmental problems	Job absenteeism, credit card debt
Axis V	
Global assessment of functioning (symptom and functional rating on 1–100 scale)	35 (major impairment of symptoms of functioning)

noses from administrative claims have demonstrated limited accuracy in mental health care. Analyses of Medicaid data from 1994 to 1995 found that up to one-quarter of beneficiaries with a utilization-based diagnosis of schizophrenia in 1994 also had a diagnosis for a nosologically incompatible condition in 1995.[2] Health services researchers and developers of risk-adjustment methods handle these inconsistencies in various ways, for example, by using algorithms to assign patients to the most frequent or potentially most severe diagnosis. Other studies have compared diagnoses from administrative data to additional sources. Lurie and colleagues (1992) compared claims-based diagnoses for schizophrenia to psychiatrists' assessments of clinical information and found claims diagnoses to have good specificity but lesser sensitivity. Another study, comparing diagnoses from Medicaid claims to diagnoses from patients' reports and structured clinical interviews, found good agreement for schizophrenia, fair agreement for bipolar disorder, and fair to poor agreement for other mental disorders (Lehman 2002).

The absence of objective physiological indicators complicates judgments about the severity of mental illness. Severity determinations rely largely on observation, interview, and structured assessment. While subjective, these methods are not necessarily unreliable. However, they do offer opportunities for gaming or manipulation if documentation of severity is subjected to financial incentives. For instance, evidence suggests that after implementation of Medicare's DRG-based prospective payment, depressive disorders were up-coded to a psychotic subtype (Kiesler and Simpkins 1992).

Instruments that rate symptoms and functioning provide the best information about severity of mental disorders, but relatively few health care organizations use them routinely. Medical records also contain information about severity, including clinical history, symptoms and functioning, and mental status exam findings (e.g., cognitive status, suicidal or homicidal ideation, capacity for self-care). However, as in other clinical areas (see Chapter 6), medical record documentation of mental health problems is inconsistent. Administrative claims provide severity information in the fifth digit of DSM-IV diagnostic codes. For example, major depressive disorder can be coded as mild, moderate, severe, severe with psychotic features, in remission, or in partial remission. However, these descriptors are often not completed. The aforementioned 1994–95 Medicaid claims from six states specified severity of major depression on only 30.2 percent of outpatient claims and 64.5 percent of inpatient claims (see Note 2).

Other Risk Factors

As noted in Chapter 3, virtually all risk-adjustment methods control for age. However, relationships between age and various mental health disorders are complex. For example, patients typically develop schizophrenia in their early to mid-20s, followed by chronic symptoms and progressive functional deterioration. In later years, deterioration can plateau and psychotic symptoms typically diminish (Carpenter and Buchanan 1995). Additionally, length of inpatient care for mental disorders has a biomodal relationship with age. On average, children and elderly patients stay longer in hospital than do working-age adults (CDC 1998).

For many mental disorders, social and environmental attributes are critical risk factors for poor outcomes. Persons with severe and persistent mental illness often cannot fully care for themselves, and the availability of formal or informal support can affect their outcomes. Clinicians commonly assess an individual's living status and the involvement of social service professionals, family, and other caregivers. Structured assessments of residential status often include categories such as independent residence, residence with family, group home (with and without staff), shelter, and homeless. The Psychiatric Severity Index attempts to quantify patients' dependence on clinical staff and the amount of support available to them (Horn et al. 1989).

Prior health care utilization can serve as a proxy for acuity and chronicity of mental illness and is significantly associated with important outcomes (Banks, Pandiani, and Bramley 2001; Hendryx, Dyck, and Srebnik 1999; Hirdes 2002). Early studies of risk adjustment in mental health included current treatment as a predictor of outcome (Ashcraft et al. 1989; Essock-Vitale 1987; Stoskopf and Horn 1991; Taube, Lee, and Forthofer 1984), but this is controversial. Interventions used for more severe conditions—such as electroconvulsive therapy, physical restraints, and antipsychotic medications—served as proxies for illness severity. In support of this practice, Stoskopf and Horn

(1991) pointed out that electroconvulsive therapy use is associated with higher inpatient costs and that nonpsychiatric DRGs include procedures. However, recent studies have heeded concerns that incorporating psychiatric procedures in risk-adjustment models could create undesirable incentives for providers. These concerns may be particularly warranted for electroconvulsive therapy and restraint use, for both practices have unusually high rates of geographical variation, suggesting disagreement over indications for use (Hermann et al. 1995; Okin 1985).

Other potential risk factors reflect a range of perspectives. Some models include attributes of psychiatric hospitalizations such as referral source (e.g., another inpatient service, emergency room, outpatient office, home), legal status on admission (voluntary versus involuntary commitment), and discharge status (e.g., elopement or discharge against medical advice). Potential indicators of functioning level are employment history, school performance, and involvement in the criminal justice system.

Examples of Risk Adjustment in Mental Health Care

In the absence of widely available models for mental health care, groups wishing to implement risk adjustment for mental health care face the challenge of developing a model *de novo* or searching the research literature for related efforts. While not comprehensive, the models described below and in Table 14.2 provide a starting point for identifying risk-adjustment methods for mental health costs, quality, and outcomes of care.

Resource Consumption for Inpatient Care

As noted in Chapter 2, DRGs were an early, high-profile risk-adjustment method, but Medicare mandated the use of mental health DRGs only for general hospital beds outside of specialized psychiatric units. DRGs include nine categories of mental disorders and five categories of substance-use disorders. Their predictive ability is considerably lower than surgical DRGs but comparable to the medical groups (Frank and Lave 1985). Mental health and substance-use disorders DRGs explain from 3 percent to 15 percent of variations in LOS, with most findings clustered at the lower end of the range. Hospital type explains a substantial proportion of the remaining variance, raising questions about whether facility type serves as a proxy for unmeasured severity differences (Horgan and Jencks 1987). Consequently, Medicare permits psychiatric units and specialty psychiatric hospitals to apply for exemptions from the prospective payment system.

Alternative methods for grouping ICD-9-CM diagnosis codes have been tested with limited success. DS (see Chapter 2) sorts ICD-9-CM diagnosis codes into subgroups of increasing severity and comorbidity (Mitchell et al. 1987). For example, stage 1 for depressive disorders consists of dysthymic disorder, a milder, chronic form of depression,[3] followed by comorbid dysthymia

TABLE 14.2

Examples of Risk Adjusters for Mental Health and Substance Abuse Care

Risk Adjuster	Outcome	Population	Major Risk Factors
Modified ADGs (from ACGs)[a]	Annual costs	Employed adults and dependents	Sociodemographics, diagnoses
Clinically Related Groups[b]	LOS	Adult inpatients	Sociodemographics, diagnoses
Computerized Psychiatric Severity Index[c]	LOS	Adult inpatients	Sociodemographics, diagnoses, symptoms, functioning
Modified DCG/HCC[d]	Service days	Veterans with SUD	Sociodemographics, diagnoses
Modified DCG/HCC[a]	Annual costs	Employed adults and dependents	Sociodemographics, diagnoses
DS[b]	LOS	Adult inpatients	Diagnoses
Hoosier Assurance Plan[e]	Costs	Persons with SPMI	Sociodemographics, diagnoses
Long-Stay Psychiatric Patient Classification System[f]	Staff time	Inpatient veterans	Symptoms, functioning

NOTE: SUD = substance-abuse disorders; SPMI = severe and persistent mental illness.
[a]Ettner et al. (2000).
[b]Mitchell and Liptzin (1987).
[c]Stoskopf and Horn (1991, 1992).
[d]Rosen et al. (in press).
[e]DeLiberty, Newman, and Ward (2001).
[f]Fries et al. (1990).

and a personality or substance-use disorder in stage 2, and major depression in stage 3. Another approach, Clinically Related Groups, separates diagnoses into hierarchies based on age distribution and clinical features. Psychotic conditions, for example, are separated into distinct diagnoses (e.g., schizophrenia and bipolar disorder) and then subdivided by age group (under 18, 18–64, and 65 and older). Other methods of risk adjusting inpatient utilization have supplemented diagnosis codes with readily available administrative data, such as age, sex, marital status, comorbidity, and number of previous hospitalizations (English et al. 1986; Taube, Lee, and Forthofer 1984). Although these efforts have generally bolstered the variance explained by DRGs, none explain more than 15 percent.

Models incorporating data collected from staff, medical records, or patients' reports attain significantly greater explanatory power (Ashcraft et al. 1989; Durbin et al. 1999; Horn et al 1989; Stoskopf and Horn 1991). The Computerized Psychiatric Severity Index assigns inpatients to one of four severity levels based on signs and symptoms, psychiatric history, complications, and psychosocial factors. This index combined with other patient data explained 33 percent of variation in LOS in an inpatient sample (Stoskopf and Horn 1992, 751). A revised version of this method forms the psychiatric component of the CSI, which provides risk adjustment within diagnostic categories (Durbin et al. 1999; see Chapter 2).

Canadian researchers have designed a risk-adjustment method to determine inpatient reimbursement—the System for Classification of Inpatient Psychiatry (Hirdes 2002). Developed by the Ontario Joint Policy and Planning Committee, a partnership between the provincial health ministry and hospital association, the classification assesses factors associated with inpatient costs attributable to nonphysician staff. Risk factor data come from the Resident Assessment Instrument–Mental Health (RAI-MH) (Hirdes et al. 2000). Following a decision tree structure, the classification divides patients into 47 groups, first by primary psychiatric diagnosis and then by approximately 80 attributes, including secondary diagnosis, medical problems, symptoms, functioning, suicidality, day of inpatient stay, and prior admissions. The System for Classification of Inpatient Psychiatry explains about 26 percent of staff costs (Hirdes 2002). The Ontario Health Ministry is currently considering implementing both the instrument and the data collection tool to reimburse inpatient psychiatric hospitals. CMS funded American investigators involved in the Canadian classification project to develop a less burdensome patient-assessment instrument and case-mix system for psychiatric inpatient care. These efforts produced the Case Mix Assessment Tool, which is nearing field tests (National Association of Reimbursement Officers 2001).

Capitation and Comprehensive Services

Several studies have evaluated whether risk-adjustment methods developed for capitation in general populations adequately predict costs for individuals with mental disorders. Analyses evaluating ACGs (and their ADGs) and DCG/HCCs found that these models generally underestimated total health care costs for individuals with mental health and substance-use disorders and overestimated costs for those without them. Models predicting only mental health and substance-use costs showed less explanatory power than models for total health care costs (Ettner et al. 1998; Ettner and Notman 1997). Adding more precise mental health and substance-use diagnostic categories somewhat improved cost predictions (Ettner et al. 2001). Another study looked specifically at "service days" (a proxy for costs) within VA hospitals for veterans with substance-use disorders. The proportion of variance in service days explained by DCGs/HCCs was lower among this population than DCGs have achieved in non-substance-use disorder populations (Rosen et al. in press). Adding specific substance-use diagnostic categories and dividing the disorders into groups based on severity failed to improve predictive performance significantly.

Some state Medicaid programs are risk adjusting reimbursement for mental health services. For example, Rhode Island adjusts for age, sex, and eligibility status, and Maryland uses ACGs. Indiana risk adjusts the case-reimbursement rates for adults with serious mental illness or chronic addictions and children or adolescents with serious emotional disorders. In the Indiana system, each group is further subdivided using hierarchical regression models to identify subgroups with similar levels of service costs in the 90 days following initial assessment. The payer assigns reimbursement rates to each subgroup based on historical costs. For example, adults with severe mental illness were subdivided into nine groups based on three diagnostic clusters and three functional levels; per case reimbursement levels range from $1,194 to $7,981 depending on the group (DeLiberty, Newman, and Ward 2001).

Clinical Outcomes

Several research studies demonstrate that rankings of facilities by mental health outcomes change after risk adjustment (Dow, Boaz, and Thornton 2001; Hendryx, Dyck, and Srebnik 1999; Kramer et al. 2001). For example, Hendryx, Dyck, and Srebnik (1999) compared patient satisfaction, functioning, and health-related quality of life across six community mental health agencies. Risk factors significantly predicting one or more outcomes included "severe diagnoses" (schizophrenia, bipolar disorder, and major depression), substance abuse, age, and baseline functioning and quality of life. Agency rankings also varied based on which outcome measure was used.

Other methods have focused on patient populations with a specific mental disorder. For example, Kramer and colleagues (2001) modeled treatment outcomes for major depression using detailed demographic and clinical data from the University of Arkansas Depression Outcome Module and the SF-36. Baseline depression severity, income, and medical comorbidity explained 26 percent of variation in depression severity at three months. Adding baseline functional status (SF-36 physical and mental health summary scores) increased the explained variance to 38 percent (Kramer et al. 2001, 294).

More than half of the state mental health authorities have implemented routine outcome measurement to assess symptoms or functioning of individuals with severe and persistent mental illness (National Association of State Mental Health Program Directors Research Institute 2002), but few states risk adjust these data. Massachusetts and Indiana stratify some results. The Vermont mental health authority has begun to risk adjust some outcomes data (Banks, Pandiani, and Bramley 2001; Banks et al. 1999; Pandiani, Banks, and Schacht 1998). Despite their frequent use, clinical process measures are rarely risk adjusted. A study of 251 process measures developed for mental health quality assessment found that only 13 percent were risk adjusted (12 measures with multivariable modeling and 21 with stratification) (Hermann et al. 2000). The NCQA stratifies several mental health measures by age, sex, and gender. Health Plan Employer Data Information Set (HEDIS) measures for mental health and substance-use disorders include the following:

- proportion of individuals with a psychiatric disorder who receive ambulatory care within 7 and 30 days of hospital discharge;

- proportion of enrollees who use mental health or substance abuse services during one-year periods; and
- proportion of individuals started on an antidepressant for major depression who

  1. continue the medication for at least 12 weeks,
  2. have three or more visits during the 12-week period, and
  3. remain on the medication for six months.

The National Association of State Mental Health Program Directors Research Institute performance measurement system, used by more than 240 psychiatric hospitals, has developed multivariable risk-adjustment models for three of its measures: 30-day readmission rates, percentage of inpatients restrained, and percentage secluded. In addition to diagnostic and sociodemographic data, risk factors include legal status, referral source, living arrangement, and average LOS. The VA's Northeast Program Evaluation Center risk adjusts inpatient process measure results by sociodemographic and diagnostic information, disability compensation, Global Assessment of Functioning Scale score, and the patient's distance from VA health services. The model explains an average of 2.7 percent (0.3 percent to 9.7 percent) of the variation in measures of timeliness, continuity, and intensity of treatment after discharge (Office of Quality and Performance 1999).

Risk adjustment also has furthered studies of organizational and financial influences on quality and outcomes. Sophisticated analytical techniques (see Chapter 11) have allowed for more carefully controlled comparisons in observational studies of patients receiving mental health care. Schoenbaum and colleagues (in press) employed instrumental variables to control for unmeasured differences; they found that patients appropriately treated for depression had better employment outcomes than patients receiving inappropriate care. Another study used propensity scores to compare guideline adherence among Medicaid enrollees with schizophrenia, finding that small differences between managed care and fee-for-service groups became insignificant after adjustment (Dickey et al. in press).

Conclusions

The mental health care system has made considerable progress on risk adjustment since DRGs were introduced two decades ago. Multivariable models have been developed to adjust comparisons of quality and outcomes of care and align reimbursement more closely with expected need for mental health services. These models have shown increasing methodological sophistication and gains in predictive ability.

Nevertheless, more work is needed. Several commercial risk-adjustment methods developed for general health care settings are inadequate for mental health care. Models focusing specifically on mental health have been developed but are not widely used. Many public- and private-sector quality-assessment initiatives in mental health care lack risk adjustment. Rankings of mental health facilities on the basis of clinical outcomes have proven sensitive to the choice of outcomes and statistical methods. Inpatient LOS has been the most intensively studied area, but this work has yet to yield a risk-adjustment method that balances acceptable predictive performance with a reasonable data collection burden.

Current methods for risk adjusting capitation payments do not adequately diminish incentives to avoid or undertreat persons with mental illness. An alternative approach gaining favor involves so-called "mixed payment" or "partial capitation" systems, which reimburse plans or providers based partially on actual costs and partially on adjusted costs. This approach preserves some incentive to contain costs but lessens the motivation to restrict enrollment or treatment (Ettner et al. 2001; Newhouse 1994).

Risk adjustment must extend into additional areas of mental health care. Despite substantial shifts in mental health utilization from inpatient to outpatient settings, few studies have focused on outpatient costs or utilization. Disorder-specific risk adjustment has proven powerful in certain settings, but studies to date have primarily examined depression and schizophrenia. Additionally, most models have addressed treatment of adult populations, although studies of child and adolescent mental health care are beginning to emerge (DeLiberty, Newman, and Ward 2001; Ettner and Notman 1997).

For risk adjustment to advance in mental health, several barriers must be overcome. Treatment often spans primary care and mental health specialty sectors. However, when mental health services are carved out of health plans, these carve outs process mental health claims separately from other claims, making it difficult to integrate data sets for risk adjustment or quality assessment. Rules protecting patient confidentiality restrict access to mental health data more than for other medical services and may tighten further as federal privacy regulations are implemented under the HIPAA mandate (see Chapters 5 and 6). State agencies have long relied on their own idiosyncratic coding schemes to reimburse mental health services, complicating risk-adjustment efforts. Impending HIPAA standards for code sets may bring order and consistency to mental health procedure codes.

As has been concluded about other care settings (such as rehabilitation, Chapter 15, and long-term care, Chapter 16), administrative data systems do not contain sufficient risk factor information to predict mental health outcomes. Risk adjustment will require additional data collection from medical records or directly from patients. In their study of depression outcomes, Kramer and colleagues (2001, 297) highlighted the tension between explanatory power and data collection burden: "By adding the SF-36 . . . an additional 10% of the variance was accounted for. . . . However, the additional burden of administering the SF-36 . . . may not offset the additional predictive power obtained."

Standardization of severity ratings for common mental health conditions would provide better data for risk adjustment at lower cost. For example, although clinicians diagnose depression consistently across the United States, their documentation of symptom severity varies greatly. Many clinicians do not use structured severity ratings. Those who do use such scales select from nearly a dozen well-known alternatives. The American College of Physicians, American Psychiatric Association, and American Academy of Family Practice cosponsored a Depression Diagnosis and Severity Measure Consensus Meeting in October 2002. Participants made progress toward envisioning a common measure, but adoption is seen as a distant goal. In addition to facilitating risk adjustment, broad acceptance of a common rating scale would provide the basis for routine measurement of depression outcomes. Influential report cards have emerged in other areas of medicine in part because a meaningful and easily collected outcome was available (e.g., mortality in cardiac care). Common metrics for depression and other mental health and substance-use disorders could similarly advance the state of the art of quality assessment and risk adjustment in mental health care.

Notes

1. While DSM-IV diagnostic codes numerically correspond to ICD-9-CM codes, there are minor differences in clinical terminology between the two systems.
2. Analyses used data from 11,684,089 Medicaid beneficiaries from six states: California, Georgia, Indiana, Mississippi, Missouri, and Pennsylvania. Among individuals with a utilization-based diagnosis of schizophrenia in 1994, 25.4 percent had at least one claim in 1995 for a nosologically incompatible condition, such as bipolar disorder, psychotic disorder not otherwise specified, or schizoaffective disorder (Hermann, unpublished data).
3. Dysthymia, a milder, chronic form of depression, illustrates the minor differences between coding systems. DSM-IV assigns dysthymia to code 300.4, while ICD-9-CM uses an older term, neurotic depression, for the same numeric code. Both diagnoses describe depressive syndromes more mild than major depressive disorder. Their differences reflect evolving conceptions of mental illness and nosology.

RISK ADJUSTMENT FOR STUDYING HEALTH CARE OUTCOMES OF PEOPLE WITH DISABILITIES

Lisa I. Iezzoni

When President George H. W. Bush signed the Americans with Disabilities Act (ADA, P.L. 101-336) on 26 July 1990, people with disabilities assumed the right, in Bush's words, to "pass through once-closed doors into a bright new era of equality, independence and freedom" (Young 1997, 231). Despite the ADA and other governmental mandates, however, people with disabilities are still often left behind, even by the health care delivery system. *Healthy People 2010*, which sets national health priorities, notes that 54 million Americans have disabilities; even so, misconceptions about them contribute to troubling health care lapses, especially an "underemphasis on health promotion and disease prevention activities" (U.S. DHHS 2000, 6–3). People with severe difficulty walking, for example, receive significantly fewer screening and preventive services, such as mammograms, Pap smears, and tobacco queries, than other people (Iezzoni et al. 2000a, 2001b). Women with disabilities are diagnosed with breast cancer at later stages than other women (Roetzheim and Chirikos 2002). Thus, "as a potentially underserved group, people with disabilities would be expected to experience disadvantages in health and well-being compared with the general population" (U.S. DHHS 2000, 6–5).

People with disabilities therefore represent a large subpopulation requiring further study. Most such studies will be observational (see Chapter 11). With relatively few exceptions, RCTs of medical treatments explicitly exclude persons with significant disabilities. Analyzing observational data generally requires risk adjustment, as noted throughout this book, but risk adjusting outcomes for persons with disabilities is complex, starting with fundamental questions about defining "disability." In addition, outcome studies of disabled persons must reach beyond standard medical concepts, such as the primacy of diagnosis and characteristics inextricably bound to individuals, to the role of societal and environmental factors.

This chapter introduces major issues raised in risk adjusting observational studies of people with disabilities. The examples focus on rehabilitation services, such as physical and occupational therapy. In certain contexts (e.g., following injuries or major joint-replacement surgery), short-term rehabilitation aims to restore persons to their baseline functioning. For most persons with long-standing disabilities, however, rehabilitation's goal shifts to maintaining baseline functioning or preventing its decline, as well as preventing secondary conditions, such as pressure ulcers.

Risk adjustment for reimbursing rehabilitation hospitalizations has received considerable attention, including the Functional Independence Measure (FIM) and function-related groups (FRG) (Stineman 1997; Stineman and Granger 1997; Stineman et al. 1994, 1996, 1997a, 1997b, 1997c; Deutsch, Braun, and Granger 1997). Starting in January 2002, CMS required IRFs to report clinical information using the IRF-Patient Assessment Instrument to risk adjust Medicare prospective payments to IRFs (CMS 2002a, 2002b). Although I touch on these measures, this chapter looks more broadly across outcomes and settings of care. Chapter 16 addresses topics relating to long-term care, including nursing homes, which sometimes provide rehabilitative services.

Defining Disability

Defining disability is complex, with multilayered personal, institutional, administrative, programmatic, and societal ramifications. Since the fourteenth century, disability has delineated categories of people meriting societal assistance—alms, food, shelter. However, "because physical and mental incapacity are conditions that can be feigned for secondary gain . . . , the concept of disability has always been based on a perceived need to detect deception" (Stone 1984, 23). Separating deserving from undeserving disabled persons fell to physicians and their theoretically objective medical evidence. The standard "medical model" of disability assumes that individuals "afflicted" with compromising health conditions must adapt their lives and expectations to their limitations.

Over the last half century, various definitions of disability have appeared for diverse purposes. Some definitions echo the traditional medical model, whereas others introduce a new concept: Disability results from social and physical environments that fail to accommodate persons with differing physical, sensory, cognitive, or emotional abilities. People are not disabled; society is (Shapiro 1994; Oliver 1996; Charlton 1998; Barnes, Mercer, and Shakespeare 1999; Williams 2001). This new "social model" spurred demands for accommodations to permit people with disabilities to participate fully in daily life throughout communities and workplaces.

Depending on the context, definitions of disability differ widely, as suggested by the following prominent examples:

- ADA, Section 3: "(A) a physical or mental impairment that substantially limits one or more of the major life activities . . . ; (B) a record of such impairment; or (C) being regarded as having such an impairment"

- The SSA (1998, 2), for determining adult eligibility for Social Security Disability Insurance (SSDI) or Supplemental Security Income (SSI): "the inability to engage in any substantial gainful activity by reason of any medically determinable physical or mental impairment(s) which can be expected to result in death or which has lasted or can be expected to last for a continuous period not less than 12 months"
- The WHO (2001, 3, 8) for the ICF: an "umbrella term for impairments, activity limitations or participation restrictions," conceiving "a person's functioning and disability . . . as a dynamic interaction between health conditions (diseases, disorders, injuries, traumas, etc.) and contextual factors," including environmental and personal attributes

Through recent court cases (e.g., *Sutton et al. v. United Air Lines, Inc.* and *Murphy v. United Parcel Service, Inc.* in 1999), the U.S. Supreme Court is constraining the ADA's reach, concentrating on delimiting "major life activities." In *Toyota Motor Manufacturing, Inc. v. Williams*, decided 8 January 2002, a unanimous court ruled against Ella Williams, who claimed that carpal tunnel syndrome prevented her from performing her job at a Toyota manufacturing plant. The justices argued that Ms. Williams was not "disabled" because she could still perform routine tasks at home, such as brushing her teeth and gardening, implicitly dismissing employment as a major life activity. (This decision prompted public groans from some celebrity wheelchair users who nonetheless still independently brush their teeth.) In the mid-1990s, the SSA considered fundamentally redesigning its disability definition for adults but abandoned this effort in 1999 partially because of its complexity. Instead, they refocused on improving current procedures (Wunderlich, Rice, and Amado 2002).

Semantic distinctions among disability definitions are sometimes elusive: "It is often difficult to communicate conceptual constructs within the same discipline, let alone across . . . professional fields, which may account for some of the misinterpretations that have been plaguing this area" (Pope and Tarlov 1991, 321). Nevertheless, at least among researchers, a general understanding now defines disability as difficulty conducting daily activities because of physical, sensory, cognitive, or emotional conditions interacting with barriers erected by the social and physical environments.

Disabling conditions are diverse in their causes, nature, timing, pace, and societal implications. Some are congenital; others are acquired. Some occur suddenly, with injury or accident; others arise slowly, with progressive chronic conditions. Some gradually limit but do not threaten life; others hasten death. Some are visible to outsiders; others are hidden. Some engender stigmatization and blame; others prompt pity and paternalism. Some are seen primarily as "diseases" (e.g., cancer, coronary artery disease, emphysema), although they can become profoundly disabling.

The stereotypical disabled person is someone rolling in a wheelchair or crossing a street tapping a white cane. However, in stating that 54 million

Americans have disabilities, *Healthy People 2010* took a broad view, encompassing myriad conditions. Among adults the most commonly reported disabling condition is difficulty walking, affecting about 19 million persons living in communities (Iezzoni et al. 2001a). The leading cause of these difficulties is arthritis, affecting about 25 percent, whereas another 13 percent blame back problems. If the prevalence of major chronic conditions remains unchanged, by the year 2049, the number of older Americans with functional limitations will rise by at least 311 percent (Boult et al. 1996, 1391). Arthritis, which affects roughly 55 percent of elderly people, will cause more physical impairments than ischemic heart disease, cancer, and dementia combined. However, large numbers of these people may not view themselves as disabled.

Being labeled as disabled depends on who is asked. Many people who are born deaf, for example, speak American Sign Language and do not view themselves as disabled; they participate fully within a distinct Deaf culture (Rockow 2001). According to the 1994–95 National Health Interview Survey–Disability Supplement, almost 20 percent of manual wheelchair users do not see themselves as disabled, although mainstream society probably does (Iezzoni et al. 2000b). While outsiders see a compromised life, people themselves disagree. Morris (1996, 62) interviewed a woman named Ruth Moore, whose spine was "crumbling," risking complete paralysis. Moore worried about her physicians' attitudes, observing:

> The neurosurgeon told me that he was only interested in quality of life and that in no way would he be looking to prolong my life if he didn't feel the quality would be acceptable. However, neither he nor anyone else has asked me what criteria *I* would use in judging what was an acceptable quality of life. I am very worried that if I get admitted unconscious or without the power of speech, he will take a decision based on *his* judgment and *his* criteria about what is an acceptable quality of life.

Finally, with civil rights came semantic sensitivities—so-called political correctness (Iezzoni 2003). Language matters. "Crippled," "lame," and "gimp" seem clearly out (unless people with disabilities use the words themselves), but what about "handicapped," "disabled," "impaired," or "physically challenged"? The phrases "confined to a wheelchair" or "wheelchair-bound" convey an image of being lashed into place—an inaccurate perception (wheelchair users do get out of their chairs). Some, for example, drive cars or ski mountainsides. The author Nancy Mairs, who uses a power wheelchair, does not view herself as immobile—the very trait prompting others to call her disabled. "Relaxed and focused, I feel emotionally far more 'up' than I generally did when I stood on two sound legs. . . . Certainly I am not mobility impaired; in fact, in my Quickie P100 with two twelve-volt batteries, I can shop till you drop at any mall you designate, I promise" (1996, 38, 39).

This discussion holds two important implications for observational studies of people with disabilities. First, clearly defining the population of interest, using precise descriptive language, is essential. The data source may constrain potential ways for defining persons with disabilities (see below). Second, findings will generalize only to populations defined using comparable criteria.

Risk Factors for Assessing Functional Outcomes

For studies of persons with disabilities, the answer to the question "risk of what?" often involves functional outcomes, including the extent to which people can perform daily activities. Risk adjusting rehabilitation outcomes is more difficult than risk adjusting outcomes of other services, such as ICU stays. In ICUs, clinicians typically control therapeutic interventions (e.g., intravenous medications, oxygen flow); these treatments are easily quantified and carefully calibrated to specific physiological indicators and the outcome is often obvious (e.g., mortality). In contrast, characterizing the rehabilitation intervention becomes difficult, especially outside institutional settings. Furthermore, outcomes depend on myriad factors, including not only patients' physical and cognitive abilities but also their underlying medical diseases, willingness to participate actively in their care, and supportive physical and social environments.

As described in Chapter 8, the first step in developing a risk-adjustment approach involves specifying conceptual models linking potential risk factors to pertinent outcomes. Here, the conceptual model must consider the chosen definition of disability. For example, the SSA's employment-centric disability definition locates all pertinent risk factors within the individual; it ignores the possibility of accommodations within a workplace. In contrast, the ICF's definition clearly recognizes that some risk factors belong to individuals, whereas other critical risk factors arise from the person's physical and social environments. This perspective encompasses a full range of risk factors (see Chapter 3).

Drawing from theoretical frameworks like the ICF, rehabilitation outcomes can range from the functioning of specific organs, structures, or body systems to the participation of persons within homes, social networks, and communities. Pertinent risk factors vary across outcomes. For example, a study whose outcome is the range of motion around a particular joint following an intervention must consider fewer risk factors than a study of posttreatment inability to perform daily activities.

Demographic Characteristics

Most risk-adjustment methods consider age and sex (see Chapter 3). Small changes in age may significantly affect pediatric outcomes, especially during infancy and early childhood. Even among elderly persons, older age is an important risk factor for functional dependence (Markello 1997). Younger stroke patients recover or return home significantly more often than do older patients (Oczkowski and Barreca 1993; Stineman et al. 1997d; Reker, O'Donnell, and Hamilton 1998; Marshall, Heisel, and Grinnell 1999). Age is less important for other outcomes. For instance, only 3 of 21 FIM-FRG impairment categories (stroke, nontraumatic brain, joint replacement) showed significant associations between age and inpatient LOS (Stineman et al. 1997b). Age bias can intervene. For example, when elderly patients have communication problems or appear unmotivated, "rehabilitation providers can easily find themselves on the slippery slope of providing less care to older persons" (Kramer 1997, JS49).

In general, women have higher rates of disabling conditions than men (Gill et al. 2001; Iezzoni et al. 2001a), but several studies have failed to find substantial associations between sex and future functional outcomes (Tinetti et al. 1995; Gill, Robison, and Tinetti 1997; Stineman et al. 1997d). Few valid causal hypotheses link race and ethnicity to rehabilitation outcomes. Tinetti and colleagues (1995), for example, found that black race was not significantly associated with future functional dependence among elderly patients. Evidence of racial disparities in treatment and quality of care raises troubling questions for risk adjustment (see Chapter 3). One study found that, even after adjusting for comorbidity and functional status, racial minorities were significantly less likely than whites to receive occupational or physical therapy (Mayer-Oakes et al. 1992), although another study of Medicare beneficiaries with stroke found no racial differences in inpatient rehabilitation services (Horner et al. 1997).

Physiological Status and Medical Diagnoses

People with disabling conditions are not necessarily "sick." Persons who are deaf or blind since early childhood, for example, may be in superb physical and mental health, requiring only routine, preventive care. Even if a specific etiology is found, whatever caused their deafness or blindness can carry few implications for their future health. Rehabilitation generally involves patients who are physiologically stable: Vital signs and internal organ function are controlled, without immediate risk of serious decompensation. Measures of physiological stability are therefore less relevant in most rehabilitation contexts, with possible exceptions of pulmonary or cardiac rehabilitation. Nevertheless, other standard medical measures, such as diagnoses, are potentially important risk factors.

In many instances, a medical disease, disorder, or condition underlies the impairment or functional limitation. In children or younger adults, single conditions predominate, while for late middle-aged and older adults, multiple coexisting conditions frequently produce the functional deficits. For instance, multiple diagnoses cause gait disorders among up to 75 percent of elderly persons (Alexander 1996). People may also have diagnoses that are truly comorbidities (i.e., unrelated to the debility) but could nonetheless compromise patients' abilities to respond to or participate in rehabilitation. Secondary conditions caused by the impairment or functional problem, such as decubitus ulcers, urinary tract infections, and incontinence, can also become risk factors.

Few argue that risks for most outcomes—from resource use to clinical events—differ by diagnosis. An exception is inpatient rehabilitation costs, which fail to track well with the standard, cost-based DRGs defined for general acute care hospitals (Langenbrunner et al. 1989; Wilkerson, Batavia, and DeJong 1992). Nevertheless, otherwise healthy patients with, for example, cerebral palsy would have very different outcomes, including long-term costs, than patients with hemispheric strokes. Furthermore, depending on the size and distribution of the cerebral infarction, stroke severity can range from limited motor difficulties to hemiparesis to compromised language and cognitive functioning. Not surprisingly, initial stroke severity is the most important predictor of subsequent outcomes (Alexander 1994).

Comorbid conditions are also potentially important risk factors. For someone undergoing rehabilitation for a spinal cord injury, for example, asthma and diabetes constitute comorbidities. Comorbid conditions can affect a person's ability to exercise or willingness to participate actively in rehabilitation. Some comorbidities could directly affect clinical outcomes. For instance, studies of cardiac rehabilitation outcomes should probably account for significant comorbid conditions, such as chronic pulmonary disease, peripheral vascular disease, or extensive degenerative joint disease. Cardiac rehabilitation studies should also consider important diagnoses that are potentially causally linked to the heart problem, such as diabetes, hypertension, and obesity, as well as the severity of the cardiac condition (e.g., left ventricular ejection fraction).

However, in some contexts, coexisting conditions are less important than the nature of the impairment or functional limitation itself. For example, in deriving Version 2.0 of the FIM-FRGs, Stineman and colleagues (1997b) found that including multiple diagnoses added little to predicting length of rehabilitation hospital stays, although their findings were limited by inadequacies of their coded diagnostic data. Another study found that, for persons with the most severe functional deficits, the number of comorbidities was not significantly associated with the risk of developing medical complications during inpatient rehabilitation (Siegler, Stineman, and Maislin 1994). In contrast, for persons with more mild functional impairments, comorbidities significantly predicted complications.

Cognitive Ability, Mental Health, and Sensory Functioning

Cognitive ability and mental health (e.g., depression, anxiety, fear) are potentially important risk factors for functional outcomes, for various reasons. For rehabilitation services requiring active understanding and participation by patients, both cognitive functioning and mental health can influence treatment intensity and adherence. In addition, these attributes may reflect debility in general and the likelihood of further progression. A review of 78 studies examining functional status declines among elderly persons living in the community found significant associations with cognitive impairment and depression (Stuck et al. 1999). Disorientation (to month, year, and address) and short-term memory loss are especially predictive of ADL dependence among older persons (Gill et al. 1997).

Depression and anxiety are significantly associated with functional dependence and secondary conditions, such as falls and incontinence (Tinetti et al. 1995), although the causal pathways may be circular: Depression and anxiety may produce functional dependence, which exacerbates depression and anxiety, and so on. Patients who are depressed or discouraged generally participate less actively in their care (Kane 1997). Since patients often enter rehabilitation following a terrifying event (an injury, stroke, fall), fear "may be as debilitating as the physical condition itself" (Kramer 1997, JS52). Although these mental health problems are important risk factors, they can often be treated effectively with medications; however, clinicians frequently neglect or avoid confronting these conditions among patients with disabling conditions. Consistent with broader societal stigmatization of both debility and mental health problems (Goffman 1963; Morris 1996; Cassell 1997; Thomson 1997), some clinicians may feel that depression is inevitable. Especially in studying outcomes for quality assessment, untreated mental health problems could represent not only risk factors, but also substandard care.

Cognitive and mental health factors are also important predictors of resource consumption in certain contexts. Cognitive FIM scores significantly predicted LOS for 5 of the 21 FIM-FRG impairment categories (stroke, traumatic brain, lower extremity fracture, joint replacement, and major multiple trauma with brain/spine injury) (Stineman et al. 1997b). Alzheimer's disease patients (virtually defined by impaired cognition) generate substantially lower costs to Medicare for the next year of care than do others (Ellis et al. 1996; Ash et al. 2000), perhaps because these persons receive fewer intensive services. Until 2002, Medicare generally refused to pay for rehabilitative services for Alzheimer's patients, arguing that they provided little benefit.

Sensory function—or dysfunction—could represent comorbid conditions (e.g., macular degeneration, age-related hearing loss). However, considering them separately highlights the importance of these often-neglected areas. For example, among persons age 65 and older, 23 percent of those without mobility difficulties reported having had vision tests, compared to 22 percent of those with major mobility problems (Iezzoni et al. 2000a). In this age group, however, 26 percent with major mobility problems had serious difficulty seeing, even using glasses or contact lenses, compared to only 5 percent without mobility problems.

Poor vision and hearing problems are major risk factors for falls and further functional declines (Tinetti et al. 1995; Cassel, Besdine, and Siegel 1999). A review of 78 studies found that visual deficits were strongly associated with functional declines among elderly persons living in communities (Stuck et al. 1999). Sensory difficulties may also contribute to mental-health-related risk factors: For example, hearing loss is associated with isolation, confusion, and depression among elderly patients (Lachs et al. 1990). Alone and together, vision and hearing deficits can precipitate communication problems with clinicians, sometimes contributing to therapists limiting care (Kramer 1997).

Sociocultural Factors, Preferences, and the Physical Environment

Especially once patients leave institutional settings, their social, home, and community environments and other personal factors will affect their rehabilitation outcomes. Among elderly patients, for example, social isolation significantly predicts future declines in functioning (Inouye et al. 1993). Higher education and strong social networks are closely linked to physical activity among elderly women (Walsh et al. 2001).

An extensive literature documents the association between worse functional status and socioeconomic disadvantage—poor education, poverty, lesser occupation (Pincus and Callahan 1985; Ross and Wu 1996; Lynch, Kaplan, and Shema 1997; Manton, Stallard, and Corder 1997; Liao et al. 1999; Breeze et al. 2001). Such attributes could also potentially affect a person's willingness and wherewithal to participate productively in rehabilitation. An hourly wage earner, for example, may be unable to attend daily therapy sessions. A sometimes vexing topic involves medicolegal considerations, such as whether an impairment relates to a job-related injury, potential workers' compensation claim, or motor vehicle accident. These issues may be relevant for risk adjustment in some situations.

Health beliefs, including patients' perceptions of control over their health outcomes, strongly influence patients' willingness to adhere to rehabilitation regimens (Merrill 1994; Chen et al. 1999). Patients' preferences and sociocultural attitudes are especially important in contexts involving assistive technologies, such as mobility aids (Gitlin, Luborsky, and Schemm 1998; Gitlin et al. 1996; Scherer 2000). Strongly held views of patients and their families influence patients' willingness to use devices, even when the potential benefits seem obvious to clinicians. Mobility and seating aids prompt particularly negative views, perhaps because they reflect, "in a tangible and objective fashion, the visible reality of the increased dependencies . . . and represent the personal need to adapt to functioning in public as an adult with impairments" (Gitlin, Luborsky, and Schemm 1998, 174).

Although certain factors are clearly linked to the targeted outcome, adjusting for them may prove inappropriate in particular contexts. For example, if people must participate actively in their rehabilitation regimen, motivation becomes a critical risk factor. However, in studies to assess quality of care, controlling for motivational level is controversial. Some argue that motivation is intrinsic to patients, whereas others believe the therapists' job is to instill motivation (Kane 1997). Motivation may also affect the outcomes of interest: For example, patients must be motivated to perform the daily activities regardless of their functional abilities (Lachs et al. 1990).

The physical environments where patients live and conduct their daily activities could significantly affect rehabilitation outcomes, especially disability and quality of life (Tabbarah, Silverstein, and Seeman 2000; Mitka 2001; Gitlin et al. 2001). Whether these environments physically accommodate persons with functional deficits and enhance their safety are key questions. Socioeconomic factors are intertwined, such as the financial wherewithal to renovate homes or move to more accessible surroundings. Personal preferences and other social forces, such as household composition and interpersonal relationships, influence the willingness to alter home environments to improve accessibility and safety (Moss 1997).

Functional Status, Disability, and Overall Health

Finally, prior functioning is the best predictor of future functioning. Therefore, appropriately, most studies of outcomes for people with disabilities use some measure of baseline functioning or more global performance (e.g., ADLs) as key risk factors. The literature on functional measures and measurement is extensive (see Chapter 3). Some approaches explicitly aim to predict specific outcomes (e.g., the FIM-FRGs predict rehabilitation hospital costs), whereas others are more generic. Measures for children may differ from those for adults (Dunbar and Diehl 1995; Haley, Dumas, and Ludlow 2001). Different clinical disciplines sometimes develop their own specific measures (e.g., functional measurement tools designed for rehabilitation nursing; Sarnecki et al. 1998; Ter Maat 1993).

Even theoretically "objective" measures of function vary by context. "Capability" indicates what persons "can do" in controlled settings, whereas "performance" assesses what a person "does do" in everyday life. Capability typically exceeds performance (Young et al. 1996). Primary care doctors frequently fail to assess accurately patients' functional limitations (Nelson et al. 1983; Calkins et al. 1991; Hoenig 1993).

This broad class of risk factors forces an important question: Whose perspective should drive this assessment, that of the patient or clinician? The answer depends on the context, especially since patients and clinicians may diverge in perceptions of functional states and their measurement (Batavia 1992; Stineman et al. 1998). Exploring this topic in depth is beyond my scope here; others have reviewed this issue at length (Lohr 1989, 1992; Gill and Feinstein 1994). Although many measures of impairment and functioning involve clinicians assessing patients, the patient's own voice is increasingly important. Patients and clinicians may hold very different views about rehabilitation and its role (Kersten et al. 2000).

Examining health-related quality of life, self-perceived activity limitations, and life satisfaction validates the perspective of the persons receiving rehabilitation (Whiteneck 1997). These measures distill the myriad social and environmental factors affecting disability into a specific and intrinsically meaningful metric—how persons with disabilities feel. People who perceive poor quality of life may be less motivated to participate actively in their care and less likely to do well, for diverse reasons. For many purposes, health-related quality of life may be the target outcome, as well as an important risk factor. Although "measures of patients' subjective well-being have been used only rarely to assess the outcomes of medical rehabilitation interventions . . . they are likely to increase in use" in future studies (Fuhrer 1997, JS59).

Administrative Data and Disability-Related Outcomes Research

Administrative databases do not link information about health conditions with insight into disability (e.g., performance of daily activities, participation in life situations, social and physical environmental barriers) (Iezzoni 2002). Most administrative data only report diagnoses and procedures. Certainly, some diagnoses allow inferences about potential physical disabilities (Table 15.1); mental health diagnoses, such as codes for schizophrenia or psychotic disorders, suggest potentially disabling conditions. Diagnoses alone, however, generally convey little about their effects on people's daily activities or the effect of social or physical environments. Administrative data reveal nothing about whether people view themselves as disabled.

These data can identify people meeting administrative definitions of disability, primarily persons eligible for Medicare and Medicaid through SSDI and SSI, respectively. These are important populations—almost 6.7 million persons in 2000—with significant health and health care concerns. However, findings from SSDI and SSI recipients may not generalize to other people with similar disabling conditions who, for whatever reason, have neither applied for nor qualified as disabled under Social Security. Nevertheless, administrative data permit certain insights that could produce useful research about people with disabilities. Findings require cautious interpretation, acknowledging important limitations in identifying study populations. Some health plans primarily or exclusively enroll people with significant functional limitations, although their populations typically represent small and nonrandom subsets of people with disabilities (Master et al. 1996; Riley 2000; Robinson and Karon 2000).

Enrollment and Eligibility

People enrolled in Medicare or Medicaid through SSDI or SSI, respectively, have fulfilled Social Security's disability criteria. Enrollment and most encounter databases note eligibility status. For adults, the SSA defines disability as the inability to perform "substantial gainful employment" because of "an impairment that results from anatomical, physiological, or psychologi-

TABLE 15.1
Examples of
ICD-9-CM
Codes
Representing
Physical
Functional
Impairments

Code	Description
7993	Debility, unspecified
438	Late effects of cerebrovascular disease
3420	Flaccid hemiplegia
3421	Spastic hemiplegia
3429	Hemiplegia, unspecified
3440	Quadriplegia
3441	Paraplegia
3442	Diplegia of upper limbs
3443	Monoplegia of lower limb
3444	Monoplegia of upper limb
34481	Other specified paralytic syndromes, locked-in state
3449	Paralysis, unspecified
34460	Cauda equina syndrome without mention of neurogenic bladder
34461	Cauda equina syndrome with neurogenic bladder
V440	Tracheostomy
V441	Gastrostomy
V460	Aspirator
V461	Dependence on respirator
V468	Other enabling machines
V469	Unspecified machine dependence
V538	Wheelchair

cal abnormalities which can be shown by medically acceptable clinical and laboratory diagnostic techniques" (SSA 1998, 3). Whether these criteria are applied consistently is debatable (U.S. General Accounting Office 1996; Kane 2000). While Social Security disability status conveys important information, researchers must use this variable carefully.

Employment is an irrelevant standard for children. Historically, the SSA's definitions of disability for children (leading to SSI eligibility) have been problematic. Until 1990, a restrictive medical definition, requiring children to have a disabling physical or mental disorder *per se* limited the number of children participating in SSI (Ettner et al. 2000). In their 1990 decision *Sullivan v. Zebley*, the U.S. Supreme Court required individual functional assessments for children who did not meet the medical definition. Around that time, the SSA expanded its list of qualifying mental impairments for children from 4 to 11 categories, including attention deficit hyperactivity disorder. The rolls of children with SSI have therefore varied widely over time (Perrin et al. 1998a; Ettner et al. 2000), leading to questions about the generalizability of populations identified by this label.

Depending on one's analytic goals, using SSDI and SSI to identify people with disabilities may be sufficient. Researchers may also seek information about the person's underlying disabling condition. The SSA retains information about the major medical reason for disability determinations and disseminates aggregated information. In 2000, for example, the most common reason was musculoskeletal problems (25 percent), followed by mental disorders (24 percent), circulatory conditions (12 percent), and cancer (10 percent) (Martin, Chin, and Harrison 2001). However, individual-level data about medical conditions are not available to researchers outside the SSA.

Using diagnoses on Medicare or Medicaid claims could yield reasonable inferences about the underlying medical condition, but this approach has limitations. Children qualifying for SSI because of mental retardation, for example, rarely generate claims specifically for mental-retardation-related services (Perrin et al. 1998a; see Chapter 13). For adults, identifying the disabling condition from among many disease codes may prove difficult. Another issue involves delays in Medicare eligibility: Adults qualifying for SSDI do not receive Medicare coverage until two years after first payment of SSDI cash benefits.[1] Medicare claims files do not contain services that people obtain during this waiting period. Because some people defer services during these two years (e.g., they cannot afford care), service use immediately upon qualifying for Medicare may be unusually high. Medicare beneficiaries age 65 years and older who entered Medicare at younger ages because of disability have 43 percent higher costs than otherwise comparable beneficiaries (Pope et al. 2000a, 106). Analyses of elderly Medicare beneficiaries should therefore consider "originally disabled" status.

Claims or Encounter Records

To produce claims or encounter records—and their associated diagnosis and procedure codes—people must first have health insurance. A nationwide survey in 2000 of persons age 16 and older with and without various disabilities found that both groups had comparable insurance rates, 90 percent and 89 percent, respectively (Harris Interactive 2000, 54). Once insured, services must be covered for claims to be filed. However, many important disability-related services are not covered, especially by private health plans and Medicare.

Disabled Medicare beneficiaries who were not also eligible for Medicaid and had two or more ADL limitations spent an average of $2,175 out-of-pocket for health care services in 1995 (Foote and Hogan 2001, 247). Many private health insurance policies exclude services for previously existing conditions for six months to a year (Pelka 1997, 147). Private plans generally set annual limits on mental health services (Gitterman, Sturm, and Scheffler 2001). Physical, speech-language, and occupational therapy are typically restricted to restoring persons to baseline functioning, rather than long-term maintenance or preventing functional declines. Commercial insurers "combine variations in cost sharing in myriad ways with variation in coverage, including or excluding physical therapy, rehabilitation, mental health, . . . and durable medical equipment" (Robinson 1999, 54).

Medicare explicitly excludes coverage for "any services that are not reasonable and necessary for the . . . diagnosis or treatment of illness or injury or to improve the functioning of a malformed body member" (42 C.F.R. Sec. 411.15[k]). This medical necessity criterion especially limits reimbursement for assistive devices: "In many cases, assistive technologies instrumental to maintaining an independent lifestyle and often essential to preventing secondary conditions do not satisfy the criteria on the Medicare screening list for durable medical equipment [DME]" (Pope and Tarlov 1991, 257). Medicare does not cover glasses or hearing aids (Cassel, Besdine, and Siegel 1999; MedPAC 2002c, 10), and it severely restricts other DME coverage by setting of use. In a nationwide survey, 28 percent of insured people with disabilities reported they had special needs (for particular therapies, equipment, medications) that were not covered by their health plan, compared to 7 percent of those without disabilities (Harris Interactive 2000, 56, 57). Thus, the services represented by claims or encounter records do not reflect fully the health needs of people with disabilities. To interpret results from administrative databases, researchers must appreciate the implications of health insurance coverage policies. Obviously, services obtained from outside sources are not included in health insurance databases.

Diagnosis Codes

Table 15.1 shows examples of ICD-9-CM codes representing physical functional impairments; numerous other codes depict low vision and deafness, mental retardation, cognitive impairments, mental illnesses, medical diseases, and other conditions underlying disability. Creative combinations of ICD-9-CM codes produce suggestive clinical stories, such as the following:

> A person with multiple sclerosis (code 340) has weakness of the legs (code 344.9, "paralysis unspecified"), which is a "condition influencing their health status" (code V49.2, "motor problems with limbs"). The person uses a wheelchair (code V53.8), has an inaccessible home (V60.1, "inadequate housing"), and is unemployed (V62.0).

Health services research studies have used diagnosis codes from claims, especially for chronic and disabling conditions, to identify persons at risk for high future costs of care (Kronick, Zhou, Dreyfus 1995; Kronick et al. 1996, 2000; Ellis et al. 1996; Iezzoni et al. 1998; Ash et al. 2000; Pope et al. 2000a). These methods are now used by Medicare and several Medicaid programs to risk adjust capitation payments (Greenwald 2000; Kronick et al. 2000; Iezzoni et al. 1998; Pope et al. 2000a).

By definition, however, diagnosis codes in administrative databases do not aim to tell stories, but rather to generate reimbursement. In particular, V codes, a potential source of insight about both disabling conditions and environmental barriers (e.g., inadequate housing), are coded infrequently. Insurers rarely pay based on V codes.[2] ICD-9-CM codes present special challenges for identifying disability. Codes for individual medical diagnoses reveal little about the severity or extent of the condition or its pace of progression. Code 340, for example, indicates multiple sclerosis but tells nothing about neurological signs or symptoms or whether the disease is in remission or advancing rapidly. Certainly, additional (secondary) diagnoses supply more details about neurological impairments (e.g., optic neuritis, "paralysis"), but physicians rarely code more than one diagnosis for outpatient visits. Incomplete coding is especially problematic for people with chronic conditions, as discussed in Chapter 5.

Although the ICF (WHO 2001) classifies functional abilities and social and environmental contexts, this coding scheme is rarely used in the United States. The WHO views the ICF as complementing ICD-9-CM—each classification offers insight into different aspects of health. Briefly, the ICF groups its alphanumeric codes into 30 chapters under four broad headings: body functions (physiological functions, including cognitive and psychological functions), body structures (anatomical parts of the body, such as organs, limbs, and their components), activities (execution of tasks or actions by individuals) and participation (involvement in life situations), and environmental factors (the physical, social, and attitudinal environment in which people live and conduct daily life). Qualifiers to ICF codes indicate the extent or magnitude of an impairment in body function or structure (from no impairment to complete impairment) and the difficulty experienced in executing activities or participating in life situations (from no difficulty to complete difficulty). Environmental factors may serve as either a barrier or facilitator, with a scale from none to complete.

A short vignette demonstrates how ICF codes, alongside diagnosis and procedure codes, can portray complex clinical scenarios and potentially enhance considerably the information retrievable from administrative databases (Iezzoni and Greenberg, in press[3,4]).

> Mr. Barnard, in his mid-40s, was diagnosed with multiple sclerosis (MS) (ICD-9-CM 340) several years ago. He now has increasing difficulty walking (ICD-9-CM 719.7, ICF d4509.3), but he can move around with only mild difficulty (ICF d465.1) using a motorized scooter (ICF e1201.+3). He retired from his job as a school bus driver (ICF d8452) and has recently qualified for Social Security Disability Insurance (ICF e5700.+4). Mr. Barnard's health insurance has lapsed (ICF e5650.4), and he cannot yet receive Medicare. He is having trouble paying for his medication (ICF d870.2), including drugs for his MS, for his hypertension (ICD-9-CM 401.9) and elevated cholesterol (ICD-9-CM 272.9). MS has also extremely affected his vision, impeding him from reading newspapers or books (ICD-9-CM 369.9, ICF b210.3, d920.4). He lives alone in a two-story house, spends much of his day watching television, and frequently feels sad (ICD-9-CM 311, ICF b152.3). He feels cut off from his old friends (ICF d7500.4).

Procedure Codes, DME, and Outpatient Pharmacy

Some procedures imply debility or potentially disabling physical impairments, such as amputation of a limb, hip arthroplasty, knee replacement, transplantation of a major organ, insertion of a tracheostomy tube (for long-term mechanical ventilation), or placement of a gastrostomy tube (for feeding). Certain treatments, like chemotherapy or radiation therapy, also suggest potentially disabling conditions. People receiving such interventions often generate high health care costs, reflecting considerable need for services (Pope et al. 2000b).

Medicare, Medicaid, and private insurers generally pay for acute care services without demur. Therefore, administrative databases should represent virtually all procedures or treatments obtained within a given time period. However, relying on procedure codes to identify people with disabilities raises important questions. First, people receiving these procedures are a nonrandom subset of all people with disabling conditions. Second, even for potentially life-prolonging interventions (e.g., gastrostomy tube placement), significant variations in procedure use are likely because of differing preferences for care, practice styles, and availability of services across patients, physicians, institutions, and geographical regions.

Third, people may have received the service prior to the time period covered by the administrative database. Although certain V codes (ICD-9-CM diagnoses) indicate selected prior procedures (e.g., "transplant status"), pertinent V codes are not always listed. Fourth, restrictive payment policies limiting physical, speech-language, or occupational therapy mean that only certain people receive these services; drawing inferences about disability based on the presence or absence of these interventions is problematic. Fifth, the presence of procedure codes reveals little about outcomes—whether the intervention improved functioning. A knee replacement, for example, may eliminate a patient's mobility difficulties and hence potential disability.

DME frequently compensates for or ameliorates functional limitations and can prolong life (Iezzoni 2003). Examples include supplemental oxygen, mechanical ventilation devices, parenteral and enteral nutrition supplies, limb prostheses, wheelchairs, walkers, and hospital beds. For Medicare, the most common single category of DME is wheelchairs, obtained by 2.7 percent of beneficiaries in 1996 (Pope et al. 2000b, 6-4). DME use provides the quintessential visible symbol of disability, at least from a societal perspective.

Identifying people with disabilities by DME claims, however, raises questions. Most importantly, as noted above, restrictive coverage policies mean that paid claims for DME (especially mobility aids) represent only a fraction of need. Medicare and private insurers often reimburse certain DME only in limited circumstances (e.g., homebound patients). In addition, as for procedure codes, DME use varies significantly based on differing personal preferences and practice styles. People may have obtained DME in a prior time period; V codes (e.g., indicating wheelchair use) are listed sporadically. Although claims for DME offer useful information, they identify only selected people with potentially disabling conditions.

As noted in Chapter 5, administrative databases from Medicaid, the VA, and private insurers offering prescription drug benefits contain outpatient pharmacy claims. Pharmacy data help identify people with specific conditions, such as diabetes, bipolar disorder, asthma, and AIDS (Fishman and Shay 1999; Lamers 1999; Gilmer et al. 2001). They suggest the severity of medical conditions: For example, people receiving insulin presumably have more refractory diabetes mellitus than those using oral hypoglycemic agents. Certain drugs suggest the pace of illness or the course of disease: For instance, multiple sclerosis patients prescribed interferon-beta probably have relapsing-remitting rather than secondary progressive disease. However, pharmacy data raise identical cautions as do procedure and DME codes. They identify selected subgroups of people, varying practice patterns compromise the generalizability of findings, and prescriptions not covered by insurance plans escape detection.

Merging administrative data with other data sources can significantly enhance the analytical utility of these files for disability-related research, as discussed in Chapter 5 (Iezzoni 2002). For example, the longitudinal MCBS contains questions that can create disability indicators (Table 15.2). The MCBS oversamples Medicare beneficiaries under age 65 and contains weights to produce national estimates. Table 15.3 shows population estimates of the numbers of Medicare beneficiaries nationwide with the disabling conditions defined on Table 15.2, using 1996 MCBS information.

Conclusions

Relatively few outcomes studies have considered persons with disabilities. Nevertheless, a small literature highlights worrisome disparities in the services they receive compared to the health care experiences of people without disabling conditions. Conducting research involving this important and growing subpopulation is therefore essential. The next 50 years will witness a threefold increase in the number of Americans with functional limitations, particularly among elderly persons. Importantly, even younger persons with substantial physical impairments, such as paraplegia or quadriplegia from spinal cord injury, are now living long, productive, and healthy lives. However, efforts to conduct this research confront significant challenges, starting with simply identifying persons with disabilities. Increasing the availability of data on functional status and social and environmental barriers will enhance opportunities to study the health care outcomes of persons with disabilities.

Notes

1. The one exception involves amyotrophic lateral sclerosis patients, who since 2001 immediately qualify for Medicare upon receiving SSDI. Many

TABLE 15.2
Using
Questions and
Responses from
the MCBS to
Define
Disabling
Conditions

Disability	Questions and Responses form the MCBS
Vision	"Do you wear eyeglasses or contact lenses?" (yes, no, blind)
	"Which statement best describes your vision (wearing glasses/contact lenses)?"
Blind	"Blind" on eyeglasses/contact lens question
Very low vision	"A lot of trouble" on vision question
Hearing	"Do you use a hearing aid?" (yes, no, deaf)
	Which statement best describes your hearing (even with a hearing aid)?"
Deaf/very hard of hearing	"Deaf" on hearing aid question OR "a lot of trouble" on hearing question
Hard of hearing	Uses hearing aid or has "a little trouble" hearing
Walking	"How much difficulty do you have walking a quarter of a mile (2 or 3 blocks)?"
	"Because of a health or physical problem, do you have any difficulty walking by yourself and without special equipment?"
Major difficulties	"Unable to walk 2–3 blocks" OR "Doesn't walk" by self without special equipment
Moderate difficulties	"A lot of difficulty" walking 2–3 blocks OR "difficulty" walking by self without equipment
Reaching overhead	"How much difficulty do you have reaching or extending your arms above shoulder level?"
Major difficulties	Reports being "unable to do" or having "a lot" of difficulty reaching
Moderate difficulties	Reports "some" difficulty reaching
Grasping and writing	"How much difficulty do you have either writing or handling and grasping small objects?"
Major difficulties	Reports being "unable to do" or having "a lot" of difficulty with hands
Moderate difficulties	Reports "some" difficulty with hands

SOURCE: Adapted from 1996 MCBS (Iezzoni et al. 2002).

amyotrophic lateral sclerosis patients had died or become significantly impaired during the two-year wait.

2. Exceptions include V581, maintenance chemotherapy, and V580, radiotherapy session, which must accompany hospital claims for these services.

3. The paper was prepared for *Health Care Financing Review*, which is publishing a special issue on measuring and classifying functional status. This issue will contain considerable detail about the ICF. Donna Pickett and Paul Placek, from NCHS, assigned the ICD-9-CM and ICF codes to the case scenario.

Disabling condition	All	Age in Years: Population Estimates, Millions (population %)[a]	
		<65	65+
All beneficiaries regardless of presence of disabling condition[b]	33.58	3.67	29.91
Vision			
Blind	0.21 (0.6)	0.04 (1.2)	0.17 (0.6)
Very low vision	2.88 (8.6)	0.45 (12.3)	2.43 (8.1)
Hearing			
Deaf/very hard of hearing	2.43 (7.2)	0.22 (6.1)	2.20 (7.4)
Hard of hearing	12.41 (37.0)	0.91 (24.9)	11.50 (38.5)
Walking			
Major difficulties	4.97 (14.8)	0.85 (23.0)	4.12 (13.8)
Moderate difficulties	5.17 (15.4)	0.97 (26.5)	4.20 (14.1)
Reaching overhead			
Major difficulties	2.94 (8.8)	0.73 (19.4)	2.24 (7.5)
Moderate difficulties	2.60 (7.8)	0.51 (13.5)	2.10 (7.0)
Grasping and writing			
Major difficulties	2.06 (6.1)	0.45 (12.1)	1.61 (5.4)
Moderate difficulties	2.50 (7.5)	0.54 (14.8)	1.96 (6.6)

TABLE 15.3

Medicare Population Estimates of Disabling Conditions by Age Using Disability Definitions from Table 15.2

DATA SOURCE: 1996 MCBS.

[a]Reweighted population estimates for Medicare beneficiaries, excluding those qualifying because of end-stage renal disease.

[b]11.3 percent of Medicare beneficiaries were under age 65.

4. ICF d4509.3 = walking, unspecified, severe difficulty; ICF d465.1 = moving around using equipment, mild difficulty; ICF e1201.+3 = assistive product and technology for personal indoor and outdoor mobility and transportation, substantial facilitator; ICF d8452 = terminating a job; ICF e5700.+4 = social security services, complete facilitator; ICF e5650.4 = economic services, complete barrier; ICF d870.2 = economic self-sufficiency, moderate difficulty; ICF b210.3 = seeing functions, severe impairment; ICF d920.4 = recreation and leisure, complete difficulty; ICF b152.3 = emotional functions, severe impairment; ICF d7500.4 = informal relationships with friends, complete difficulty.

RISK ADJUSTMENT FOR STUDYING LONG-TERM CARE

Dan Berlowitz and Amy K. Rosen

Long-term care consists of "an array of health care, personal care, and social services generally provided over a sustained period of time to persons with chronic conditions and with functional limitations" (Institute of Medicine 2001d, 27). For many patients, it represents one end of the care spectrum that begins with acute care for a new condition, transitions to postacute care for ongoing treatment and rehabilitation, and ends with long-term care for any remaining impairment or disability (Kramer 2002). While informal caregivers such as family and friends provide substantial amounts of long-term care, public and private institutions and organizations also play essential roles. Long-term-care settings include nursing homes, community-based residential care, and assisted living facilities, as well as people's homes through home health and hospice care agencies. These settings, however, may also provide other types of care, especially postacute care. Understanding and improving care provided in these myriad settings is increasingly important to consumers, regulators, managers, and clinicians. Many audiences therefore seek information requiring risk-adjustment methods specific to long-term care.

The rationale and basic framework for risk adjustment in long-term care parallel those in other care settings. Risk adjustment for long-term care, however, raises important conceptual and methodological issues that differ from those in acute and routine outpatient care. Here, we examine risk adjustment for long-term care, emphasizing how it differs from other health care settings. We also describe current applications of risk adjustment to quality improvement. Our examples primarily involve nursing homes and home health care, the two settings that have received the greatest attention. Risk adjustment for other long-term-care settings and populations needs much more development, although many of the same methodological issues apply. Relevant outcomes and predictors of these outcomes will likely differ for hospice care or when examining children receiving long-term care.

Impetus for Long-Term-Care Risk Adjustment

Interest in long-term-care risk adjustment has grown recently, reflecting the convergence of three forces: the aging population and increased demand for long-term care, concerns about costs of long-term care and refining payment policies, and persistent questions about quality of care.

Among people aged 18 and over in 1994, approximately 9 million used formal or informal long-term care (Spector et al. 1998). Frail elderly persons constitute the majority of these long-term-care users. As the baby boomers age, elderly persons have become the fastest-growing segment of the U.S. population. The number of people aged 85 and over, the "oldest old," is projected to increase from 4.2 million in 2000 to 5.8 million in 2010. Assuming no changes in age-specific rates of disability, the demand for long-term-care services should soar. The Congressional Budget Office projects that the nursing home population, now totaling approximately 1.6 million residents, will increase 50 percent between 1990 and 2010, double by 2030, and triple by 2050 (Binstock and Spector 1997). Smaller families and growing rates of childlessness will likely decrease the pool of informal caregivers in future decades, increasing reliance on formal providers (Wolf 2001). A detailed understanding of the aging population and its expected health care needs will be critical to managing what will likely be increasingly scarce long-term-care resources.

As demand for long-term care escalates, expenditures will rapidly increase. Home health care expenditures, which totaled $32.4 billion in 2000 ($9.2 billion through Medicare and $6 billion through Medicaid), are projected to more than double to $70.8 billion by 2011. In 2000, nursing home expenditures totaled $92.2 billion ($9.5 billion from Medicare and $44.4 billion from Medicaid) and are expected to rise to $166.4 billion by 2011 (Heffler et al. 2002; CMS 2002e).

To promote efficiency and control costs, long-term care has pursued various payment strategies, including risk adjustment (Table 16.1). Prospective payment for Medicare beneficiaries in nursing homes began in 1998, and most state Medicaid programs now use prospective or mixed (combined prospective and retrospective) reimbursement systems (Chen and Shea 2002; Fries 1990). Medicare currently risk adjusts nursing home payments using RUG III (Fries et al. 1994). Medicare's prospective payment system for home care, HHRG, was implemented in 2001 (CMS 2002a). Central to both prospective payment systems are risk-adjustment methods that allocate resources to providers based on the clinical characteristics of patients. Providers caring for sicker patient populations receive higher payments, thereby providing an incentive to care for those patients requiring the most resources. However, this may generate potentially complex incentives. For example, these payment approaches could reward poor quality by paying more for patients whose functional status declines because of inadequate care (Butler and Schlenker 1989). Whether these reimbursement systems will maintain quality, ensure access, and reduce costs remains uncertain (Chen and Shea 2002).

Concerns about quality of long-term care will only grow as resource constraints persist. In 1986, a landmark report from the Institute of Medicine,

Method	Payment Episode	No. of Groups	Description
RUGs III	Day	44	Assigns patient to one of seven categories: • Special rehabilitation • Extensive services (e.g., ventilatory support, parenteral feeding) • Special care (e.g., quadriplegia, pressure ulcer, tube feeding) • Clinically complex (e.g., oxygen therapy, chemotherapy, terminal illness) • Impared cognition (impaired short-term memory, decision making, orientation) • Behavioral problem (daily inappropriate behavior) • Reduced physical functions (high ADL dependence) Additional subdivisions based on ADL deficits, depression, receipt of nursing rehabilitation
HHRGs	60 days	80	Scores patients on each of three domains: • Clinical severity (four levels) including diagnoses, wounds, elimination patterns, intravenous therapy • Fuctional status (five levels) including six ADLs • Service utilization (four levels) including recent hospitalization or rehabilitation

TABLE 16.1

Medicare's Methods for Risk Adjusting Nursing Home and Home Health Care Payments

Improving the Quality of Care in Nursing Homes, motivated the major regulatory reforms of the Omnibus Budget Reconciliation Act of 1987. Since then, nursing home practices have changed significantly, and studies have demonstrated some improvement in the quality of care (Institute of Medicine 2001d; Berlowitz et al. 2000; Hawes et al. 1997). Yet, questions remain about nursing home quality, fueled by well-publicized cases of flagrant abuse and governmental investigations (U.S. General Accounting Office 1998, 1999b). Quality problems have also been identified in home health care, where the lack of oversight of health workers is particularly worrisome (Jette, Smith, and McDermott 1996). Work force concerns, such as problems recruiting and retaining employees who often receive low wages, overlie worries about quality of nursing home and home health care.

Performance monitoring based on valid, reliable, and timely data is widely viewed as central to efforts to assess and improve the quality of long-term care (Institute of Medicine 2001d). As in other settings, risk adjustment is an essential component of many quality measures. Studies have demonstrated that clinically and statistically credible risk-adjustment methods can be developed for long-term care, that different providers see very different populations of patients, and that risk adjustment alters judgments of provider performance (Berlowitz et al. 1996a; Mukamel 1997; Arling et al. 1997; Mukamel and Brower 1998; Porell and Caro 1998; Rosen et al. 2001b). Risk adjustment is also important to determine whether efforts to improve the quality of long-term care are succeeding (Berlowitz et al. 2001a). Changes in the long-term-care population over time may complicate efforts to determine whether improvements in outcomes are due to improved care or differences in patient mix. Thus, risk adjustment is necessary to evaluate temporal trends in care.

Data for Risk Adjustment in Long-Term Care

As in other settings, data for risk adjustment in long-term care come from various sources, including administrative databases, medical records, and patients' reports. However, as noted in Chapter 5, "administrative" databases in long-term care settings, particularly those reimbursed by Medicare and Medicaid, offer much richer clinical insight than standard, ICD-9-CM code–based acute care hospital or outpatient data sets (Berlowitz, Brandeis, and Moskowitz 1997). Much of the risk-adjustment work in long-term care has relied on these specialized administrative databases, which have often followed congressional mandate, starting with the MDS requirements within the 1987 Omnibus Budget Reconciliation Act. The 1997 Balanced Budget Act carried significant new ramifications for data reporting and documentation prompted by fundamental changes in payment policies, notably implementing prospective payment for home health agencies and skilled nursing facilities, as well as rehabilitation (see Chapter 15) and long-term-care hospitals (see Table 1.1). In particular, as shown in Table 16.2, Medicare currently requires the following:

1. The MDS, conceived in response to the 1987 Omnibus Budget Reconciliation Act; it is collected using the Resident Assessment Instrument administered quarterly in nursing homes; with more than 300 items, it includes cognitive and sensory function, mood and behavior, physical functioning, performance of daily activities, and other health factors (Morris et al. 1990; Morris, Murphy, and Nonemaker 1995). MDS is the basis for calculating nursing home prospective payment using RUG III (Fries et al. 1994; Swan and Newcomer 2000); and
2. The OASIS, collected during home health care visits (more than 100 items); it includes living arrangements, supportive assistance, sensory and physical functioning, emotional and behavioral status, equipment management, and other factors (Shaughnessy, Schlenker, and Hittle 1995; Shaughnessy et al. 1997, 2002; HCFA 1997). OASIS is the basis for calculating home care prospective payment using HHRG.

Long-term-care databases are structured very differently from hospital databases because they must account for patients receiving care over extended periods. Administrative databases for acute care hospitalizations capture all information about particular hospitalizations (e.g., admission and discharge dates, discharge diagnoses, discharge disposition) in the associated record. In contrast, long-term-care databases are typically cross-sectional, describing patients' status on specific dates or events. Individual records in a long-term-care administrative database generally do not reflect a patient's entire experience over time.

The content of long-term-care databases also differs from those data sets relying exclusively on ICD-9-CM diagnosis codes. As suggested above, long-term-care databases generally provide a more comprehensive picture of patients' clinical situations, often with detailed descriptions of their abilities to perform ADL. Databases compiled from MDS and OASIS may contain dozens of clinical indicators; however, information on diagnoses and procedures may be limited. Relying on assessments by care providers of patients' functional status raises questions about the accuracy and reliability of the data. While some reports question the quality of MDS data in nursing homes (MedPAC 2001; U.S. General Accounting Office 2002), others argue that data reliability is well established (Berg et al. 2002; Morris et al. 1990, 1997; Hawes et al. 1995). More information on data accuracy is necessary to assess the credibility of these data sets.

Regulatory Monitoring and Reimbursement

Databases used for risk adjustment in long-term care have been developed for two primary purposes. The first purpose is regulatory monitoring and reimbursement. As shown in Table 16.2, these include databases created by the VA and New York state for RUG II (Schneider et al. 1988), a predecessor of RUG III, and the national On-Line Survey and Certification Assessment Reporting System (OSCAR). These particular databases typically include limited clinical information. Furthermore, OSCAR contains facility-level data rather than information on individual residents. Studies using OSCAR to examine the association of provider characteristics and risk-adjusted outcomes must rely on facility-level variables describing patient characteristics and outcomes. Examples include investigations that have adjusted prevalence rates of pressure ulcers (Zinn, Aaronson, and Rosko 1993) or institutional deficiency citations by a regulatory oversight body (Harrington et al. 2001) in nursing homes by the percentage of residents with dependent ADL and rates of antipsychotic medication use by dementia or psychiatric diagnoses (Hughes, Lapane, and Mor 2000).

Using facility-level data like OSCAR for risk adjustment may sometimes bias conclusions, a situation analogous to the ecological fallacy in epidemiological research. For example, in one study, rankings of nursing homes on their risk-adjusted pressure ulcer rate differed depending on whether patient-level data were used or whether these same data were first combined into facility-level measures (Fries, Morris, and Skarupski 1998). Additionally, many

TABLE 16.2

Databases Used in Long-Term Care Risk Adjustment

Database	Source	Purpose	Frequency of Assessment
RUGs II	VA, New York state	Nursing home reimbursements	Admission/semiannual
OSCAR	CMS	Storage of survey and certification data on nursing homes	Approximately annually
MDS	CMS	Uniform clinical assessments of nursing home residents	Admission, every 90 days, or with significant change in status
OASIS	CMS	Outcome-based quality improvement	Admission, every 60 days, and discharge

concerns arise regarding the quality of OSCAR data (Ray 2000). Thus, facility-level data on patient outcomes and risk factors from OSCAR will probably be increasingly supplanted by MDS data, although institutional characteristics from OSCAR will remain useful.

Clinical Management, Quality Assessment, and Improvement

The second reason for developing long-term-care databases is to assist clinical management, quality assessment, and improvement efforts (Table 16.2). These databases usually contain the detailed clinical information necessary for managing and evaluating patients' outcomes. The MDS was developed specifically to ensure uniform resident assessment systems in nursing homes as mandated in the 1987 Omnibus Budget Reconciliation Act; it is required for all residents of nursing homes receiving Medicare or Medicaid reimbursement (Morris et al. 1990). Data on MDS assessments are routinely transmitted to CMS. MDS information is sufficiently detailed to allow the development of complex risk-adjustment models (Berlowitz et al. 2001b; Berg et al. 2002).

In contrast, for home care, OASIS was not designed to improve the assessment process. Instead, from the outset, OASIS aimed to support a reporting system that could inform outcome-based quality improvement (Shaughnessy, Crisler, and Schlenker 1998; Shaughnessy et al. 2002). Initial design of OASIS anticipated developing risk-adjustment methods to assist outcome comparisons.

Given their cross-sectional structure, a strength of long-term-care databases is their ability to detect changes in health status over time by linking

Unit of Assessment	Assessors	Data Elements	Limitations
Patient	Clinical staff	ADLs, behavior problems, selected diagnoses, treatments	Clinical content limited Data accuracy uncertain Many patients lost to follow-up because of long interval between assessments
Nursing home	State surveyors	Facilities characteristics, resident characteristics, staffing levels, survey deficiencies, complaints	No data on individual patients Data accuracy uncertain "Gaming" at time of nursing home survey
Patient	Clinical staff	300 data elements covering 15 clinical domains including ADLs, diagnoses, and cognitive patterns	Data accuracy uncertain Currently limited availability
Patient	Clinical staff	107 items including history, clinical status, and ADLs	Data accuracy uncertain Currently limited availability

multiple records for individual patients. Thus, within a given time period, an index assessment describes baseline status for specific patients, which can then be linked to later (outcome) assessments; the outcome assessments may serve as the index assessment for a subsequent time period (Figure 16.1). Changes in health status between the index and outcome assessments may then be used as outcome events in developing risk-adjustment models, with characteristics from the index assessment serving as predictor variables (i.e., risk factors). Examples include occurrence of a pressure ulcer in patients without previous ulcers, changes in ADL function, and development of contractures (Arling et al. 1997; Berlowitz et al. 1996a; Mukamel 1997; Shaughnessy et al. 2002).

In calculating rates for these "change" events, some cases are inevitably missed. For example, pressure ulcers are not counted if they develop and then heal or the patient is discharged before the next cross-sectional assessment. Thus, these rates are not "true" incidence rates, although this term is commonly used.

Each database described above is useful for examining risk-adjusted outcomes in nursing homes or home health care settings. However, linking several databases offers important benefits (Lipowski and Bigelow 1996). Numerous studies have combined OSCAR with MDS data, allowing the examination of facility characteristics associated with risk-adjusted outcomes. A noteworthy example is the Systematic Assessment of Geriatric Drug Use via Epidemiology (SAGE) database that not only has MDS and OSCAR data but also has combined this with information on medications and Medicare utilization

FIGURE 16.1

Using Cross-Sectional Assessments from Specific Dates as Index and Outcome Data Sources when Monitoring Changes in Health Status

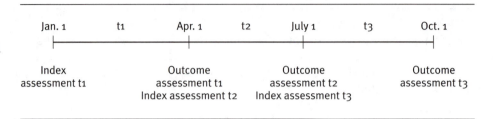

(Bernabei et al. 1999). Medication data could provide additional details on comorbidities and disease severity for risk-adjustment models.

Outcome Measures

As noted throughout this book, a fundamental first question in defining risk requires specifying the outcome: Risk of what? Because of prospective payment, perhaps dollars are the best-known outcome for nursing home and home health care risk adjustment. Both RUG and HHRG use payment levels to define risk. However, as elsewhere in health care, using clinical outcomes to judge quality is important for long-term-care services (Kane 1998).

No global outcome measure captures all aspects of long-term care. Nevertheless, the detailed clinical and functional status information contained in patient-level long-term-care databases permits construction of various outcome measures that can provide a broader view of quality than is generally possible with other administrative data sources, such as acute care hospital discharge abstract files. These include functional status change, continence, pressure ulcers, dehydration, contractures, and falls. Good performance on one of these outcome measures does not necessarily guarantee good performance on other measures, emphasizing the need to examine multiple outcomes (Mukamel 1997).

Although the use of multiple outcome measures is desirable, the specific outcomes must be tailored to the unique situation of the population and setting being studied. Outcomes relevant to the frail elderly may not be appropriate for children receiving long-term care for chronic disabilities. Special considerations arise when measuring the quality of end-of-life care, where patient preferences and expectations are central (Donaldson and Field 1998). Satisfaction may be a useful outcome measure for many long-term-care patients, but it is difficult to capture in populations with high degrees of cognitive impairment. Screening tools do exist to identify nursing home patients able to participate in satisfaction surveys (Simmons et al. 1997), and studies examining the quality of nursing home care have used satisfaction as an outcome measure (Schnelle et al. 1999). Mortality, which is widely used to evaluate acute hospital care, may be less relevant for long-term-care settings and in particular hospice care; death often represents the final stages of disease progression and not the quality of care. Ideally, studies using mortality as an outcome would also incorporate other clinical outcomes as well as patient preferences.

Even when examining the same construct, selecting relevant outcome measures depends on the long-term-care setting. Functional decline is often studied in nursing homes, whereas home care typically considers improvement. The literature offers little consensus on these choices. One study identified six different definitions of ADL decline in nursing home residents that have been used in research projects (Rosen et al. 1999). The percentage of patients declining and judgments of facility performance varied considerably depending on which of these definitions was used.

As described in Chapter 8, empirical derivation of risk-adjustment methods often involves regressing outcomes on various predictor variables or risk factors. This requires clearly specifying the outcome measures. However, constructing long-term-care outcome indicators can be difficult, with little consensus about specific definitions. For example, analysts have used both incidence and prevalence rates of pressure ulcers as outcome measures. Prevalence rates are generally easier to calculate and comprehend. However, they may include cases in which the condition developed outside long-term-care settings so they do not represent current quality of care.

Functional status is usually described by ADL or IADL. Each activity measure, such as dependence in toileting, eating, or walking, may be examined individually, or they may be combined into an overall index. Change in ADL or IADL can be viewed as continuous variables or by setting some dichotomous threshold (either people worsen or they do not). If dichotomized, the focus may be on whether patients decline, stabilize, or improve. To create scales from multiple ADL and IADL questions, researchers often simply count the number of activity limitations (e.g., 0, 1, or >1 ADL difficulty). Finch, Kane, and colleagues developed a summary numerical ADL and IADL scale (Finch, Kane, and Philip 1995; Kane et al. 1996, 2000) by asking experts to assign weights to different activities and levels of limitations. The scale using only ADL ranges from 0 to 5,350, whereas that combining ADL and IADL extends from 0 to 6,614, with 0 indicating optimal functioning. For a study of postacute care for elderly Medicare beneficiaries, Kane and colleagues (2000) transformed these numerical values to a 0-to-100 scale, where 100 represented no disability. Hadley and collaborators (2000) mapped this algorithm to the MCBS questions (see Chapter 5; the MCBS questions do not match perfectly) to create a continuous functional status score for their study of posthospitalization home care. Continuous scores offer advantages over counts of ADL or IADL difficulties. Scores can give different ADL and IADL different weights and avoid making dichotomous judgments about impairments. Different functional status measures would require different risk-adjustment methods.

Risk Factors for Long-Term-Care Outcomes

Risk-adjustment models for long-term care must account for important patient characteristics that increase the probability of the outcome of interest and that are likely to be distributed unevenly among providers. These characteristics encompass the range of risk factors described in Chapter 3. The relative importance of these different dimensions of risk for predicting outcomes differs between long-term and acute care settings, even for identical outcomes (e.g., costs of care). In addition, significant predictors vary across long-term-care outcomes. Developing appropriate risk-adjustment models across the many outcomes and settings of long-term care is daunting. As elsewhere in health care, different risk-adjusted quality indicators may offer different pictures of the relative quality of care for specific providers, hindering consumers' ability to form overall judgments about quality.

In long-term care, the most important risk factor typically is functional status. As noted in Chapter 3, many different disease processes, such as cardiorespiratory conditions, cancer, dementia, or musculoskeletal problems, cause functional deficits. In long-term care, the specific underlying disease is often less important for predicting outcomes than the extent of functional impairment. Consequently, risk-adjustment methods for both clinical and cost outcomes of long-term care generally rely heavily on functional status measures.

The limited role of diagnostic data in long-term-care risk adjustment is well documented. ADL are important components of RUG III and HHRG, whereas RUG III ignore diagnoses entirely, and HHRG use only diabetes, neurological disorders, and orthopedic conditions. For clinical outcomes, initial risk-adjustment models developed for nursing homes generally did not include diagnoses, largely because of data limitations (e.g., the minimal clinical content of the reimbursement databases used in these efforts) (Berlowitz et al. 1996a; Mukamel 1997).

As databases with diagnostic information have become increasingly available, more comprehensive evaluations are now possible. Usually, as anticipated by clinical judgment, only a few diagnoses are significantly associated with specific outcomes. For example, for predicting pressure ulcer development, diabetes, peripheral vascular disease, and recent hip fracture are the only significant diagnostic predictors (Berlowitz et al. 2001b). Broader measures of comorbidity, such as number of diagnoses, are not associated with pressure ulcer development. Schizophrenia is associated with declining mental status but not with incontinence; schizophrenia reduces ADL decline, possibly because these patients tend to be younger (Porell et al. 1998). Rosen and colleagues (2000) found that adding specific diagnoses, such as neurological diseases, minimally improved predictions of functional decline, with c-statistics increasing from 0.66 to 0.68.

While measures of functional status are important in predicting outcomes, there is little consensus on how to represent ADL as predictor(s) in a risk-adjustment model for a clinical outcome. Many of the considerations described above for functional status as an outcome are also relevant when it is the predictor. A first decision is often which ADL to include. For example, the MDS includes ten ADL, along with measures for bathing and continence. These variables are highly correlated so that paradoxical results may arise if models include too many ADL. Generally, selection of specific ADL for risk-adjustment models should rely on plausible clinical linkages with the outcome, such as immobility causing pressure ulcer development. Closely examining the statistical performance of models that include different combinations of ADL is also helpful. Alternatively, researchers may use an ADL scale as described above (Finch, Kane, and Philip 1995; Kane et al. 1996, 2000; Hadley et al. 2000) or one developed specifically for the MDS (Morris, Fries, and Morris 1999). Researchers could then compare the statistical performance of risk-adjustment models including individual ADL to that of models using ADL scales.

Another decision involves how to scale ADL variables in the risk-adjustment model. One option is to treat each ADL as a continuous variable. Berlowitz and colleagues (1996a, 2001b) used this approach in developing risk-adjustment models for pressure ulcer development in nursing home patients based on bivariable analyses revealing that each one-point increase in the five-point mobility and transfer scales produced proportional increases in the rate of pressure ulcer development. Mukamel (1997), in contrast, used a categorical approach in her pressure ulcer model, with dummy variables for each level of the mobility and transfer scales. A third approach is to consider each ADL as dichotomous (dependent/not dependent) and sum the number of dependent ADL for each patient (Porell et al. 1998). None of these approaches for using ADL is necessarily superior. Choosing an approach must rely on thorough examination of the empirical analyses alongside clinical input.

Examining other potential risk factors requires careful thought. Cognitive impairment is common in long-term care and is often reasonable to evaluate in risk-adjustment models. Age is inconsistently associated with outcomes, possibly reflecting the relatively compressed range typically seen in long-term care. Patient-centered information obtained from surveys, while likely to be valuable, has generally not been used for risk adjustment, probably because of difficulties collecting these data in populations with frequently compromised cognition. Special considerations in home health care include social supports, socioeconomic status, and physical environmental factors.

Studies clearly demonstrate that risk-adjustment models encompassing multiple dimensions of risk can be developed for long-term care. Nonetheless, two questions arise about the wisdom of this approach. First, many potential risk factors used in models to evaluate providers' performance are themselves products of the quality of care. Including these risk factors raises the possibility of "overadjusting" or "adjusting out" the quality of care and compromising provider comparisons. Figure 16.2 provides an example for the outcome pressure ulcer development. If a nursing home provides poor care, many patients will experience declining ADL function. Consequently, many patients will also develop a pressure ulcer. The unadjusted rate of pressure ulcer development will be high; however, after adjusting for patients' poor functional status, the adjusted rate appears better. This is only an issue for long-staying patients whose baseline status for the time interval used in the risk-adjustment model probably differs from their status on admission. As with hospital care, status at the time of admission does not reflect the quality of nursing home care, so it is an acceptable risk factor.[1] How great a problem this is for long-term-care risk adjustment remains uncertain. Proposed solutions include omitting as predictors those variables linked to the quality of care or using only admission assessments (Mukamel 1997; Arling et al. 1997).

The second concern is that some risk factors do not necessarily result in poor outcomes when high-quality care is provided (Zimmerman et al. 1995). As the risk factor does not predict outcomes equally among all providers, difficulties could arise in comparing performance (Zaslavsky 2001).[2] For example, in high-quality nursing homes, the effects of immobility on pressure ulcer development may be mitigated by frequent repositioning. This may not be the case in poor-quality nursing homes. Diabetes, in contrast, due to co-existing neuropathy and vascular disease, is likely to be similarly important among all patients. Once again, the extent of this concern for long-term-care risk adjustment is uncertain.

Time Frame

Considering the windows of observation (see Chapter 4) is especially crucial in long-term care, which sees two broad types of patients: those who are admitted following an acute event, with high hopes of recovery, and those who stay long term, with little chance of improvement. Patients admitted to long-term care solely for postacute care need different quality measures than do chronic, debilitated patients (Kramer 2002). However, even new admissions anticipating lengthy stays are likely to differ from established, long-staying patients in important ways. As a result of their recent illness or surgery, they probably have metabolic derangements, new functional impairments, or side effects from medications. Although these conditions probably have considerable effects on outcomes, long-term-care data sets do not adequately capture some sequelae of acute illnesses. Consequently, risk-adjustment models have frequently considered new admission (or "type of assessment" within MDS) as a predictor variable to capture elements of disease severity.

Long-staying patients may require intermittent hospitalizations for acute medical events. Capturing these hospitalizations is important; strategies

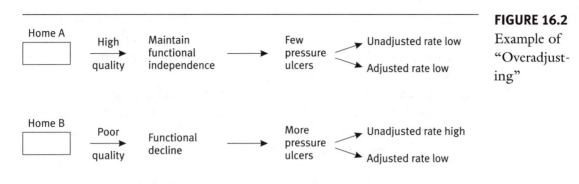

FIGURE 16.2
Example of "Overadjusting"

NOTE: Here, a poorly performing nursing home appears better following risk adjustment. Home A has good unadjusted and adjusted rates of pressure ulcer development. Home B has a high unadjusted rate, but after adjusting for the functional dependence of its patients, home B's adjusted rate appears better.

include linking hospital databases or identifying "readmission assessments" in the long-term-care database. Often, these patients are excluded from the analysis because of uncertainty about whether changes in health status reflect care administered by the hospital or the long-term-care provider.

Time intervals between consecutive records in long-term-care databases may vary for each patient. For example, in the MDS, most records involve 90-day intervals, but shorter intervals occur when the patient's health status significantly changes. Because many outcomes are more likely to appear with longer follow-up, comparing outcomes in patients assessed at different intervals (i.e., 90-day versus shorter time frames) may be inappropriate. In using the MDS to examine pressure ulcer development, Berlowitz and colleagues (2001b) first defined an index assessment in each calendar quarter and then sought outcomes from as close as possible to 90 days afterward. They only examined information from 45 to 135 days following the index evaluation to ensure that all patients had relatively similar intervals between assessments.

Censoring observations occurs when long-term-care patients are discharged or die before the outcomes are assessed (e.g., within the standard 90-day interval). This issue frequently arises for new admissions, many of whom stay in nursing homes or home care only briefly. Thus, persons with censored observations likely differ importantly from those with complete, periodic assessments. The amount of potential bias may depend on the periodicity and timing of the assessments. For example, in VA databases, assessments are performed when patients are admitted, then every April 1 and October 1. In measuring health status between admission and the next assessment, time intervals can range from days to up to six months depending on the date of admission; for long-staying patients, it is exactly six months. Changes for patients admitted and then discharged before the next April 1 or October 1 cannot be analyzed. In examining rates of pressure ulcer development, patients with less than two months between assessments had the lowest rate (Table 16.3; Berlowitz et al. 1996b). These patients were all admitted in February, March, August, or September, and they did not differ from patients admitted in other months. However, patients admitted in those months and remaining for an April 1 or October 1 outcome assessment were significantly less functionally impaired than patients with two to four or four to six months between assessments. This likely arose through the selective discharge of healthier patients after two months, with only "sicker" patients remaining. This is further suggested by the large drop in the number of patients as the time between assessments increases, indicating the censoring of many patients. Including the time between assessments among the independent predictors can help address this problem.

Because of extended time frames during which people receive care, some individuals may be included several times when creating a sample for modeling. For example, MDS assessments are performed every 90 days; therefore, an individual may contribute four records when researchers evaluate care over a year. Because observations for patients included more than once are likely correlated, statistical modeling should account for this by using such methods as generalized estimating equations. This approach is often preferable to randomly selecting one observation per patient, as it provides a larger sample size for modeling. Furthermore, for some outcomes, randomly selecting one observation falsely elevates the observed rate in the resulting sample.[3] In one study, results from generalized estimating equations were very similar to risk-adjusted models obtained through a standard logistic regression (Berlowitz et al. 2001a).

Examples of Risk Adjustment in Long-Term Care

Providing performance feedback is central to current efforts by CMS for improving quality in nursing homes and home care. Very different approaches toward risk adjustment are used, as suggested by several examples. CMS's research on risk-adjusted quality indicators for long-term care is active and ongoing, especially with Medicare's widespread public dissemination of nursing home results starting in November 2002 (Harris and Clauser 2002). Information from every nursing home is now available online for ten resident characteristics derived from the MDS. More comprehensive quality measures will be disseminated in six states as part of a CMS demonstration project. New methods may already have supplanted those described below and are generally posted on the CMS or Medicare Internet web sites.

Medicare Nursing Home Quality Assessment

Under contract from CMS, researchers at the Center for Health System Research and Analysis at the University of Wisconsin–Madison have developed a set of nursing home quality indicators based on MDS data (Zimmerman et al. 1995). The quality indicators were developed through a process combining clinical input, empirical analyses, and field testing. Researchers began with an initial pool of 175 indicators, finally selecting 30 items. Importantly, these quality indicators are not intended to measure quality directly; rather, they

	Time Between Assessments for Patients Remaining for an Outcome Assessment			TABLE 16.3
	0 to 2 Months	2 to 4 Months	4 to 6 Months	Effect of Censoring Patient
No. of patients	11,860	5,013	2,994	Assessments on
% develops pressure ulcer	4.0	5.2	5.1	Pressure Ulcer
% incontinent	38.6	45.9	44.2	Rates and
% immobile	54.5	61.1	58.5	Associated Risk
% dependent in transfer	28.2	32.0	31.0	Factors[*]

[*]No differences existed among the groups in functional status if one only examines residents at the time of admission. However, the table demonstrates significant differences among those residents remaining in long-term care for their outcome assessment. Note should also be made of the large decrease in numbers of residents, indicating the extent of the occurence.

may indicate potential problems that need further investigation, such as by state surveyors or nursing home staff. This limits their utility for consumers.

Given their goals and the concerns about overadjusting described above, these quality indicators do not use comprehensive risk adjustment. Instead, they stratify patients, typically dividing them into low- and high-risk groups based on the presence of any one of several risk factors. Rates are then reported for the entire population, as well as for each of the subgroups. Thresholds, either absolute or relative, are set for each group, and rates exceeding the threshold are considered suspect. Nursing homes often exceed the threshold for one risk group but not for another (Arling et al. 1997), suggesting that problems with care are not specific to a condition but vary depending on the characteristics of the patients.

These nursing home quality indicators have undergone further review and refinement (Harris and Clauser 2002); full results of this review are still pending (U.S. General Accounting Office 2002). While still based on the MDS, they now employ a broader range of risk-adjustment techniques that include multivariable regression models. Additionally, quality indicators may be adjusted by an admission profile for each nursing home, recognizing that some facilities admit sicker patients. For example, the pressure ulcer prevalence measure is adjusted by the percentage of admissions with a deep (stage 3 or 4) pressure ulcer. Based on conceptual and empirical reviews, a total of 22 quality indicators were recommended, including weight loss incidence, pressure ulcer incidence or worsening, deterioration in mood, and prevalence of daily physical restraints (Berg et al. 2002). Ten of these measures are included in the November 2002 release on the Medicare Nursing Home Compare web site. This release has been criticized by the U.S. General Accounting Office (2002) on the grounds that it is premature, accuracy of the MDS remains uncertain, and the risk-adjustment techniques may be inadequate, similar to the concerns raised with the initial release of Medicare hospital mortality rates (see Chapter 1). Several reviewers recommended against the use of facility-level risk adjustment, as described above for the pressure ulcer prevalence measure. Views of various concerned parties diverge on the need for further evaluation and research related to risk-adjustment techniques. Debate about the merits of CMS's nursing home quality measures will likely continue.

Medicare Home Care Quality Assessment

CMS has also sponsored efforts to develop risk-adjusted outcome measures for home care based on OASIS (Shaughnessy et al. 2002). As described above, OASIS was created to assist outcome-based quality improvement. Therefore, its quality measures intend to provide accurate performance data to support improvement activities. The researchers first specified outcomes and then identified risk factors for each of these outcomes; these data items were then incorporated into OASIS. The initial demonstration projects used 41 outcome measures.

The researchers developed risk-adjustment models for these outcomes through a detailed process starting with 149 potential predictors. They used bivariable testing to screen risk factors, then incorporated candidate risk factors into multivariable logistic regression models. They estimated each model several times, revising subsequent models based on clinical input, and evaluated model performance in derivation and validation samples. Final models include from 20 to more than 50 risk factors encompassing multiple dimensions, including functional status, social supports, diagnoses, and care needs. Models are used to compare home health care agencies' current performance to a national reference and to an agency's performance in the prior year. Results from the demonstration projects have shown that quality-improvement programs incorporating these risk-adjusted data can significantly improve patient outcomes, such as reducing hospitalization rates (Shaughnessy et al. 2002). The researchers continue to refine their risk-adjustment models by evaluating new predictors and examining alternative statistical techniques. Detailed descriptions of their risk-adjustment approaches are available (Shaughnessy and Hittle 2002).

Conclusions

Considerable progress has been made in developing risk-adjustment strategies for long-term care. Detailed clinical information is available through existing databases for many long-term care patients, and this information is currently used in quality measurement and improvement. Both the accuracy and content of these databases are likely to improve, as is their utility for risk adjustment. As with other health care settings, information on patient satisfaction and preferences will become increasingly crucial to assessing care. The growing demand for long-term care will also continue to strain the health care system, and care for frail elderly patients will increasingly rely on alternative long-term-care settings. The means to assess quality and equitably distribute resources among many potential long-term-care settings will be critical. This will require risk-adjustment models applicable across the long-term-care spectrum and will likely challenge the next generation of researchers in long-term-care risk adjustment.

Notes

1. Especially in areas with nursing home shortages, concerns nevertheless arise about "selection bias"—whether some nursing homes specifically avoid patients at potentially high risk of developing problems that could reflect poorly on the facility. In addition, nursing homes with particular trouble recruiting and retaining even low-level staff may refuse to admit patients who require considerable assistance even for the most basic activities. All these issues likely relate in complex ways to the quality of nursing homes.

2. Zaslavsky (2001) provides a more detailed description of why it may be problematic when the effect of a given risk factor on the outcome varies by provider. Briefly, consider two providers. For each provider, the association between disease severity and the outcome rate may be described by a line, with "sicker" patients having a higher rate. The lines for the two providers are not parallel when the effect of risk factor varies. No single value will then characterize the difference in performance among providers, as it differs for healthier and sicker patients.

3. To understand how randomly selecting one observation per patient may falsely elevate the observed rate, consider an outcome, such as development of a pressure ulcer or contracture, that precludes the patient from being included in the sample once it develops. Suppose data on long-staying patients are collected from three consecutive periods. There will be three observations for a patient never developing the condition, one of which will be selected for the sample. In contrast, a patient developing the condition during the second period will have only two observations. Thus, in randomly selecting an observation, the cases are more likely to be selected. The observed rate in the final sample will then be higher than in each of the time periods from which observations were selected. This could affect model calibration when applied to individual time periods.

FINAL OBSERVATIONS

Lisa I. Iezzoni

The three editions of this book span almost a decade, which—in the American health care system of recent years—seems like an eternity. As we prepared the first edition, President Clinton's health care reform proposals preoccupied the public discourse, with bold assertions about protecting the best in American medicine (White House Domestic Policy Council 1993, 100):

> If we reformed everything else in health care, but failed to preserve and enhance the high quality of our medical care, we will have taken a step backward, not forward. Quality is something that we simply can't leave to chance.

"Report cards" on provider performance were to inform consumers and purchasers alike. As Dennis S. O'Leary (1993, 487), president of the Joint Commission on Accreditation of Healthcare Organizations, stated then, "Report card day is coming in the health care world." Report cards aimed to help individuals and organizations make informed choices and facilitate oversight of health care quality, as Clinton's proposed "managed competition" took hold. Of course, Clinton's health care reform package imploded spectacularly within the year.

Three years later, as we completed the second edition, managed care was ascendant. Health care "reform" had become balkanized through countless, divergent regional initiatives (Iglehart 1994). "Performance profiling" intended to direct vigorous competition, both for individual providers and managed care plans. Plans and providers thus would battle based on "value," an amalgam of cost and quality. A suspicious public suspected that touting performance profiling was merely a ruse: All the much-maligned managed care companies ostensibly cared about was controlling costs. Managed care plans did explicitly use performance profiles to inform contracting decisions and target individual physicians for in-depth review (Goldfield and Boland 1996). At least for New York state CABG surgeons, public reporting of individual performance data had become routine, and other clinicians anticipated (feared) they would be next. As Blumenthal and Epstein (1996, 1329) observed:

> It seems fair to say that in the area of quality measurement and reporting, physicians can expect little relief from the feeling that they increasingly work in a fishbowl and are being judged by groups and

measures with which they have little familiarity. Managing this reality is one of the greatest challenges confronting the profession at the current time.

Now, as we finish the third edition, managed care has retreated, side-lined largely by consumers' persistent demands for options and choices. Costs are again rising dramatically, the number of uninsured persons continues to expand, several authoritative Institute of Medicine (1999, 2001a, 2002c) reports have raised pointed and troubling questions about the quality of U.S. health care, and some politicians are cautiously reawakening long-dormant proposals for universal coverage. Meanwhile, the new mantra is "pay for performance." This phrase has a hard-headed ring not shared by the perhaps euphemistic report cards and performance profiling. However, at least its intention is crystal clear.

Risk Adjustment as a Common Thread

Risk adjustment links the three defining concepts from these recent mini-eras in our health care system—report cards to support managed competition, performance profiling to inform "unmanaged" competition, and pay for performance to control intractably rising costs. In fact, in operational terms, these three phrases mean the same thing. All involve comparing how well patients do across clinicians, hospitals, health plans, or other providers, and meaningful comparisons generally require risk adjustment.

As noted throughout this book, risk adjustment is well developed for certain purposes, such as setting selected prospective payment rates and evaluating outcomes of specific interventions, like ICU care and CABG surgery. Using even imperfect risk-adjustment methods for internal quality-improvement activities is well accepted and has proven remarkably effective for individual hospitals and entire health care systems, such as the VHA (see Chapter 8). Even reasonable physicians may hesitate to change or examine critically their practices when shown information they see as flawed. Therefore, hospitals or other provider groups need risk-adjusted information to promote a productive dialog with their clinical staffs. Once clinicians believe the information, they begin discussing ways to improve.

Problems can arise when comparisons of risk-adjusted data move beyond the safe confines of individual practice settings into the external world. As noted in Chapter 2, clinicians and purchasers, for example, may define even basic terms differently. Table 17.1 summarizes common views held by many clinicians and purchasers that are almost diametrically opposed. At the bottom line, clinicians worry about being treated unfairly or punitively based on data they view as fundamentally flawed. In contrast, purchasers want providers to assume responsibility for the cost and quality of their "product," arguing

Clinicians
- The risk adjustment method is not clinically credible; therefore, comparing risk-adjusted outcomes across clinicians is neither valid nor meaningful.
- The risk-adjusted data focus on limited outcomes (e.g., in-hospital mortality for specific conditions) and do not target quality concerns most relevant to either patients or clinicians.
- Those reviewing the risk-adjusted data do not understand the limitations of the risk adjuster, data, or analytic techniques; they therefore draw inappropriate conclusions and make unwarranted decisions.
- Collecting the data is logistically burdensome and expensive, adding another administrative expense to an already stressed system.
- The data do not provide useful information about how exactly to change care to improve outcomes.
- These imperfect data are used wrongly to threaten clinicians or make punitive decisions (e.g., withdrawing health plan contracts, reducing payments.)
- When risk-adjusted data are widely reported by the media or through the Internet, few caveats are presented about their limitations; the general public therefore receives erroneous impressions about clinicians' performance, and reputations suffer.

Purchasers
- Given double-digit inflation of health care costs, clinicians must be held accountable for what they produce.
- Several Institute of Medicine reports confirm that health care quality is often poor and life-threatening medical errors are much too common.
- Purchasers and consumers require information to make informed decisions about where to obtain health care.
- Some risk-adjusted outcomes measures, such as CABG mortality predictions, are well developed and a good place to start.
- Other complex industries must justify their outputs and quality of their products—health care is no different.
- The dollars spent on risk-adjustment data are trivial compared to the total cost of health care.
- Clinicians should invest in health informatics technologies to improve their care; computerized information systems could easily generate data for risk adjustment.
- Given the relative dearth of information available about clinicians' performance, we must start somewhere, even with imperfect data.

TABLE 17.1

Common Concerns of Clinicians and Purchasers

against waiting for that chimerical "perfect" risk-adjustment methodology that will probably never materialize.

Sometimes, the rhetoric of today's debates about performance measures evokes the memory of Ernest Amory Codman from early in the last century (see Chapter 1): "Comparisons are odious, but comparison is necessary in science. Until we freely make therapeutic comparisons, we cannot claim that a given hospital is efficient, for efficiency implies that the results have been looked into" (Codman 1934, xxiii). The difference today is the huge size of the stakes. Although concerns about fairness of risk-adjusted prospective payment remain, this area is often treated as an arcane concern amenable to technical patches (e.g., adopting partial capitation, special payments for "outliers"). The more heated exchanges involve using risk-adjusted outcomes information to draw inferences about quality of care.

With relatively few exceptions, little objective independent information is available about what most risk-adjusted outcome results actually mean. Do worse risk-adjusted outcomes truly reflect worse quality of care? This dearth of information suggests several important considerations for initiatives using risk-adjusted information as a quality indicator, for example, to create pay-for-performance programs or publish performance profiles on the Internet.

First, participants should acknowledge that they are jointly conducting an applied experiment. In an experiment—compared to endeavors using well-accepted, rigorous methods with clearly understood benefits—evaluation is critical. Some initiatives have recognized this concern. For example, New York state officials site visited CABG programs with alarmingly high risk-adjusted mortality rates to see first hand whether problems existed (Hannan et al. 1990). If providers, payers, and purchasers all recognize the experimental nature of their undertaking, tensions may ease. They could work together to learn how to use the risk-adjusted data in a productive fashion.

Second, as in all controversies, participants must understand better the goals and concerns of each other. American businesses, for example, often use quality to hone their competitive edge. Clinicians, in turn, have spent years debating quality measurement, returning continually to the difficulty of capturing complexities surrounding individual patients. For almost a century, emphasizing the idiosyncrasies of individual cases has led clinicians to reject efforts to standardize patient care or even documentation (see Chapter 6). Physicians typically do not believe that single numerical scores or categories adequately represent complex clinical scenarios. In addition, focusing on such outcomes as costs, short-term mortality, and LOS neglects many outcomes (such as functional status and quality of life) that reflect the goals not only of clinicians but also of patients.

Clinicians could learn more about the desire of purchasers and payers to quantify quality, to permit more prudent, better-informed decisions. These groups reasonably no longer accept vague promises about quality monitoring without concrete evidence of results. In turn, purchasers and payers should involve clinicians in designing risk-adjusted quality indicators. However, this does not guarantee complete acceptance of the methods. Several Cleveland Clinic physicians, for example, rejected risk-adjustment methods developed with in-depth clinical involvement (see Chapter 1).

Third, given the uncertainty surrounding what risk-adjusted outcomes information really means, weighing what actions these data can reasonably support becomes critical. The need of purchasers to act aggressively to control costs must be balanced against legitimate questions about the validity of inferences about comparative provider quality from risk-adjusted data. At a minimum, adopting appropriate and statistically rigorous analytical techniques is essential (see Chapters 10 through 12). For example, given reservations about the accuracy of their administrative data, California's first report card used conservative significance levels to avoid overcalling outlier providers. Using the data to direct punitive actions against providers seems inappropriate without objective evidence that the data are valid (see Chapter 9). Even if the information appears methodologically sound, publicity surrounding release of provider-specific findings can have untoward consequences (e.g., clinicians avoiding high-risk patients) that must be monitored.

Fourth, with increasingly constrained health care resources, concerns about costs and trade-offs inevitably arise. New electronic data systems may mitigate questions about spending large sums on capturing risk-factor information, as in the VHA. Nevertheless, moving to completely computerized information systems is years away for many health care settings, especially private physicians' offices and many small hospitals. Over the next several years, strategies for installing informatics technologies throughout the health care system will likely attract considerable attention. Improving patient care and administrative efficiency will motivate computerization; risk adjustment will benefit downstream from these efforts. This electronic transformation, however, will cost millions, if not billions, of dollars system wide.

Finally, as an Institute of Medicine committee observed (Donaldson and Lohr 1994, 95):

> The public interest is materially served when society is given as much information on costs, quality, and value for health care dollar expended as can be given accurately and provided with educational materials that aid interpretation of that information. . . . Public disclosure is acceptable *only* when it: (1) involves information and analytic results that come from studies that have been well conducted, (2) is based on data that can be shown to be reliable and valid for the purposes intended, and (3) is accompanied by appropriate educational material.

While this proposal urges a cool, scholarly approach, nowadays little in the health care marketplace retains a detached, academic demeanor. Especially with the easy access of the Internet, information about providers' performance will be disseminated swiftly and widely in the future. Despite an ostensibly laudable goal of assisting consumers by revealing information, a fundamental irony has emerged—commercial sources typically offer no details about their proprietary methods for risk adjusting outcomes or measuring quality. They are "black boxes."

Krumholz and colleagues (2002) reviewed report cards for individual hospitals posted on its Internet site by one company, a publicly traded firm with more than $7 million in revenues in 2000. The researchers compared the company's ratings of hospital quality, which used Medicare administrative data to assign hospitals one to five stars (five stars are best) based on their risk-adjusted 30-day mortality, with ratings the researchers derived from clinically detailed information. The company's stars did "convey some important information in aggregate, but provide little meaningful discrimination between individual hospitals' performance in a manner sufficient for a public interested in making informed hospital choices" (Krumholz et al. 2002, 1283). Although the researchers could not evaluate the company's secret methodology, they nevertheless argued, "Risk models based on administrative data can lead to substantial misclassification of hospitals when compared with models based on higher-quality data" (Krumholz et al. 2002, 1285). As their bottom line, Krumholz and colleagues (2002, 1287) observed:

> The necessary and often overlooked caveat associated with such reports cards is that the public (and health care professionals) often become focused on identifying "winners and losers" rather than using these data to inform quality improvement efforts. . . . Current outcome-based report card efforts are better used as a tool for quality improvement, rather than as a publicly reported means of discriminating between hospital performance.

Many factors will determine the future environment of generating and disseminating risk-adjusted outcomes information, such as pay-for-performance schemes, posting of performance profiles on the Internet, and growing financial pressures on providers and the entire health care system. The only guarantee is that risk-adjusted outcomes information will continue to raise many questions—and perhaps generate fractious debates—for the foreseeable future. However, we are not the first to confront such issues.

Striking historical precedents anticipate precisely the controversies of our times about measuring provider performance and promoting change. I therefore close the book by returning to Florence Nightingale, William Farr, and hospital mortality statistics and the story begun in Chapter 1 (excerpted from Iezzoni 1996).

Epilogue: Nightingale, Farr, and Hospital Death Rates

In 1863, Florence Nightingale published the third edition of her *Notes on Hospitals*, proposing reforms that she believed would improve the quality of hospitals and patient outcomes. To bolster her arguments about the direction of reforms, she included a table listing 1861 death rates at 106 hospitals in England (see Table 1.2). Nightingale (1863, 4) drew attention to the startling mortality rates at 24 London hospitals:

> We have 24 London hospitals, affording a mortality of no less than 90.84 per cent., very nearly every bed yielding a death in the course

of the year. . . . Here we have at once a hospital problem demanding solution . . .

Facts such as these (and it is not the first time that they have been placed before the public) have sometimes raised grave doubts as to the advantages to be derived from hospitals at all, and have led many an one to think that in all probability a poor sufferer would have a much better chance of recovery if treated at home.

Subtly embedded within Nightingale's commentary, although obvious from the table itself, is the method employed for calculating these death rates—a method that raised questions about interpreting these figures. Taken verbatim from his *24th Annual Report of the Registrar-General*, William Farr (Figure 17.1) had calculated the death rates as (total number of deaths at the hospital in 1861)/(number of patients at the hospital on April 8, 1861). Thus, the numerator reflected figures from an entire year, whereas the denominator encompassed a single day. Farr had computed death rates per occupied hospital bed—or deaths per person-year in hospital—not death rates per total number of hospitalized patients. Not surprisingly, ostensible hospital death rates fell considerably when calculated as the annual number of deaths divided by the total number of inpatients treated during the year. Using this method, mortality rates for 1861 in the "general wards" at 14 London hospitals averaged 9.7 percent (Statistical Society 1865).

Cynical modern observers might think that Farr and Nightingale intentionally skewed statistics to bolster political arguments. In the 1860s, however, little consensus existed on statistical techniques, let alone how to calculate hospital death rates. Victorian statisticians emphasized subject matter rather than methods, accepting "men of little mathematical ability" into their field (Eyler 1979, 19). Today's standard statistical techniques and approaches toward error and uncertainty (see Chapters 10 through 12) were decades away.

Hospitals calculated death rates in different ways to suit their particular goals (Woodward 1974; Bristowe and Holmes 1864). Changing specification of the numerator allowed hospitals to modulate their apparent death rates. According to the 1863 Privy Council report (Bristowe and Holmes 1864, 527):

In the majority of hospitals, it is . . . the custom to reckon among their deaths those who have been brought dead to the institution; but there are many hospitals where such cases are not reckoned, and there are some indeed where even those who die within 24 hours are, on the ground that they were moribund at the time of admission, excluded from computation.

Admission practices affected death rate comparisons between urban and provincial hospitals. Many provincial hospitals explicitly refused patients with phthisis (consumption), fevers, and the "dead or dying," whereas urban

FIGURE 17.1
William Farr

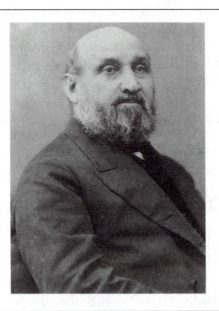

SOURCE: Courtesy of the Boston Medical Library in the Francis A. Countway Library of Medicine.

facilities took everyone. Urban facilities objected to comparisons with outlying hospitals that excluded such patients. As the 1846 Glasgow Royal Infirmary report stated, "The reception of moribund cases greatly swells the number of deaths recorded in the Hospital, and very materially increases the proportionate mortality thereby producing misconceptions in the public mind" (Woodward 1974, 135).

Farr and Nightingale faced criticism primarily because of their denominator. Nonetheless, in the mid-nineteenth century, some viewed the number of "deaths per bed" as a useful indicator of a hospital's productivity—another way of showing charitable donors that they were getting their money's worth.

Today's media would swiftly decry hospital mortality rates of more than 90 percent. My review of indices to *The Times* from 1861 through 1865, however, found few articles about hospitals and none about controversies over Nightingale's book and hospital mortality statistics. Nevertheless, a raucous debate immediately erupted in the London *Medical Times and Gazette* and the *Lancet*, with men practicing at urban hospitals as the major critics (Eyler 1979).

An anonymous reviewer (1864a, 129) of *Notes on Hospitals* began, "It is sad to see a work of so much value—full of such useful information— disfigured by a few serious and elementary mistakes. Much as all Medical men must appreciate the philanthropic labour of its authoress, it is a false kindness to pass erroneous views without protest." The reviewer observed that, since the mortality rate table came from the Registrar-General, "perhaps

Miss Nightingale can hardly be held responsible for it," but he nonetheless excoriated the methodology (Anonymous 1864a, 129):

> The inmates of a single day are balanced with the deaths of a whole year, and no wonder the results are "striking enough." It is to be hoped there are valid reasons for giving to the world what seems to us a simple piece of arithmetical legerdemain. Surely it is the very essence of percentages and of averages (both, we believe, fruitful sources of error), that the figures dealt with should stand on one and the same bottom, and that deaths for one year should be compared with admissions or discharges for that period, and no other. There is something audacious in the last column of this table, where twenty-four London Hospitals are accredited with a "mortality per cent. on inmates" of 90.84. No doubt it will be said this is the quotient of the figures employed; but we entirely deny their validity and the accuracy of the impression thus conveyed. The problem as here put is exactly that so often asked of forward schoolboys—What is the quotient of a hundred apples divided by fifteen red herrings?

John Bristowe, a prominent London physician, slyly caricatured Farr's arithmetic choices, showing that hospital "recovery" rates calculated using Farr's methods would range from 899.5 percent to 953 percent (1864, 492). Timothy Holmes (1864, 365), a London surgeon, indicated that, by Farr's method, one hospital had a mortality rate of 130 percent.

Another anonymous critic (1864b, 187) objected to the absence of risk adjustment, viewing comparisons between inner-city and rural hospitals as hopelessly flawed. "Any comparison which ignores the difference between the apple-cheeked farm-laborers who seek relief at Stoke Pogis (probably for rheumatism and sore legs), and the wizzened [sic], red-herring-like mechanics of Soho or Southwark, who come from a London Hospital, is fallacious." Bristowe (1864, 492) concurred:

> Has Dr. Farr . . . really overlooked the differences in relative severity of cases admitted into his different classes of Hospitals, the different relative length of stay of their inmates, the different numbers of patients treated in them in relation to the numbers of constantly-occupied beds? Has he no suspicion that his death-rate is determined almost wholly by these causes?

Bristowe (1864, 491) also questioned how the public would interpret Farr's death rates: "That Dr. Farr understands the mathematical meaning of his figures no one will doubt; but that the majority of his readers understand them neither in this sense nor in any other, and are utterly mislead by them, is certain." Bristowe (1864, 492) directly challenged the motivations of Farr and Nightingale, stating that when they "try to mislead others into the belief that the unhealthiness of Hospitals is in proportion to Dr. Farr's death-rates of Hospitals, we are bound to protest against the whole matter as an unfounded and mischievous delusion."

Two weeks after the first review of *Notes on Hospitals*, the *Medical Times and Gazette* published Farr's response. He took exception to an anonymous reviewer "who could treat a lady roughly" (Farr 1864a, 186), although he later accurately acknowledged that Nightingale was "well able to defend herself" (Farr 1864b, 421). Farr argued that, if hospitals would provide accurate figures concerning cases treated and deaths, few disputes would arise. In several back-and-forth rebuttals of his critics over about two months, Farr did not refute specific attacks on his calculation. Instead, he emphasized fundamental reservations about most death rate calculations (Farr 1864a, 186):

> This [Farr's approach] is one method; there is another which is less correct, but more common. The deaths are divided by the mean number of cases admitted and discharged. . . . The defect of this method lies in this: it does not take the element of time into account, which is important, as it so happens that cases are scarcely ever admitted as in-patients of Hospitals at their origin, and that many cases are discharged from Hospital before they have terminated.

Farr (1864a, 186) wanted to hold constant the window of observation, saying, for example, that it was unfair to compare death rates at St. Thomas's in London, with an average inpatient stay of 39 days, with rates at two Dublin hospitals, with average stays of 27 days. At least, Farr argued, his calculation clearly specified what it aimed to capture.

At the end of the heated letter exchange between Farr and his critics, however, Bristowe made perhaps the key point: "If Dr. Farr had made his calculations about Hospitals in a tentative spirit, with the object of ascertaining whether they were likely to lead to any useful results, he would have acted in a way to which no exception could have been taken" (Bristowe 1864, 492).

One year later, when the Statistical Society, with Farr as treasurer, published hospital death rates for 1863, they calculated death rates as (annual deaths)/(annual admissions + [patients at the beginning – those at the end of the year]) (Statistical Society 1865). The publication noted that hospital stays were long, averaging 30 days for 14 London hospitals. Despite this methodological shift, Farr continued using statistics to urge reform, writing to Nightingale in 1864, "What are figures worth if they do no good to men's bodies or souls?" (Diamond and Stone 1981, 70).

References

Adler, G. S. 1994. "A Profile of the Medicare Current Beneficiary Survey." *Health Care Financing Review* 15 (4): 153–63.

———. 1995. "Medicare Beneficiaries Rate Their Medical Care: New Data from the MCBS (Medicare Current Beneficiary Survey)." *Health Care Financing Review* 16 (4): 175–87.

Adler, N. E., and K. Newman. 2002. "Socioeconomic Disparities in Health: Pathways and Policies. Inequality in Education, Income, and Occupation Exacerbates the Gaps Between the Health 'Haves' and 'Have-Nots.' " *Health Affairs (Millwood)* 21 (2): 60–76.

Agresti, A., and B. A. Coull. 1998. "Approximate Is Better than 'Exact' for Interval Estimation of Binomial Proportions." *The American Statistician* 52: 119–26.

Akaike, H. 1973. "Information Theory and an Extension of the Maximum Likelihood Principle." In *Second International Symposium on Information Theory*, edited by B. N. Petrov and F. Csaki. Budapest: Akademia Kiado.

Alessandrini, E. A., K. N. Shaw, W. B. Bilker, D. F. Schwarz, and L. M. Bell. 2001. "Effects of Medicaid Managed Care on Quality: Childhood Immunizations." *Pediatrics* 107 (6): 1335–42.

Alexander, M. P. 1994. "Stroke Rehabilitation Outcome. A Potential Use of Predictive Variables to Establish Levels of Care." *Stroke* 25 (1): 128–34.

Alexander, N. B. 1996. "Gait Disorders in Older Adults." *Journal of the American Geriatric Society* 44 (4): 434–51.

Almond, R. G., L Charles, J. W. Tukey, and D. Yan. 2000. "Displays for Comparing a Given State to Many Others." *The American Statistician* 54: 89–93.

Alonso, J., C. Black, J. C. Norregaard, E. Dunn, T. F. Andersen, M. Espallargues, P. Bernth-Petersen, and G. F. Anderson. 1998. "Cross-Cultural Differences in the Reporting of Global Functional Capacity: An Example in Cataract Patients." *Medical Care* 36 (6): 868–78.

American College of Surgeons. 1918. "Standard of Efficiency for the First Hospital Survey of the College." *Bulletin of American College of Surgeons* 3: 1–4.

American Heritage® Dictionary of the English Language, Fourth Edition. 2000. [Online information; retrieved 11/8/2002.] New York: Dell Publishing Company. http://www.bartleby.com/61/84/RO258400.htm.

American Psychiatric Association. 1994. *Diagnostic and Statistical Manual of Mental Disorders,* 4th ed. Washington, DC: APA Press.

Anderson, G., and J. R. Knickman. 2001. "Changing the Chronic Care System to Meet People's Needs." *Health Affairs (Millwood)* 20 (6): 146–60.

Anderson, R. N. 2002. "Deaths: Leading Causes for 2000. National Vital Statistics Report." Vol. 50, No. 16. Hyattsville, MD: National Center for Health Statistics.

Anderson, R. N., A. M. Minino, D. L. Hoyert, and H. M. Rosenberg. 2001. "Comparability of Cause of Death Between ICD-9 and ICD-10: Preliminary Estimates." *National Vital Statistics Report* 49 (2): 1–32.

Andresen, E. M., D. L. Patrick, W. B. Carter, and J. A. Malmgren. 1995. "Comparing the Performance of Health Status Measures for Healthy Older Adults." *Journal of the American Geriatric Society* 43 (9): 1030–34.

Angrist, J. D., G. W. Imbens, and D. Rubin. 1996. "Identification of Causal Effects Using Instrumental Variables." *Journal of the American Statistical Association* 91: 444–55.

Anonymous. 1864a. "Reviews. Notes on Hospitals. By Florence Nightingale." *Medical Times and Gazette* Jan. 30: 129–30.

———. 1864b. "Untitled. Response to Letter by William Farr." *Medical Times and Gazette* Feb. 13: 187–88.

Applegate, W. B., J. P. Blass, and T. F. Williams. 1990. "Instruments for the Functional Assessment of Older Patients." *New England Journal of Medicine* 322 (17): 1207–14.

Arling, G., S. L. Karon, F. Sainfort, D. R. Zimmerman, and R. Ross. 1997. "Risk Adjustment of Nursing Home Quality Indicators." *Gerontologist* 37 (6): 757–66.

Arozullah, A. M., J. Daley, W. G. Henderson, and S. F. Khuri. 2000. "Multifactorial Risk Index for Predicting Postoperative Respiratory Failure in Men After Major Noncardiac Surgery. The National Veterans Administration Surgical Quality Improvement Program." *Annals of Surgery* 232 (2): 242–53.

Arozullah, A. M., S. F. Khuri, W. G. Henderson, and J. Daley. 2001. "Development and Validation of a Multifactorial Risk Index for Predicting Postoperative Pneumonia After Major Noncardiac Surgery." *Annals of Internal Medicine* 135 (10): 847–57.

Ash, A. 1996. "Identifying Poor-Quality Hospitals with Mortality Rates. Often There's More Noise than Signal." *Medical Care* 34 (8): 735–36.

Ash, A. S., and S. Byrne-Logan. 1998. "How Well Do Models Work? Predicting Health Care Costs." In *Proceedings of the Section on Statistics in Epidemiology, American Statistical Association*, 42–49. Alexandria, VA: American Statistical Association.

Ash, A. S., R. P. Ellis, G. C. Pope, J. Z. Ayanian, D. W. Bates, H. Burstin, L. I. Iezzoni, E. MacKay, and W. Yu. 2000. "Using Diagnoses to Describe Populations and Predict Costs." *Health Care Financing Review* 21 (3): 7–28.

Ash, A., F. Porell, L. Gruenberg, E. Sawitz, and A. Beiser. 1989. "Adjusting Medicare Capitation Payments Using Prior Hospitalization Data." *Health Care Financing Review* 10 (4): 17–29.

Ash, A. S., M. A. Posner, J. Speckman, S. Franco, A. C. Yacht, and L. Bramwell. In press. "Using Risk Adjustment to Examine Mortality Trends Following Hospitalization for Heart Attack in Medicare." *Health Services Research*.

Ash, A., and M. Shwartz. 1999. "R^2: A Useful Measure of Model Performance when Predicting a Dichotomous Outcome." *Statistics in Medicine* 18 (4): 375–84.

Ash, A., M. Shwartz, S. M. Payne, and J. D. Restuccia. 1990. "The Self-Adapting Focused Review System. Probability Sampling of Medical Records to Monitor Utilization and Quality of Care." *Medical Care* 28 (11): 1025–39.

Ash, A. S., Y. Zhao, R. P. Ellis, and M. S. Kramer. 2001. "Finding Future High-Cost Cases: Comparing Prior Cost Versus Diagnosis-Based Methods." *Health Services Research* 36 (6, Part II): 194–206.

Ashcraft, M. L., B. E. Fries, D. R. Nerenz, S. P. Falcon, S. V. Srivastava, C. Z. Lee, S. E. Berki, and P. Errera. 1989. "A Psychiatric Patient Classification System. An Alternative to Diagnosis-Related Groups." *Medical Care* 27 (5): 543–57.

Atkinson, A. C. 1985. *Plots, Transformations, and Regression: An Introduction to Graphical Methods of Diagnostic Regression Analysis.* Oxford, UK: Clarendon Press.

Au, D. H., M. B. McDonell, D. C. Martin, and S. D. Fihn. 2001. "Regional Variations in Health Status." *Medical Care* 39 (8): 879–88.

Averill, R. F. 1999. "Honest Mistake or Fraud? Meeting the Coding Compliance Challenge." *Journal of AHIMA* 70 (5): 16–21.

Averill, R. F., T. E. McGuire, B. E. Manning, D. A. Fowler, S. D. Horn, P. S. Dickson, M. J. Coye, D. L. Knowlton, and J. A. Bender. 1992. "A Study of the Relationship Between Severity of Illness and Hospital Cost in New Jersey Hospitals." *Health Services Research* 27 (5): 587–606.

Averill, R. F., R. L. Mullin, B. A. Steinbeck, N. I. Goldfield, and T. M. Grant. 1998. "Development of the ICD-10 Procedure Coding System (ICD-10-PCS)." *Journal of AHIMA* 69 (5): 65–72.

Ayanian, J. Z., and A. M. Epstein. 1991. "Differences in the Use of Procedures Between Women and Men Hospitalized for Coronary Heart Disease." *New England Journal of Medicine* 325 (4): 221–25.

Bailar, J. C., and F. Mosteller. 1986. *Medical Use of Statistics.* Waltham, MA: NEJM Books.

Baker, D. W., D. Einstadter, C. L. Thomas, S. S. Husak, N. H. Gordon, and R. D. Cebul. 2002a. "Mortality Trends During a Program that Publicly Reported Hospital Performance." *Medical Care* 40 (10): 879–90.

Baker, D. W., J. A. Gazmararian, M. V. Williams, T. Scott, R. M. Parker, D. Green, J. Ren, and J. Peel. 2002b. "Functional Health Literacy and the Risk of Hospital Admission Among Medicare Managed Care Enrollees." *American Journal of Public Health* 92 (8): 1278–83.

Banks, S. M., J. A. Pandiani, and J. Bramley. 2001. "Approaches to Risk-Adjusting Outcome Measures Applied to Criminal Justice Involvement After Community Service." *Journal of Behavioral Health Services & Research* 28 (3): 235–46.

Banks, S. M., J. A. Pandiani, L. Schacht, and L. Gauvin. 1999. "A Risk-Adjusted Measure of Hospitalization Rates for Evaluating Community Mental Health Program Performance." *Administration and Policy in Mental Health* 26 (4): 269–79.

Barnes, C., G. Mercer, and T. Shakespeare. 1999. *Exploring Disability. A Sociological Introduction.* Cambridge, UK: Polity Press.

Batavia, A. L. 1992. "Assessing the Function of Functional Assessment: A Consumer Perspective." *Disability and Rehabilitation* 14: 156–60.

Bazos, D. A., W. B. Weeks, E. S. Fisher, H. A. DeBlois, E. Hamilton, and M. J. Young. 2001. "The Development of a Survey Instrument for Community Health Improvement." *Health Services Research* 36 (4): 773–92.

Beers, M. H., M. Munekata, and M. Storrie. 1990. "The Accuracy of Medication Histories in the Hospital Medical Records of Elderly Persons." *Journal of the American Geriatric Society* 38 (11): 1183–87.

Bennett, C. L., S. Greenfield, H. Aronow, P. Ganz, N. J. Vogelzang, and R. M. Elashoff. 1991. "Patterns of Care Related to Age of Men with Prostate Cancer." *Cancer* 67 (10): 2633–41.

Benson, K., and A. J. Hartz. 2000. "A Comparison of Observational Studies and Randomized, Controlled Trials." *New England Journal of Medicine* 342 (25): 1878–86.

Berg, K., V. Mor, J. Morris, K. M. Murphy, T. Moore, and Y. Harris. 2002. "Identification and Evaluation of Existing Nursing Home Quality Indicators." *Health Care Financing Review* 23 (4): 19–36.

Berger, M. M., A. Marazzi, J. Freeman, and R. Chiolero. 1992. "Evaluation of the Consistency of Acute Physiology and Chronic Health Evaluation (APACHE II) Scoring in a Surgical Intensive Care Unit." *Critical Care Medicine* 20 (12): 1681–87.

Bergner, M. 1989. "Quality of Life, Health Status, and Clinical Research." *Medical Care* 27 (3, Suppl.): S148–S156.

Berkman, L. 2002. *The Epidemiology Monitor* 2 (July).

Berlowitz, D. R., A. S. Ash, G. H. Brandeis, H. K. Brand, J. L. Halpern, and M. A. Moskowitz. 1996a. "Rating Long-Term Care Facilities on Pressure Ulcer Development: Importance of Case-Mix Adjustment." *Annals of Internal Medicine* 124 (6): 557–63.

Berlowitz, D. R., H. Q. Bezerra, G. H. Brandeis, B. Kader, and J. J. Anderson. 2000. "Are We Improving the Quality of Nursing Home Care: The Case of Pressure Ulcers." *Journal of the American Geriatric Society* 48 (1): 59–62.

Berlowitz, D. R., G. H. Brandeis, H. K. Brand, J. Halpern, A. S. Ash, and M. A. Moskowitz. 1996b. "Evaluating Pressure Ulcer Occurrence in Long-Term Care: Pitfalls in Interpreting Administrative Data." *Journal of Clinical Epidemiology* 49 (3): 289–92.

Berlowitz, D. R., G. H. Brandeis, J. N. Morris, A. S. Ash, J. J. Anderson, B. Kader, and M. A. Moskowitz. 2001b. "Deriving a Risk-Adjustment Model for Pressure Ulcer Development Using the Minimum Data Set." *Journal of the American Geriatric Society* 49 (7): 866–71.

Berlowitz, D. R., G. H. Brandeis, and M. A. Moskowitz. 1997. "Using Administrative Databases to Evaluate Long-Term Care." *Journal of the American Geriatric Society* 45 (5): 618–23.

Berlowitz, D. R., G. J. Young, G. H. Brandeis, B. Kader, and J. J. Anderson. 2001a. "Health Care Reorganization and Quality Of Care: Unintended Effects on Pressure Ulcer Prevention." *Medical Care* 39 (2): 138–46.

Bernabei, R., G. Gambassi, K. Lapane, A. Sgadari, F. Landi, C. Gatsonis, L. Lipsitz, and V. Mor. 1999. "Characteristics of the SAGE Database: A New Resource for Research on Outcomes in Long-Term Care. SAGE (Systematic Assessment of

Geriatric Drug Use via Epidemiology) Study Group." *Journal of Gerontology: Medical Sciences* 54A (1): M25–M33.

Berwick, D. M. 1989. "E. A. Codman and the Rhetoric of Battle: A Commentary." *Milbank Quarterly* 67 (2): 262–67.

———. 1996. "This Year of 'How': New Systems for Delivering Health Care." *Quality Connections* 5 (1): 1–4.

———. 2002. "A User's Manual for the IOM's 'Quality Chasm' Report." *Health Affairs (Millwood)* 21 (3): 80–90.

Best, W. R., S. F. Khuri, M. Phelan, K. Hur, W. G. Henderson, J. G. Demakis, and J. Daley. 2002. "Identifying Patient Preoperative Risk Factors and Postoperative Adverse Events in Administrative Databases: Results from the Department of Veterans Affairs National Surgical Quality Improvement Program." *Journal of the American College of Surgeons* 194 (3): 257–66.

Bickell, N. A., K. S. Pieper, K. L. Lee, D. B. Mark, D. D. Glower, D. B. Pryor, and R. M. Califf. 1992. "Referral Patterns for Coronary Artery Disease Treatment: Gender Bias or Good Clinical Judgment?" *Annals of Internal Medicine* 116 (10): 791–97.

Bierman, A. S., T. A. Bubolz, E. S. Fisher, and J. H. Wasson. 1999. "How Well Does a Single Question About Health Predict the Financial Health of Medicare Managed Care Plans?" *Effective Clinical Practice* 2 (2): 56–62.

Billings, J., L. Zeitel, J. Lukomnik, T. S. Carey, A. E. Blank, and L. Newman. 1993. "Impact of Socioeconomic Status on Hospital Use in New York City." *Health Affairs (Millwood)* 12 (1): 162–73.

Bindman, A. B., D. Keane, and N. Lurie. 1990. "Measuring Health Changes Among Severely Ill Patients. The Floor Phenomenon." *Medical Care* 28 (12): 1142–52.

Binstock, R. H., and W. D. Spector. 1997. "Five Priority Areas for Research on Long-Term Care." *Health Services Research* 32 (5): 715–30.

Black, C., N. P. Roos, and L. Roos. 1999. "From Health Statistics to Health Information Systems: A New Path for the 21st Century." Paper commissioned by the National Committee for Vital and Health Statistics for a Workshop on Developing the 21st Century Vision for Health Statistics, Draft.

Blumberg, M. S. 1991. "Biased Estimates of Expected Acute Myocardial Infarction Mortality Using MedisGroups Admission Severity Groups." *Journal of the American Medical Association* 265 (22): 2965–70.

Blumberg, M. S., and G. S. Binns. 1989. "Risk-Adjusted 30-Day Mortality of Fresh Acute Myocardial Infarctions: The Technical Report." Chicago: Hospital Research and Educational Trust, American Hospital Association.

Blumenthal, D., and A. M. Epstein. 1996. "Quality of Health Care. Part 6: The Role of Physicians in the Future of Quality Management." *New England Journal of Medicine* 335 (17): 1328–31.

Bogardus, S. T., Jr., V. Towle, C. S. Williams, M. M. Desai, and S. K. Inouye. 2001. "What Does the Medical Record Reveal About Functional Status? A Comparison of Medical Record and Interview Data." *Journal of General Internal Medicine* 16 (11): 728–36.

Boult, C., M. Altmann, D. Gilbertson, C. Yu, and R. L. Kane. 1996. "Decreasing

Disability in the 21st Century: The Future Effects of Controlling Six Fatal and Nonfatal Conditions." *American Journal of Public Health* 86 (10): 1388–93.

Bowden, R. J., and D. A. Turkington. 1984. *Instrumental Variables.* Cambridge, UK: Cambridge University Press.

Bowlin, S. J., B. D. Morrill, A. N. Nafziger, C. Lewis, and T. A. Pearson. 1996. "Reliability and Changes in Validity of Self-Reported Cardiovascular Disease Risk Factors Using Dual Response: The Behavioral Risk Factor Survey." *Journal of Clinical Epidemiology* 49 (5): 511–17.

Box, G. E. P., W. G. Hunter, and J. S. Hunter. 1978. *Statistics for Experimenters: An Introduction to Design, Data Analysis, and Model Building.* New York: John Wiley.

Bradbury, A. 1990. "Computerized Medical Records: The Need for a Standard." *Journal of the American Medical Records Association* 61 (3): 25–37.

Brailer, D. J., E. Kroch, M. V. Pauly, and J. Huang. 1996. "Comorbidity-Adjusted Complication Risk: A New Outcome Quality Measure." *Medical Care* 34 (5): 490–505.

Brannen, A. L., II, L. J. Godfrey, and W. E. Goetter. 1989. "Prediction of Outcome from Critical Illness. A Comparison of Clinical Judgment with a Prediction Rule." *Archives of Internal Medicine* 149 (5): 1083–86.

Braveman, P., and E. Tarimo. 2002. "Social Inequalities in Health Within Countries: Not Only an Issue for Affluent Nations." *Social Science and Medicine* 54 (11): 1621–35.

Breeze, E., A. E. Fletcher, D. A. Leon, M. G. Marmot, R. J. Clarke, and M. J. Shipley. 2001. "Do Socioeconomic Disadvantages Persist into Old Age? Self-Reported Morbidity in a 29-Year Follow-up of the Whitehall Study." *American Journal of Public Health* 91 (2): 277–83.

Breiman. L., J. H. Friedman, R. A. Olshen, and C. J. Stone. 1984. *Classification and Regression Trees.* Belmont, CA: Wadsworth International Group.

Brewster, A. C., R. C. Bradbury, and C. M. Jacobs. 1985. "Measuring the Effect of Illness Severity on Revenue Under DRGs." *Healthcare Financial Management* 39 (7): 52–53, 56–60.

Brewster, A. C., B. G. Karlin, L. A. Hyde, C. M. Jacobs, R. C. Bradbury, and Y. M. Chae. 1985. "MEDISGRPS: A Clinically Based Approach to Classifying Hospital Patients at Admission." *Inquiry* 22 (4): 377–87.

Bright, R. A., J. Avorn, and D. E. Everitt. 1989. "Medicaid Data as a Resource for Epidemiologic Studies: Strengths and Limitations." *Journal of Clinical Epidemiology* 42 (10): 937–45.

Brinkley, J. 1986. "U.S. Releasing Lists of Hospitals with Abnormal Mortality Rates." *New York Times,* 12 March, 1.

Bristowe, J. S. 1864. "Hospital Mortality." *Medical Times and Gazette* April 30; 491–92.

Bristowe, J. S., and T. Holmes. 1864. "Report on the Hospitals of the United Kingdom." In *Sixth Report of the Medical Officer of the Privy Council, 1863*, edited by G. E. Eyre and W. Spottiswoode. London: Her Majesty's Stationery Office.

Brown, F. 1989. *ICD-9-CM Coding Handbook, Without Answers.* Chicago: American Hospital Publishing, Division of Quality Control Management, American Hospital Association.

Bryk, A. S., and S. W. Raudenbush. 1992. *Hierarchical Linear Models: Applications and Data Analysis Methods.* Newbury Park, CA: Sage.

Burns, R. B., E. P. McCarthy, K. M. Freund, S. L. Marwill, M. Shwartz, A. Ash, and M. A. Moskowitz. 1996. "Black Women Receive Less Mammography even with Similar Use of Primary Care." *Annals of Internal Medicine* 125 (3): 173–82.

Burnum, J. F. 1989. "The Misinformation Era: The Fall of the Medical Record." *Annals of Internal Medicine* 110 (6): 482–84.

Butler, P. A., and R. E. Schlenker. 1989. "Case-mix Reimbursements for Nursing Homes: Objectives and Achievements." *Milbank Quarterly* 67 (1) 103–36.

Bye, B. V., and G. F. Riley. 1989. "Eliminating the Medicare Waiting Period for Social Security Disabled-Worker Beneficiaries." *Social Security Bulletin* 52 (5): 2–15.

Bye, B., G. Riley, and J. Lubitz. 1987. "Medicare Utilization by Disabled-Worker Beneficiaries: A Longitudinal Analysis." *Social Security Bulletin* 50 (12): 13–28.

Bye, B. V., J. M. Dykacz, J. C. Hennessey, and G. F. Riley. 1991. "Medicare Costs Prior to Retirement for Disabled-Worker Beneficiaries." *Social Security Bulletin* 54 (4): 2–23.

Calkins, D. R., L. V. Rubenstein, P. D. Cleary, A. R. Davies, A. M. Jette, A. Fink, J. Kosecoff, R. T. Young, R. H. Brook, and T. L. Delbanco. 1991. "Failure of Physicians to Recognize Functional Disability in Ambulatory Patients." *Annals of Internal Medicine* 114 (6): 451–54.

Campbell, J. R., P. Carpenter, C. Sneiderman, S. Cohn, C. G. Chute, and J. Warren. 1997. "Phase II Evaluation of Clinical Coding Schemes: Completeness, Taxonomy, Mapping, Definitions, and Clarity. CPRI Work Group on Codes and Structures." *Journal of the American Medical Information Association* 4 (3): 238–51.

Capdeville, M., J. H. Lee, and A. L. Taylor. 2001. "Effect of Gender on Fast-Track Recovery After Coronary Artery Bypass Graft Surgery." *Journal of Cardiothoracic and Vascular Anesthesia* 15 (2): 146–51.

Carpenter, C. E., M. D. Rosko, D. Z. Louis, and E. J. Yuen. 1999. "Severity of Illness and Profitability: A Patient Level Analysis." *Health Services Management Research* 12 (4): 217–26.

Carpenter, W. T., and R. W. Buchanan. 1995. "Schizophrenia." In *Comprehensive Textbook of Psychiatry/VI*, edited by H. Kaplan and B. Sadock. Baltimore: Williams & Wilkins.

Carson, S. S., and P. B. Bach. 2001. "Predicting Mortality in Patients Suffering from Prolonged Critical Illness: An Assessment of four Severity-of-Illness Measures." *Chest* 120 (3): 928–33.

Carter, G. M., J. P. Newhouse, and D. A. Relles. 1990. "How Much Change in the Case Mix Index is DRG Creep?" Santa Monica, CA: RAND.

———. 1991. "Has DRG Creep Crept up? Decomposing the Case Mix Index Change Between 1987 and 1988." R-3826-HCFA. Santa Monica, CA: RAND.

Case, R. B., A. J. Moss, N. Case, M. McDermott, and S. Eberly. 1992. "Living Alone After Myocardial Infarction. Impact on Prognosis." *Journal of the American Medical Association* 267 (4): 515–19.

Casella, G. 1985. "An Introduction to Empirical Bayes Data Analysis." *The American Statistician* 39 (2): 83–87.

Cassel, C. K., R. W. Besdine, and L. C. Siegel. 1999. "Restructuring Medicare for the Next Century: What Will Beneficiaries Really Need?" *Health Affairs (Millwood)* 18 (1): 118–31.

Cassel, E. J. 1997. *Doctoring. The Nature of Primary Care Medicine.* New York: Oxford University Press.

Cave, D. G. 1995. "Profiling Physician Practice Patterns Using Diagnostic Episode Clusters." *Medical Care* 33 (5): 463–86.

Centers for Disease Control and Prevention. 2000. "Unrealized Prevention Opportunities. Reducing the Health and Economic Burden of Chronic Disease. National and State Perspectives." Atlanta: CDC.

Centers for Disease Control and Prevention, National Center for Health Statistics. 1998. "Average Length of Stay for Discharges from Short-Stay Hospitals, by Age and First-Listed Diagnosis: United States 1998." [Online report; retrieved 9/24/02.] http://www.cdc.gov/nchs/data/hdasd/sr13_148t9.pdf.

Centers for Medicare & Medicaid Services. 2002a. "Overview of the Prospective Payment System for Inpatient Rehabilitation Hospitals and Rehabilitation Units." [Online information; retrieved 4/22/02.] http://www.cms.gov/providers/irfpps/ default.asp.

———. 2002b. "IRF-PAI Data Specifications in Effect for January 2002." [Online information; retrieved 4/22/02.] http://www.cms.gov/providers/irfpps. irfpai.asp.

———. 2002c. "The State Children's Health Insurance Program Annual Enrollment Survey." [Online information; retrieved 7/18/02.] http://www.cms.hhs. gov/schip.

———. 2002d. "Quality of Care—National Projects. Medicare Health Outcomes Survey." [Online information; retrieved 7/1/02.] http://www.cms.gov/ surveys/hos/.

———. 2002e. "National Health Expenditure Projections." [Online information; retrieved 11/15/02.] http://www.cms.hhs.gov/statistics/nhe/projections-2001.

———. 2002f. "HH-PPS Case-Mix Overview." [Online information; retrieved 7/11/02.] http://www.cms.gov/medlearn/hhppsch3.pdf.

Centor, R. M., and J. S. Schwartz. 1985. "An Evaluation of Methods for Estimating the Area Under the Receiver Operating Characteristic (ROC) Curve." *Medical Decision Making* 5 (2): 149–56.

Chamberlain, J. M., K. M. Patel, U. E. Ruttimann, and M. M. Pollack. 1998. "Pediatric Risk of Admission (PRISA): A Measure of Severity of Illness for Assessing the Risk of Hospitalization from the Emergency Department." *Annals of Emergency Medicine* 32 (2): 161–69.

Chambers, J. M., and T. J. Hastie. 1992. "Statistical Models in S." Pacific Grove, CA: Wadsworth & Brooks/Cole.

Chambers, L. W., L. A. Macdonald, P. Tugwell, W. W. Buchanan, and G. Kraag. 1982. "The McMaster Health Index Questionnaire as a Measure of Quality of Life for Patients with Rheumatoid Disease." *Journal of Rheumatology* 9 (5): 780–84.

Chan, A. W., D. L. Bhatt, D. P. Chew, M. J. Quinn, D. J. Moliterno, E. J. Topol, and S. G. Ellis. 2002. "Early and Sustained Survival Benefit Associated with Statin Therapy at the Time of Percutaneous Coronary Intervention." *Circulation* 105 (6): 691–96.

Chan, L., J. N. Doctor, R. F. MacLehose, H. Lawson, R. A. Rosenblatt, L. M. Baldwin, and A. Jha. 1999. "Do Medicare Patients with Disabilities Receive Preventive Services? A Population-Based Study." *Archives of Physical Medicine and Rehabilitation* 80 (6): 642–46.

Chang, R. W. 1989. "Individual Outcome Prediction Models for Intensive Care Units." *Lancet* 2 (8655): 143–46.

Charlson, M. E., P. Pompei, K. L. Ales, and C. R. MacKenzie. 1987. "A New Method of Classifying Prognostic Comorbidity in Longitudinal Studies: Development and Validation." *Journal of Chronic Disease* 40 (5): 373–83.

Charlton, J. I. 1998. *Nothing About Us Without Us: Disability Oppression and Empowerment.* Berkeley, CA: University of California Press.

Chassin, M. R. 2002. "Achieving and Sustaining Improved Quality: Lessons from New York State and Cardiac Surgery." *Health Affairs (Millwood)* 21 (4): 40–51.

Chassin, M. R., E. L. Hannan, and B. A. DeBuono. 1996. "Benefits and Hazards of Reporting Medical Outcomes Publicly." *New England Journal of Medicine* 334 (6): 394–98.

Chen, C. Y., P. S. Neufeld, C. A. Feely, and C. S. Skinner. 1999. "Factors Influencing Compliance with Home Exercise Programs Among Patients with Upper-Extremity Impairment." *American Journal of Occupational Health* 53 (2): 171–80.

Chen, F. G., K. F. Koh, and M. H. Goh. 1993. "Validation of APACHE II Score in a Surgical Intensive Care Unit." *Singapore Medical Journal* 34 (4): 322–24.

Chen, J., M. J. Radford, Y. Wang, T. A. Marciniak, and H. M. Krumholz. 1999. "Do 'America's Best Hospitals' Perform Better for Acute Myocardial Infarction?" *New England Journal of Medicine* 340 (4): 286–92.

Chen, L. W., and D. G. Shea. 2002. "Does Prospective Payment Really Contain Nursing Home Costs?" *Health Services Research* 37 (2): 251–71.

Clancy, C. M., and J. M. Eisenberg. 1997. "Outcomes Research at the Agency for Health Care Policy and Research." *Disease Management and Clinical Outcomes* 1 (3): 72–80.

Clapesattle, H. 1941. *The Doctors Mayo.* Minneapolis, MN: The University of Minneapolis.

Clark, R. E., S. K. Ricketts, and G. J. McHugo. 1996. "Measuring Hospital Use Without Claims: A Comparison of Patient and Provider Reports." *Health Services Research* 31 (2): 153–69.

Cleary, P. D. 1997. "Subjective and Objective Measures of Health: Which Is Better When?" *Journal of Health Service Research and Policy* 2 (1): 3–4.

Cleary, P. D., and R. Angel. 1984. "The Analysis of Relationships Involving Dichotomous Dependent Variables." *Journal of Health and Social Behavior* 25 (3): 334–48.

Cleary, P. D., S. Edgman-Levitan, M. Roberts, T. W. Moloney, W. McMullen, J. D. Walker, and T. L. Delbanco. 1991. "Patients Evaluate Their Hospital Care: A National Survey." *Health Affairs (Millwood)* 10 (4): 254–67.

Cleary, P. D., S. Edgman-Levitan, J. D. Walker, M. Gerteis, and T. L. Delbanco. 1993. "Using Patient Reports to Improve Medical Care: A Preliminary Report from 10 Hospitals." *Quality Management in Health Care* 2 (1): 31–38.

Cleveland, W. S. 1979. "Robust Locally Weighted Regression and Smoothing Scatterplots." *Journal of the American Statistical Association* 74: 829–36.

————. 1993. *Visualizing Data*. Summit, NJ: Hobart Press.

Clinical Assessment of the Reliability of the Examination (CARE). 2002. [Online article; retrieved 11/12/02.] http://www.carestudy.com/CareStudy/Default. asp.

Clough, R. A., B. J. Leavitt, J. R. Morton, S. K. Plume, F. Hernandez, W. Nugent, S. J. Lahey, C. S. Ross, and G. T. O'Connor. 2002. "The Effect of Comorbid Illness on Mortality Outcomes in Cardiac Surgery." *Archives of Surgery* 137 (4): 428–32.

Codman, E. A. 1917. "Case-Records and Their Value." *Bulletin of American College of Surgeons* 3: 24–27.

————. 1934. *The Shoulder: Rupture of the Supraspinatus Tendon and Other Lesions in or About the Subacromial Bursa*. Boston: Thomas Todd.

Coffey, R. M., T. Mark, E. King, H. Harwood, D. McKusick, J. Genuardi, J. Dilonardo, and J. Buck. 2000. "National Estimates of Expenditures for Mental Health and Substance Abuse Treatment, 1997." Rockville, MD: U.S. DHHS Substance Abuse and Mental Health Services Administration.

Cohen, I. B. 1984. "Florence Nightingale." *Scientific American* 250 (3): 128–37.

Cohen, J. A. 1960. "A Coeffecient of Agreement for Normal Scales." *Educational and Psychological Measurement* 20 (1): 37–46.

Cohen, M. M., and L. MacWilliam. 1995. "Measuring the Health of the Population." *Medical Care* 33 (12, Suppl.): DS21–DS42.

Collins, T., J. Daley, W. H. Henderson, and S. F. Khuri. 1999. "Risk Factors for Prolonged Length of Stay After Major Elective Surgery." *Annals of Surgery* 230 (2): 251–59.

Collins, T. C., M. Johnson, J. Daley, W. G. Henderson, S. F. Khuri, and H. S. Gordon. 2001. "Preoperative Risk Factors for 30-Day Mortality After Elective Surgery for Vascular Disease in Department of Veterans Affairs Hospitals: Is Race Important?" *Journal of Vascular Surgery* 34 (4): 634–40.

Collins, T. C., M. Johnson, W. Henderson, S. F. Khuri, and J. Daley. 2002. "Lower Extremity Nontraumatic Amputation Among Veterans with Peripheral Arterial Disease: Is Race an Independent Factor?" *Medical Care* 40 (1, Suppl.): I106–I116.

Concato, J., N. Shah, and R. I. Horwitz. 2000. "Randomized, Controlled Trials, Observational Studies, and the Hierarchy of Research Designs." *New England Journal of Medicine* 342 (25): 1887–92.

Conklin, J. E., J. V. Lieberman, C. A. Barnes, and D. Z. Louis. 1984. "Disease Staging: Implications for Hospital Reimbursement and Management." *Health Care Financing Review* (Suppl.): 13–22.

Connors, A. F., Jr., T. Speroff, N. V. Dawson, C. Thomas, F. E. Harrell, Jr., D. Wagner, N. Desbiens, L. Goldman, A. W. Wu, R. M. Califf, W. J. Fulkerson, Jr., H. Vidaillet, S. Broste, P. Bellamy, J. Lynn, and W. A. Knaus. 1996. "The Effectiveness of Right Heart Catheterization in the Initial Care of Critically Ill Patients. SUPPORT Investigators." *Journal of the American Medical Association* 276 (11): 889–97.

Cooper, G. S., Z. Yuan, K. C. Stange, L. K. Dennis, S. B. Amini, and A. A. Rimm. 2000. "Agreement of Medicare Claims and Tumor Registry Data for Assessment of Cancer-Related Treatment." *Medical Care* 38 (4): 411–21.

Cooper, J. K. 1998. "Measuring the Health of Seniors." *Archives of Family Medicine* 7 (5): 415–16.

Cooper, J. K., T. Kohlmann, J. A. Michael, S. C. Haffer, and M. Stevic. 2001. "Health Outcomes. New Quality Measure for Medicare." *International Journal for Quality in Health Care* 13 (1): 9–16.

Cooper-Patrick, L., J. J. Gallo, J. J. Gonzales, H. T. Vu, N. R. Powe, C. Nelson, and D. E. Ford. 1999. "Race, Gender, and Partnership in the Patient-Physician Relationship." *Journal of the American Medical Association* 282 (6): 583–89.

Corbie-Smith, G., S. B. Thomas, M. V. Williams, and S. Moody-Ayers. 1999. "Attitudes and Beliefs of African Americans Toward Participation in Medical Research." *Journal of General Internal Medicine* 14 (9): 537–46.

Covinsky, K. E., G. E. Rosenthal, M. M. Chren, A. C. Justice, R. H. Fortinsky, R. M. Palmer, and C. S. Landefeld. 1998. "The Relation Between Health Status Changes and Patient Satisfaction in Older Hospitalized Medical Patients." *Journal of General Internal Medicine* 13 (4): 223–29.

Cox, D. R. 1972. "Regression Models and Life-Tables (with Discussion)." *Journal of the Royal Statistical Society* 34 (Series B, 2): 187–220.

Cox, D. R., and N. Wermuth. 1992. "A Comment on the Coefficient of Determination for Binary Responses." *The American Statistician* 46 (1): 1–4.

Cuffel, B. J., E. P. Fischer, R. R. Owen, Jr., and G. R. Smith, Jr. 1997. "An Instrument for Measurement of Outcomes of Care for Schizophrenia. Issues in Development and Implementation." *Evaluation and the Health Professions* 20 (1): 96–108.

Culler, S. D., C. M. Callahan, and F. D. Wolinsky. 1995. "Predicting Hospital Costs Among Older Decedents over Time." *Medical Care* 33 (11): 1089–1105.

Cumming, R. B., D. Knutson, B. A. Cameron, and B. Derrick. 2002. "A Comparative Analysis of Claims-Based Methods of Health Risk Assessment for Commercial Populations. Society of Actuaries." [Online article; retieval 5/24/02.] soa.org/sections/riskadjfinalreport1.pdf.

Currie, RJ. 2002. "Report Summary. Health Care and Health: Experience with a Population-Based Information System. University of Manitoba." [Online article; retieval 10/30/02.] http://www.umanitoba.ca/centres/mchp/medcare.htm.

Cutler, D. M. 2001. "Declining Disability Among the Elderly." *Health Affairs (Millwood)* 20 (6): 11–27.

D'Agostino, R. B., Jr. 1998. "Propensity Score Methods for Bias Reduction in the Comparison of a Treatment to a Non-Randomized Control Group." *Statistics in Medicine* 17 (19): 2265–81.

Daley, J., M. G. Forbes, G. J. Young, M. P. Charns, J. O. Gibbs, K. Hur, W. Henderson, and S. F. Khuri. 1997b. "Validating Risk-Adjusted Surgical Outcomes: Site Visit Assessment of Process and Structure. National VA Surgical Risk Study." *Journal of the American College of Surgeons* 185 (4): 341–51.

Daley, J., W. G. Henderson, and S. F. Khuri. 2001. "Risk-Adjusted Surgical Outcomes." *Annual Review of Medicine* 52: 275–87.

Daley, J., S. Jencks, D. Draper, G. Lenhart, N. Thomas, and J. Walker. 1988. "Predicting Hospital-Associated Mortality for Medicare Patients. A Method for Patients with Stroke, Pneumonia, Acute Myocardial Infarction, and Congestive Heart Failure." *Journal of the American Medical Association* 260 (24): 3617–24.

Daley, J., S. F. Khuri, W. Henderson, K. Hur, J. O. Gibbs, G. Barbour, J. Demakis, G. Irvin, J. F. Stremple, F. Grover, G. McDonald, E. Passaro, P. J. Fabri, J. Spencer, K. Hammermeister, J. B. Aust, and C. Oprian. 1997a. "Risk Adjustment of the Postoperative Morbidity Rate for the Comparative Assessment of the Quality of Surgical Care: Results of the National Veterans Affairs Surgical Risk Study." *Journal of the American College of Surgeons* 185 (4): 328–40.

Danis, M., J. Garrett, R. Harris, and D. L. Patrick. 1994. "Stability of Choices About Life-Sustaining Treatments." *Annals of Internal Medicine* 120 (7): 567–73.

Davis, R. B., L. I. Iezzoni, R. S. Phillips, P. Reiley, G. A. Coffman, and C. Safran. 1995. "Predicting In-Hospital Mortality. The Importance of Functional Status Information." *Medical Care* 33 (9): 906–21.

Degnan, D., R. Harris, J. Ranney, D. Quade, J. A. Earp, and J. Gonzalez. 1992. "Measuring the Use of Mammography: Two Methods Compared." *American Journal of Public Health* 82 (10): 1386–88.

DeLew, N. 2000. "Medicare: 35 Years of Service." *Health Care Financing Review* 22 (1): 75–103.

DeLiberty, R. N., F. L. Newman, and E. O. Ward. 2001. "Risk Adjustment in the Hoosier Assurance Plan: Impact on Providers." *Journal of Behavioral Health Services & Research* 28 (3): 301–18.

Derogatis, L. R. 1994. "SCL-90-R, Brief Symptom Inventory, and Matching Clinical Rating Scales." In *Psychological Testing, Treatment Planning, and Outcome Assessment*, edited by M. E. Maruisch. New York: Erlbaum.

Deutsch, A., S. Braun, and C. V. Granger. 1997. "The Functional Independence Measure." *Journal of Rehabilitation Outcomes Measures* 1: 67–71.

Deyo, R. A., D. C. Cherkin, and M. A. Ciol. 1992. "Adapting a Clinical Comorbidity Index for Use with ICD-9-CM Administrative Databases." *Journal of Clinical Epidemiology* 45 (6): 613–19.

D'Hoore, W., A. Bouckaert, and C. Tilquin. 1996. "Practical Considerations on the Use of the Charlson Comorbidity Index with Administrative Data Bases." *Journal of Clinical Epidemiology* 49 (12): 1429–33.

Diamond, M., and M. Stone. 1981. "Nightingale on Quetelet. Part I. The Passionate Statistician." *Journal of the Royal Statistical Society* 144: 66–79.

Dick, R. S., E. Steen, and D. E. Detmer. 1997. *The Computer-Based Patient Record: An Essential Technology for Health Care, Revised Edition.* Washington, DC: National Academy Press, Institute of Medicine, Committee on Improving the Patient Record.

Dickey, B., R. C. Hermann, and S. V. Eisen. 1998. "Assessing the Quality of Psychiatric Care: Research Methods and Application in Clinical Practice." *Harvard Review of Psychiatry* 6 (2): 88–96.

Dickey, B. D., S. Normand, R. C. Hermann, S. V. Eisen, D. Cortes, P. Cleary, and N. Ware. In press. "Guideline Recommendations for Treatment of Schizophrenia: The Impact of Managed Care." *Archives of General Psychiatry.*

DiFranza, J. R., and R. A. Lew. 1996. "Morbidity and Mortality in Children Associated with the Use of Tobacco Products by Other People." *Pediatrics* 97 (4): 560–68.

DiSalvo, T. G., S. L. Normand, P. J. Hauptman, E. Guadagnoli, R. H. Palmer, and B. J. McNeil. 2001. "Pitfalls in Assessing the Quality of Care for Patients with Cardiovascular Disease." *American Journal of Medicine* 111 (4): 297–303.

Dixon, W. J., and F. J. Massey. 1969. *Introduction to Statistical Analysis.* 3d ed. New York: McGraw-Hill.

Dixon, W. J., and J. W. Tukey. 1968. "Approximate Behavior of the Distribution of Winsorized *t*. (For a Proof of the Properties of Statistical Tests with Winsorized Data)." *Technometrics* 10.

Dolan, P. 1996. "The Effect of Experience of Illness on Health State Valuations." *Journal of Clinical Epidemiology* 49 (5): 551–64.

Donabedian, A. 1980. *Explorations in Quality Assessment and Monitoring. Volume 1. The Definition of Quality and Approaches to Its Assessment.* Chicago: Health Administration Press.

———. 1989. "The End Results of Health Care: Ernest Codman's Contribution to Quality Assessment and Beyond." *Milbank Quarterly* 67 (2): 233–56.

Donaldson, M. S., and M. J. Field. 1998. "Measuring Quality of Care at the End of Life." *Archives of Internal Medicine* 158 (2): 121–28.

Donaldson, M. S., and K. N. Lohr. 1994. *Health Data in the Information Age. Use, Disclosure and Privacy.* Washington, DC: National Academy Press.

Dow, M. G., T. L. Boaz, and D. Thornton. 2001. "Risk Adjustment of Florida Mental Health Outcomes Data: Concepts, Methods, and Results." *Journal of Behavioral Health Services & Research* 28 (3): 258–72.

Draper, N. R., and H. Smith. 1981. *Applied Regression Analysis,* 2d ed. New York: John Wiley.

Druss, B. G., M. Schlesinger, T. Thomas, and H. Allen. 2000. "Chronic Illness and Plan Satisfaction Under Managed Care." *Health Affairs (Millwood)* 19 (1): 203–09.

Duan, N. 1983. "Smearing Estimate: A Nonparametric Retransformation Method." *Journal of the American Statistical Association* 78 (383): 605–10.

Dubois, R. W., and R. H. Brook. 1988. "Preventable Deaths: Who, How Often, and Why?" *Annals of Internal Medicine* 109 (7): 582–89.

Dubois, R. W., R. H. Brook, and W. H. Rogers. 1987. "Adjusted Hospital Death Rates: A Potential Screen for Quality of Medical Care." *American Journal of Public Health* 77 (9): 1162–66.

Dubois, R. W., W. H. Rogers, J. H. Moxley, III, D. Draper, and R. H. Brook. 1987. "Hospital Inpatient Mortality: Is It a Predictor of Quality?" *New England Journal of Medicine* 317 (26): 1674–80.

Duggan, A. K., B. Starfield, and C. DeAngelis. 1990. "Structured Encounter Form: The Impact on Provider Performance and Recording of Well-Child Care." *Pediatrics* 85 (1): 104–13.

Dunbar, L. J., and B. C. Diehl. 1995. "Developing a Patient Classification System for the Pediatric Rehabilitation Setting." *Rehabilitation Nursing* 20: 328–32.

Duncan, G. J., J. Brooks-Gunn, and P. K. Klebanov. 1994. "Economic Deprivation and Early Childhood Development." *Child Development* 65 (2, Special No.): 296–318.

Durbin, J., P. Goering, G. Pink, and M. Murray. 1999. "Classifying Psychiatric Inpatients: Seeking Better Measures." *Medical Care* 37 (4): 415–23.

Eddy, D. M. 1984. "Variations in Physician Practice: The Role of Uncertainty." *Health Affairs (Millwood)* 3 (2): 74–89.

Edlavitch, S. A., M. Feinleib, and C. Anello. 1985. "A Potential Use of the National Death Index for Postmarketing Drug Surveillance." *Journal of the American Medical Association* 253 (9): 1292–95.

Edwards, N., D. Honemann, D. Burley, and M. Navarro. 1994. "Refinement of the Medicare Diagnosis-Related Groups to Incorporate a Measure of Severity." *Health Care Financing Review* 16 (2): 45–64.

Efron, B. 1979. "Another Look at the Jacknife." *Annals of Statistics* 7: 1–26.

Efron, B., and C. Morris. 1972. "Limiting the Risk of Bayes and Empirical Bayes Estimators—Part II: The Empirical Bayes Case." *Journal of the American Statistical Association* 67 (337): 130–39.

———. 1973. "Stein's Estimation Rule and Its Competitors—An Empirical Bayes Approach." *Journal of the American Statistical Association* 68 (341): 117–30.

———. 1975. "Data Analysis Using Stein's Estimator and Its Generalizations." *Journal of the American Statistical Association* 70 (350): 311–19.

———. 1977. "Stein's Paradox in Statistics." *Scientific American* 236 (5): 119–27.

Eisen, S. V., M. C. Grob, and A. A. Klein. 1986. "BASIS: The Development of a Self-Report Measure for Psychiatric Inpatient Evaluation." *Psychiatric Hospital* 17 (4): 165–71.

Eisenberg, D. M., R. B. Davis, S. L. Ettner, S. Appel, S. Wilkey, M. Van Rompay, and R. C. Kessler. 1998. "Trends in Alternative Medicine Use in the United States, 1990–1997: Results of a Follow-up National Survey." *Journal of the American Medical Association* 280 (18): 1569–75.

Eisenberg, D. M., R. C. Kessler, C. Foster, F. E. Norlock, D. R. Calkins, and T. L. Delbanco. 1993. "Unconventional Medicine in the United States. Prevalence, Costs, and Patterns of Use." *New England Journal of Medicine* 328 (4): 246–52.

Eisenberg, J. M. 2002. "Measuring Quality: Are We Ready to Compare the Quality of Care Among Physician Groups?" *Annals of Internal Medicine* 136 (2): 153–54.

Elad, Y., W. J. French, D. M. Shavelle, L. S. Parsons, M. J. Sada, and N. R. Every. 2002. "Primary Angioplasty and Selection Bias In Patients Presenting Late (>12 h) after Onset of Chest Pain and ST Elevation Myocardial Infarction." *Journal of the American College of Cardiologists* 39 (5): 826–33.

Elixhauser, A., R. M. Andrews, and S. Fox. 1993. "Clinical Classifications for Health Policy Research: Discharge Statistics by Principal Diagnosis and Procedure. (AHCPR Publication No. 93–0043)." Rockville, MD: Agency for Health Care Policy and Research, Public Health Service.

Elixhauser, A., and E. McCarthy. 1996. "Clinical Classifications for Health Policy Research, Version 2: Hospital Inpatient Statistics (AHCPR Publication No. 96–0017). Healthcare Cost and Utilization Project (HCUP-3) Research Note 1." Rockville, MD: Agency for Health Care Policy and Research.

Elixhauser, A., C. Steiner, D. R. Harris, and R. M. Coffey. 1998. "Comorbidity Measures for Use with Administrative Data." *Medical Care* 36 (1): 8–27.

Elliott, M. N., R. Swartz, J. Adams, K. L. Spritzer, and R. D. Hays. 2001. "Case-Mix

Adjustment of the National CAHPS Benchmarking Data 1.0: A Violation of Model Assumptions?" *Health Services Research* 36 (3): 555–73.

Ellis, R. P., and A. Ash. 1995. "Refinements to the Diagnostic Cost Group (DCG) Model." *Inquiry* 32 (4): 418–29.

Ellis, R. P., G. C. Pope, L. Iezzoni, J. Z. Ayanian, D. W. Bates, H. Burstin, and A. S. Ash. 1996. "Diagnosis-Based Risk Adjustment for Medicare Capitation Payments." *Health Care Financing Review* 17 (3): 101–28.

Elmore, J. G., and A. R. Feinstein. 1992. "A Bibliography of Publications on Observer Variability (Final Statement)." *Journal of Clinical Epidemiology* 45 (6): 567–80.

Endicott, J., R. L. Spitzer, J. L. Fleiss, and J. Cohen. 1976. "The Global Assessment Scale. A Procedure for Measuring Overall Severity of Psychiatric Disturbance." *Archives of General Psychiatry* 33 (6): 766–71.

English, J. T., S. S. Sharfstein, D. J. Scherl, B. Astrachan, and I. L. Muszynski. 1986. "Diagnosis-Related Groups and General Hospital Psychiatry: The APA Study." *American Journal of Psychiatry* 143 (2): 131–39.

Epping-Jordan, A., and T. Ustun. 2000. "The WHODAS II: Leveling the Playing Field for All Disorders." *WHO Mental Health Bulletin* 6: 4–5.

Epstein, A. M., J. Z. Ayanian, J. H. Keogh, S. J. Noonan, N. Armistead, P. D. Cleary, J. S. Weissman, J. A. David-Kasdan, D. Carlson, J. Fuller, D. Marsh, and R. M. Conti. 2000. "Racial Disparities in Access to Renal Transplantation—Clinically Appropriate or Due to Underuse or Overuse?" *New England Journal of Medicine* 343 (21): 1537–44.

Epstein, A. M., and E. J. Cumella. 1988. "Capitation Payment: Using Predictors for Medical Utilization to Adjust Rates." *Health Care Financing Review* 10 (1): 51–69.

Epstein, S. E., A. A. Quyymi, and R. O. Bonow. 1989. "Sudden Cardiac Death Without Warning. Possible Mechanisms and Implications for Screening Asymptomatic Populations." *New England Journal of Medicine* 321 (5): 320–24.

Erickson, L. C., P. H. Wise, E. F. Cook, A. Beiser, and J. W. Newburger. 2000. "The Impact of Managed Care Insurance on Use of Lower-Mortality Hospitals by Children Undergoing Cardiac Surgery in California." *Pediatrics* 105 (6): 1271–78.

Essock-Vitale, S. 1987. "Patient Characteristics Predictive of Treatment Costs on Inpatient Psychiatric Wards." *Hospital and Community Psychiatry* 38 (3): 263–69.

Ettner, S. L., and R. G. Frank. 1998. "The Use of Risk Adjustment to Set Capitation Rates." In *Mental Health, United States, 1998*, edited by R. Manderscheid and M. L. Henderson. Washington, DC: Government Printing Office.

Ettner, S. L., R. G. Frank, T. Mark, and M. W. Smith. 1999. "Risk Adjustment of Capitation Payments to Behavioral Health Care Carve-outs: How Well Do Existing Methodologies Account for Psychiatric Disability?" *Health Care Management Science* 3 (2): 159–69.

Ettner, S. L., R. G. Frank, T. G. McGuire, and R. C. Hermann. 2001. "Risk Adjustment Alternatives in Paying for Behavioral Health Care Under Medicaid." *Health Services Research* 36 (4): 793–811.

Ettner, S. L., R. G. Frank, T. G. McGuire, J. P. Newhouse, and E. H. Notman. 1998. "Risk Adjustment of Mental Health and Substance Abuse Payments." *Inquiry* 35 (2): 223–39.

Ettner, S. L., K. Kuhlthau, T. J. McLaughlin, J. M. Perrin, and S. L. Gortmaker. 2000. "Impact of Expanding SSI on Medicaid Expenditures of Disabled Children." *Health Care Financing Review* 21 (3): 185–201.

Ettner, S. L., and E. H. Notman. 1997. "How Well Do Ambulatory Care Groups Predict Expenditures on Mental Health and Substance Abuse Patients?" *Administration and Policy in Mental Health* 24 (4): 339–57.

Evans, R. G., M. L. Barer, and T. R. Marmor. 1994. *Why Are Some People Healthy and Others Not? The Determinants of Health of Populations.* New York: Aldine de Gryter.

Evans, R. G., and J. F. Mustard. 1995. "Forward." *Medical Care* 33 (Suppl.): DS5–DS6.

Eyler, J. M. 1979. *Victorian Social Medicine. The Ideas and Methods of William Farr.* Baltimore: The Johns Hopkins University Press.

Fan, V. S., D. Au, P. Heagerty, R. A. Deyo, M. B. McDonell, and S. D. Fihn. 2002. "Validation of Case-Mix Measures Derived from Self-Reports of Diagnoses and Health." *Journal of Clinical Epidemiology* 55 (4): 371–80.

Farr, W. *24th Annual Report of the Registrar-General.* [Further information on this publication not available.]

———. 1864a. "Miss Nightingale's Notes on Hospitals." *Medical Times and Gazette* (Feb. 13): 186–87.

———. 1864b. "Mortality in Hospitals." *Lancet* (April 9): 420–22.

Feigl, P., G. Glaefke, L. Ford, P. Diehr, and J. Chu. 1988. "Studying Patterns of Cancer Care: How Useful Is the Medical Record?" *American Journal of Public Health* 78 (5): 526–33.

Feinstein, A. R. 1967. *Clinical Judgement.* Baltimore: Williams & Wilkins.

———. 1987. *Clinimetrics.* New Haven, CT: Yale University Press.

———. 1992. "Benefits and Obstacles for Development of Health Status Assessment Measures in Clinical Settings." *Medical Care* 30 (5, Suppl.): MS50–MS56.

Feinstein, A. R., C. K. Wells, and S. D. Walter. 1990. "A Comparison of Multivariable Mathematical Methods for Predicting Survival—I. Introduction, Rationale, and General Strategy." *Journal of Clinical Epidemiology* 43 (4): 339–47.

Ferreira, F. L., D. P. Bota, A. Bross, C. Melot, and J. L. Vincent. 2001. "Serial Evaluation of the SOFA Score to Predict Outcome in Critically Ill Patients." *Journal of the American Medical Association* 286 (14): 1754–58.

Ferris, T. G., E. F. Crain, E. Oken, L. Wang, S. Clark, and C. A. Camargo, Jr. 2001. "Insurance and Quality of Care for Children with Acute Asthma." *Ambulatory Pediatrics* 1 (5): 267–74.

Ferris, T. G., D. Saglam, R. S. Stafford, N. Causino, B. Starfield, L. Culpepper, and D. Blumenthal. 1998. "Changes in the Daily Practice of Primary Care for Children." *Archives of Pediatric and Adolescent Medicine* 152 (2): 227–33.

Fetter, R. B., Y. Shin, J. L. Freeman, R. F. Averill, and J. D. Thompson. 1980. "Case Mix Definition by Diagnosis-Related Groups." *Medical Care* 18 (2, Suppl.): 1–53.

Fihn, S. D. 2000. "Does VA Health Care Measure Up?" *New England Journal of Medicine* 343 (26): 1963–65.

Finch, M., R. L. Kane, and I. Philip. 1995. "Developing a New Metric for ADLs." *Journal of the American Geriatric Society* 43 (8): 877–84.

Fine, E. M., D. E. Singer, B. H. Hanusa, J. R. Lave, and W. N. Kaoor. 1993. "Validation of a Pneumonia Prognostic Index Using the MedisGroups Comparative Hospital Database." *American Journal of Medicine* 94: 153–59.

Fine, M. J., B. H. Hanusa, J. R. Lave, D. E. Singer, R. A. Stone, L. A. Weissfeld, C. M. Coley, T. J. Marrie, and W. N. Kapoor. 1995. "Comparison of a Disease-Specific and a Generic Severity of Illness Measure for Patients with Community-Acquired Pneumonia." *Journal of General Internal Medicine* 10 (7): 359–68.

Finkelstein, J. A., R. W. Brown, L. C. Schneider, S. T. Weiss, J. M. Quintana, D. A. Goldmann, and C. J. Homer. 1995. "Quality of Care for Preschool Children with Asthma: The Role of Social Factors and Practice Setting." *Pediatrics* 95 (3): 389–94.

First, B. 1994. "M.D. Advance Data No. 237." U.S. Government Printing Office Publication No. 301–060/80012. Washington, DC: U.S. Government Printing Office.

Fiscella, K., and P. Franks. 2001. "Impact of Patient Socioeconomic Status on Physician Profiles: A Comparison of Census-Derived and Individual Measures." *Medical Care* 39 (1): 8–14.

Fisher, E. S., F. S. Whaley, W. M. Krushat, D. J. Malenka, C. Fleming, J. A. Baron, and D. C. Hsia. 1992. "The Accuracy of Medicare's Hospital Claims Data: Progress Has Been Made, but Problems Remain." *American Journal of Public Health* 82 (2): 243–48.

Fishman, P. A., and D. K. Shay. 1999. "Development and Estimation of a Pediatric Chronic Disease Score Using Automated Pharmacy Data." *Medical Care* 37 (9): 874–83.

Flanders, W. D., G. Tucker, A. Krishnadasan, D. Martin, E. Honig, and W. M. McClellan. 1999. "Validation of the Pneumonia Severity Index. Importance of Study-Specific Recalibration." *Journal of General Internal Medicine* 14 (6): 333–40.

Flegal, K. M., M. D. Carroll, C. L. Ogden, and C. L. Johnson. 2002. "Prevalence and Trends in Obesity Among US Adults, 1999–2000." *Journal of the American Medical Association* 288 (14): 1723–27.

Foote, S. M., and C. Hogan. 2001. "Disability Profile and Health Care Costs of Medicare Beneficiaries Under Age Sixty-Five." *Health Affairs (Millwood)* 20 (6): 242–53.

Forrest, C. B., and R. J. Reid. 2001. "Prevalence of Health Problems and Primary Care Physicians' Specialty Referral Decisions." *Journal of Family Practice* 50 (5): 427–32.

Forrest, C. B., L. Simpson, and C. Clancy. 1997. "Child Health Services Research. Challenges and Opportunities." *Journal of the American Medical Association* 277 (22): 1787–93.

Fowler, E. J., and G. F. Anderson. 1996. "Capitation Adjustment for Pediatric Populations." *Pediatrics* 98 (1): 10–17.

Fowles, J. B., A. G. Lawthers, J. P. Weiner, D. W. Garnick, D. S. Petrie, and R. H. Palmer. 1995. "Agreement Between Physicians' Office Records and Medicare Part B Claims Data." *Health Care Financing Review* 16 (4): 189–99.

Fowles, J. B., K. Rosheim, E. J. Fowler, C. Craft, and L. Arrichiello. 1999. "The Validity of Self-Reported Diabetes Quality of Care Measures." *International Journal for Quality in Health Care* 11 (5): 407–12.

Fowles, J. B., J. P. Weiner, D. Knutson, E. Fowler, A. M. Tucker, and M. Ireland. 1996. "Taking Health Status into Account when Setting Capitation Rates: A Comparison of Risk-Adjustment Methods." *Journal of the American Medical Association* 276 (16): 1316–21.

Frank, E., R. F. Prien, R. B. Jarrett, M. B. Keller, D. J. Kupfer, P. W. Lavori, A. J. Rush, and M. M. Weissman. 1991. "Conceptualization and Rationale for Consensus Definitions of Terms in Major Depressive Disorder. Remission, Recovery, Relapse, and Recurrence." *Archives of General Psychiatry* 48 (9): 851–55.

Frank, R. G., and J. R. Lave. 1985. "The Psychiatric DRGs. Are They Different?" *Medical Care* 23 (10): 1148–55.

Franks, P., and K. Fiscella. 2002. "Effect of Patient Socioeconomic Status on Physician Profiles for Prevention, Disease Management, and Diagnostic Testing Costs." *Medical Care* 40 (8): 717–24.

Freeman, J. L., R. B. Fetter, H. Park, K. C. Schneider, J. L. Lichtenstein, J. S. Hughes, W. A. Bauman, C. C. Duncan, D. H. Freeman, Jr., and G. R. Palmer. 1995. "Diagnosis-Related Group Refinement with Diagnosis- and Procedure-Specific Comorbidities and Complications." *Medical Care* 33 (8): 806–27.

Friedman, C., and G. Hripcsak. 1999. "Natural Language Processing and Its Future in Medicine." *Academic Medicine* 74 (8): 890–95.

Fries, B. E. 1990. "Comparing Case-Mix Systems for Nursing Home Payment." *Health Care Financing Review* 11 (4): 103–19.

Fries, B. E., J. N. Morris, and K. Skarupski. 1998. "Facility Report Cards and the Ecological Fallacy." *Canadian Journal of Quality and Health Care* 14 (2): 18–22.

Fries, B. E., D. R. Nerenz, S. P. Falcon, M. L. Ashcraft, and C. Z. Lee. 1990. "A Classification System for Long-Staying Psychiatric Patients." *Medical Care* 28 (4): 311–23.

Fries, B. E., D. P. Schneider, W. J. Foley, M. Gavazzi, R. Burke, and E. Cornelius. 1994. "Refining a Case-Mix Measure for Nursing Homes: Resource Utilization Groups (RUG-III)." *Medical Care* 32 (7): 668–85.

Fuchs, V. R. 1999. "Health Care for the Elderly: How Much? Who Will Pay for It?" *Health Affairs (Millwood)* 18 (1): 1121.

Fuhrer, M. J. 1997. "Response and Commentary. Comments on: Rehabilitation Care and Outcomes from the Patient's Perspective." *Medical Care* 35: JS58–JS60.

Garnick, D. W., A. M. Hendricks, C. B. Cornstock, and D. B. Pryor. 1996. "A Guide to Using Administrative Data for Medical Effectiveness Research." *Journal of Outcomes Management* 3 (1): 18–23.

Gatsonis, C. A., A. M. Epstein, J. P. Newhouse, S. T. Normand, and B. J. McNeil. 1995. "Variations in the Utilization of Coronary Angiography for Elderly Patients with an Acute Myocardial Infarction." *Medical Care* 33 (6): 625–42.

Gelfand, A., and A. F. M. Smith. 1990. "Sampling-Based Approaches to Calculating

Marginal Densities." *Journal of the American Statistical Association* 85: 398–409.

Gelman, A., and D. Nolan. 2002. "You Can Load a Die, but You Can't Bias a Coin." *The American Statistician* 56: 308–11.

Gesensway, D. 2001. "Reasons for Sex-Specific and Gender-Specific Study of Health Topics." *Annals of Internal Medicine* 135 (10): 935–38.

Gfroerer, J. C., and A. L. Hughes. 1991. "The Feasibility of Collecting Drug Abuse Data by Telephone." *Public Health Reports* 106 (4): 384–93.

Ghali, W. A., P. D. Faris, P. D. Galbraith, C. M. Norris, M. J. Curtis, L. D. Saunders, V. Dzavik, L. B. Mitchell, and M. L. Knudtson. 2002. "Sex Differences in Access to Coronary Revascularization After Cardiac Catheterization: Importance of Detailed Clinical Data." *Annals of Internal Medicine* 136 (10): 723–32.

Ghali, W. A., R. E. Hall, A. K. Rosen, A. S. Ash, and M. A. Moskowitz. 1996. "Searching for an Improved Clinical Comorbidity Index for Use with ICD-9-CM Administrative Data." *Journal of Clinical Epidemiology* 49 (3): 273–78.

Gibbons, J. D. 1993. "Nonparametric Measures of Association." University Paper Series on Quantitative Applications in the Social Sciences, Series No. 07–091. Newbury Park, CA: Sage.

Gibbs, J., K. Clark, S. Khuri, W. Henderson, K. Hur, and J. Daley. 2001. "Validating Risk-Adjusted Surgical Outcomes: Chart Review of Process of Care." *International Journal for Quality in Health Care* 13 (3): 187–96.

Gibbs, J., W. Cull, W. Henderson, J. Daley, K. Hur, and S. F. Khuri. 1999. "Preoperative Serum Albumin Level as a Predictor of Operative Mortality and Morbidity: Results from the National VA Surgical Risk Study." *Archives of Surgery* 134 (1): 36–42.

Gilden, D. 2002. Personal communication, 7 Oct. Cambridge, MA: JEN Associates, Inc.

Gill, T. M., M. M. Desai, E. A. Gahbauer, T. R. Holford, and C. S. Williams. 2001. "Restricted Activity Among Community-Living Older Persons: Incidence, Precipitants, and Health Care Utilization." *Annals of Internal Medicine* 135 (5): 313–21.

Gill, T. M., and A. R. Feinstein. 1994. "A Critical Appraisal of the Quality of Quality-of-Life Measurements." *Journal of the American Medical Association* 272 (8): 619–26.

Gill, T. M., J. T. Robison, and M. E. Tinetti. 1997. "Predictors of Recovery in Activities of Daily Living Among Disabled Older Persons Living in the Community." *Journal of General Internal Medicine* 12 (12): 757–62.

Gilmer, T., R. Kronick, P. Fishman, and T. G. Ganiats. 2001. "The Medicaid Rx Model: Pharmacy-Based Risk Adjustment for Public Programs." *Medical Care* 39 (11): 1188–1202.

Gitlin, L. N., M. Corcoran, L. Winter, A. Boyce, and W. W. Hauck. 2001. "A Randomized, Controlled Trial of a Home Environmental Intervention: Effect on Efficacy and Upset in Caregivers and on Daily Function of Persons with Dementia." *Gerontologist* 41 (1): 4–14.

Gitlin, L. N., M. R. Luborsky, and R. L. Schemm. 1998. "Emerging Concerns of Older Stroke Patients About Assistive Device Use." *Gerontologist* 38 (2): 169–80.

Gitlin, L. N., R. L. Schemm, L. Landsberg, and D. Burgh. 1996. "Factors Predicting

Assistive Device Use in the Home by Older People Following Rehabilitation." *Journal of Aging and Health* 8 (4): 554–75.

Gitterman, D. P., R. Sturm, and R. M. Scheffler. 2001. "Toward Full Mental Health Parity and Beyond." *Health Affairs (Millwood)* 20 (4): 68–76.

Goffman, E. 1963. *Stigma: Notes on the Management of Spoiled Identity.* New York: Simon and Schuster.

Golden, W. 2001. "Integrating Health Status into the Quality Equation." *International Journal for Quality in Health Care* 13 (1): 5–6.

Goldfarb, M. G., and R. M. Coffey. 1992. "Change in the Medicare Case-Mix Index in the 1980s and the Effect of the Prospective Payment System." *Health Services Research* 27 (3): 385–415.

Goldfield, N., and R. Averill. 2000. "On 'Risk-Adjusting Acute Myocardial Infarction Mortality: Are APR-DRGs the Right Tool?'" *Health Services Research* 34 (7): 1491–95.

Goldfield, N., and P. Boland, eds. 1996. *Physician Profiling and Risk Adjustment.* Gaithersburg, MD: Aspen.

Goldstein, H., and D. J. Spiegelhalter. 1996. "League Tables and Their Limitations: Statistical Issues in Comparisons of Institutional Performance." *Journal of the Royal Statistical Society* 159 (Part 3): 385–443.

Gonnella, J. S., M. C. Hornbrook, and D. Z. Louis. 1984. "Staging of Disease. A Case-Mix Measurement." *Journal of the American Medical Association* 251 (5): 637–44.

Gonnella, J. S., D. Z. Louis, C. Zeleznik, and B. J. Turner. 1990. "The Problem of Late Hospitalization: A Quality and Cost Issue." *Academic Medicine* 65 (5): 314–19.

Gordon, H. S., and G. E. Rosenthal. 1999. "The Relationship of Gender and In-Hospital Death: Increased Risk of Death in Men." *Medical Care* 37 (3): 318–24.

Gordon, N. P., R. A. Hiatt, and D. I. Lampert. 1993. "Concordance of Self-Reported Data and Medical Record Audit for Six Cancer Screening Procedures." *Journal of the National Cancer Institute* 85 (7): 566–70.

Gostin, L. O. 2001. "National Health Information Privacy: Regulations Under the Health Insurance Portability and Accountability Act." *Journal of the American Medical Association* 285 (23): 3015–21.

Gostin, L. O., and J. Hadley. 1998. "Health Services Research: Public Benefits, Personal Privacy, and Proprietary Interests." *Annals of Internal Medicine* 129 (10): 833–35.

Grady, D., S. M. Rubin, D. B. Petitti, C. S. Fox, D. Black, B. Ettinger, V. L. Ernster, and S. R. Cummings. 1992. "Hormone Therapy to Prevent Disease and Prolong Life in Postmenopausal Women." *Annals of Internal Medicine* 117 (12): 1016–37.

Gray, J. E., D. K. Richardson, M. C. McCormick, K. Workman-Daniels, and D. A. Goldmann. 1992. "Neonatal Therapeutic Intervention Scoring System: A Therapy-Based Severity-of-Illness Index." *Pediatrics* 90 (4): 561–67.

Green, J., and N. Wintfeld. 1995. "Report Cards on Cardiac Surgeons: Assessing New York State's Approach." *New England Journal of Medicine* 332 (18): 1229–32.

Greenfield, S., G. Apolone, B. J. McNeil, and P. D. Cleary. 1993. "The Importance of Co-Existent Disease in the Occurrence of Postoperative Complications and One-Year Recovery in Patients Undergoing Total Hip Replacement. Comorbidity and Outcomes After Hip Replacement." *Medical Care* 31 (2): 141–54.

Greenfield, S., D. M. Blanco, R. M. Elashoff, and P. A. Ganz. 1987. "Patterns of Care Related to Age of Breast Cancer Patients." *Journal of the American Medical Association* 257 (20): 2766–70.

Greenfield, S., S. H. Kaplan, R. Kahn, J. Ninomiya, and J. L. Griffith. 2002. "Profiling Care Provided by Different Groups of Physicians: Effects of Patient Case-Mix (Bias) and Physician-Level Clustering on Quality Assessment Results." *Annals of Internal Medicine* 136 (2): 111–21.

Greenfield, S., L. Sullivan, K. A. Dukes, R. Silliman, R. D'Agostino, and S. H. Kaplan. 1995. "Development and Testing of a New Measure of Case Mix for Use in Office Practice." *Medical Care* 33 (4, Suppl.): AS47–AS55.

Greenfield, S., L. Sullivan, R. A. Silliman, K. Dukes, and S. H. Kaplan. 1994. "Principles and Practice of Case Mix Adjustment: Applications to End-Stage Renal Disease." *American Journal of Kidney Disease* 24 (2): 298–307.

Greenland, S. 2000a. "An Introduction to Instrumental Variables for Epidemiologists." *International Journal of Epidemiology* 29 (4): 722–29.

———. 2000b. "When Should Epidemiologic Regressions Use Random Coefficients?" *Biometrics* 56 (3): 915–21.

———. 2000c. "Principles of Multilevel Modelling." *International Journal of Epidemiology* 29 (1): 158–67.

Greenwald, L. M. 2000. "Medicare Risk-Adjusted Capitation Payments: From Research to Implementation." *Health Care Financing Review* 21 (3): 1–5.

Greenwald, L. M., A. Esposito, M. J. Ingber, and J. M. Levy. 1998. "Risk Adjustment for the Medicare Program: Lessons Learned from Research and Demonstrations." *Inquiry* 35 (2): 193–209.

Gross, R., N. Bentur, A. Elhayany, M. Sherf, and L. Epstein. 1996. "The Validity of Self-Reports on Chronic Disease: Characteristics of Underreporters and Implications for the Planning of Services." *Public Health Review* 24 (2): 167–82.

Grover, F. L., J. C. Cleveland, Jr., and L. W. Shroyer. 2002. "Quality Improvement in Cardiac Care." *Archives of Surgery* 137 (1): 28–36.

Grover, F. L., K. E. Hammermeister, and C. Burchfiel. 1990. "Initial Report of the Veterans Administration Preoperative Risk Assessment Study for Cardiac Surgery." *Annals of Thoracic Surgery* 50 (1): 12–26.

Grover, F. L., R. R. Johnson, A. L. Shroyer, G. Marshall, and K. E. Hammermeister. 1994. "The Veterans Affairs Continuous Improvement in Cardiac Surgery Study." *Annals of Thoracic Surgery* 58 (6): 1845–51.

Grover, F. L., A. L. Shroyer, and K. E. Hammermeister. 1996. "Calculating Risk and Outcome: The Veterans Affairs Database." *Annals of Thoracic Surgery* 62 (5, Suppl.): S6–11.

Grover, F. L., A. L. Shroyer, K. Hammermeister, F. H. Edwards, T. B. Ferguson, Jr., S. W. Dziuban, Jr., J. C. Cleveland, Jr., R. E. Clark, and G. McDonald. 2001. "A Decade's Experience with Quality Improvement in Cardiac Surgery Using the Veterans Affairs and Society of Thoracic Surgeons National Databases." *Annals of Surgery* 234 (4): 464–72.

Gruenberg, L., E. Kaganova, and M. C. Hornbrook. 1996. "Improving the AAPCC (Adjusted Average per Capita Cost) with Health-Status Measures from the MCBS (Medicare Current Beneficiary Survey)." *Health Care Financing Review* 17 (3): 59–75.

Guadagnoli, E., C. Shapiro, J. H. Gurwitz, R. A. Silliman, J. C. Weeks, C. Borbas, and S. B. Soumerai. 1997. "Age-Related Patterns of Care: Evidence Against Ageism in the Treatment of Early-Stage Breast Cancer." *Journal of Clinical Oncology* 15 (6): 2338–44.

Gum, P. A., M. Thamilarasan, J. Watanabe, E. H. Blackstone, and M. S. Lauer. 2001. "Aspirin Use and All-Cause Mortality Among Patients Being Evaluated for Known or Suspected Coronary Artery Disease: A Propensity Analysis." *Journal of the American Medical Association* 286 (10): 1187–94.

Hadley, J., D. Rabin, A. Epstein, S. Stein, and C. Rimes. 2000. "Posthospitalization Home Health Care Use and Changes in Functional Status in a Medicare Population." *Medical Care* 38 (5): 494–507.

Hadorn, D. C., D. Draper, W. H. Rogers, E. B. Keeler, and R. H. Brook. 1992. "Cross-Validation Performance of Mortality Prediction Models." *Statistics in Medicine* 11 (4): 475–89.

Hahn, R. A. 1992. "The State of Federal Health Statistics on Racial and Ethnic Groups." *Journal of the American Medical Association* 267 (2): 268–71.

Hahn, R. A., J. Mulinare, and S. M. Teutsch. 1992. "Inconsistencies in Coding of Race and Ethnicity Between Birth and Death in US Infants. A New Look at Infant Mortality, 1983 Through 1985." *Journal of the American Medical Association* 267 (2): 259–63.

Hahn, R. A., and D. F. Stroup. 1994. "Race and Ethnicity in Public Health Surveillance: Criteria for the Scientific Use of Social Categories." *Public Health Report* 109 (1): 7–15.

Hakim, R. B., P. J. Boben, and J. B. Bonney. 2000. "Medicaid and the Health of Children." *Health Care Financing Review* 22 (1): 133–40.

Haley, S. M., H. M. Dumas, and L. H. Ludlow. 2001. "Variation by Diagnostic and Practice Pattern Groups in the Mobility Outcomes of Inpatient Rehabilitation Programs for Children And Youth." *Physical Therapy* 81 (8): 1425–36.

Halfon, N., and M. Hochstein. 2002. "Life Course Health Development: An Integrated Framework for Developing Health, Policy, and Research." *Milbank Quarterly* 80 (3): 433–79.

Hamel, M. B., R. B. Davis, J. M. Teno, W. A. Knaus, J. Lynn, F. Harrell, Jr., A. N. Galanos, A. W. Wu, and R. S. Phillips. 1999a. "Older Age, Aggressiveness of Care, and Survival for Seriously Ill, Hospitalized Adults. SUPPORT Investigators. Study to Understand Prognoses and Preferences for Outcomes and Risks of Treatments." *Annals of Internal Medicine* 131 (10): 721–28.

Hamel, M. B., J. Lynn, J. M. Teno, K. E. Covinsky, A. W. Wu, A. Galanos, N. A. Desbiens, and R. S. Phillips. 2000. "Age-Related Differences in Care Preferences, Treatment Decisions, and Clinical Outcomes of Seriously Ill Hospitalized Adults: Lessons from SUPPORT." *Journal of the American Geriatric Society* 48 (5, Suppl.): S176–S182.

Hamel, M. B., J. M. Teno, L. Goldman, J. Lynn, R. B. Davis, A. N. Galanos, N. Desbiens, A. F. Connors, Jr., N. Wenger, and R. S. Phillips. 1999b. "Patient Age and

Decisions to Withhold Life-Sustaining Treatments from Seriously Ill, Hospitalized Adults. SUPPORT Investigators. Study to Understand Prognoses and Preferences for Outcomes and Risks of Treatment." *Annals of Internal Medicine* 130 (2): 116–25.

Hamilton, M. 1967. "Development of a Rating Scale for Primary Depressive Illness." *British Journal of Social Clinical Psychology* 6 (4): 278–96.

Hammermeister, K. E., A. L. Shroyer, G. K. Sethi, and F. L. Grover. 1995. "Why It Is Important to Demonstrate Linkages Between Outcomes of Care and Processes and Structures of Care." *Medical Care* 33 (10, Suppl.): OS5–OS16.

Hanley, J. A., and B. J. McNeil. 1982. "The Meaning and Use of the Area Under a Receiver Operating Characteristic (ROC) Curve." *Radiology* 143 (1): 29–36.

———. 1983. "A Method of Comparing the Area under Receiver Operating Characteristic Curves Derived from the Same Cases." *Radiology* 148 (3): 839–43

Hannan, E. L., H. R. Bernard, J. F. O'Donnell, and H. Kilburn, Jr. 1989. "A Methodology for Targeting Hospital Cases for Quality of Care Record Reviews." *American Journal of Public Health* 79 (4): 430–36.

Hannan, E. L., H. Kilburn Jr., M. L. Lindsey, and R. Lewis. 1992. "Clinical Versus Administrative Data Bases for CABG Surgery: Does It Matter?" *Medical Care* 30 (10): 892–907.

Hannan, E. L., H. Kilburn, Jr., J. F. O'Donnell, G. Lukacik, and E. P. Shields. 1990. "Adult Open Heart Surgery in New York State: An Analysis of Risk Factors and Hospital Mortality Rates." *Journal of the American Medical Association* 264 (21): 2768–74.

Hannan, E. L., H. Kilburn, Jr., M. Racz, E. Shields, and M. R. Chassin. 1994. "Improving the Outcomes of Coronary Artery Bypass Surgery in New York State." *Journal of the American Medical Association* 271 (10): 761–66.

Hannan, E. L., M. J. Racz, J. G. Jollis, and E. D. Peterson. 1997. "Using Medicare Claims Data to Assess Provider Quality for CABG Surgery: Does It Work Well Enough?" *Health Services Research* 31 (6): 659–78.

Hannan, E. L., M. Racz, R. E. Kavey, J. M. Quaegebeur, and R. Williams. 1998. "Pediatric Cardiac Surgery: The Effect of Hospital and Surgeon Volume on In-Hospital Mortality." *Pediatrics* 101 (6): 963–69.

Hannan, E. L., A. L. Siu, D. Kuman, H. Kilburn, and M. R. Chassin. 1995. "The Decline in Coronary Artery Bypass Graft Surgery Mortality in New York State." *Journal of the American Medical Association* 273 (3): 209–13.

Hannan, E. L., M. van Ryn, J. Burke, D. Stone, D. Kumar, D. Arani, W. Pierce, S. Rafii, T. A. Sanborn, S. Sharma, J. Slater, and B. A. DeBuono. 1999. "Access to Coronary Artery Bypass Surgery by Race/Ethnicity and Gender Among Patients Who Are Appropriate for Surgery." *Medical Care* 37 (1): 68–77.

Harada, N. D., V. M. Villa, and R. Andersen. 2002. "Satisfaction with VA and Non-VA Outpatient Care Among Veterans." *American Journal of Medical Quality* 17 (4): 155–64.

Hargraves, J. L., I. B. Wilson, A. Zaslavsky, C. James, J. D. Walker, G. Rogers, and P. D. Cleary. 2001. "Adjusting for Patient Characteristics when Analyzing Reports from Patients About Hospital Care." *Medical Care* 39 (6): 635–41.

Harrell, F. E. 2001. *Regression Modeling Strategies, with Applications to Linear Models, Logistic Regression, and Survival Analysis.* New York: Springer.

Harrell, F. E., Jr., K. L. Lee, R. M. Califf, D. B. Pryor, and R. A. Rosati. 1984. "Regression Modelling Strategies for Improved Prognostic Prediction." *Statistics in Medicine* 3 (2): 143–52.

Harrell, F. E., Jr., K. L. Lee, and B. G. Pollock. 1988. "Regression Models in Clinical Studies: Determining Relationships Between Predictors and Response." *Journal of the National Cancer Institute* 80 (15): 1198–1202.

Harrington, C., S. Woolhandler, J. Mullan, H. Carrillo, and D. U. Himmelstein. 2001. "Does Investor Ownership of Nursing Homes Compromise the Quality of Care?" *American Journal of Public Health* 91 (9): 1452–55.

Harris Interactive, Inc. 2000. "2000 N. O. D./Harris Survey of Americans with Disabilities." Conducted for the National Organization on Disability. New York: Harris Interactive, Inc.

Harris, K. M., and D. K. Remler. 1998. "Who Is the Marginal Patient? Understanding Instrumental Variables Estimates of Treatment Effects." *Health Services Research* 33 (5, Part I): 1337–60.

Harris, Y., and S. B. Clauser. 2002. "Achieving Improvement Through Nursing Home Quality Measurement." *Health Care Financing Review* 23 (4): 5–18.

Hartley, C., A. Cozens, A. D. Mendelow, and J. C. Stevenson. 1995. "The APACHE II Scoring System in Neurosurgical Patients: A Comparison with Simple Glasgow Coma Scoring." *British Journal of Neurosurgery* 9 (2): 179–87.

Hartz, A. J., M. S. Gottlieb, E. M. Kuhn, and A. A. Rimm. 1993. "The Relationship Between Adjusted Hospital Mortality and the Results of Peer Review." *Health Services Research* 27 (6): 765–77.

Hartz, A. J., C. Guse, P. Sigmann, H. Krakauer, R. S. Goldman, and T. C. Hagen. 1994. "Severity of Illness Measures Derived from the Uniform Clinical Data Set (UCDSS)." *Medical Care* 32 (9): 881–901.

Hawes, C., V. Mor, C. D. Phillips, B. E. Fries, J. N. Morris, E. Steele-Friedlob, A. M. Greene, and M. Nennstiel. 1997. "The OBRA-87 Nursing Home Regulations and Implementation of the Resident Assessment Instrument: Effects on Process Quality." *Journal of the American Geriatric Society* 45 (8): 977–85.

Hawes, C., J. N. Morris, C. D. Phillips, V. Mor, B. E. Fries, and S. Nonemaker. 1995. "Reliability Estimates for the Minimum Data Set for Nursing Home Resident Assessment and Care Screening (MDS)." *Gerontologist* 35 (2): 172–78.

Headley, J., R. Theriault, and T. L. Smith. 1992. "Independent Validation of APACHE II Severity of Illness Score for Predicting Mortality in Patients with Breast Cancer Admitted to the Intensive Care Unit." *Cancer* 70 (2): 497–503.

Health Care Financing Administration, U.S. Department of Health and Human Services. 1997. "Medicare and Medicaid Programs: Revision of Conditions of Participation for Home Health Agencies and Use of Outcome Assessment Information Set (OASIS); Proposed Rules. 42 CFR Part 484." *Federal Register* 11004–64.

Healthcare Cost and Utilization Project (HCUP), Agency for Healthcare Research and Quality. 2001. "1988–99: A Federal-State-Industry Partnership in Health Data." [Online information; retrieved 8/1/02.] http://www.ahrq.gov/data/hcup/hcup-pkt.htm.

Heard, C. M., J. E. Fletcher, and M. C. Papo. 1998. "A Report of the Use of the

Dynamic Objective Risk Assessment (DORA) Score in the Changing Pediatric Intensive Care Environment." *Critical Care Medicine* 26 (9): 1593–95.

Heffler, S., S. Smith, G. Won, M. K. Clemens, S. Keehan, and M. Zezza. 2002. "Health Spending Projections for 2001–2011: The Latest Outlook. Faster Health Spending Growth and a Slowing Economy Drive the Health Spending Projection for 2001 up Sharply." *Health Affairs (Millwood)* 21 (2): 207–18.

Heiat, A., C. P. Gross, and H. M. Krumholz. 2002. "Representation of the Elderly, Women, and Minorities in Heart Failure Clinical Trials." *Archives of Internal Medicine* 162 (15): 1682–88.

Hendryx, M. S., A. Beigel, and A. Doucette. 2001. "Introduction: Risk-Adjustment Issues in Mental Health Services." *Journal of Behavioral Health Services & Research* 28 (3): 225–34.

Hendryx, M. S., D. G. Dyck, and D. Srebnik. 1999. "Risk-Adjusted Outcome Models for Public Mental Health Outpatient Programs." *Health Services Research* 34 (1, Part I): 171–95.

Hermann, R. C., R. A. Dorwart, C. W. Hoover, and J. Brody. 1995. "Variation in ECT Use in the United States." *American Journal of Psychiatry* 152 (6): 869–75.

Hermann, R. C., S. L. Ettner, and R. A. Dorwart. 1998. "The Influence of Psychiatric Disorders on Patients' Ratings of Satisfaction with Health Care." *Medical Care* 36 (5): 720–27.

Hermann, R. C., H. S. Leff, R. H. Palmer, D. Yang, T. Teller, S. Provost, C. Jakubiak, and J. Chan. 2000. "Quality Measures for Mental Health Care: Results from a National Inventory." *Medical Care Research and Review* 57 (2, Suppl.): 136–54.

Hermann, R. C., and R. H. Palmer. 2002. "Common Ground: A Framework for Selecting Core Quality Measures for Mental Health and Substance Abuse Care." *Psychiatric Services* 53 (3): 281–87.

Higgins, T. L., F. G. Estafanous, F. D. Loop, G. J. Beck, J. M. Blum, and L. Paranandi. 1992. "Stratification of Morbidity and Mortality Outcome by Preoperative Risk Factors in Coronary Artery Bypass Patients. A Clinical Severity Score." *Journal of the American Medical Association* 267 (17): 2344–48.

Hilden, J. 1991. "The Area Under the ROC Curve and Its Competitors." *Medical Decision Making* 11 (2): 95–101.

Hirdes, J. P. 2002. Personal communication, 16 June.

Hirdes, J. P., M. Marhaba, T. F. Smith, L. Clyburn, L. Mitchell, R. A. Lemick, N. C. Telegdi, E. Perez, P. Prendergast, T. Rabinowitz, and K. Yamauchi. 2000. "Development of the Resident Assessment Instrument—Mental Health (RAI-MH)." *Hospital Quarterly* 4 (2): 44–51.

Hoaglin, D.C., and B. Iglewicz. 1987. "Fine-Tuning Some Resistant Rules for Outlier Labeling." *Journal of the American Statistical Association* 82 (400): 1147–49.

Hoenig, H. 1993. "Educating Primary Care Physicians in Geriatric Rehabilitation." *Clinics in Geriatric Medicine* 9: 883–93.

Hofer, T. P. 2001. "Adjustment of Physician Profiles for Patient Socioeconomic Status Using Aggregate Geographic Data." *Medical Care* 39 (1): 4–7.

Hofer, T. P., and R. A. Hayward. 1996. "Identifying Poor-Quality Hospitals. Can Hospital Mortality Rates Detect Quality Problems for Medical Diagnoses?" *Medical Care* 34 (8): 737–53.

Hofer, T. P., R. A. Hayward, S. Greenfield, E. H. Wagner, S. H. Kaplan, and W. G. Manning. 1999. "The Unreliability of Individual Physician 'Report Cards' for Assessing the Costs and Quality of Care of a Chronic Disease." *Journal of the American Medical Association* 281 (22): 2098–2105.

Holmes, T. 1864. "Mortality in Hospitals." *Lancet* (March 26): 365–66.

Homer, C. J., P. Szilagyi, L. Rodewald, S. R. Bloom, P. Greenspan, S. Yazdgerdi, J. M. Leventhal, D. Finkelstein, and J. M. Perrin. 1996. "Does Quality of Care Affect Rates of Hospitalization for Childhood Asthma?" *Pediatrics* 98 (1): 18–23.

Horbar, J. D. 1999. "The Vermont Oxford Network: Evidence-Based Quality Improvement for Neonatology." *Pediatrics* 103 (1, Suppl. E): 350–59.

Horbar, J. D., L. Onstad, and E. Wright. 1993. "Predicting Mortality Risk for Infants Weighing 501 to 1500 grams at Birth: A National Institutes of Health Neonatal Research Network Report." *Critical Care Medicine* 21 (1): 12–18.

Horgan, C., and S. F. Jencks. 1987. "Research on Psychiatric Classification and Payment Systems." *Medical Care* 25 (9, Suppl.): S22–S36.

Horn, S. D., A. F. Chambers, P. D. Sharkey, and R. A. Horn. 1989. "Psychiatric Severity of Illness. A Case Mix Study." *Medical Care* 27 (1): 69–84.

Horn, S. D., P. D. Sharkey, J. M. Buckle, J. E. Backofen, R. F. Averill, and R. A. Horn. 1991. "The Relationship Between Severity of Illness and Hospital Length of Stay and Mortality." *Medical Care* 29 (4): 305–17.

Horn, S. D., P. D. Sharkey, and J. Gassaway. 1996. "Managed Care Outcomes Project: Study, Design, Baseline Patient Characteristics, and Outcome Measures." *American Journal of Managed Care* 3: 237–47.

Horn, S. D., A. Torres, Jr., D. Willson, J. M. Dean, J. Gassaway, and R. Smout. 2002. "Development of a Pediatric Age- and Disease-Specific Severity Measure." *Journal of Pediatrics* 141 (4): 496–503.

Hornbrook, M. C. 1982. "Hospital Case Mix: Its Definition, Measurement and Use. Part II: Review of Alternative Measures." *Medical Care Review* 39 (2): 73–123.

———. 1999. "Commentary: Improving Risk-Adjustment Models for Capitation Payment and Global Budgeting." *Health Services Research* 33 (6): 1745–51.

Hornbrook, M. C., and M. J. Goodman. 1995. "Assessing Relative Health Plan Risk with the RAND-36 Health Survey." *Inquiry* 32 (1): 56–74.

———. 1996. "Chronic Disease, Functional Health Status, and Demographics: A Multi-Dimensional Approach to Risk Adjustment." *Health Services Research* 31 (3): 283–307.

Hornbrook, M. C., M. J. Goodman, M. D. Bennett, and M. R. Greenlick. 1991. "Assessing Health Plan Case Mix in Employed Populations: Self-Reported Health Status Models." *Advances in Health Economics and Health Service Research* 12: 233–72.

Hornbrook, M. C., M. J. Goodman, P. A. Fishman, and R. T. Meenan. 1998b. "Health-Based Payment and Computerized Patient Record Systems." *Effective Clinical Practice* 1 (2): 66–72.

Hornbrook, M. C., M. J. Goodman, P. A. Fishman, R. T. Meenan, M. O'Keefe-Rosetti, and D. J. Bachman. 1998a. "Building Health Plan Databases to Risk

Adjust Outcomes and Payments." *International Journal for Quality in Health Care* 10: 531–38.

Hornbrook, M. C., A. V. Hurtado, and R. E. Johnson. 1985. "Health Care Episodes: Definition, Measurement and Use." *Medical Care Review* 42 (2): 163–218.

Horner, R. D., H. Hoenig, R. Sloane, L. V. Rubenstein, and K. L. Kahn. 1997. "Racial Differences in the Utilization of Inpatient Rehabilitation Services Among Elderly Stroke Patients." *Stroke* 28: 19–25.

Horner, R. D., E. Z. Oddone, K. M. Stechuchak, S. C. Grambow, J. Gray, S. F. Khuri, W. G. Henderson, and J. Daley. 2002. "Racial Variations in Postoperative Outcomes of Carotid Endarterectomy: Evidence from the Veterans Affairs National Surgical Quality Improvement Program." *Medical Care* 40 (1, Suppl.): 35–43.

Hornsby, J. A. 1917. "The Hospital Problem of Today—What Is It?" *Bulletin of American College of Surgeons* 3: 4–11.

Hosmer, D. W., and S. Lemeshow. 1989. *Applied Logistic Regression.* New York: John Wiley & Sons.

———. 1995. "Confidence Interval Estimates of an Index of Quality Performance Based on Logistic Regression Models." *Statistics in Medicine* 14 (19): 2161–72.

Howard, D. 2000. "The Impact of Waiting Time on Liver Transplant Outcomes." *Health Services Research* 35 (5, Part II): 1117–34.

Hripcsak, G., G. J. Kuperman, and C. Friedman. 1998. "Extracting Findings from Narrative Reports: Software Transferability and Sources of Physician Disagreement." *Methods in Medicine* 37 (1): 1–7.

Hsia, D. C., C. A. Ahern, B. P. Ritchie, L. M. Moscoe, and W. M. Krushat. 1992. "Medicare Reimbursement Accuracy Under the Prospective Payment System, 1985 to 1988." *Journal of the American Medical Association* 268 (7): 896–99.

Hsia, D. C., W. M. Krushat, A. B. Fagan, J. A. Tebbutt, and R. P. Kusserow. 1988. "Accuracy of Diagnostic Coding for Medicare Patients Under the Prospective-Payment System." *New England Journal of Medicine* 318 (6): 352–55.

Hughes, C. M., K. L. Lapane, and V. Mor. 2000. "Influence of Facility Characteristics on Use of Antipsychotic Medications in Nursing Homes." *Medical Care* 38 (12): 1164–73.

Hughes, J. S., and A. S. Ash. 1997. "Reliability of Risk-Adjusted Methods." *Risk Adjustment for Measuring Healthcare Outcomes,* 2d ed., edited by L. I. Iezzoni, 365–90. Chicago: Health Administration Press.

Hughes, J. S., L. I. Iezzoni, J. Daley, and L. Greenberg. 1996. "How Severity Measures Rate Hospitalized Patients." *Journal of General Internal Medicine* 11 (5): 303–11.

Hunt, S. M., and J. McEwen. 1980. "The Development of a Subjective Health Indicator." *Sociology of Health and Illness* 2 (3): 231–46.

Hwang, W., H. T. Ireys, and G. F. Anderson. 2001. "Comparison of Risk Adjusters for Medicaid-Enrolled Children with and without Chronic Health Conditions." *Ambulatory Pediatrics* 1 (4): 217–24.

Iezzoni, L. I. 1995. "Risk Adjustment for Medical Effectiveness Research: An Overview of Conceptual and Methodological Considerations." *Journal of Investigative Medicine* 43 (2): 136–50.

———. 1996. "100 Apples Divided by 15 Red Herrings: A Cautionary Tale from the Mid-19th Century on Comparing Hospital Mortality Rates." *Annals of Internal Medicine* 124 (12): 1079–85.

———. 1997. "The Risks of Risk Adjustment." *Journal of the American Medical Association* 278 (19): 1600–07.

———. 2002. "Using Administrative Data to Study Persons with Disabilities." *Milbank Quarterly* 80 (2): 347–79.

———. 2003. *When Walking Fails.* Berkeley, CA: University of California Press.

Iezzoni, L. I., A. S. Ash, G. A. Coffman, and M. A. Moskowitz. 1992c. "Predicting In-Hospital Mortality. A Comparison of Severity Measurement Approaches." *Medical Care* 30 (4): 347–59.

Iezzoni, L. I., A. S. Ash, M. Shwartz, J. Daley, J. S. Hughes, and Y. D. Mackiernan. 1995b. "Predicting Who Dies Depends on How Severity Is Measured: Implications for Evaluating Patient Outcomes." *Annals of Internal Medicine* 123 (10): 763–70.

———. 1996e. "Judging Hospitals by Severity-Adjusted Mortality Rates: The Influence of the Severity-Adjustment Method." *American Journal of Public Health* 86 (10): 1379–87.

Iezzoni, L. I., A. S. Ash, M. Shwartz, and Y. D. Mackiernan. 1997. "Differences in Procedure Use, In-Hospital Mortality, and Illness Severity by Gender for Acute Myocardial Infarction Patients: Are Answers Affected by Data Source and Severity Measure?" *Medical Care* 35 (2): 158–71.

Iezzoni, L. I., J. Z. Ayanian, D. W. Bates, and H. Burstin. 1998. "Paying More Fairly for Medicare Capitated Care." *New England Journal of Medicine* 339 (26): 1933–38.

Iezzoni, L. I., S. Burnside, L. Sickles, M. A. Moskowitz, E. Sawitz, and P. A. Levine. 1988. "Coding of Acute Myocardial Infarction. Clinical and Policy Implications." *Annals of Internal Medicine* 109 (9): 745–51.

Iezzoni, L. I., and J. Daley. 1992. "A Description and Clinical Assessment of the Computerized Severity Index." *QRB Quality Review Bulletin* 18 (2): 44–52.

Iezzoni, L. I., J. Daley, T. Heeren, S. M. Foley, J. S. Hughes, E. S. Fisher, C. C. Duncan, and G. A. Coffman. 1994a. "Using Administrative Data to Screen Hospitals for High Complication Rates." *Inquiry* 31 (1): 40–55.

Iezzoni, L. I., J. Daley, T. Heeren, S. M. Foley, E. S. Fisher, C. Duncan, J. S. Hughes, and G. A. Coffman. 1994b. "Identifying Complications of Care Using Administrative Data." *Medical Care* 32 (7): 700–15.

Iezzoni, L. I., R. B. Davis, R. H. Palmer, M. Cahalane, M. B. Hamel, K. Mukamal, R. S. Phillips, N. J. Banks, and D. T. Davis, Jr. 1999. "Does the Complications Screening Program Flag Cases with Process of Care Problems? Using Explicit Criteria to Judge Processes." *International Journal for Quality in Health Care* 11 (2): 107–18.

Iezzoni, L. I., R. B. Davis, J. Soukup, and B. O'Day. 2002. "Satisfaction with Quality and Access to Health Care Among People with Disabling Conditions." *International Journal for Quality in Health Care* 14 (5): 369–81.

Iezzoni, L. I., S. M. Foley, J. Daley, J. Hughes, E. S. Fisher, and T. Heeren. 1992a. "Comorbidities, Complications, and Coding Bias. Does the Number of Diagnosis Codes Matter in Predicting In-Hospital Mortality?" *Journal of the American Medical Association* 267: 2197–2203.

Iezzoni, L. I., and L. G. Greenberg. In press. "Capturing and Classifying Functional Status Information in Administrative Databases." *Health Care Financing Review.*

Iezzoni, L. I., E. K. Hotchkin, A. S. Ash, M. Shwartz, and Y. Mackiernan. 1993. "MedisGroups Data Bases. The Impact of Data Collection Guidelines on Predicting In-Hospital Mortality." *Medical Care* 31 (3): 277–83.

Iezzoni, L. I., E. P. McCarthy, R. B. Davis, L. Harris-David, and B. O'Day. 2001b. "Use of Screening and Preventive Services Among Women with Disabilities." *American Journal of Medical Quality* 16 (4): 135–44.

Iezzoni, L. I., E. P. McCarthy, R. B. Davis, and H. Siebens. 2000a. "Mobility Impairments and Use of Screening and Preventive Services." *American Journal of Public Health* 90: 955–61.

———. 2001a. "Mobility Difficulties Are Not Only a Problem of Old Age." *Journal of General Internal Medicine* 16: 235–43.

———. 2000b. "Mobility Problems and Perceptions of Disability by Self- and Proxy-Respondents." *Medical Care* 38: 1051–57.

Iezzoni, L. I., and M. A. Moskowitz. 1986. "Clinical Overlap among Medical Diagnosis-Related Groups." *Journal of the American Medical Association* 255 (7): 927–29.

———. 1988. "A Clinical Assessment of MedisGroups." *Journal of the American Medical Association* 260 (21): 3159–63.

Iezzoni, L. I., M. A. Moskowitz, and A. S. Ash. 1988. "The Ability of MedisGroups and Its Clinical Variables to Predict Cost and In-Hospital Death." Boston: Health Care Research Unit, Boston University Medical Center.

Iezzoni, L. I., J. D. Restuccia, M. Shwartz, D. Schaumburg, G. A. Coffman, B. E. Kreger, J. R. Butterly, and H. P. Selker. 1992b. "The Utility of Severity of Illness Information in Assessing the Quality of Hospital Care. The Role of the Clinical Trajectory." *Medical Care* 30 (5): 428–44.

Iezzoni, L. I., M. Shwartz, A. S. Ash, J. S. Hughes, J. Daley, and Y. D. Mackiernan. 1995a. "Using Severity-Adjusted Stroke Mortality Rates to Judge Hospitals." *International Journal for Quality in Health Care* 7 (2): 81–94.

Iezzoni, L. I., M. Shwartz, A. S. Ash, J. S. Hughes, J. Daley, and Y. D. Mackiernan. 1996a. "Severity Measurement Methods and Judging Hospital Death Rates for Pneumonia." *Medical Care* 34 (1): 11–28.

———. 1996b. "Using Severity Measures to Predict the Likelihood of Death for Pneumonia Inpatients." *Journal of General Internal Medicine* 11 (1): 23–31.

Iezzoni, L. I., M. Shwartz, A. S. Ash, J. S. Hughes, J. Daley, Y. D. Mackiernan, and D. Stone. 1995c. *Evaluating Severity Adjustors for Patient Outcome Studies: Final Report.* Prepared for the Agency for Health Care Policy and Research under Grant No. RO1-HS06742. Boston: Beth Israel Hospital.

Iezzoni, L. I., M. Shwartz, A. S. Ash, and Y. D. Mackiernan. 1996c. "Does Severity Explain Differences in Hospital Length of Stay for Pneumonia Patients?" *Journal of Health Service Research and Policy* 1 (2): 65–76.

———. 1996d. "Predicting In-Hospital Mortality for Stroke Patients: Results Differ Across Severity-Measurement Methods." *Medical Decision Making* 16 (4): 348–56.

Iezzoni, L. I., M. Shwartz, S. Burnside, A. S. Ash, E. Sawitz, and M. A. Moskowitz. 1989. "Diagnostic Mix, Illness Severity, and Costs at Teaching and Non-Teaching Hospitals." PB 89 184675/AS. Springfield, VA: U.S. Department of Commerce, National Technical Information Service.

Iezzoni, L. I., M. Shwartz, M. A. Moskowitz, A. S. Ash, E. Sawitz, and S. Burnside. 1990. "Illness Severity and Costs of Admissions at Teaching and Nonteaching Hospitals." *Journal of the American Medical Association* 264 (11): 1426–31.

Iglehart, J. K. 1994. "Health Care Reform: The States." *New England Journal of Medicine* 330 (1): 75–79.

Ingelfinger, J. A., F. Mosteller, L. A. Thibodeau, and J. H. Ware. 1987. *Biostatistics in Clinical Medicine*. New York: Macmillan.

Inouye, S. K., D. R. Wagner, D. Acampora, R. I. Horwitz, L. M. Cooney, Jr., L. D. Hurst, and M. E. Tinetti. 1993. "A Predictive Index for Functional Decline in Hospitalized Elderly Medical Patients." *Journal of General Internal Medicine* 8 (12): 645–52.

Institute of Medicine. 1977a. *Reliability of Hospital Discharge Abstracts*. Washington, DC: National Academy of Sciences.

———. 1977b. *Reliability of Medicare Hospital Discharge Records*. Washington, DC: National Academy of Sciences.

———. 1986. *Improving the Quality of Care in Nursing Homes*. Washington, DC: National Academy of Sciences.

———. 2001b. *The Interplay of Biological, Behavioral, and Societal Influences*. Washington, DC: National Academy Press.

———. 2002c. *Leadership by Example: Coordinating Government Roles in Improving Health Care Quality*. Washington, DC: National Academy of Sciences.

———. 2001d. *Improving the Quality of Long-Term Care*. Washington, DC: National Academy Press.

Institute of Medicine, Committee on the Consequences of Uninsurance. 2001c. *Coverage Matters: Insurance and Health Care*. Washington, DC: National Academy Press.

———. 2002a. *Care Without Coverage. Too Little, Too Late*. Washington, DC: National Academy Press.

Institute of Medicine, Committee on Maintaining Privacy and Security in Health Care Applications of the National Information Infrastructure. 1997. *For the Record. Protecting Electronic Health Information*. Washington, DC: National Academy Press.

Institute of Medicine, Committee on Quality of Health Care in America. 2000. *To Err Is Human: Building a Safer Health System*. Washington, DC: National Academy Press.

———. 2001a. *Crossing the Quality Chasm: A New Health System for the 21st Century*. Washington, DC: National Academy Press.

Institute of Medicine, Committee on Understanding and Eliminating Racial Disparities in Health Care. 2002b. In *Unequal Treatment:Confronting Racial and Ethnic Disparities in Health Care*, edited by B. D. Smedley, A. Y. Stith, and A. R. Nelson. Washington, DC: National Academy of Sciences.

The International Neonatal Network. 1993. "The CRIB (Clinical Risk Index for Babies) Score: A Tool for Assessing Initial Neonatal Risk and Comparing Performance of Neonatal Intensive Care Units." *Lancet* 342: 193–98.

Ioannidis, J. P., A. B. Haidich, M. Pappa, N. Pantazis, S. I. Kokori, M. G. Tektonidou, D. G. Contopoulos-Ioannidis, and J. Lau. 2001. "Comparison of Evidence of Treatment Effects in Randomized and Nonrandomized Studies." *Journal of the American Medical Association* 286 (7): 821–30.

IsHak, W., T. Burt, and L. Sederer, eds. 2002. *Outcome Measurement in Psychiatry: A Critical Review.* Washington, DC: American Psychiatric Publishing.

Israel, R. A. 1978. "The International Classification of Diseases: Two Hundred Years of Development." *Public Health Reports* 93 (2): 150–52.

Jacobs, A. K., J. M. Johnston, A. Haviland, M. M. Brooks, S. F. Kelsey, D. R. Holmes, Jr., D. P. Faxon, D. O. Williams, and K. M. Detre. 2002. "Improved Outcomes for Women Undergoing Contemporary Percutaneous Coronary Intervention: A Report from the National Heart, Lung, and Blood Institute Dynamic Registry." *Journal of the American College of Cardiologists* 39 (10): 1608–14.

Jencks, S. F., C. Horgan, H. H. Goldman, and C. A. Taube. 1987. "Bringing Excluded Psychiatric Facilities Under the Medicare Prospective Payment System. A Review of Research Evidence and Policy Options." *Medical Care* 25 (9, Suppl.): S1–S51.

Jencks, S. F., and G. R. Wilensky. 1992. "The Health Care Quality Improvement Initiative: A New Approach to Quality Assurance in Medicare." *Journal of the American Medical Association* 268 (7): 900–03.

Jencks, S. F., D. K. Williams, and T. L. Kay. 1988. "Assessing Hospital-Associated Deaths from Discharge Data: The Role of Length of Stay and Comorbidities." *Journal of the American Medical Association* 260 (15): 2240–46.

Jenkins, K. J., K. Gauvreau, J. W. Newburger, T. L. Spray, J. H. Moller, and L. I. Iezzoni. 2002. "Consensus-Based Method for Risk Adjustment for Surgery for Congenital Heart Disease." *Journal of Thoracic and Cardiovascular Surgery* 123 (1): 110–18.

Jenkins, K. J., J. W. Newburger, J. E. Lock, R. B. Davis, G. A. Coffman, and L. I. Iezzoni. 1995. "In-Hospital Mortality for Surgical Repair of Congenital Heart Defects: Preliminary Observations of Variation by Hospital Caseload." *Pediatrics* 95 (3): 323–30.

Jenkins, P. C., M. F. Flanagan, K. J. Jenkins, J. D. Sargent, C. E. Canter, R. E. Chinnock, R. N. Vincent, A. N. Tosteson, and G. T. O'Connor. 2000. "Survival Analysis and Risk Factors for Mortality in Transplantation and Staged Surgery for Hypoplastic Left Heart Syndrome." *Journal of the American College of Cardiologists* 36 (4): 1178–85.

Jette, A. M., K. W. Smith, and S. M. McDermott. 1996. "Quality of Medicare-Reimbursed Home Health Care." *Gerontologist* 36 (4): 492–501.

Jha, A., D. L. Patrick, R. F. MacLehose, J. N. Doctor, and L. Chan. 2002. "Dissatisfaction with Medical Services Among Medicare Beneficiaries with Disabilities." *Archives of Physical Medicine and Rehabilitation* 83 (10): 1335–41.

Johnson, R. E., M. C. Hornbrook, and G. A. Nichols. 1994. "Replicating the Chronic Disease Score (CDS) from Automated Pharmacy Data." *Journal of Clinical Epidemiology* 47 (10): 1191–99.

Junger, A., J. Engel, M. Benson, S. Bottger, C. Grabow, B. Hartmann, A. Michel, R. Rohrig, K. Marquardt, and G. Hempelmann. 2002. "Discriminative Power on Mortality of a Modified Sequential Organ Failure Assessment Score for Complete Automatic Computation in an Operative Intensive Care Unit." *Critical Care Medicine* 30 (2): 338–42.

Justice, A. C., L. H. Aiken, H. L. Smith, and B. J. Turner. 1996. "The Role of Functional Status in Predicting Inpatient Mortality with AIDS: A Comparison with Current Predictors." *Journal of Clinical Epidemiology* 49 (2): 193–201.

Justice, A. C., K. E. Covinsky, and J. A. Berlin. 1999. "Assessing the Generalizability of Prognostic Information." *Annals of Internal Medicine* 130 (6): 515–24.

Kaboli, P. J., M. J. Barnett, S. M. Fuehrer, and G. E. Rosenthal. 2001. "Length of Stay as a Source of Bias in Comparing Performance in VA and Private Sector Facilities: Lessons Learned from a Regional Evaluation of Intensive Care Outcomes." *Medical Care* 39 (9): 1014–24.

Kahn, K. L., D. Draper, E. B. Keeler, W. H. Rogers, L. V. Rubenstein, J. Kosecoff, M. J. Sherwood, E. J. Reinisch, M. F. Carney, C. J. Kamberg, S. S. Bentow, K. B. Wells, H. Allen, D. Reboussin, C. P. Roth, C. Chew, and R. H. Brook. 1992. *The Effects of the DRG-Based Prospective Payment System on Quality of Care for Hospitalized Medicare Patients.* Publication No. R-3931-HCFA. Santa Monica, CA: RAND.

Kahn, R. S., B. Zuckerman, H. Bauchner, C. J. Homer, and P. H. Wise. 2002. "Women's Health After Pregnancy and Child Outcomes at Age 3 Years: A Prospective Cohort Study." *American Journal of Public Health* 92 (8): 1312–18.

Kalbfleisch, J. D., and R. L. Prentiss. 1980. *The Statistical Analysis of Failure Time Data.* New York: John Wiley.

Kane, R. L. 1997. "Improving Outcomes on Rehabilitation. A Call to Arms (and Legs)." *Medical Care* 35 (6, Suppl.): JS21–JS27.

———. 1998. "Assuring Quality in Nursing Home Care." *Journal of the American Geriatric Society* 46 (2): 232–37.

———. 2000. "Choosing and Using an Assessment Tool." In *Assessing Older Persons: Measures, Meaning, and Practical Applications,* edited by R. L. Kane and R. A. Kane, 1–13. New York: Oxford University Press.

Kane, R. L., Q. Chen, M. Finch, L. Blewett, R. Burns, and M. Moskowitz. 2000. "The Optimal Outcomes of Post-Hospital Care Under Medicare." *Health Services Research* 35 (3): 615–61.

Kane, R. L., M. Finch, L. Blewett, Q. Chen, R. Burns, and M. Moskowitz. 1996. "Use of Post-Hospital Care by Medicare Patients." *Journal of the American Geriatric Society* 44 (3): 242–50.

Kaplan, S. H., S. Greenfield, and J. E. Ware, Jr. 1989. "Assessing the Effects of Physician-Patient Interactions on the Outcomes of Chronic Disease." *Medical Care* 27 (3, Suppl.): S110–S127.

Kaplan, S. H., and J. R. Ware. 1989. "The Patient's Role in Health Care and Quality Assessment." In *Providing Quality Care: The Challenge to Clinicians,* edited by N. Goldfield and D. B. Nash, 25–70. Philadelphia: American College of Physicians.

Kapur, K., A. S. Young, and D. Murata. 2000. "Risk Adjustment for High Utilizers of

Public Mental Health Care." *Journal of Mental Health Policy and Economics* 3 (3): 129–37.

Katz, J. N., L. C. Chang, O. Sangha, A. H. Fossel, and D. W. Bates. 1996. "Can Comorbidity be Measured by Questionnaire Rather than Medical Record Review?" *Medical Care* 34 (1): 73–84.

Katz, S. J., J. K. Zemencuk, and T. P. Hofer. 2000. "Breast Cancer Screening in the United States and Canada, 1994: Socioeconomic Gradients Persist." *American Journal of Public Health* 90 (5): 799–803.

Keeler, E. B., K. L. Kahn, D. Draper, M. J. Sherwood, L. V. Rubenstein, E. J. Reinisch, J. Kosecoff, and R. H. Brook. 1990. "Charges in Sickness at Admission Following the Introduction of the Prospective Payment System." *Journal of the American Medical Association* 264 (15): 1962–68.

Keeler, E. B., L. V. Rubenstein, K. L. Kahn, D. Draper, E. R. Harrison, M. J. McGinty, W. H. Rogers, and R. H. Brook. 1992. "Hospital Characteristics and Quality of Care." *Journal of the American Medical Association* 268 (13): 1709–14.

Kelly-Hayes, M., A. M. Jette, P. A. Wolf, R. B. D'Agostino, and P. M. Odell. 1992. "Functional Limitations and Disability Among Elders in the Framingham Study." *American Journal of Public Health* 82 (6): 841–45.

Kennedy, J., and C. Erb. 2002. "Prescription Noncompliance Due to Cost Among Adults with Disabilities in the United States." *American Journal of Public Health* 92 (7): 1120–24.

Kersten, P., S. George, L. McLellan, J. A. Smith, and M. A. Mullee. 2000. "Disabled People and Professionals Differ in Their Perceptions of Rehabilitation Needs." *Journal of Public Health and Medicine* 22 (3): 393–99.

Kessler, R. C., K. A. McGonagle, S. Zhao, C. B. Nelson, M. Hughes, S. Eshleman, H. U. Wittchen, and K. S. Kendler. 1994. "Lifetime and 12-Month Prevalence of DSM-III-R Psychiatric Disorders in the United States. Results from the National Comorbidity Survey." *Archives of General Psychiatry* 51 (1): 8–19.

Khuri, S. F., J. Daley, and W. G. Henderson. 1999. "The Measurement of Quality in Surgery." *Advances in Surgery* 33: 113–40.

Khuri, S. F., J. Daley, W. Henderson, G. Barbour, P. Lowry, G. Irvin, J. Gibbs, F. Grover, K. Hammermeister, J. F. Stremple, J. B. Aust, J. Demakis, D. Deykin, G. McDonald, and participants in the National Veterans Administration Surgical Risk Study. 1995. "The National Veterans Administration Surgical Risk Study: Risk Adjustment for the Comparative Assessment of the Quality of Surgical Care." *Journal of the American College of Surgeons* 180 (5): 519–31.

Khuri, S. F., J. Daley, W. Henderson, K. Hur, J. Demakis, J. B. Aust, V. Chong, P. J. Fabri, J. O. Gibbs, F. Grover, K. Hammermeister, G. Irvin, III, G. McDonald, E. Passaro, Jr., L. Phillips, F. Scamman, J. Spencer, and J. F. Stremple. 1998. "The Department of Veterans Affairs' NSQIP: The First National, Validated, Outcome-Based, Risk-Adjusted, and Peer-Controlled Program for the Measurement and Enhancement of the Quality of Surgical Care. National VA Surgical Quality Improvement Program." *Annals of Surgery* 228 (4): 491–507.

Khuri, S. F., J. Daley, W. Henderson, K. Hur, J. O. Gibbs, G. Barbour, J. Demakis, G. Irvin, III, J. F. Stremple, F. Grover, G. McDonald, E. Passaro, Jr., P. J. Fabri, J. Spencer, K. Hammermeister, and J. B. Aust. 1997. "Risk Adjustment of the Postoperative Mortality Rate for the Comparative Assessment of the

Quality of Surgical Care: Results of the National Veterans Affairs Surgical Risk Study." *Journal of the American College of Surgeons* 185 (4): 315–27.

Khuri, S. F., J. Daley, W. Henderson, K. Hur, M. Hossain, D. Soybel, K. W. Kizer, J. B. Aust, R. H. Bell, V. Chong, J. Demakis, P. J. Fabri, J. O. Gibbs, F. Grover, K. Hammermeister, G. McDonald, E. Passaro, L. Phillips, F. Scamman, J. Spencer, J. F. Stremple, R. H. Bell, Jr., and E. Passaro, Jr. 1999. "Relation of Surgical Volume to Outcome in Eight Common Operations: Results from the VA National Surgical Quality Improvement Program." *Annals of Surgery* 230 (3): 414–29; discussion 429–32.

Khuri, S. F., S. F. Najjar, J. Daley, B. Krasnicka, M. Hossain, W. G. Henderson, J. B. Aust, B. Bass, M. J. Bishop, J. Demakis, R. DePalma, P. J. Fabri, A. Fink, J. Gibbs, F. Grover, K. Hammermeister, G. McDonald, L. Neumayer, R. H. Roswell, J. Spencer, and R. H. Turnage. 2001. "Comparison of Surgical Outcomes Between Teaching and Nonteaching Hospitals in the Department of Veterans Affairs." *Annals of Surgery* 234 (3): 370–82.

Kiesler, C. A., and C. Simpkins. 1992. "Changes in Diagnostic Case Mix in Psychiatric Care in General Hospitals, 1980–85." *General Hospital Psychiatry* 14 (3): 156–61.

Klabunde, C. N., J. L. Warren, and J. M. Legler. 2002. "Assessing Comorbidity Using Claims Data: An Overview." *Medical Care* 40 (8, Suppl.): IV-26–IV-35.

Klemm, J. D. 2000. "Medicaid Spending: A Brief History." *Health Care Financing Review* 22 (1): 105–12.

Knaus, W. A. 2002. "APACHE 1978–2001. The Development of a Quality Assurance System Based on Prognosis: Milestones and Personal Reflections." *Archives of Surgery* 137 (1): 37–41.

Knaus, W. A., E. A. Draper, D. P. Wagner, and J. E. Zimmerman. 1985. "APACHE II: A Severity of Disease Classification System." *Critical Care Medicine* 13 (10): 818–29.

———. 1986. "An Evaluation of Outcome from Intensive Care in Major Medical Centers." *Annals of Internal Medicine* 104 (3): 410–18.

Knaus, W. A., F. E. Harrell, Jr., J. Lynn, L. Goldman, R. S. Phillips, A. F. Connors, Jr., N. V. Dawson, W. J. Fulkerson, Jr., R. M. Califf, N. Desbiens, L. Norman, O. Peter, R. K. Bellamy, P. E. Hakim, B. Rosemarie, and D. P. Wagner. 1995. "The SUPPORT Prognostic Model. Objective Estimates of Survival for Seriously Ill Hospitalized Adults. Study to Understand Prognoses and Preferences for Outcomes and Risks of Treatments." *Annals of Internal Medicine* 122 (3): 191–203.

Knaus, W. A., D. P. Wagner, E. A. Draper, J. E. Zimmerman, M. Bergner, P. G. Bastos, C. A. Sirio, D. J. Murphy, T. Lotring, and A. Damiano. 1991. "The APACHE III Prognostic System. Risk Prediction of Hospital Mortality for Critically Ill Hospitalized Adults." *Chest* 100 (6): 1619–36.

Knaus, W. A., D. P. Wagner, and J. Lynn. 1991. "Short-Term Mortality Predictions for Critically Ill Hospitalized Adults: Science and Ethics." *Science* 254 (5030): 389–94.

Knaus, W. A., D. P. Wagner, J. E. Zimmerman, and E. A. Draper. 1993. "Variations in Mortality and Length of Stay in Intensive Care Units." *Annals of Internal Medicine* 118 (10): 753–61.

Knaus, W. A., J. E. Zimmerman, D. P. Wagner, E. A. Draper, and D. E. Lawrence. 1981. "APACHE—Acute Physiology and Chronic Health Evaluation: A Physiologically Based Classification System." *Critical Care Medicine* 9 (8): 591–97.

Korn, E. L., and R. Simon. 1991. "Explained Residual Variation, Explained Risk, and Goodness of Fit." *The American Statistician* 45 (3): 201–06.

Krakauer, H. R. C. Bailey, K. J. Skellan, J. D. Stewart, A. J. Hartz, E. M. Kuhn, and A. A. Rimm. 1992. "Evaluation of the HCFA Model for the Analysis of Mortality Following Hospitalization." *Health Services Research* 27 (3): 317–35.

Kramer, A. M. 1997. "Rehabilitation Care and Outcomes from the Patient's Perspective." *Medical Care* 35 (6, Suppl.): JS48–JS57.

———. 2002. "Quality of Post-Acute and Long-Term Care: Defining the Terms and Issues." Chapel Hill, NC: Carolina Health Summit, School of Public Health, The University of North Carolina.

Kramer, T. L., R. B. Evans, R. Landes, M. Mancino, B. M. Booth, and G. R. Smith. 2001. "Comparing Outcomes of Routine Care for Depression: The Dilemma of Case-Mix Adjustment." *Journal of Behavioral Health Services & Research* 28 (3): 287–300.

Krauss, N. A., S. Machlin, and B. L. Kass. 1999. "Research Findings No. 7: Use of Health Care Services, 1996." Agency for Healthcare Research and Quality. [Online article; retrieved 12/19/02.] http://www.meps.ahrq.gov/papers/rf7_99-0018/rf7.htm.

Kravitz, R. L., R. D. Hays, C. D. Sherbourne, M. R. DiMatteo, W. H. Rogers, L. Ordway, and S. Greenfield. 1993. "Recall of Recommendations and Adherence to Advice Among Patients with Chronic Medical Conditions." *Archives of Internal Medicine* 153 (16): 1869–78.

Kressin, N. R., J. A. Clark, J. Whittle, M. East, E. D. Peterson, B. H. Chang, A. K. Rosen, X. S. Ren, L. G. Alley, L. Kroupa, T. C. Collins, and L. A. Petersen. 2002. "Racial Differences in Health-Related Beliefs, Attitudes, and Experiences of VA Cardiac Patients: Scale Development and Application." *Medical Care* 40 (1, Suppl.): I72–85.

Krieger, J., and D. L. Higgins. 2002. "Housing and Health: Time Again for Public Health Action." *American Journal of Public Health* 92 (5): 758–68.

Krieger, N., P. Waterman, J. T. Chen, M. J. Soobader, S. V. Subramanian, and R. Carson. 2002. "Zip Code Caveat: Bias Due to Spatiotemporal Mismatches between Zip Codes and US Census-Defined Geographic Areas—The Public Health Disparities Geocoding Project." *American Journal of Public Health* 92 (7): 1100–02.

Kriegsman, D. M., B. W. Penninx, J. T. van Eijk, A. J. Boeke, and D. J. Deeg. 1996. "Self-Reports and General Practitioner Information on the Presence of Chronic Diseases in Community Dwelling Elderly. A Study on the Accuracy of Patients' Self-Reports and on Determinants of Inaccuracy." *Journal of Clinical Epidemiology* 49 (12): 1407–17.

Kronick, R., T. Dreyfus, L. Lee, and Z. Zhou. 1996. "Diagnostic Risk Adjustment for Medicaid: The Disability Payment System." *Health Care Financing Review* 17 (3): 7–33.

Kronick, R., T. Gilmer, T. Dreyfus, and L. Lee. 2000. "Improving Health-Based

Payment for Medicaid Beneficiaries: CDPS." *Health Care Financing Review* 21 (3): 29–64.

Kronick, R., Z. Zhou, and T. Dreyfus. 1995. "Making Risk Adjustment Work for Everyone." *Inquiry* 32 (1): 41–55.

Krousel-Wood, M. A., A. Abdoh, and R. Re. 1996. "Comparing Comorbid-Illness Indices Assessing Outcome Variation: The Case of Prostatectomy." *Journal of General Internal Medicine* 11 (1): 32–38.

Krumholz, H. M., P. S. Douglas, M. S. Lauer, and R. C. Pasternak. 1992. "Selection of Patients for Coronary Angiography and Coronary Revascularization Early After Myocardial Infarction: Is There Evidence for a Gender Bias?" *Annals of Internal Medicine* 116 (10): 785–90.

Krumholz, H. M., S. S. Rathore, J. Chen, Y. Wang, and M. J. Radford. 2002. "Evaluation of a Consumer-Oriented Internet Health Care Report Card: The Risk of Quality Ratings Based on Mortality Data." *Journal of the American Medical Association* 287 (10): 1277–87.

Kruse, J. A., M. C. Thill-Baharozian, and R. W. Carlson. 1988. "Comparison of Clinical Assessment with APACHE II for Predicting Mortality Risk in Patients Admitted to a Medical Intensive Care Unit." *Journal of the American Medical Association* 260 (12): 1739–42.

Ku, L., M. R. Ellwood, and J. Klemm. 1990. "Deciphering Medicaid Data: Issues and Needs." *Health Care Financing Review* Dec. (Annual Suppl.): 35–45.

Kuhlthau, K., T. G. Ferris, A. C. Beal, S. L. Gortmaker, and J. M. Perrin. 2001. "Who Cares for Medicaid-Enrolled Children with Chronic Conditions?" *Pediatrics* 108 (4): 906–12.

Kuhlthau, K., J. M. Perrin, S. L. Ettner, T. J. McLaughlin, and S. L. Gortmaker. 1998. "High-Expenditure Children with Supplemental Security Income." *Pediatrics* 102: 610–15.

Kuperman, G. J., R. M. Gardner, and T. A. Pryor. 1991. *HELP: A Dynamic Hospital Information System*. New York: Springer.

Kurtz, D. L. 1943. *Unit Medical Records in Hospital and Clinic*. New York: Columbia University Press.

Kutner, N. G., M. G. Ory, D. I. Baker, K. B. Schechtman, M. C. Hornbrook, and C. D. Mulrow. 1992. "Measuring the Quality of Life of the Elderly in Health Promotion Intervention Clinical Trials." *Public Health Report* 107 (5): 530–39.

Lachs, M. S., A. R. Feinstein, L. M. Cooney, Jr., M. A. Drickamer, R. A. Marottoli, F. C. Pannill, and M. E. Tinetti. 1990. "A Simple Procedure for General Screening for Functional Disability in Elderly Patients." *Annals of Internal Medicine* 112 (9): 699–706.

Lamers, L. M. 1999. "Pharmacy Cost Groups. A Risk-Adjuster for Capitation Payment Based on the Use of Prescription Drugs." *Medical Care* 37 (8): 824–30.

Lamont, E. B., D. S. Lauderdale, R. L. Schilsky, and N. A. Christakis. 2002. "Construct Validity of Medicare Chemotherapy Claims: The Case of 5FU." *Medical Care* 40 (3): 201–11.

Lamoreaux, J. 1996. "The Organizational Structure for Medical Information Management in the Department of Veterans Affairs. An Overview of Major Health Care Databases." *Medical Care* 34 (3, Suppl.): MS31–MS44.

Landis, J. R., and G. G. Koch. 1977. "The Measurement of Observer Agreement for Categorical Data." *Biometrics* 33 (1): 159–74.

Landon, B., L. I. Iezzoni, A. S. Ash, M. Shwartz, J. Daley, J. S. Hughes, and Y. D. Mackiernan. 1996. "Judging Hospitals by Severity-Adjusted Mortality Rates: The Case of CABG Surgery." *Inquiry* 33 (2): 155–66.

Langenbrunner, J. C., J. P. Willis, S. F. Jencks, A. Dobson, and L. I. Iezzoni. 1989. "Developing Payment Refinements and Reforms Under Medicare for Excluded Hospitals." *Health Care Financing Review* 10 (3): 91–106.

Lantz, P. M., J. S. House, J. M. Lepkowski, D. R. Williams, R. P. Mero, and J. Chen. 1998. "Socioeconomic Factors, Health Behaviors, and Mortality: Results from a Nationally Representative Prospective Study of U.S. Adults." *Journal of the American Medical Association* 279 (21): 703–08.

Lantz, P. M., J. W. Lynch, J. S. House, J. M. Lepkowski, R. P. Mero, M. A. Musick, and D. R. Williams. 2001. "Socioeconomic Disparities in Health Change in a Longitudinal Study of US Adults: The Role of Health-Risk Behaviors." *Social Science and Medicine* 53 (1): 29–40.

Lasker, R. D., and M. S. Marquis. 1999. "The Intensity of Physicians' Work in Patient Visits—Implications for the Coding of Patient Evaluation and Management Services." *New England Journal of Medicine* 341 (5): 337–41.

Lave, J. R., C. L. Pashos, G. F. Anderson, D. Brailer, T. Bubolz, D. Conrad, D. A. Freund, S. H. Fox, E. Keeler, J. Lipscomb, H. S. Luft, and G. Provenzano. 1994. "Costing Medical Care: Using Medicare Administrative Data." *Medical Care* 32 (7, Suppl.): JS77–89.

LaVeist, T. A. 1994. "Beyond Dummy Variables and Sample Selection: What Health Services Researchers Ought to Know About Race as a Variable." *Health Services Research* 29 (1): 1–16.

———. 2000. "On the Study of Race, Racism, and Health: A Shift from Description to Explanation." *International Journal of Health Services* 30 (1): 217–19.

LaVeist, T. A., K. J. Nickerson, and J. V. Bowie. 2000. "Attitudes About Racism, Medical Mistrust, and Satisfaction with Care Among African American and White Cardiac Patients." *Medical Care Research and Review* 57 (1, Suppl.): 146–61.

Lawthers, A. G., E. P. McCarthy, R. B. Davis, L. E. Peterson, R. H. Palmer, and L. I. Iezzoni. 2000. "Identification of In-Hospital Complications from Claims Data. Is It Valid?" *Medical Care* 38 (8): 785–95.

Le Gall, J. R., S. Lemeshow, and F. Saulnier. 1993. "A New Simplified Acute Physiology Score (SAPS II) Based on a European/North American Multicenter Study." *Journal of the American Medical Association* 270 (24): 2957–63.

Lehman, A. F. 2002. Personal communication, 2 Aug. 2

Lemeshow, S., and D. W. Hosmer, Jr. 1982. "A Review of Goodness of Fit Statistics for Use in the Development of Logistic Regression Models." *American Journal of Epidemiology* 115 (1): 92–106.

Lemeshow, S., J. Klar, D. Teres, J. S. Avrunin, S. H. Gehlbach, J. Rapoport, and M. Rue. 1994. "Mortality Probability Models for Patients in the Intensive Care Unit for 48 or 72 Hours: A Prospective, Multicenter Study." *Critical Care Medicine* 22 (9): 1351–58.

Lemeshow, S., and J. R. Le Gall. 1994. "Modeling the Severity of Illness of ICU

Patients. A Systems Update." *Journal of the American Medical Association* 272 (13): 1049–55.

Lemeshow, S., D. Teres, J. S. Avrunin, and R. W. Gage. 1988. "Refining Intensive Care Unit Outcome Prediction by Using Changing Probabilities of Mortality." *Critical Care Medicine* 16 (5): 470–77.

Lemeshow, S., D. Teres, J. Klar, J. S. Avrunin, S. H. Gehlbach, and J. Rapoport. 1993. "Mortality Probability Models (MPM II) Based on an International Cohort of Intensive Care Unit Patients." *Journal of the American Medical Association* 270 (20): 2478–86.

Lemeshow, S. D. Teres, H. Pastides, J. S. Avrunin, and J. S. Steingrub. 1985. "A Method for Predicting Survival and Mortality of ICU Patients Using Objectively Derived Weights." *Critical Care Medicine* 13 (7): 519–25.

Leteurtre, S., A. Martinot, A. Duhamel, F. Gauvin, B. Grandbastien, T. V. Nam, F. Proulx, J. Lacroix, and F. Leclerc. 1999. "Development of a Pediatric Multiple Organ Dysfunction Score: Use of Two Strategies." *Medical Decision Making* 19 (4): 399–410.

Liao, Y., D. L. McGee, J. S. Kaufman, G. Cao, and R. S. Cooper. 1999. "Socioeconomic Status in the Last Years of Life." *American Journal of Public Health* 89: 569–72.

Lieu, T. A., P. Lozano, J. A. Finkelstein, F. W. Chi, N. G. Jensvold, A. M. Capra, C. P. Quesenberry, J. V. Selby, and H. J. Farber. 2002. "Racial/Ethnic Variation in Asthma Status and Management Practices Among Children in Managed Medicaid." *Pediatrics* 109 (5): 857–65.

Lillard, L. A., and M. M. Farmer. 1997. "Linking Medicare and National Survey Data." *Annals of Internal Medicine* 127 (8, Part II): 691–95.

Lipowski, E. E., and W. E. Bigelow. 1996. "Data Linkages for Research on Outcomes of Long-Term Care." *Gerontologist* 36 (4): 441–47.

Little, R. J. A., and D. B. Rubin. 1987. *Statistical Analysis with Missing Data.* New York: John Wiley & Sons.

Lloyd-Jones, D. M., D. O. Martin, M. G. Larson, and D. Levy. 1998. "Accuracy of Death Certificates for Coding Coronary Heart Disease as the Cause of Death." *Annals of Internal Medicine* 129 (12): 1020–26.

Localio, A. R., B. H. Hamory, A. C. Fisher, and T. R. TenHave. 1997. "The Public Release of Hospital and Physician Mortality Data in Pennsylvania. A Case Study." *Medical Care* 35 (3): 272–86.

Lohr, K. 1989. "Advances in Health Status Assessment, Conference Proceedings." *Medical Care* 27 (Suppl.): S1–S294.

———. 1992. "Advances in Health Status Assessment: Fostering the Application of Health Status Measures in Clinical Settings: Proceedings of a Conference." *Medical Care* 30 (5, Suppl.): MS1–MS293.

Louis, D. Z., E. J. Yuen, M. Braga, A. Cicchetti, C. Rabinowitz, C. Laine, and J. S. Gonnella. 1999. "Impact of a DRG-Based Hospital Financing System on Quality and Outcomes of Care in Italy." *Health Services Research* 34 (1, Part II): 405–15.

Ludwigs, U., and J. Hulting. 1995. "Acute Physiology and Chronic Health Evaluation II Scoring System in Acute Myocardial Infarction: A Prospective Validation Study." *Critical Care Medicine* 23 (5): 854–59.

Luft, H. S., and B. W. Brown, Jr. 1993. "Calculating the Probability of Rare Events: Why Settle for an Approximation?" *Health Services Research* 28 (4): 419–39.

Luft, H. S., and S. S. Hunt. "Evaluating Individual Hospital Quality Through Outcome Statistics." *Journal of the American Medical Association* 255 (20): 2780–84.

Luft, H. S., and P. S. Romano. 1993. "Chance, Continuity, and Change in Hospital Mortality Rates. Coronary Artery Bypass Graft Patients in California Hospitals, 1983 to 1989." *Journal of the American Medical Association* 270 (3): 331–37.

Lumley, T., P. Diehr, S. Emerson, and L. Chen. 2002. "The Importance of the Normality Assumption in Large Public Health Data Sets." *Annual Review of Public Health* 23: 151–69.

Lurie, N., M. Popkin, M. Dysken, I. Moscovice, and M. Finch. 1992. "Accuracy of Diagnoses of Schizophrenia in Medicaid Claims." *Hospital and Community Psychiatry* 43 (1): 69–71.

Lynch, J. W., G. A. Kaplan, and S. J. Shema. 1997. "Cumulative Impact of Sustained Economic Hardship on Physical, Cognitive, Psychological, and Social Functioning." *New England Journal of Medicine* 337 (26): 1889–95.

Lyons, T. F., and B. C. Payne. 1974. "The Relationship of Physicians' Medical Recording Performance to Their Medical Care Performance." *Medical Care* 12 (8): 714–20.

Mairs, N. 1996. *Waist-High in the World*. Boston: Beacon Press.

Malkin, J. D., M. S. Broder, and E. Keeler. 2000. "Do Longer Postpartum Stays Reduce Newborn Readmissions? Analysis Using Instrumental Variables." *Health Services Research* 35 (5, Part II): 1071–91.

Mangione, C. M., E. R. Marcantonio, L. Goldman, E. F. Cook, M. C. Donaldson, D. J. Sugarbaker, R. Poss, and T. H. Lee. 1993. "Influence of Age on Measurement of Health Status in Patients Undergoing Elective Surgery." *Journal of the American Geriatric Society* 41 (4): 377–83.

Mangione, C. M., R. S. Phillips, J. M. Seddon, M. G. Lawrence, E. F. Cook, R. Dailey, and L. Goldman. 1992. "Development of the 'Activities of Daily Vision Scale.' A Measure of Visual Functional Status." *Medical Care* 30 (12): 1111–26.

Mansfield, B. G. 1986. "How Bad Are Medical Records? A Review of the Notes Received by a Practice." *Journal of the Royal College of General Practitioners* 36 (290): 405–06.

Manton, K. G., L. Corder, and E. Stallard. 1993. "Changes in the Use of Personal Assistance and Special Equipment, from 1982 to 1989: Results from the 1982 and 1989 NLTCS." *Gerontologist* 33 (2): 168–76.

———. 1997. "Chronic Disability Trends in Elderly United States Populations: 1982–1994." *Proceedings of the National Academy of Science U S A* 94 (6): 2593–98.

Manton, K. G., and X. Gu. 2001. "Changes in the Prevalence of Chronic Disability in the United States Black and Nonblack Population Above Age 65 from 1982 to 1999." *Proceedings of the National Academy of Science U S A* 98 (11): 6354–59.

Manton, K. G., E. Stallard, and L. Corder. 1997. "Education-Specific Estimates of Life Expectancy and Age-Specific Disability in the U.S. Elderly Population." *Journal of Aging and Health* 9 (4): 419–50.

Mapi Research Institute. 2002. "The Quality of Life Instrument Database." [Online information; retrieved 9/24/02.] http://www.qolid.org.

Mark, D. B., L. K. Shaw, E. R. DeLong, R. M. Califf, and D. B. Pryor. 1994. "Absence of Sex Bias in the Referral of Patients for Cardiac Catheterization." *New England Journal of Medicine* 330 (16): 1101–06.

Markello, S. J. 1997. "Measuring Case Mix, Severity, and Complexity in Geriatric Patients Undergoing Rehabilitation. Small Working Group II Report." *Medical Care* 35 (6, Suppl.): JS118–JS120.

Markens, S., S. A. Fox, B. Taub, and M. L. Gilbert. 2002. "Role of Black Churches in Health Promotion Programs: Lessons from the Los Angeles Mammography Promotion in Churches Program." *American Journal of Public Health* 92 (5): 805–10.

Marmot, M. 2002. "The Influence of Income on Health: Views of an Epidemiologist. Does Money Really Matter? Or Is It a Marker for Something Else?" *Health Affairs (Millwood)* 21 (2): 31–46.

Marshall, G., F. L. Grover, W. G. Henderson, and K. E. Hammermeister. 1994. "Assessment of Predictive Models for Binary Outcomes: An Empirical Approach Using Operative Death from Cardiac Surgery." *Statistics in Medicine* 13 (15): 1501–11.

Marshall, G., W. G. Henderson, T. E. Moritz, A. L. Shroyer, F. L. Grover, and K. E. Hammermeister. 1995. "Statistical Methods and Strategies for Working with Large Data Bases." *Medical Care* 33 (10, Suppl.): OS35–OS42.

Marshall, S. C., B. Heisel, and D. Grinnell. 1999. "Validity of the PULSES Profile Compared with the Functional Independence Measure for Measuring Disability in a Stroke Rehabilitation Center." *Archives of Physical Medicine and Rehabilitation* 80 (7): 760–65.

Martin, L., C. Chin, and C. A. Harrison. 2001. "Annual Statistical Report on the Social Security Disability Insurance Program, 2000." [Online article; retrieved 12/28/01.] http://www.ssa.gov/statistical/di_asr/2000/index.html.

Master, R., T. Dreyfus, S. Connors, C. Tobias, Z. Zhou, and R. Kronick. 1996. "The Community Medical Alliance: An Integrated System of Care in Greater Boston for People with Severe Disability and AIDS." *Managed Care Quarterly* 4 (2): 26–37.

Mathias, S. D., S. K. Fifer, and D. L. Patrick. 1994. "Rapid Transition of Quality of Life Measures for International Clinical Trials: Avoiding Errors in the Minimalist Approach." *Quality of Life Research* 3 (6): 403–12.

Mavroudis, C., and J. P. Jacobs. 2002. "Congenital Heart Disease Outcome Analysis: Methodology and Rationale." *Journal of Thoracic and Cardiovascular Surgery* 123 (1): 6–7.

Mayer-Oakes, S. A., H. Hoenig, K. A. Atchison, J. E. Lubben, F. De Jong, and S. O. Schweitzer. 1992. "Patient-Related Predictors of Rehabilitation Use for Community-Dwelling Older Americans." *Journal of the American Geriatrics Society* 40 (4): 336–42.

McBean, A. M., J. D. Babish, and J. L. Warren. 1993. "Determination of Lung Cancer Incidence in the Elderly Using Medicare Claims Data." *American Journal of Epidemiology* 137 (2): 226–34.

McCabe, J. 1988. "The Uniform Health-Care Information Act: Current Status, Part

II." [Interview by Joan Banach.] *Journal of the American Medical Record Association* 59 (10): 23–25.

McCarthy, E. P., R. B. Burns, S. S. Coughlin, K. M. Freund, J. Rice, S. L. Maxwell, A. Ash, M. Shwartz, and M. A. Moskowitz. 1998. "Mammography Use Helps to Explain Differences in Breast Cancer Stage at Diagnosis Between Older Black and White Women." *Annals of Internal Medicine* 126 (9): 729–36.

McCarthy, E. P., R. B. Burns, K. M. Freund, A. S. Ash, M. Shwartz, S. L. Marwill, and M. A. Moskowitz. 2000b. "Mammography Use, Breast Cancer Stage at Diagnosis, and Survival Among Older Women." *Journal of the American Geriatric Society* 48 (10): 1226–33.

McCarthy, E. P., L. I. Iezzoni, R. B. Davis, R. H. Palmer, M. Cahalane, M. B. Hamel, K. Mukamal, R. S. Phillips, and D. T. Davies, Jr. 2000a. "Does Clinical Evidence Support ICD-9-CM Diagnosis Coding of Complications?" *Medical Care* 38 (8): 868–76.

McClellan, M., B. J. McNeil, and J. P. Newhouse. 1994. "Does More Intensive Treatment of Acute Myocardial Infarction in the Elderly Reduce Mortality? Analysis Using Instrumental Variables." *Journal of the American Medical Association* 272 (11): 859–66.

McClellan, M. B., and J. P. Newhouse. 2000. "Overview of the Special Supplement Issue." *Health Services Research* 35 (5, Part II): 1061–69.

McCullagh, P., and J. A. Nelder. 1989. *Generalized Linear Models,* 2d ed. London: Chapman and Hall.

McDiarmid, M. A., R. Bonanni, and M. Finocchiaro. 1991. "Poor Agreement of Occupational Data Between a Hospital-Based Cancer Registry and Interview." *Journal of Occupational Medicine* 33 (6): 726–29.

McDonald, C. J. 1997. "The Barriers to Electronic Medical Record Systems and How to Overcome them." *Journal of the American Medical Information Association* 4 (3): 213–21.

McDowell, I., and C. Newell. 1987. *Measuring Health: A Guide to Rating Scales and Questionnaires.* New York: Oxford University Press.

McKenney, N. R., and C. E. Bennett. 1994. "Issues Regarding Data on Race and Ethnicity: The Census Bureau Experience." *Public Health Report* 109 (1): 16–25.

McMahon, L. F., Jr., and H. L. Smits. 1986. "Can Medicare Prospective Payment Survive the ICD-9-CM Disease Classification System?" *Annals of Internal Medicine* 104 (4): 562–66.

McNeil, B. J., S. H. Pedersen, and C. Gatsonis. 1992. "Current Issues in Profiling Quality of Care." *Inquiry* 29 (3): 298–307.

Mechanic, D. 1998. "Emerging Trends in Mental Health Policy and Practice." *Health Affairs (Millwood)* 17 (6): 82–98.

———. 2002. "Disadvantage, Inequality, and Social Policy. Major Initiatives Intended to Improve Population Health May Also Increase Health Disparities." *Health Affairs (Millwood)* 21 (2): 48–59.

Medicare Payment Advisory Commission. 1998. *Report to the Congress: Medicare Payment Policy. Volume II: Analytical Papers.* Washington, DC: U.S. Government Printing Office.

————. 2000. *Report to the Congress: Improved Risk Adjustment in Medicare.* Washington, DC: U.S. Government Printing Office.

————. 2001. *Report to the Congress: Medicare Payment Policy.* Washington, DC: U.S. Government Printing Office.

————. 2002a. *Report to the Congress: Medicare Payment Policy.* Washington, DC: U.S. Government Printing Office.

————. 2002b. *Report to the Congress. Applying Quality Improvement Standards in Medicare.* Washington, DC: U.S. Government Printing Office.

————. 2002c. "Report to the Congress: Assessing Medicare Benefits." Washington, DC: U.S. Government Printing Office.

Meenan, R. F. 1986. "New Approaches to Outcome Assessment: The AIMS Questionnaire for Arthritis." *Advances in Internal Medicine* 31: 167–85.

Meistrell, M., and C. Schlehuber. 1996. "Adopting a Corporate Perspective on Databases. Improving Support for Research and Decision Making." *Medical Care* 34 (3, Suppl.): MS91–MS102.

Melton, L. J., III. 1997. "The Threat to Medical-Records Research." *New England Journal of Medicine* 337 (20): 1466–70.

Merrill, B. A. 1994. "A Global Look at Compliance in Health/Safety and Rehabilitation." *Journal of Orthopaedic and Sports Physical Therapy* 19: 242–48.

Mesler, D. E., S. Byrne-Logan, E. P. McCarthy, A. S. Ash, and M. A. Moskowitz. 1999. "How Much Better Can We Predict Dialysis Patient Survival Using Clinical Data?" *Health Services Research* 34 (1, Part II): 365–75.

Messite, J., and S. D. Stellman. 1996. "Accuracy of Death Certificate Completion: The Need for Formalized Physician Training." *Journal of the American Medical Association* 275 (10): 794–96.

Metlay, J. P., R. Schulz, Y. H. Li, D. E. Singer, T. J. Marrie, C. M. Coley, L. J. Hough, D. S. Obrosky, W. N. Kapoor, and M. J. Fine. 1997. "Influence of Age on Symptoms at Presentation in Patients with Community-Acquired Pneumonia." *Archives of Internal Medicine* 157 (13): 1453–59.

Meux, E. 1994. "Encrypting Personal Identifiers." *Health Services Research* 29 (2): 247–56.

Meux, E. F., S. A. Stith, and A. Zach. 1990. "Report of Results from the OSHPD Reabstracting Project: An Evaluation of the Reliability of Selected Patient Discharge Data, July Through December 1988." Sacramento, CA: Office of Statewide Health Planning and Development.

Meyer, A. A., W. J. Messick, P. Young, C. C. Baker, S. Fakhry, F. Muakkassa, E. J. Rutherford, L. M. Napolitano, and R. Rutledge. 1992. "Prospective Comparison of Clinical Judgment and APACHE II Score in Predicting the Outcome in Critically Ill Surgical Patients." *Journal of Trauma* 32 (6): 747–53.

Minkovitz, C. S., P. J. O'Campo, Y. H. Chen, and H. A. Grason. 2002. "Associations Between Maternal and Child Health Status and Patterns of Medical Care Use." *Ambulatory Pediatrics* 2 (2): 85–92.

Mitchell, J. B., T. Bubolz, J. E. Paul, C. L. Pashos, J. J. Escarce, L. H. Muhlbaier, J. M. Wiesman, W. W. Young, R. S. Epstein, and J. C. Javitt. 1994. "Using Medicare Claims for Outcomes Research." *Medical Care* 32 (7, Suppl.): JS38–JS51.

Mitchell, J. B., B. Dickey, B. Liptzin, and L. I. Sederer. 1987. "Bringing Psychiatric Patients into the Medicare Prospective Payment System: Alternatives to DRGs." *American Journal of Psychiatry* 144 (5): 610–15.

Mitka, M. 2001. "Home Modifications to Make Older Living Easier." *Journal of the American Medical Association* 286 (14): 1699–1700.

Montague, T. J., R. M. Ikuta, R. Y. Wong, K. S. Bay, K. K. Teo, and N. J. Davies. 1991. "Comparison of Risk and Patterns of Practice in Patients Older and Younger than 70 Years with Acute Myocardial Infarction in a Two-Year Period (1987–1989)." *American Journal of Cardiology* 68 (9): 843–47.

Mor, V., V. Wilcox, W. Rakowski, and J. Hiris. 1994. "Functional Transitions Among the Elderly: Patterns, Predictors, and Related Hospital Use." *American Journal of Public Health* 84 (8): 1274–80.

Morales, L. S., M. N. Elliott, R. Weech-Maldonado, K. L. Spritzer, and R. D. Hays. 2001. "Differences in CAHPS Adult Survey Reports and Ratings by Race and Ethnicity: An Analysis of the National CAHPS Benchmarking Data 1.0." *Health Services Research* 36 (3): 595–617.

Morgan, R. O., B. A. Virnig, C. A. DeVito, and N. A. Persily. 1997. "The Medicare-HMO Revolving Door—The Healthy Go in and the Sick Go out." *New England Journal of Medicine* 337 (3): 169–75.

Morris, J. 1996. *Pride Against Prejudice. Transforming Attitudes to Disability.* London: The Women's Press.

Morris, J. N., B. E. Fries, and S. A. Morris. 1999. "Scaling ADLs Within the MDS." *Journal of Gerontology: Medical Sciences* 54A (11): M546–M553.

Morris, J. N., C. Hawes, B. E. Fries, C. D. Phillips, V. Mor, S. Katz, K. Murphy, M. L. Drugovich, and A. S. Friedlob. 1990. "Designing the National Resident Assessment Instrument for Nursing Homes." *Gerontologist* 30 (3): 293–307.

Morris, J. N., K. Murphy, and S. Nonemaker. 1995. "Long Term Care Resident Assessment Instrument User's Manual. Version 2.0." Baltimore, MD: Health Care Financing Administration.

Morris, J. N., S. Nonemaker, K. Murphy, C. Hawes, B. E. Fries, V. Mor, and C. Phillips. 1997. "A Commitment to Change: Revision of HCFA's RAI." *Journal of the American Geriatric Society* 45 (8): 1011–16.

Moss, P. 1997. "Negotiating Spaces in Home Environments: Older Women Living with Arthritis." *Social Science and Medicine* 45 (1): 23–33.

Mosteller, F., and J. W. Tukey. 1977. *Data Analysis and Regression: A Second Course in Statistics.* Reading, MA: Addison-Wesley.

Mosteller, F., J. E. Ware, Jr., and S. Levine. 1989. "Finale Panel: Comments on the Conference on Advances in Health Status Assessment." *Medical Care* 27 (3, Suppl.): S282–S294.

Mukamel, D. B. 1997. "Risk-Adjusted Outcome Measures and Quality of Care in Nursing Homes." *Medical Care* 35 (4): 367–85.

Mukamel, D. B., and C. A. Brower. 1998. "The Influence of Risk Adjustment Methods on Conclusions About Quality of Care in Nursing Homes Based on Outcome Measures." *Gerontologist* 38 (6): 695–703.

Muldoon, J. H., J. M. Neff, and J. C. Gay. 1997. "Profiling the Health Service Needs of Populations Using Diagnosis-Based Classification Systems." *Journal of Ambulatory Care Management* 20 (3): 1–18.

Mulley, A.G. 1989. "E. A. Codman and the End Results Idea: A Commentary." *Milbank Quarterly* 67 (2): 257–61.

Mustard, C. A., and N. Frohlich. 1995. "Socioeconomic Status and the Health of the Population." *Medical Care* 33 (12, Suppl.): DS43–DS54.

Nagelkerke, N. J. D. 1991. "A Note on a General Definition of the Coefficient of Determination." *Biometrika* 78 (3): 691–92.

Narrow, W. E., D. S. Rae, L. N. Robins, and D. A. Regier. 2002. "Revised Prevalence Estimates of Mental Disorders in the United States: Using a Clinical Significance Criterion to Reconcile 2 Surveys' Estimates." *Archives of General Psychiatry* 59 (2): 115–23.

National Association of Reimbursement Officers. 2001. "The PsychPPS Project Work Plan Is Released." Alexandria, VA: NARO News.

National Association of State Mental Health Program Directors Research Institute. 2002. *Implementation of the NASMHPD Framework of Mental Health Performance Measures by States to Measure Community Performance: 2001.* Alexandria, VA: National Association of State Mental Health Program Directors Research Institute.

National Cancer Institute. 2002a. "About SEER. Website: National Cancer Institute. About SEER." [Online information; retrieved 3/14/02.] seer.cancer.gov/AboutSEER.html.

National Cancer Institute, Applied Research Program. 2002b. "SEER-Medicare Database." [Online information; retrieved 3/14/02.] healthservices.cancer.gov/SEERMed/seermedicare.html.

National Committee on Vital and Health Statistics. 1980. "Uniform Hospital Discharge Data Minimum Data Set." DHWQ Publication No. (PHS) 80–1157. Hyattsville, MD: U.S. DHEW.

National Committee on Vital and Health Statistics, Subcommittee on Ambulatory and Hospital Care Statistics. 1992. "Proposed Revision to the Uniform Hospital Discharge Data Set." Washington, DC: National Committee on Vital and Health Statistics.

National Health Service Information Authority. 1998. "Information and IT for the NHS: Information Strategy and Development." [Online information; retrieved 04/08/2003.] http://www.doh.gov.uk/ipu/develop/index.htm.

———. 2002. "Frequently Asked Questions (FAQs). Purpose of SNOMED Clinical Terms and Clinical Terminologies in General." [Online information; retrieved 8/7/02.] http://www.nhsia.nhs.uk/terms/pages/snomedct/sno_faqp1.asp.

National Public Radio. 2002. "NPR/Kaiser/Kennedy School Poll on Health Care." [Online article; retrieved 6/6/02.] http://www.npr.org/news/specials/healthcarepoll/index.html.

Naylor, C. D. 2002. "Public Profiling of Clinical Performance." *Journal of the American Medical Association* 287 (10): 1323–25.

Nelson, E., B. Conger, R. Douglass, D. Gephart, J. Kirk, R. Page, A. Clark, K. Johnson, K. Stone, J. Wasson, and M. Zubkoff. 1983. "Functional Health Status Levels of Primary Care Patients." *Journal of the American Medical Association* 249 (24): 3331–38.

Nerenz, D. R. 1996. "Who Has the Responsibility for a Population's Health?" *Milbank Quarterly* 74: 43–49.

Neter, J., and W. Wasserman. 1974. *Applied Linear Statistical Models: Regression, Analysis of Variance, and Experimental Design*. Homewood, IL: R. D. Irwin.

Neter, J., W. Wasserman, and M. H. Kutner. 1990. *Applied Linear Statistical Models: Regression, Analysis of Variance, and Experimental Design*. 3d ed. Homewood, IL: R. D. Irwin.

Neuhauser, D. 1990. "Ernest Amory Codman, M.D., and End Results of Medical Care." *International Journal of Technology Assessment in Health Care* 6 (2): 307–25.

Newby, L. K., A. Kristinsson, M. V. Bhapkar, P. E. Aylward, A. P. Dimas, W. W. Klein, D. K. McGuire, D. J. Moliterno, F. W. Verheugt, W. D. Weaver, and R. M. Califf. 2002. "Early Statin Initiation and Outcomes in Patients with Acute Coronary Syndromes." *Journal of the American Medical Association* 287 (23): 3087–95.

Newhouse, J. P. 1994. "Patients at Risk: Health Reform and Risk Adjustment." *Health Affairs (Millwood)* 13 (1): 132–46.

———. 1998. "Risk Adjustment: Where Are We Now?" *Inquiry* 35 (2): 122–31.

Newhouse, J. P., and M. McClellan. 1998. "Econometrics in Outcomes Research: The Use of Instrumental Variables." *Annual Review of Public Health* 19: 17–34.

Ngo-Metzger, Q., M. P. Maasagli, B. R. Clarridge, M. Manocchia, R. B. Davis, L. I. Iezzoni, and R. S. Phillips. 2003. "Linguistic and Cultural Barriers to Care." *Journal of General Internal Medicine* 18 (1): 44–52.

Nightingale, F. 1863. *Notes on Hospitals*. 3d ed. London: Longman, Green, Longman, Roberts, and Green.

Normand, S. N. L. T., M. E. Glickman, and C. A. Gatsonis. 1997. "Statistical Methods for Profiling Providers of Medical Care: Issues and Applications." *Journal of the American Statistical Association* 92: 803–14.

Normand, S. L. T., M. E. Glickman, and T. J. Ryan. 1996. "Modeling Mortality Rates for Elderly Heart Attack Patients: Profiling Hospitals in the Cooperative Cardiovascular Project." In *Case Studies in Bayesian Statistics. Volume 3*. New York: Springer.

Normand, S. T., M. E. Glickman, R. G. Sharma, and B. J. McNeil. 1996. "Using Admission Characteristics to Predict Short-Term Mortality from Myocardial Infarction in Elderly Patients. Results from the Cooperative Cardiovascular Project." *Journal of the American Medical Association* 275 (17): 1322–28.

O'Connor, G. T., J. R. Morton, M. J. Diehl, E. M. Olmstead, L. H. Coffin, D. G. Levy, C. T. Maloney, S. K. Plume, W. Nugent, and D. J. Malenka. 1993. "Differences Between Men and Women in Hospital Mortality Associated with Coronary Artery Bypass Graft Surgery. The Northern New England Cardio-vascular Disease Study Group." *Circulation* 88 (5, Part I): 2104–10.

Oczkowski, W. J., and S. Barreca. 1993. "The Functional Independence Measure: Its use to Identify Rehabilitation Needs in Stroke Survivors." *Archives of Physical Medicine and Rehabilitation* 74 (1): 1291–94.

Office of Management and Budget, The Executive Office of the President. 2002. "Revisions to the Standards for the Collection of Federal Data on Race and Ethnicity." [Online information; retrieved 8/9/02.] http://www.whitehouse.gov/omb/fedreg/ombdir15.html.

Office of Quality and Performance. 1999. "Department of Veternans Affairs National

Mental Health Program Performance Monitoring System: Fiscal Year 1999 Report." West Haven, CT: VA.

Office of Technology Assessment, U.S. Congress. 1994. "Identifying Health Technologies that Work: Searching for Evidence." OTA-H-608. Washington, DC: U.S. Government Printing Office.

O'Gara, S. 1990. "Data Sets and Coding Guidelines: Sequencing vs. Classification Rules." *Journal of the American Medical Records Association* 61 (2): 20–21.

Okin, R. L. 1985. "Variation Among State Hospitals in Use of Seclusion and Restraint." *Hospital and Community Psychiatry* 36 (6): 648–52.

O'Leary, D. S. 1993. "The Measurement Mandate: Report Card Day Is Coming." *Joint Commission Journal on Quality Improvement* 19 (11): 487–91.

Oliver, M. 1996. *Understanding Disability: From Theory to Practice.* New York: St. Martin's Press.

Osswald, B. R., E. H. Blackstone, U. Tochtermann, P. Schweiger, G. Thomas, C. F. Vahl, and S. Hagl. 2001. "Does the Completeness of Revascularization Affect Early Survival After Coronary Artery Bypass Grafting in Elderly Patients?" *European Journal of Cardiothoracic Surgery* 20 (1): 120–25.

Otten, M. W., S. M. Teutsch, D. F. Williamson, and J. S. Marks. 1990. "The Effect of Known Risk Factors on the Excess Mortality of Black Adults in the United States." *Journal of the American Medical Association* 263 (6): 845–50.

Owens, P. L., E. H. Bradley, S. M. Horwitz, C. M. Viscoli, W. N. Kernan, L. M. Brass, P. M. Sarrel, and R. I. Horwitz. 2002. "Clinical Assessment of Function Among Women with a Recent Cerebrovascular Event: A Self-Reported Versus Performance-Based Measure." *Annals of Internal Medicine* 136 (11): 802–11.

Pandiani, J. A., S. M. Banks, and L. M. Schacht. 1998. "Using Incarceration Rates to Measure Mental Health Program Performance." *Journal of Behavioral Health Services & Research* 25 (3): 300–11.

Panju, A. A., B. R. Hemmelgarn, G. H. Guyatt, and D. L. Simel. 1998. "The Rational Clinical Examination. Is this Patient Having a Myocardial Infarction?" *Journal of the American Medical Association* 280 (14): 1256–63.

Park, R. E., R. H. Brook, J. Kosecoff, J. Keesey, L. Rubenstein, E. Keeler, K. L. Kahn, W. H. Rogers, and M. R. Chassin. 1990. "Explaining Variations in Hospital Death Rates. Randomness, Severity of Illness, Quality of Care." *Journal of the American Medical Association* 264 (4): 484–90.

Parsons, J. A., S. Baum, and T. P. Johnson. 2000. "Inclusion of Disabled Populations in Social Surveys: Review and Recommendations." Chicago: Survey Research Laboratory, College of Urban Planning and Public Affairs, University of Illinois at Chicago.

Patrician, P. A. 2002. "Multiple Imputation for Missing Data." *Research in Nursing and Health* 25 (1): 76–84.

Patrick, D. L., and R. A. Deyo. 1989. "Generic and Disease-Specific Measures in Assessing Health Status and Quality of Life." *Medical Care* 27 (3, Suppl.): S217–S232.

Payne, S. M., R. D. Cebul, M. E. Singer, J. Krishnaswamy, and K. Gharrity. 2000. "Comparison of Risk-Adjustment Systems for the Medicaid-Eligible Disabled Population." *Medical Care* 38 (4): 422–32.

Payne, T. H., G. R. Murphy, and A. A. Salazar. 1992. "How Well Does ICD9 Represent Phrases Used in the Medical Record Problem List?" *Proceedings of the Annual Symposium for Computer Applications to Medical Care*: 654–57.

Pear, R. 2002. "Medicare Is Now Covering Treatment for Alzheimer's." *The New York Times,* 31 March, A1.

Pearl, R. 1921. "Modern Methods in Handling Hospital Statistics." *Bulletin of the Johns Hopkins Hospital* 32 (364): 184–94.

Pearson, G. A., J. Stickley, and F. Shann. 2001. "Calibration of the Paediatric Index of Mortality in UK Paediatric Intensive Care Units." *Archives of Disease in Children* 84 (2): 125–28.

Pelka, F. 1997. *The ABC-CLIO Companion to the Disability Rights Movement.* Santa Barbara, CA: ABC-CLIO.

Pennsylvania Health Care Cost Containment Council (PHC4). 1996. "Focus on Heart Attack in Western Pennsylvania." Harrisburg, PA: Pennsylvania Health Care Cost Containment Council.

Perls, T. 2002. "Genetic and Environmental Influences on Exceptional Longevity and the AGE Nomogram." *Annals of the New York Academy of Science* 959: 1–13.

Perls, T. T., J. Wilmoth, R. Levenson, M. Drinkwater, M. Cohen, H. Bogan, E. Joyce, S. Brewster, L. Kunkel, and A. Puca. 2002. "Life-Long Sustained Mortality Advantage of Siblings of Centenarians." *Proceedings of the National Academy of Science U S A* 99 (12): 8442–47.

Perrin, J. M., S. L. Ettner, T. J. McLaughlin, S. L. Gortmaker, S. R. Bloom, and K. Kuhlthau. 1998b. "State Variations in Supplemental Security Income Enrollment for Children and Adolescents." *American Journal of Public Health* 88 (6): 928–31.

Perrin, J. M., C. J. Homer, D. M. Berwick, A. D. Woolf, J. L. Freeman, and J. E. Wennberg. 1989. "Variations in Rates of Hospitalization of Children in Three Urban Communities." *New England Journal of Medicine* 320 (18): 1183–87.

Perrin, J. M., K. Kuhlthau, S. L. Ettner, T. J. McLaughlin, and S. L. Gortmaker. 1998a. "Previous Medicaid Status of Children Newly Enrolled in Supplemental Security Income." *Health Care Financing Review* 19: 117–27.

Perrin, J. M., K. A. Kuhlthau, S. L. Gortmaker, A. C. Beal, and T. G. Ferris. 2002. "Generalist and Subspecialist Care for Children with Chronic Conditions." *Ambulatory Pediatrics* 2 (6): 462–69.

Perrin, J. M., K. Kuhlthau, T. J. McLaughlin, S. L. Ettner, and S. L. Gortmaker. 1999. "Changing Patterns of Conditions Among Children Receiving Supplemental Security Income Disability Benefits." *Archives of Pediatric and Adolescent Medicine* 153 (1): 80–84.

Petersen, L. A. 2002. "Racial Differences in Trust: Reaping What We Have Sown?" *Medical Care* 40 (2): 81–84.

Petersen, L. A., S. M. Wright, E. D. Peterson, and J. Daley. 2002. "Impact of Race on Cardiac Care and Outcomes in Veterans with Acute Myocardial Infarction." *Medical Care* 40 (1, Suppl.): 86–96.

Peterson, E. D., S. M. Wright, J. Daley, and G. E. Thibault. 1994. "Racial Variation in Cardiac Procedure Use and Survival Following Acute Myocardial Infarction in the Department of Veterans Affairs." *Journal of the American Medical Association* 271 (15): 1175–80.

Petitti, D. B. 1998. "Hormone Replacement Therapy and Heart Disease Prevention:

Experimentation Trumps Observation." *Journal of the American Medical Association* 280 (7): 650–52.

Pham, A. 1996a. "3 HMOs Win Top Marks in Survey." *Boston Globe,* 22 Oct., C1, C5.

———. 1996b. "Insurer Rejects Rating." *Boston Globe,* 18 Oct., C1, C3.

Phibbs, C. S., J. M. Bronstein, E. Buxton, and R. H. Phibbs. 1996. "The Effects of Patient Volume and Level of Care at the Hospital of Birth on Neonatal Mortality." *Journal of the American Medical Association* 276 (13): 1054–59.

Phillips, R. S., M. B. Hamel, J. M. Teno, P. Bellamy, S. K. Broste, R. M. Califf, H. Vidaillet, R. B. Davis, L. H. Muhlbaier, and A. F. Connors, Jr. 1996. "Race, Resource Use, and Survival in Seriously Ill Hospitalized Adults. The SUPPORT Investigators." *Journal of General Internal Medicine* 11 (7): 387–96.

Picard, R. R., and K. N. Berk. 1990. "Data Splitting." *The American Statistician* 40 (2): 140–47.

Pincus, T., and L. F. Callahan. 1985. "Formal Education as a Marker for Increased Mortality and Morbidity in Rheumatoid Arthritis." *Journal of Chronic Disease* 38 (12): 973–84.

Pine, M., B. Jones, and Y. B. Lou. 1998. "Laboratory Values Improve Predictions of Hospital Mortality." *International Journal for Quality in Health Care* 10 (6): 491–501.

Pinker, R. 1966. *English Hospital Statistics 1861–1938.* London: Heinemann Educational Books.

Pollack, M. M., T. T. Cuerdon, K. M. Patel, U. E. Ruttimann, P. R. Getson, and M. Levetown. 1994. "Impact of Quality-of-Care Factors on Pediatric Intensive Care Unit Mortality." *Journal of the American Medical Association* 272 (12): 941–46.

Pollack, M. M., M. A. Koch, D. A. Bartel, I. Rapoport, R. Dhanireddy, A. A. El-Mohandes, K. Harkavy, and K. N. Subramanian. 2000. "A Comparison of Neonatal Mortality Risk Prediction Models in Very Low Birth Weight Infants." *Pediatrics* 105 (5): 1051–57.

Pollack, M. M., K. M. Patel, and U. E. Ruttimann. 1996. "PRISM III: An Updated Pediatric Risk of Mortality Score." *Critical Care Medicine* 24 (5): 743–52.

———. 1997. "The Pediatric Risk of Mortality III—Acute Physiology Score (PRISM III-APS): A Method of Assessing Physiologic Instability for Pediatric Intensive Care Unit Patients." *Journal of Pediatrics* 131 (4): 575–81.

Pollack, M. M., U. E. Ruttimann, and P. R. Getson. 1987. "Accurate Prediction of the Outcome of Pediatric Intensive Care. A New Quantitative Method." *New England Journal of Medicine* 316 (3): 134–39.

———. 1988. "Pediatric Risk of Mortality (PRISM) Score." *Critical Care Medicine* 16 (11): 1110–16.

Pope, A. M., and A. R. Tarlov. 1991. *Disability in America: Toward a National Agenda for Prevention.* Washington, DC: National Academy Press, Institute of Medicine.

Pope, G. C., K. W. Adamache, E. G. Walsh, and R. K. Khander. 1998. "Evaluating Alternative Risk Adjusters for Medicare." *Health Care Financing Review* 20 (2): 109–29.

Pope, G. C., R. P. Ellis, A. S. Ash, J. Z. Ayanian, D. W. Bates, H. Burstin, L. I. Iezzoni, E. Marcantonio, and B. Wu. 2000b. "Diagnostic Cost Group Hierarchical Condition Category Models for Medicare Risk Adjustment." Final Report. Prepared for the Health Care Financing Administration Under Contract No. 500–95-048. Waltham, MA: Health Economics Research.

Pope, G. C., R. P. Ellis, A. S. Ash, C. F. Liu, J. Z. Ayanian, D. W. Bates, H. Burstin, L. I. Iezzoni, and M. J. Ingber. 2000a. "Principal Inpatient Diagnostic Cost Group Model for Medicare Risk Adjustment." *Health Care Financing Review* 21 (3): 93–118.

Porath, A., N. Eldar, I. Harman-Bohem, and G. Gurman. 1994. "Evaluation of the APACHE II Scoring System in an Israeli Intensive Care Unit." *Israeli Journal of Medical Science* 30 (7): 514–20.

Porell, F., and F. G. Caro. 1998. "Facility-Level Outcome Performance Measures for Nursing Homes." *Gerontologist* 38 (6): 665–83.

Porell, F., F. G. Caro, A. Silva, and M. Monane. 1998. "A Longitudinal Analysis of Nursing Home Outcomes." *Health Services Research* 33 (4, Part I): 835–65.

Poses, R. M., D. K. McClish, W. R. Smith, C. Bekes, and W. E. Scott. 1996. "Prediction of Survival of Critically Ill Patients by Admission Comorbidity." *Journal of Clinical Epidemiology* 49 (7): 743–47.

Poses, R. M., D. K. McClish, W. R. Smith, E. C. Huber, F. L. Clemo, B. P. Schmitt, D. Alexander, E. M. Racht, and C. C. Colenda, III. 2000. "Results of Report Cards for Patients with Congestive Heart Failure Depend on the Method Used to Adjust for Severity." *Annals of Internal Medicine* 133 (1): 10–20.

Potosky, A. L., R. M. Merrill, G. F. Riley, S. H. Taplin, W. Barlow, B. H. Fireman, and R. Ballard-Barbash. 1997. "Breast Cancer Survival and Treatment in Health Maintenance Organization and Fee-for-Service Settings." *Journal of the National Cancer Institute* 89 (22): 1683–91.

Potosky, A. L., R. M. Merrill, G. F. Riley, S. H. Taplin, W. Barlow, B. H. Fireman, and J. D. Lubitz. 1999. "Prostate Cancer Treatment and Ten-Year Survival Among Group/Staff HMO and Fee-for-Service Medicare Patients." *Health Services Research* 34 (2): 525–46.

Potosky, A. L., G. F. Riley, J. D. Lubitz, R. M. Mentnech, and L. G. Kessler. 1993. "Potential for Cancer Related Health Services Research Using a Linked Medicare-Tumor Registry Database." *Medical Care* 31: 732–48.

Potosky, A. L., J. L. Warren, E. R. Riedel, C. N. Klabunde, C. C. Earle, and C. B. Begg. 2002. "Measuring Complications of Cancer Treatment Using the SEER-Medicare Data." *Medical Care* 40 (8, Suppl.): IV-62–IV-68.

Pritchard, R. S., E. S. Fisher, J. M. Teno, S. M. Sharp, D. J. Reding, W. A. Knaus, J. E. Wennberg, and J. Lynn. 1998. "Influence of Patient Preferences and Local Health System Characteristics on the Place of Death. SUPPORT Investigators. Study to Understand Prognoses and Preferences for Risks and Outcomes of Treatment." *Journal of the American Geriatrics Society* 46 (10): 1242–50.

Prospective Payment Assessment Commission. 1996. "Report to the Congress. Medicare and the American Health Care System." Washington, DC: ProPAC.

Provost, C., and P. Hughes. 2000. "35 Years of Service." *Health Care Financing Review* 22 (1): 141–74.

Quan, H., G. A. Parsons, and W. A. Ghali. 2002. "Validity of Information on Comorbidity Derived from ICD-9-CM Administrative Data." *Medical Care* 40 (8): 675–85.

Ramasubbu, K., H. Gurm, and D. Litaker. 2001. "Gender Bias in Clinical Trials: Do Double Standards Still Apply?" *Journal of Women's Health and Gender Based Medicine* 10 (8): 757–64.

Ramsey, G. A., and R. C. Kingswood. 1923. "Case Records." *Bulletin of American College of Surgeons* 7: 22–24.

Rathore, S. S., Y. Wang, M. J. Radford, D. L. Ordin, and H. M. Krumholz. 2002. "Sex Differences in Cardiac Catheterization After Acute Myocardial Infarction: The Role of Procedure Appropriateness." *Annals of Internal Medicine* 137 (6): 487–93.

Rattner, S. L., D. Z. Louis, C. Rabinowitz, J. E. Gottlieb, T. J. Nasca, F. W. Markham, R. P. Gottlieb, J. W. Caruso, J. L. Lane, J. Veloski, M. Hojat, and J. S. Gonnella. 2001. "Documenting and Comparing Medical Students' Clinical Experiences." *Journal of the American Medical Association* 286 (9): 1035–40.

Ray, W. A. 2000. "Improving Quality of Long-Term Care. *Medical Care* 38 (12): 1151–53.

Ray, W. A., and M. R. Griffin. 1989. "Use of Medicaid Data for Pharmacoepidemiology." *American Journal of Epidemiology* 129 (4): 837–49.

Raymond, B., and C. Dold. 2002. "Clinical Information Systems: Achieving the Vision." Oakland, CA: Kaiser Permanente Institute for Health Policy.

Reid, B. 1991. "The Impact of Different Coding Systems on DRG Assignment and Data." *Health Policy* 17 (2): 133–49.

Reker, D. M., J. C. O'Donnell, and B. B. Hamilton. 1998. "Stroke Rehabilitation Outcome Variation in Veterans Affairs Rehabilitation Units: Accounting for Case-Mix." *Archives of Physical Medicine and Rehabilitation* 35: 235–43.

Ren, X. S., B. C. Amick, and D. R. Williams. 1999. "Racial/Ethnic Disparities in Health: The Interplay Between Discrimination and Socioeconomic Status." *Ethnicity and Disease* 9 (2): 151–65.

Research Data Assistance Center. 2002. [Online information; retrieved 1/10/02.] http://www.resdac.umn.edu/medicaid.htm.

Rice, N., and P. C. Smith. 2001. "Capitation and Risk Adjustment in Health Care Financing: An International Progress Report." *Milbank Quarterly* 79 (1): 81–113.

Richardson, D. K., J. D. Corcoran, G. J. Escobar, and S. K. Lee. 2001. "SNAP-II and SNAPPE-II: Simplified Newborn Illness Severity and Mortality Risk Scores." *Journal of Pediatrics* 138 (1): 92–100.

Richardson, D. K., J. E. Gray, M. C. McCormick, K. Workman, and D. A. Goldmann. 1993a. "Score for Neonatal Acute Physiology: A Physiologic Severity Index for Neonatal Intensive Care." *Pediatrics* 91 (3): 617–23.

Richardson, D. K., C. S. Phibbs, J. E. Gray, M. C. McCormick, K. Workman-Daniels, and D. A. Goldmann. 1993b. "Birth Weight and Illness Severity: Independent Predictors of Neonatal Mortality." *Pediatrics* 91 (5): 969–75.

Richardson, D. K., B. L. Shah, I. D. Frantz, III, F. Bednarek, L. P. Rubin, and M. C. McCormick. 1999. "Perinatal Risk and Severity of Illness in Newborns at 6 Neonatal Intensive Care Units." *American Journal of Public Health* 89 (4): 511–16.

Richardson, D. K., W. O. Tarnow-Mordi, and G. J. Escobar. 1998. "Neonatal Risk Scoring Systems. Can they Predict Mortality and Morbidity?" *Clinical Perinatology* 25 (3): 591–611.

Richardson, D., W. O. Tarnow-Mordi, and S. K. Lee. 1999. "Risk Adjustment for Quality Improvement." *Pediatrics* 103 (1, Suppl. E): 255–65.

Riley, G. F. 2000. "Risk Adjustment for Health Plans Disproportionately Enrolling Frail Medicare Beneficiaries." *Health Care Financing Review* 21 (3): 135–48.

Riley, G. F., A. L. Potosky, C. N. Klabunde, J. L. Warren, and R. Ballard-Barbash. 1999. "Stage at Diagnosis and Treatment Patterns Among Older Women with Breast Cancer: An HMO and Fee-for-Service Comparison." *Journal of the American Medical Association* 281 (8): 720–26.

Riley, G. F., A. L. Potosky, J. D. Lubitz, and M. L. Brown. 1994. "Stage of Cancer at Diagnosis for Medicare HMO and Fee-for-Service Enrollees." *American Journal of Public Health* 84 (10): 1598–1604.

Riley, G. F., A. L. Potosky, J. D. Lubitz, and L. G. Kessler. 1995. "Medicare Payments from Diagnosis to Death for Elderly Cancer Patients by Stage at Diagnosis." *Medical Care* 33 (8): 828–41.

Riley, G., C. Tudor, Y. P. Chiang, and M. Ingber. 1996. "Health Status of Medicare Enrollees in HMOs and Fee-for-Service in 1994." *Health Care Financing Review* 17 (4): 65–76.

Ripley, B. D., and W. N. Venable. 1994. *Modern Applied Statistics with S-Plus.* New York: Springer.

Roberts, R. O., E. J. Bergstrahl, L. Schmidt, and S. J. Jacobsen. 1996. "Comparison of Self-Reported and Medical Record Health Care Utilization Measures." *Journal of Clinical Epidemiology* 49 (9): 989–95.

Robinson, J., and S. L. Karon. 2000. "Modeling Costs of PACE Populations." *Health Care Financing Review* 21: 149–70.

Robinson, J. C. 1999. *The Corporate Practice of Medicine: Competition and Innovation in Health Care.* Berkeley, CA: University of California Press.

Roblin, D. W. 1998. "Physician Profiling Using Outpatient Pharmacy Data as a Source for Case Mix Measurement and Risk Adjustment." *Journal of Ambulatory Care Management* 21 (4): 68–84.

Roblin, D. W., D. K. Richardson, E. Thomas, F. Fitzgerald, R. Veintimilla, P. Hulac, G. Bemis, and L. Leon. 2000. "Variation in the Use of Alternative Levels of Hospital Care for Newborns in a Managed Care Organization." *Health Services Research* 34 (7): 1535–53.

Rockow, K. 2001. *Working with Deaf and Hard of Hearing Patients. A Guide for Medical Professionals.* Allston, MA: D.E.A.F, Inc.

Roetzheim, R. G., and T. N. Chirikos. 2002. "Breast Cancer Detection and Outcomes in a Disability Beneficiary Population." *Journal of Health Care for the Poor and Underserved* 13 (4): 461–476.

Rogers, G., and D. P. Smith. 1999. "Reporting Comparative Results from Hospital Patient Surveys." *International Journal for Quality in Health Care* 11 (3): 251–59.

Rogers, M. Y. 1999. "Getting Started with Geographic Information Systems (GIS): A Local Health Department Perspective." *Journal of Public Health Management and Practice* 5 (4): 22–33.

Romano, P. S. 2000. "Should Health Plan Quality Measures Be Adjusted for Case Mix?" *Medical Care* 38 (10): 977–80.

Romano, P. S., and B. K. Chan. 2000. "Risk-Adjusting Acute Myocardial Infarction Mortality: Are APR-DRGs the Right Tool?" *Health Services Research* 34 (7): 1469–89.

Romano, P. S., B. K. Chan, M. E. Schembri, and J. A. Rainwater. 2002. "Can Administrative Data Be Used to Compare Postoperative Complication Rates Across Hospitals?" *Medical Care* 40 (10): 856–76.

Romano, P., and H. S. Luft. 1992. "Getting the Most out of Messy Data: Problems and Approaches for Dealing with Large Administrative Data Sets." In *Medical Effectiveness Research Data Methods,* edited by M. L. Grady and H. A. Schwartz, 57–75. AHCPR Publication No. 92–0056. Rockville, MD: Agency for Health Care Policy and Research.

Romano, P. S., H. S. Luft, J. A. Rainwater, and A. P. Zach. 1997. "Report on Heart Attack 1991–1993. Volume Two: Technical Guide." Sacramento, CA: California Office of Statewide Health Planning and Development.

Romano, P. S., and D. H. Mark. 1994. "Bias in the Coding of Hospital Discharge Data and Its Implications for Quality Assessment." *Medical Care* 32: 81–90.

Romano, P. S., L. L. Roos, and J. G. Jollis. 1993. "Adapting a Clinical Comorbidity Index for Use with ICD-9-CM Administrative Data: Differing Perspectives." *Journal of Clinical Epidemiology* 46 (10): 1075–79.

Romano, P. S., M. E. Schembri, and J. A. Rainwater. 2002. "Can Administrative Data Be Used to Ascertain Clinically Significant Postoperative Complications?" *American Journal of Medical Quality* 17 (4): 145–54.

Romm, F. J., and S. M. Putnam. 1981. "The Validity of the Medical Record." *Medical Care* 19 (3): 310–15.

Roos, L. L., R. Walld, A. Wajda, R. Bond, and K. Hartford. 1996. "Record Linkage Strategies, Outpatient Procedures, and Administrative Data." *Medical Care* 34 (6): 570–82.

Roos, L. L., Jr., J. P. Nicol, and S. M. Cageorge. 1987. "Using Administrative Data for Longitudinal Research: Comparisons with Primary Data Collection." *Journal of Chronic Disease* 40 (1): 41–49.

Roos, N. P., C. D. Black, N. Frohlich, C. Decoster, M. M. Cohen, D. J. Tataryn, C. A. Mustard, F. Toll, K. C. Carriere, C. A. Burchill, L. MacWilliam, and B. Bogdanovic. 1995. "A Population-Based Health Information System." *Medical Care* 33 (12, Suppl.): DS13–DS20.

Roos, N. P., and E. Shapiro. 1995a. "A Productive Experiment with Administrative Data." *Medical Care* 33 (12, Suppl.): DS7–DS12.

———. 1995b. "Using the Information System to Assess Change: The Impact of Downsizing the Acute Sector." *Medical Care* 33 (12, Suppl.): DS109–DS126.

Roos, N. P., J. E. Wennberg, and K. McPherson. 1988. "Using Diagnosis-Related Groups for Studying Variations in Hospital Admissions." *Health Care Financing Review* 9 (4): 53–62.

Rose, J. H., E. E. O'Toole, N. V. Dawson, C. Thomas, A. F. Connors, Jr., N. S. Wenger, R. S. Phillips, M. B. Hamel, H. J. Cohen, and J. Lynn. 2000. "Age Differences in Care Practices and Outcomes for Hospitalized Patients with Cancer." *Journal of the American Geriatric Society* 48 (5, Suppl.): S25–S32.

Rosen, A. K., A. S. Ash, J. M. Geraci, E. P. McCarthy, and M. A. Moskowitz. 1995. "Postoperative Adverse Events of Cholecystectomy in the Medicare Population." *American Journal of Medical Quality* 10 (1): 29–37.

Rosen, A. K., D. R. Berlowitz, J. J. Anderson, A. S. Ash, L. E. Kazis, and M. A. Moskowitz. 1999. "Functional Status Outcomes for Assessment of Quality in Long-Term Care." *International Journal for Quality in Health Care* 11 (1): 37–46.

Rosen, A. K., J. M. Geraci, A. S. Ash, K. J. McNiff, and M. A. Moskowitz. 1992. "Postoperative Adverse Events of Common Surgical Procedures in the Medicare Population." *Medical Care* 30 (9): 753–65.

Rosen, A. K., R. L. Houchens, T. B. Gibson, and A. Mayer-Oakes. 1998. "Developing Episodes of Care for Adult Asthma Patients: A Cautionary Tale." *American Journal of Medical Quality* 13 (1): 25–35.

Rosen, A. K., S. Loveland, J. J. Anderson, J. A. Rothendler, C. S. Hankin, C. C. Rakovski, M. A. Moskowitz, and D. R. Berlowitz. 2001a. "Evaluating Diagnosis-Based Case-Mix Measures: How Well Do they Apply to the VA Population?" *Medical Care* 39 (7): 692–704.

Rosen, A. K., S. A. Loveland, J. J. Anderson, C. S. Hankin, J. N. Breckenridge, and D. R. Berlowitz. 2002. "Diagnostic Cost Groups (DCGs) and Concurrent Utilization Among Patients with Substance Abuse Disorders." *Health Services Research* 37 (4): 1079–1102.

Rosen, A. K., and A. Mayer-Oakes. 1998. "Developing a Tool for Analyzing Medical Care Utilization of Adult Asthma Patients in Indemnity and Managed Care Plans: Can an Episodes of Care Framework Be Used?" *American Journal of Medical Quality* 13 (4): 203–12.

———. 1999. "Episodes of Care: Theoretical Frameworks Versus Current Operational Realities." *Joint Commission Journal on Quality Improvement* 25 (3): 111–28.

Rosen, A., J. Wu, B. H. Chang, D. Berlowitz, A. Ash, and M. Moskowitz. 2000. "Does Diagnostic Information Contribute to Predicting Functional Decline in Long-Term Care?" *Medical Care* 38 (6): 647–59.

Rosen, A., J. Wu, B. H. Chang, D. Berlowitz, C. Rakovski, A. Ash, and M. Moskowitz. 2001b. "Risk Adjustment for Measuring Health Outcomes: An Application in VA Long-Term Care." *American Journal of Medical Quality* 16 (4): 118–27.

Rosenbach, M. L. 1995. "Access and Satisfaction Within the Disabled Medicare Population." *Health Care Financing Review* 17 (2): 147–67.

Rosenbaum, P. 1989. "Optimal Matching in Observational Studies." *Journal of the American Statistical Association* 84: 1024–32.

Rosenbaum, P. R., and D. B. Rubin. 1983. "The Central Role of the Propensity Score in Observational Studies of Casual Effect." *Biometrika* 76: 41–55.

———. 1984. "Reducing Bias in Observational Studies Using Subclassification on the Propensity Score." *Journal of the American Statistical Association* 79: 516–24.

———. 1985. "Constructing a Control Group Using Multivariate Matched Sampling Methods that Incorporate the Propensity Score." *The American Statistician* 39: 33–38.

Rosenblatt, A., and C. C. Attkisson. 1993. "Assessing Outcomes for Sufferers of Severe Mental Disorder: A Conceptual Framework and Review." *Evaluation and Program Planning* 16 (4): 347–63.

Rosenkranz, S. L., and H. S. Luft. 1997. "Expenditure Models for Prospective Risk Adjustment: Choosing the Measure Appropriate for the Problem." *Medical Care Research and Review* 54 (2): 123–43.

Ross, C. E., and C. L. Wu. 1996. "Education, Age, and the Cumulative Advantage in Health." *Journal of Health and Social Behavior* 37 (1): 104–20.

Rowan, K. M., J. H. Kerr, E. Major, K. McPherson, A. Short, and M. P. Vessey. 1993. "Intensive Care Society's APACHE II Study in Britain and Ireland—II: Outcome Comparisons of Intensive Care Units After Adjustment for Case Mix by the American APACHE II Method." *British Medical Journal* 307 (6910): 977–81.

———. 1994. "Intensive Care Society's Acute Physiology and Chronic Health Evaluation (APACHE II) Study in Britain and Ireland: A Prospective, Multicenter, Cohort Study Comparing Two Methods for Predicting Outcome for Adult Intensive Care Patients." *Critical Care Medicine* 22 (9): 1392–1401.

Rubenstein, L. V., D. R. Calkins, S. Greenfield, A. M. Jette, R. F. Meenan, M. A. Nevins, L. Z. Rubenstein, J. H. Wasson, and M. E. Williams. 1989. "Health Status Assessment for Elderly Patients. Report of the Society of General Internal Medicine Task Force on Health Assessment." *Journal of the American Geriatric Society* 37 (6): 562–69.

Ruberman, W., E. Weinblatt, J. D. Goldberg, and B. S. Chaudhary. 1984. "Psychosocial Influences on Mortality After Myocardial Infarction." *New England Journal of Medicine* 311 (9): 552–59.

Rubin, D. B. 1974. "Estimating Causal Effects of Treatments in Randomized and Nonrandomized Studies." *Journal of Educational Psychology* 66: 688–701.

———. 1977. "Assignment to Treatment Group on the Basis of a Covariate." *Journal of Educational Statistics* 2: 1–26.

———. 1978. "Bayesian Inference for Causal Effects: The Role of Randomization." *Annals of Statistics* 7: 34–58.

———. 1987. *Multiple Imputation for Nonresponse in Surveys.* New York: John Wiley & Sons.

———. 1997. "Estimating Causal Effects from Large Data Sets Using Propensity Scores." *Annals of Internal Medicine* 127 (8, Part II): 757–63.

Rubin, D. B., and N. Thomas. 1996. "Matching Using Estimated Propensity Scores: Relating Theory to Practice." *Biometrics* 52 (1): 249–64.

Rutledge, R., S. Fakhry, E. Rutherford, F. Muakkassa, and A. Meyer. 1993. "Comparison of APACHE II, Trauma Score, and Injury Severity Score as Predictors of Outcome in Critically Injured Trauma Patients." *American Journal of Surgery* 166 (3): 244–47.

Ruttimann, U. E., M. M. Pollack, and D. H. Fiser. 1996. "Prediction of Three Outcome States from Pediatric Intensive Care." *Critical Care Medicine* 24 (1): 78–85.

Sackett, D. L., W. S. Richardson, W. Rosenberg, and R. B Hayes. 1997. *Evidence-Based Medicine: How to Practice and Teach EBM.* New York: Churchill Livingstone.

Safran, D. G. 2001. "Measuring, Monitoring and Reporting Functional Health Outcomes: Opportunities and Challenges in a Bold National Initiative." *International Journal for Quality in Health Care* 13 (1): 7–8.

Safran, D. G., and W. H. Rogers. 2002. "Survey-Based Measures of Physician-Level Performance. Prepared for The National Committee for Quality Assurance." Washington, DC: NCQA.

Saha, S., G. D. Stettin, and R. F. Redberg. 1999. "Gender and Willingness to Undergo Invasive Cardiac Procedures." *Journal of General Internal Medicine* 14 (2): 122–25.

Sarnecki, A. J., S. Haas, K. A. Stevens, and J. A. Willemsen. 1998. "Design and Implementation of a Patient Classification System for Rehabilitation Nursing." *Rehabilitation Nursing* 18: 244–48.

Schafer, J. L. 1997. *Analysis of Incomplete Multivariate Data*. New York: Chapman and Hall.

———. 1999. "Multiple Imputation: A Primer." *Statistical Methods in Medical Research* 8: 3–15.

Schafer, J. L., and M. K. Olsen. 1998. "Multiple Imputation for Multivariate Missing-Data Problems: A Data Analyst's Perspective." Working paper, The Pennsylvania State University, Harrisburg, PA, 9 March.

Scherer, M. J. 2000. *Living in the State of Stuck. How Technology Impacts the Lives of People with Disabilities,* 3d ed. Cambridge, MA: Brookline Books.

Schillinger, D., K. Grumbach, J. Piette, F. Wang, D. Osmond, C. Daher, J. Palacios, G. D. Sullivan, and A. B. Bindman. 2002. "Association of Health Literacy with Diabetes Outcomes." *Journal of the American Medical Association* 288 (4): 475–82.

Schlesinger, M., B. Druss, and T. Thomas. 1999. "No Exit? The Effect of Health Status on Dissatisfaction and Disenrollment from Health Plans." *Health Services Research* 34 (2): 547–76.

Schmidt, R. M., and L. K. White. 2002. "Internists and Adolescent Medicine." *Archives of Internal Medicine* 162 (14): 1550–56.

Schneider, D. P., B. E. Fries, W. J. Foley, M. Desmond, and W. J. Gormley. 1988. "Case Mix for Nursing Home Payment: Resource Utilization Groups, Version II." *Health Care Financing Review* 10 (Suppl.): 39–52.

Schneider, E. C., P. D. Cleary, A. M. Zaslavsky, and A. M. Epstein. 2001b. "Racial Disparity in Influenza Vaccination: Does Managed Care Narrow the Gap Between African Americans and Whites?" *Journal of the American Medical Association* 286 (12): 1455–60.

Schneider, E. C., L. L. Leape, J. S. Weissman, R. N. Piana, C. Gatsonis, and A. M. Epstein. 2001a. "Racial Differences in Cardiac Revascularization Rates: Does 'Overuse' Explain Higher Rates Among White Patients?" *Annals of Internal Medicine* 135 (5): 328–37.

Schneider, E. C., A. M. Zaslavsky, and A. M. Epstein. 2002. "Racial Disparities in the Quality of Care for Enrollees in Medicare Managed Care." *Journal of the American Medical Association* 287 (10): 1288–94.

Schnelle, J. F., J. G. Ouslander, J. Buchanan, G. Zellman, D. Farley, S. H. Hirsch, and D. B. Reuben. 1999. "Objective and Subjective Measures of the Quality of Managed Care in Nursing Homes." *Medical Care* 37 (4): 375–83.

Schoenbaum, M., J. Unutzer, D. McCaffrey, N. Duan, C. D. Sherbourne, and K. B. Wells. In press. "The Effects of Primary Care Depression Treatment on Patients' Clinical Status and Employment." *Health Services Research.*

Schulman, K. A., L. E. Rubenstein, F. D. Chesley, and J. M. Eisenberg. 1995. "The Roles of Race and Socioeconomic Factors in Health Services Research." *Health Services Research* 30 (1, Part II): 179–95.

Selker, H. P. 1993. "Systems for Comparing Actual and Predicted Mortality Rates: Characteristics to Promote Cooperation in Improving Hospital Care." *Annals of Internal Medicine* 118 (10): 820–22.

Selker, H. P., J. L. Griffith, S. Patil, W. J. Long, and R. B. D'Agostino. 1995. "A Comparison of Performance of Mathematical Predictive Methods for Medical Diagnosis: Identifying Acute Cardiac Ischemia Among Emergency Department Patients." *Journal of Investigative Medicine* 43 (5): 468–76.

Shahian, D. M., S. L. Normand, D. F. Torchiana, S. M. Lewis, J. O. Pastore, R. E. Kuntz, and P. I. Dreyer. 2001. "Cardiac Surgery Report Cards: Comprehensive Review and Statistical Critique." *Annals of Thoracic Surgery* 72 (6): 2155–68.

Shapiro, J. P. 1994. *No Pity. People with Disabilities Forging a New Civil Rights Movement.* New York: Times Books.

Shapiro, M. F., R. E. Park, J. Keesey, and R. H. Brook. 1994. "The Effect of Alternative Case-Mix Adjustments on Mortality Differences Between Municipal and Voluntary Hospitals in New York City." *Health Services Research* 29 (1): 95–112.

Shaughnessy, P. W., K. S. Crisler, and R. E. Schlenker. 1998. "Outcome-Based Quality Improvement in Home Health Care: The OASIS Indicators." *Quality Management in Health Care* 7 (1): 58–67.

Shaughnessy, P. W., K. S. Crisler, R. E. Schlenker, and A. G. Arnold. 1997. "Outcomes Across the Care Continuum. Home Health Care." *Medical Care* 35 (11, Suppl.): NS115–NS123.

Shaughnessy, P. W., and D. F. Hittle. 2002. "Overview of Risk Adjustment and Outcome Measures for Home Health Agency OBQI Reports: Highlights of Current Approaches and Outline of Planned Enhancements." Denver, CO: University of Colorado Health Sciences Center.

Shaughnessy, P. W., D. F. Hittle, K. S. Crisler, M. C. Powell, A. A. Richard, A. M. Kramer, R. E. Schlenker, J. F. Steiner, N. S. Donelan-McCall, J. M. Beaudry, K. L. Mulvey-Lawlor, and K. Engle. 2002. "Improving Patient Outcomes of Home Health Care: Findings from Two Demonstration Trials of Outcome-Based Quality Improvement." *Journal of the American Geriatric Society* 50 (8): 1354–64.

Shaughnessy, P. W., R. E. Schlenker, and D. F. Hittle. 1995. "Case Mix of Home Health Patients Under Capitated and Fee-for-Service Payment." *Health Services Research* 30: 79–113.

Shavelle, D. M., L. Parsons, M. J. Sada, W. J. French, and N. R. Every. 2002. "Is There a Benefit to Early Angiography in Patients with ST-Segment Depression Myocardial Infarction? An Observational Study." *American Heart Journal* 143 (3): 488–96.

Shaw, L. J., D. D. Miller, J. C. Romeis, D. Kargl, L. T. Younis, and B. R. Chaitman. 1994. "Gender Differences in the Noninvasive Evaluation and Management of Patients with Suspected Coronary Artery Disease." *Annals of Internal Medicine* 120 (7): 559–66.

Sheehy, K. H. 1991. "White Paper: Coding and Classification Systems—Implications for the Profession." *Journal of the American Medical Records Association* 62 (2): 44–49.

Shenkman, E. A., and J. R. Breiner. 2001. "Characteristics of Risk Adjustment Systems." Working Paper Series #2 Division of Child Health Services Research and Evaluation. Institute for Child Health Policy, University of Florida, Gainesville.

Sherbourne, C. D., L. S. Meredith, W. Rogers, and J. E. Ware, Jr. 1992. "Social Support and Stressful Life Events: Age Differences in Their Effects on Health-Related Quality of Life Among the Chronically Ill." *Quality of Life Research* 1 (4): 235–46.

Sherbourne, C. D., and A. L. Stewart. 1991. "The MOS Social Support Survey." *Social Science and Medicine* 32 (6): 705–14.

Shi, L., and B. Starfield. 2000. "Primary Care, Income Inequality, and Self-Rated Health in the United States: A Mixed-Level Analysis." *International Journal of Health Services* 30 (3): 541–55.

Shields, A. E., J. A. Finkelstein, C. Comstock, and K. B. Weiss. 2002. "Process of Care for Medicaid-Enrolled Children with Asthma: Served by Community Health Centers and Other Providers." *Medical Care* 40 (4): 303–14.

Shortell, S. M., J. E. Zimmerman, D. M. Rousseau, R. R. Gillies, D. P. Wagner, E. A. Draper, W. A. Knaus, and J. Duffy. 1994. "The Performance of Intensive Care Units: Does Good Management Make a Difference?" *Medical Care* 32 (5): 508–25.

Shrout, P. E., and J. L. Fleiss. 1979. "Intraclass Correlation: Uses in Assessing Rater Reliability." *Psychological Bulletin* 86 (2): 420–28.

Shroyer, A. L., I. Dauber, R. H. Jones, J. Daley, F. L. Grover, and K. E. Hammermeister. 1994. "Provider Perceptions in Using Outcomes Data to Improve Clinical Practice." *Annals of Thoracic Surgery* 58 (6): 1877–80.

Shroyer, A. L., M. J. London, G. K. Sethi, G. Marshall, F. L. Grover, and K. E. Hammermeister. 1995. "Relationships Between Patient-Related Risk Factors, Processes, Structures, and Outcomes of Cardiac Surgical Care. Conceptual Models." *Medical Care* 33 (10, Suppl.): OS26–OS34.

Shwartz, M., A. S. Ash, J. Anderson, L. I. Iezzoni, S. M. Payne, and J. D. Restuccia. 1994. "Small Area Variations in Hospitalization Rates: How Much You See Depends on How You Look." *Medical Care* 32 (3): 189–201.

Shwartz, M., L. I. Iezzoni, A. S. Ash, and Y. D. Mackiernan. 1996a. "Do Severity Measures Explain Differences in Length of Hospital Stay? The Case of Hip Fracture." *Health Services Research* 31 (4): 365–85.

Shwartz, M., L. I. Iezzoni, M. A. Moskowitz, A. S. Ash, and E. Sawitz. 1996b. "The Importance of Comorbidities in Explaining Differences in Patient Costs." *Medical Care* 34 (8): 767–82.

Shwartz, M., R. Saitz, K. Mulvey, and P. Brannigan. 1999. "The Value of Acupuncture Detoxification Programs in a Substance Abuse Treatment System." *Journal of Substance Abuse Treatment* 17 (4): 305–12.

Siegler, E. L., M. G. Stineman, and G. Maislin. 1994. "Development of Complications During Rehabilitation." *Archives of Internal Medicine* 154 (19): 2185–90.

Silber, J. H., P. R. Rosenbaum, L. F. Koziol, N. Sutaria, R. R. Marsh, and O. Even-Shoshan. 1999. "Conditional Length of Stay." *Health Services Research* 34 (1, Part II): 349–63.

Silber, J. H., P. R. Rosenbaum, S. V. Williams, R. N. Ross, and J. S. Schwartz. 1997. "The Relationship Between Choice of Outcome Measure and Hospital Rank in General Surgical Procedures: Implications for Quality Assessment." *International Journal for Quality in Health Care* 9 (3): 193–200.

Silliman, R. A., and T. L. Lash. 1999. "Comparison of Interview-Based and Medical-Record Based Indices of Comorbidity Among Breast Cancer Patients." *Medical Care* 37 (4): 339–49.

Simborg, D. W. 1981. "DRG Creep: A New Hospital-Acquired Disease." *New England Journal of Medicine* 304 (26): 1602–04.

Simmons, S. F., J. F. Schnelle, G. C. Uman, A. D. Kulvicki, K. O. Lee, and J. G. Ouslander. 1997. "Selecting Nursing Home Residents for Satisfaction Surveys." *Gerontologist* 37 (4): 543–50.

Slee, V. N. 1978. "The International Classification of Diseases: Ninth Revision (ICD-9)." *Annals of Internal Medicine* 88 (3): 424–26.

Smoller, J. W., R. Y. McLean, M. W. Otto, and M. H. Pollack. 1998. "How Do Clinicians Respond to Patients Who Miss Appointments?" *Journal of Clinical Psychiatry* 59 (6): 330–38.

Snedecor, G. W., and W. G. Cochran. 1980. *Statistical Methods*, 7th ed. Ames, IA: Iowa State University Press.

Social Security Administration, Office of Disability. 1998. "Disability Evaluation Under Social Security." S.S.A. Publication No. 64–039. Washington, DC: U.S. Government Printing Office.

Société Française d'Anesthésie et de Réanimation. 2002. "Scoring Systems for ICU and Surgical Patients." [Online article; retrieved 8/3/02.] http://www.sfar.org/scores2/scores2.html.

Somogyi-Zalud, E., Z. Zhong, M. B. Hamel, and J. Lynn. 2002. "The Use of Life-Sustaining Treatments in Hospitalized Persons Aged 80 and Older." *Journal of the American Geriatric Society* 50 (5): 930–34.

Spector, W. D., J. A. Fleishman, L. E. Pezzin, and B. C. Spillman. 1998. "The Characteristics of Long-Term Care Users." Paper Prepared for the Institute of Medicine Committee on Improving Quality in Long-Term Care. Washington, DC: Institute of Medicine.

Spitzer, J. J. 1982. "A Primer on Box-Cox Estimation." *Reviews of Economics and Statistics* 64 (2): 307–13.

Stafford, R. S., D. Saglam, N. Causino, B. Starfield, L. Culpepper, W. D. Marder, and D. Blumenthal. 1999. "Trends in Adult Visits to Primary Care Physicians in the United States." *Archives of Family Medicine* 8 (1): 26–32.

Stampfer, M. J., and G. A. Colditz. 1991. "Estrogen Replacement Therapy and Coronary Heart Disease: A Quantitative Assessment of the Epidemiologic Evidence." *Preventive Medicine* 20 (1): 47–63.

Starfield, B. 1992. "Effects of Poverty on Health Status." *Bulletin of the New York Academy of Medicine* 68 (1): 17–24.

Starfield, B., M. Bergner, M. Ensminger, A. Riley, S. Ryan, B. Green, P. McGauhey,

A. Skinner, and S. Kim. 1993. "Adolescent Health Status Measurement: Development of the Child Health and Illness Profile." *Pediatrics* 91 (2): 430–35.

Starfield, B., J. Weiner, L. Mumford, and D. Steinwachs. 1991. "Ambulatory Care Groups: A Categorization of Diagnoses for Research and Management." *Health Services Research* 26 (1): 53–74.

Statistical Society. 1865. "Statistics of Metropolitan and Provincial General Hospitals for 1863." *Journal of the Statistical Society of London* 28: 527–35.

Stearns, S. C., M. G. Kovar, K. Hayes, and G. G. Koch. 1996. "Risk Indicators for Hospitalization During the Last Year of Life." *Health Services Research* 31 (1): 49–69.

Steen, P. M. 1994. "Approaches to Predictive Modeling." *Annals of Thoracic Surgery* 58 (6): 1836–40.

Steen, P. M., A. C. Brewster, R. C. Bradbury, E. Estabrook, and J. A. Young. 1993. "Predicted Probabilities of Hospital Death as a Measure of Admission Severity of Illness." *Inquiry* 30 (2): 128–41.

Stein, C. 1955. "Inadmissibility of the Usual Estimator for the Mean of a Multivariate Normal Distribution." In *Proceedings of the 3rd Berkeley Symposium on Mathmatical Statistics and Probability. Volume 1*, 197. Berkeley, CA: University of California Press.

Steingart, R. M., M. Packer, P. Hamm, M. E. Coglianese, B. Gersh, E. M. Geltman, J. Sollano, S. Katz, L. Moye, L. L. Basta, S. J. Lewis, S. S. Gottlieb, V. Bernstein, P. McEwan, K. Jacobson, E. J. Brown, M. L. Kukin, N. E. Kantrowitz, and M. A. Pfefer for the Survival and Ventricular Enlargement Investigators. 1994. "Sex Differences in the Management of Coronary Artery Disease." *New England Journal of Medicine* 325 (4): 226–30.

Steinwachs, D. M. 1989. "Application of Health Status Assessment Measures in Policy Research." *Medical Care* 27 (3, Suppl.): S12–S26.

Steinwachs, D. M., M. E. Stuart, S. Scholle, B. Starfield, M. H. Fox, and J. P. Weiner. 1998. "A Comparison of Ambulatory Medicaid Claims to Medical Records: A Reliability Assessment." *American Journal of Medical Quality* 13 (2): 63–69.

Steinwald, B., and L. A. Dummit. 1989. "Hospital Case-Mix Change: Sicker Patients or DRG Creep?" *Health Affairs (Millwood)* 8 (2): 35–47.

Stenestrand, U., and L. Wallentin. 2001. "Early Statin Treatment Following Acute Myocardial Infarction and 1-Year Survival." *Journal of the American Medical Association* 285 (4): 430–36.

———. 2002. "Early Revascularisation and 1-Year Survival in 14-Day Survivors of Acute Myocardial Infarction: A Prospective Cohort Study." *Lancet* 359: 1805–11.

Stewart, A. L., S. Greenfield, R. D. Hays, K. Wells, W. H. Rogers, S. D. Berry, E. A. McGlynn, and J. E. Ware, Jr. 1989. "Functional Status and Well-Being of Patients with Chronic Conditions. Results from the Medical Outcomes Study." *Journal of the American Medical Association* 262 (7): 907–13.

Stewart, A. L., R. D. Hays, and J. E. Ware, Jr. 1988. "The MOS Short-Form General Health Survey. Reliability and Validity in a Patient Population." *Medical Care* 26 (7): 724–35.

———. 1992. "Methods of Validating MOS Health Measures." In *Measuring Func-*

tioning and Well-Being. The Medical Outcomes Study Approach, edited by A. L. Stewart and J. E. Ware, Jr., 309–24. Durham, NC: Duke University Press.

Stewart, A. L., and J. E. Ware, Jr. 1992. *Measuring Functioning and Well-Being: The Medical Outcomes Study Approach.* Durham, NC: Duke University Press.

Stineman, M. G. 1997. "Measuring Casemix, Severity, and Complexity in Geriatric Patients Undergoing Rehabilitation." *Medical Care* 35 (6, Suppl.): JS90–JS105.

Stineman, M. G., J. J. Escarce, J. E. Goin, B. B. Hamilton, C. V. Granger, and S. V. Williams. 1994. "A Case-Mix Classification System for Medical Rehabilitation." *Medical Care* 32 (4): 366–79.

Stineman, M. G., J. E. Goin, C. V. Granger, R. Fiedler, and S. V. Williams. 1997c. "Discharge Motor FIM-Function Related Groups." *Archives of Physical Medicine and Rehabilitation* 78 (9): 980–85.

Stineman, M. G., J. E. Goin, C. J. Tassoni, C. V. Granger, and S. V. Williams. 1997a. "Classifying Rehabilitation Inpatients by Expected Functional Gain." *Medical Care* 35 (9): 963–73.

Stineman, M. G., and C. V. Granger. 1997. "A Modular Case-Mix Classification System for Medical Rehabilitation Illustrated." *Health Care Financing Review* 19 (1): 87–103.

Stineman, M. G., G. Maislin, R. C. Fiedler, and C. V. Granger. 1997d. "A Prediction Model for Functional Recovery in Stroke." *Stroke* 28 (3): 550–56.

Stineman, M. G., G. Maislin, M. Nosek, R. Fiedler, and C. V. Granger. 1998. "Comparing Consumer and Clinician Values for Alternative Functional States: Application of a New Feature Trade-off Consensus Building Tool." *Archives of Physical Medicine and Rehabilitation* 79 (12): 1522–29.

Stineman, M. G., J. A. Shea, A. Jette, C. J. Tassoni, K. J. Ottenbacher, and R. Fiedler. 1996. "The Functional Independence Measure: Tests for Scaling Assumptions, Structure, and Reliability Across 20 Diverse Impairment Categories." *Archives of Physical Medicine and Rehabilitation* 77: 1101–08.

Stineman, M. G., C. J. Tassoni, J. J. Escarce, J. E. Goin, C. V. Granger, R. C. Fiedler, and S. V. Williams. 1997b. "Development of Function-Related Groups Version 2.0: A Classification System for Medical Rehabilitation." *Health Services Research* 32 (4): 529–48.

Stone, D. A. 1984. *The Disabled State.* Philadelphia: Temple University Press.

Stoskopf, C., and S. D. Horn. 1991. "The Computerized Psychiatric Severity Index as a Predictor of Inpatient Length of Stay for Psychoses." *Medical Care* 29 (3): 179–95.

———. 1992. "Predicting Length of Stay for Patients with Psychoses." *Health Services Research* 26 (6): 743–66.

Streiner, D. L., and G. R. Norman. 1995. *Health Status Measurements Scales. A Practical Guide to Their Development and Use,* 2d ed. Oxford, UK: Oxford University Press.

Stuck, A. E., J. M. Walthert, N. Thorsten, C. J. Bula, C. Hohnmann, and J. C. Beck. 1999. "Risk Factors for Functional Status Decline in Community-Living Elderly People: A Systematic Literature Review." *Social Science and Medicine* 48 (4): 445–69.

Stukenborg, G. J., D. P. Wagner, and A. F. Connors, Jr. 2001. "Comparison of the

Performance of Two Comorbidity Measures, with and without Information from Prior Hospitalizations." *Medical Care* 39 (7): 727–39.

Sullivan, L. M., K. A. Dukes, L. Harris, R. S. Dittus, S. Greenfield, and S. H. Kaplan. 1995. "A Comparison of Various Methods of Collecting Self-Reported Health Outcomes Data Among Low-Income and Minority Patients." *Medical Care* 33 (4, Suppl.): AS183–AS194.

Svensson, C. K. 1989. "Representation of American Blacks in Clinical Trials of New Drugs." *Journal of the American Medical Association* 261 (2): 263–65.

Swan, J., and R. Newcomer. 2000. "Residential Care Supply, Nursing Home Licensing, and Case Mix in Four States." *Health Care Financing Review* 21 (3): 203–29.

Tabbarah, M., M. Silverstein, and T. Seeman. 2000. "A Health and Demographic Profile of Noninstitutionalized Older Americans Residing in Environments with Home Modifications." *Journal of Aging and Health* 12 (2): 204–28.

Task Force for the Handbook of Psychiatric Measures. 2000. *Handbook of Psychiatric Measures*. Washington, DC: American Psychiatric Association.

Taube, C., E. S. Lee, and R. N. Forthofer. 1984. "DRGs in Psychiatry. An Empirical Evaluation." *Medical Care* 22 (7): 597–610.

Teno, J. M., R. B. Hakim, W. A. Knaus, N. S. Wenger, R. S. Phillips, A. W. Wu, P. Layde, A. F. Connors, Jr., N. V. Dawson, and J. Lynn. 1995. "Preferences for Cardiopulmonary Resuscitation: Physician-Patient Agreement and Hospital Resource Use. The SUPPORT Investigators." *Journal of General Internal Medicine* 10 (4): 179–86.

Teno, J. M., J. Lynn, R. S. Phillips, D. Murphy, S. J. Youngner, P. Bellamy, A. F. Connors, Jr., N. A. Desbiens, W. Fulkerson, and W. A. Knaus. 1994. "Do Formal Advance Directives Affect Resuscitation Decisions and the Use of Resources for Seriously Ill Patients? SUPPORT Investigators. Study to Understand Prognoses and Preferences for Outcomes and Risks of Treatments." *Journal of Clinical Ethics* 5 (1): 23–30.

Teres, D., and S. Lemeshow. 1993. "Using Severity Measures to Describe High Performance Intensive Care Units." *Critical Care Clinics* 9 (3): 543–54.

———. 1994. "Why Severity Models Should Be Used with Caution." *Critical Care Clinics* 11 (3): 525–51.

Ter Maat, M. 1993. "An Appropriate Nursing Skill Mix: Survey of Acuity Systems in Rehabilitation Hospitals." *Rehabilitation Nursing* 18 (4): 244–48.

Thomas, J. W., and M. L. Ashcraft. 1989. "Measuring Severity of Illness: A Comparison of Interrater Reliability Among Severity Methodologies." *Inquiry* 26 (4): 483–92.

———. 1991. "Measuring Severity of Illness: Six Severity Systems and Their Ability to Explain Cost Variations." *Inquiry* 28 (1): 39–55.

Thomas, J. W., M. L. F. Ashcraft, and J. Zimmerman. 1986. "An Evaluation of Alternative Severity of Illness Measures for Use by University Hospitals: Volume II, Technical Report." Ann Arbor, MI: Department of Health Services Management and Policy, School of Public Health, University of Michigan.

Thomas, J. W., and T. P. Hofer. 1999. "Accuracy of Risk-Adjusted Mortality Rate as a Measure of Hospital Quality of Care." *Medical Care* 37 (1): 83–92.

Thomas, N., N. T. Longford, and J. E. Rolph. 1994. "Empirical Bayes Methods for Estimating Hospital-Specific Mortality Rates." *Statistics in Medicine* 13 (9): 889–903.

Thomson, R. G. 1997. *Extraordinary Bodies. Figuring Physical Disability in American Culture and Literature*. New York: Columbia University Press.

Thorpe, J. M., and S. R. Machlin. 2001. "Health Care Expenses in the US Civilian Non-Institutionalized Population, 1997." Research Findings. Publication No. 01-R086. Rockville, MD: Agency for Healthcare Research and Quality.

Tinetti, M. E., S. K. Inouye, T. M. Gill, and J. T. Doucette. 1995. "Shared Risk Factors for Falls, Incontinence, and Functional Dependence: Unifying the Approach to Geriatric Syndromes." *Journal of the American Medical Association* 273: 1348–53.

Tinetti, M. E., T. F. Williams, and R. Mayewski. 1986. "Fall Risk Index for Elderly Patients Based on Number of Chronic Disabilities." *American Journal of Medicine* 80 (3): 429–34.

Todorov, A., and C. Kirchner. 2000. "Bias in Proxies' Reports of Disability: Data from the National Health Interview Survey on Disability." *American Journal of Public Health* 90 (8): 1248–53.

Tsevat, J., E. F. Cook, M. L. Green, D. B. Matchar, N. V. Dawson, S. K. Broste, A. W. Wu, R. S. Phillips, R. K. Oye, and L. Goldman. 1995. "Health Values of the Seriously Ill. SUPPORT Investigators." *Annals of Internal Medicine* 122 (7): 514–20.

Tucker, A, J. Weiner, and C. Abrams. 2002. "Health-Based Risk Adjustment: Application to Premium Development and Profiling." In *Financial Strategy for Managed Care Organizations: Rate Setting, Risk Adjustment, and Competitive Advantage*, edited by C. W. Wrightson, 165–225. Chicago: Health Administration Press.

Tufte, E. R. 1983. *The Visual Display of Quantitative Information*. Chesire, CT: Graphics Press.

Tukey, J. W. 1977. *Exploratory Data Analysis*. Reading, MA: Addison-Wesley.

Udvarhelyi, I. S., C. Gatsonis, A. M. Epstein, C. L. Pashos, J. P. Newhouse, and B. J. McNeil. 1992. "Acute Myocardial Infarction in the Medicare Population. Process of Care and Clinical Outcomes." *Journal of the American Medical Association* 268 (18): 2530–36.

U.S. Department of Health and Human Services. 2000. "Healthy People 2010. Second Edition. With Understanding and Improving Health and Objectives for Improving Health." Washington, DC: U.S. Government Printing Office.

U.S. Department of Veterans Affairs. 2002. "Veteran Data and Information Web Site." [Online information; retieval 7/18/02.] http://www.va.gov/vetdata/index.htm.

U.S. Food and Drug Administration, Center for Drug Evaluation and Research. 2003. "The National Drug Code Directory." [Online directory; retrieved 4/2/2003.] http://www.fda.gov/cder/ndc/.

U.S. General Accounting Office. 1992. "FDA Needs to Ensure More Study of Gender Differences in Prescription Drug Testing." Washington, D.C.: U.S. GAO.

———. 1996. "S.S.A. Disability. Program Redesign Necessary to Encourage Return to Work. GAO/HEHS-96–62,. Washington, D.C.: U.S. GAO.

———. 1998. "California Nursing Homes: Care Problems Persist Despite Federal and State Oversight: Report to the Special Committee on Aging. GAO/HEHS-98–202." Washington, DC: U.S. Senate.

———. 1999a. "Medical Records Privacy. Access Needed for Health Research, but Oversight of Privacy Protections Is Limited." GAO/HEHS-99–55. Washington, DC: U.S. GAO.

———. 1999b. "Nursing Homes: Additional Steps Needed to Strengthen Enforcement of Federal Standards: Report to the Special Committee on Aging." GAO/HEHS-99–46. Washington, DC: U.S. Senate.

———. 2001. "Record Linkage and Privacy. Issues in Creating New Federal Research and Statistical Information." GAO-01–126SP. Washington, DC: U.S. GAO.

———. 2002. "Nursing Homes: Public Reporting of Quality Indicators Has Merit, but National Implementation Is Premature." GAO-03–187. Report to Congressional Requestors. Washington, DC: U.S. GAO.

van den Akker, M., F. Buntinx, J. F. Metsemakers, S. Roos, and J. A. Knottnerus. 1998. "Multimorbidity in General Practice: Prevalence, Incidence, and Determinants of Co-Occurring Chronic and Recurrent Diseases." *Journal of Clinical Epidemiology* 51 (5): 367–75.

Van Ruiswyk, J., A. Hartz, E. Kuhn, H. Krakauer, M. Young, and A. Rimm. 1993. "A Measure of Mortality Risk for Elderly Patients with Acute Myocardial Infarction." *Medical Decision Making* 13 (2): 152–60.

Vassar, M. J., and J. W. Holcroft. 1994. "The Case Against Using the APACHE System to Predict Intensive Care Unit Outcome in Trauma Patients." *Critical Care Clinics* 10 (1): 117–26.

Vassar, M. J., C. L. Wilkerson, P. J. Duran, C. A. Perry, and J. W. Holcroft. 1992. "Comparison of APACHE II, TRISS, and a Proposed 24-Hour ICU Point System for Prediction of Outcome in ICU Trauma Patients." *Journal of Trauma* 32 (4): 490–99.

Velanovich, V., M. Gabel, E. M. Walker, T. J. Doyle, R. M. O'Bryan, W. Szymanski, J. J. Ferrara, and F. R. Lewis, Jr. 2002. "Causes for the Undertreatment of Elderly Breast Cancer Patients: Tailoring Treatments to Individual Patients." *Journal of the American College of Surgeons* 194 (1): 8–13.

Vidaver, R. M., B. Lafleur, C. Tong, R. Bradshaw, and S. A. Marts. 2000. "Women Subjects in NIH-Funded Clinical Research Literature: Lack of Progress in Both Representation and Analysis by Sex." *Journal of Women's Health and Gender Based Medicine* 9 (5): 495–504.

Vincent, J. L., A. de Mendonca, F. Cantraine, R. Moreno, J. Takala, P. M. Suter, C. L. Sprung, F. Colardyn, and S. Blecher. 1998. "Use of the SOFA Score to Assess the Incidence of Organ Dysfunction/Failure in Intensive Care Units: Results of a Multicenter, Prospective Study. Working Group on 'Sepsis-Related Problems' of the European Society of Intensive Care Medicine." *Critical Care Medicine* 26 (11): 1793–1800.

Vincent, J. L., R. Moreno, J. Takala, S. Willatts, A. De Mendonca, H. Bruining, C. K. Reinhart, P. M. Suter, and L. G. Thijs. 1996. "The SOFA (Sepsis-Related Organ Failure Assessment) Score to Describe Organ Dysfunction/Failure. On Behalf of the Working Group on Sepsis-Related Problems of the European Society of Intensive Care Medicine." *Intensive Care Medicine* 22 (7): 707–10.

Virnig, B. A., A. Ash, S. Kind, and D. E. Mesler. 2000. "Survival Analysis Using Medicare Data: Examples and Methods." *Health Services Research* 35: 85–101.

Vladeck, B. C. 1984. "Medicare Hospital Payment by Diagnosis-Related Groups." *Annals of Internal Medicine* 100 (4): 576–91.

Vogel, R. A., and E. J. Topol. 1996. "Practice Guidelines and Physician Scorecards: Grading the Graders." *Cleveland Clinics Journal of Medicine* 63 (2): 124–28.

Von Korff, M., E. H. Wagner, and K. Saunders. 1992. "A Chronic Disease Score from Automated Pharmacy Data." *Journal of Clinical Epidemiology* 45 (2): 197–203.

Wagner, D. P., W. A. Knaus, and E. A. Draper. 1986. "Physiologic Abnormalities and Outcome from Acute Disease. Evidence for a Predictable Relationship." *Archives of Internal Medicine* 146 (7): 1389–96.

Wagner, D. P., W. A. Knaus, F. E. Harrell Jr., J. E. Zimmerman, and C. Watts. 1994. "Daily Prognostic Estimates for Critically Ill Adults in Intensive Care Units: Results from a Prospective, Multicenter, Inception Cohort Analysis." *Critical Care Medicine* 22 (9): 1359–72.

Wald, J. S., D. Rind, C. Safran, H. Kowaloff, R. Barker, and W. V. Slack. 1995. "Patient Entries in the Electronic Medical Record: An Interactive Interview Used in Primary Care." In *Proceedings of the Annual Symposium for Computer Applications to Medical Care*: 147–51.

Walker, H. M. 1929. *Studies in the History of Statistical Method*. Baltimore: Williams & Wilkins.

Walsh, J. M., A. R. Pressman, J. A. Cauley, and W. S. Browner. 2001. "Predictors of Physical Activity in Community-Dwelling Elderly White Women." *Journal of General Internal Medicine* 16 (11): 721–27.

Wang, P. S., R. L. Bohn, E. Knight, R. J. Glynn, H. Mogun, and J. Avorn. 2002. "Noncompliance with Antihypertensive Medications: The Impact of Depressive Symptoms and Psychosocial Factors." *Journal of General Internal Medicine* 17 (7): 504–11.

Wang, P. S., O. Demler, and R. C. Kessler. 2002. "Adequacy of Treatment for Serious Mental Illness in the United States." *American Journal of Public Health* 92 (1): 92–98.

Ware, J. E., Jr. 1995. "The Status of Health Assessment 1994." *Annual Review of Public Health* 16: 327–54.

Ware, J. E., S. D. Keller, B. Gandek, J. E. Brazier, and M. Sullivan. 1995. "Evaluating Translations of Health Status Questionnaires: Methods from the IQOLA Project. International Quality of Life Assessment." *International Journal of Technology Assessment in Health Care* 11 (3): 525–51.

Warren, J. L., L. C. Harlan, A. Fahey, B. A. Virnig, J. L. Freeman, C. N. Klabunde, G. S. Cooper, and K. B. Knopf. 2002b. "Utility of the SEER-Medicare Data to Identify Chemotherapy Use." *Medical Care* 40 (8, Suppl.): IV-55–IV-61.

Warren, J. L., C. N. Klabunde, D. Schrag, P. B. Bach, and G. F. Riley. 2002a. "Overview of the SEER-Medicare Data: Content, Research Applications, and Generalizability to the United States Elderly Population." *Medical Care* 40 (8, Suppl.): IV-3–IV-18.

Watanabe, C. T., C. Maynard, and J. L. Ritchie. 2001. "Comparison of Short-Term

Outcomes Following Coronary Artery Stenting in Men Versus Women."
American Journal of Cardiology 88 (8): 848–52.

Waterstraat, F. L., J. Barlow, and F. Newman. 1990. "Diagnostic Coding Quality and Its Impact on Healthcare Reimbursement: Research Prospectives." *Journal of the Amerian Medical Records Association* 61 (9): 52–59.

Weech-Maldonado, R., L. S. Morales, K. Spritzer, M. Elliott, and R. D. Hays. 2001. "Racial and Ethnic Differences in Parents' Assessments of Pediatric Care in Medicaid Managed Care." *Health Services Research* 36 (3): 575–94.

Weed, L. L. 1968. "Medical Records that Guide and Teach." *New England Journal of Medicine* 278 (11): 593–600.

———. 1971. "Quality Control and the Medical Record." *Archives of Internal Medicine* 127 (1): 101–05.

Weigel, K. M., and C. A. Lewis. 1991. "Forum: In Sickness and in Health—The Role of the ICD in the United States Health Care Data and ICD-10." *Topics in Health Records Management* 12 (1): 70–82.

Weinberger, M., E. Z. Oddone, G. P. Samsa, and P. B. Landsman. 1996. "Are Health-Related Quality-of-Life Measures Affected by the Mode of Administration?" *Journal of Clinical Epidemiology* 49 (2): 135–40.

Weiner, J. P., A. Dobson, S. L. Maxwell, K. Coleman, B. Starfield, and G. F. Anderson. 1996a. "Risk-Adjusted Medicare Capitation Rates Using Ambulatory and Inpatient Diagnoses." *Health Care Financing Review* 17 (3): 77–99.

Weiner, J. P., B. H. Starfield, N. R. Powe, M. E. Stuart, and D. M. Steinwachs. 1996b. "Ambulatory Care Practice Variation Within a Medicaid Program." *Health Services Research* 30 (6): 751–70.

Weiner, J. P., B. H. Starfield, D. M. Steinwachs, and L. M. Mumford. 1991. "Development and Application of a Population-Oriented Measure of Ambulatory Care Case-Mix." *Medical Care* 29 (5): 452–72.

Weiner, J. P., A. M. Tucker, A. M. Collins, H. Fakhraei, R. Lieberman, C. Abrams, G. R. Trapnell, and J. G. Folkemer. 1998. "The Development of a Risk-Adjusted Capitation Payment System: The Maryland Medicaid Model." *Journal of Ambulatory Care Management* 21 (4): 29–52.

Weingart, S. N., R. B. Davis, R. H. Palmer, M. Cahalane, M. B. Hamel, K. Mukamal, R. S. Phillips, D. T. Davies, Jr., and L. I. Iezzoni. 2002. "Discrepancies Between Explicit and Implicit Review: Physician and Nurse Assessments of Complications and Quality." *Health Services Research* 37 (2): 483–98.

Weingart, S. N., K. Mukamal, R. B. Davis, D. T. Davies, Jr., R. H. Palmer, M. Cahalane, M. B. Hamel, R. S. Phillips, and L. I. Iezzoni. 2001. "Physician-Reviewers' Perceptions and Judgments About Quality of Care." *International Journal for Quality in Health Care* 13 (5): 357–65.

Wenger, N. S., M. L. Pearson, K. A. Desmond, E. R. Harrison, L. V. Rubenstein, W. H. Rogers, and K. L. Kahn. 1995. "Epidemiology of Do-Not-Resuscitate Orders. Disparity by Age, Diagnosis, Gender, Race, and Functional Impairment." *Archives of Internal Medicine* 155 (19): 2056–62.

Wennberg, D. E., F. L. Lucas, J. D. Birkmeyer, C. E. Bredenberg, and E. S. Fisher. 1998. "Variation in Carotid Endarterectomy Mortality in the Medicare Population: Trial Hospitals, Volume, and Patient Characteristics." *Journal of the American Medical Association* 279 (16): 1278–81.

Wennberg, J. E., E. S. Fisher, and J. S. Skinner. 2002. "Geography and the Debate over Medicare Reform." *Health Affairs Web Exclusive*, 13 Feb., W96–W114 [Online article; retrieved 4/3/2003.] http://www.healthaffairs.org.

Wennberg, J., and A. Gittelsohn. 1973. "Small Area Variations in Health Care Delivery." *Science* 182 (117): 1102–08.

Westat. 2001. "Annual Report of the National CAHPS Benchmarking Database 2000. What Consumers Say About the Quality of Their Health Plans and Medical Care." AHRQ Publication No. 01–0005. Rockville, MD: U.S. Department of Health and Human Services, Agency for Healthcare Research and Quality.

Westgren, M., M. Divon, J. Greenspoon, and R. Paul. 1986. "Missing Hospital Records: A Confounding Variable in Retrospective Studies." *American Journal of Obstetrics and Gynecology* 155 (2): 269–71.

White House Domestic Policy Council. 1993. "Health Security: The President's Report to the American People." Washington, DC: White House Domestic Policy Council.

Whiteneck, G. G. 1997. "Disablement Outcomes in Geriatric Rehabilitation. Report: Group D." *Medical Care* 35 (6, Suppl.): JS45–JS47.

Whiting-O'Keefe, Q. E., C. Henke, and D. W. Simborg. 1984. "Choosing the Correct Unit of Analysis in Medical Care Experiments." *Medical Care* 22 (12): 1101–14.

Wilkerson, D. L., A. L. Batavia, and G. DeJong. 1992. "Use of Functional Status Measures for Payment of Medical Rehabilation Services." *Archives of Physical Medicine and Rehabilitation* 73 (2): 111–20.

Williams, D. R. 1994. "The Concept of Race in Health Services Research: 1966 to 1990." *Health Services Research* 29 (3): 261–74.

———. 1996. "Race/Ethnicity and Socioeconomic Status: Measurement and Methodological Issues." *International Journal of Health Services* 26 (3): 483–505.

———. 1999. "The Monitoring of Racial/Ethnic Status in the USA: Data Quality Issues." *Ethnicity and Health* 4 (3): 121–37.

Williams, G. 2001. "Theorizing Disability." In *Handbook of Disability Studies*, edited by K. D. Seelman, G. L. Albrecht, and M. Bury, 123–44. Thousand Oaks, CA: Sage.

Williams, J. F., J. E. Zimmerman, D. P. Wagner, M. Hawkins, and W. A. Knaus. 1995. "African-American and White Patients Admitted to the Intensive Care Unit: Is There a Difference in Therapy and Outcome?" *Critical Care Medicine* 23 (4): 626–36.

Williams, R. B., J. C. Barefoot, R. M. Califf, T. L. Haney, W. B. Saunders, D. B. Pryor, M. A. Hlatky, I. C. Siegler, and D. B. Mark. 1992. "Prognostic Importance of Social and Economic Resources Among Medically Treated Patients with Angiographically Documented Coronary Artery Disease." *Journal of the American Medical Association* 267 (4): 520–24.

Willson, D. F., S. D. Horn, J. O. Hendley, R. Smout, and J. Gassaway. 2001. "Effect of Practice Variation on Resource Utilization in Infants Hospitalized for Viral Lower Respiratory Illness." *Pediatrics* 108 (4): 851–55.

Wilson, P., S. R. Smoley, and D. Werdegar. 1996. "Second Report of the California Hospital Outcomes Project. Acute Myocardial Infarction. Volume Two: Technical Appendix." Sacramento, CA: Office of Statewide Health Planning and Development.

Winship, C., and S. L. Morgan. 1999. "The Estimation of Causal Effects from Observational Data." *Annual Review of Sociology* 25: 659–707.

Wolf, D. A. 2001. "Population Change: Friend or Foe of the Chronic Care System?" *Health Affairs (Millwood)* 20 (6): 28–42.

Wong, D. T., S. L. Crofts, M. Gomez, G. P. McGuire, and R. J. Byrick. 1995. "Evaluation of Predictive Ability of APACHE II System and Hospital Outcome in Canadian Intensive Care Unit Patients." *Critical Care Medicine* 23 (7): 1177–83.

Wood, D., C. Donald-Sherbourne, N. Halfon, M. B. Tucker, V. Ortiz, J. S. Hamlin, N. Duan, R. M. Mazel, M. Grabowsky, P. Brunell, and H. Freeman. 1995. "Factors Related to Immunization Status Among Inner-City Latino and African-American Preschoolers." *Pediatrics* 96 (2, Part I): 295–301.

Wood, W. D., and D. F. Beardmore. 1986. "Prospective Payment for Outpatient Mental Health Services: Evaluation of Diagnosis-Related Groups." *Community Mental Health Journal* 22 (4): 286–93.

Wood, W. R., R. P. Ament, and E. J. Kobrinski. 1981. "A Foundation for Hospital Case Mix Measurement." *Inquiry* 18 (3): 247–54.

Woodward, J. H. 1974. *To Do the Sick No Harm. A British Voluntary Hospital System to 1875*. London: Routledge & Kegan Paul.

Working Group on Risk and High Blood Pressure. 1985. "An Epidemiologic Approach to Describing Risk Associated with Blood Pressure Levels." *Hypertension* 7 (4): 641–51.

World Health Organization. 2001. *International Classification of Functioning, Disability and Health*. Geneva: WHO.

———. 2002. "The International Statistical Classification of Diseases and Related Health Problems, Tenth Revision." [Online article; retrieved 8/1/02.] http://www.who.int/whosis/icd10/.

Writing Group for the Women's Health Initiative Investigators. 2002. "Risks and Benefits of Estrogen Plus Progestin in Healthy Postmenopausal Women: Principal Results from the Women's Health Initiative Randomized Controlled Trial." *Journal of the American Medical Association* 288; 321–33.

Wunderlich, G. S., D. P. Rice, and N. L. Amado, eds., for the Institute of Medicine. 2002. *The Dynamics of Disability. Measuring and Monitoring Disability for Social Security Programs*. Washington, DC: National Academy Press.

Yates, J. F. 1982. "External Correspondence: Decompositions of the Mean Probability Score." *Organizational Behavior and Human Performance* 30: 132–56.

Young, G. J., M. P. Charns, J. Daley, M. G. Forbes, W. Henderson, and S. F. Khuri. 1997. "Best Practices for Managing Surgical Services: The Role of Coordination." *Health Care Management and Review* 22 (4): 72–81.

Young, J. M. 1997. "Equality of Opportunity. The Making of Americans with Disabilities Act." Washington, DC: National Council on Disability.

Young, N. L., J. I. Williams, K. K. Yoshida, C. Bombardier, and J. G. Wright. 1996. "The Context of Measuring Disability: Does It Matter Whether Capability or

Performance Is Measured?" *Journal of Clinical Epidemiology* 49 (10): 1097–1101.

Zapka, J. G., C. Bigelow, T. Hurley, L. D. Ford, J. Egelhofer, W. M. Cloud, and E. Sachsse. 1996. "Mammography Use Among Sociodemographically Diverse Women: The Accuracy of Self-Report." *American Journal of Public Health* 86 (7): 1016–21.

Zaslavsky, A. M. 2001. "Statistical Issues in Reporting Quality Data: Small Samples and Casemix Variation." *International Journal for Quality in Health Care* 13 (6): 481–88.

Zaslavsky, A. M., N. D. Beaulieu, B. E. Landon, and P. D. Cleary. 2000. "Dimensions of Consumer-Assessed Quality of Medicare Managed-Care Health Plans." *Medical Care* 38 (2): 162–74.

Zaslavsky, A. M., and M. J. Buntin. 2002. "Using Survey Measures to Assess Risk Selection Among Medicare Managed Care Plans." *Inquiry* 39 (2): 138–51.

Zaslavsky, A. M., L. Zaborski, and P. D. Cleary. 2000. "Does the Effect of Respondent Characteristics on Consumer Assessments Vary Across Health Plans?" *Medical Care Research and Review* 57 (3): 379–94.

———. 2002. "Factors Affecting Response Rates to the Consumer Assessment of Health Plans Study Survey." *Medical Care* 40 (6): 485–99.

Zelmer, J., S. Virani, and R. Alvarez. 1999. "Recent Developments in Health Information: An International Perspective." Paper commissioned by the National Committee for Vital and Health Statistics for a Workshop on Developing the 21st Century Vision for Health Statistics. [Online paper; retrieved 4/8/2003.] Washington, DC: U.S. Department of Health and Human Services. http://www.ncvhs.hhs.gov/hsvision/CP-zelmer.pdf.

Zemencuk, J. K., R. A. Hayward, K. A. Skarupski, and S. J. Katz. 1999. "Patients' Desires and Expectations for Medical Care: A Challenge to Improving Patient Satisfaction." *American Journal of Medical Quality* 14 (1): 21–27.

Zhao, Y. A. S. Ash, J. Haughton, and B. McMillan. In press. "Identify High Cost Cases through Predictive Modeling." *Disease Management and Health Outcomes.*

Zhao, Y., R. P. Ellis, A. S. Ash, D. Calabrese, J. Z. Ayanian, and J. P. Slaughter. 2001. "Measuring Population Health Risk Using Inpatient Diagnoses and Outpatient Pharmacy Data." *Health Services Research* 36 (6): 180–93.

Zimmerman, D. R., S. L. Karon, G. Arling, B. R. Clark, T. Collins, R. Ross, and F. Sainfort. 1995. "Development and Testing of Nursing Home Quality Indicators." *Health Care Financing Review* 16 (4): 107–27.

Zinn, J. S., W. E. Aaronson, and M. D. Rosko. 1993. "Variations in the Outcomes of Care Provided in Pennsylvania Nursing Homes. Facility and Environmental Correlates." *Medical Care* 31 (6): 475–87.

Zuckerman, Z. E., B. Starfield, C. Hochreiter, and B. Kovasznay. 1975. "Validating the Content of Pediatric Outpatient Medical Records by Means of Tape-Recording Doctor-Patient Encounters." *Pediatrics* 56 (3): 407–11.

Glossary of Acronyms

ACGs	Adjusted Clinical Groups (formerly Ambulatory Care Groups)
ADGs	Ambulatory Diagnosis Groups (from ACGs)
ADLs	activities of daily living
AHRQ	Agency for Healthcare Research and Quality (formerly Agency for Health Care Policy and Research, or AHCPR)
AIDS	acquired immunodeficiency syndrome
AIM	Acuity Index Method
AMI	acute myocardial infarction
ANOVA	analysis of variance
APACHE	Acute Physiology and Chronic Health Evaluation
APC	Ambulatory Payment Classification
APR-DRGs	All Patient Refined Diagnosis Related Groups
APS	Acute Physiology Score (from APACHE)
ASA	American Society of Anesthesiologists
BUN	blood urea nitrogen
CABG	coronary artery bypass graft
CAHPS	Consumer Assessment of Health Plans Study
CDC	Centers for Disease Control and Prevention
CDPS	Chronic Illness and Disability Payment System (formerly Disability Payment System)
CHF	congestive heart failure
CI	confidence interval
CMGs	Case-Mix Groups
CMI	Case-Mix Index
CMS	Centers for Medicare & Medicaid Services (formerly HCFA)
CPT	*Current Procedural Terminology*
CRIB	Clinical Risk Index for Babies
CSI	Comprehensive Severity Index (formerly Computerized Severity Index)

CSP	Complications Screening Program
CV	coefficient of variation
DCG/HCC	diagnostic cost group/hierarchical condition category
DME	durable medical equipment
DNR	do not resuscitate
DRGs	diagnosis related groups
DS	Disease Staging
DSM	*Diagnostic and Statistical Manual of Mental Disorders*
ECG	electrocardiogram
ERGs	episode risk groups
ETGs	Episode Treatment Groups
FY	fiscal year
GLM	generalized linear model
HCFA	Health Care Financing Administration (renamed CMS in 2001)
HCPCS	*Healthcare Common Procedure Coding System* (formerly *HCFA Common Procedure Coding System*)
HCUP	Healthcare Cost and Utilization Project
HHRGs	Home Health Resource Groups
HIPAA	Health Insurance Portability and Accountability Act of 1996
HIV	human immunodeficiency virus
HMO	health maintenance organization
IADLs	instrumental activities of daily living
ICC	intraclass correlation coefficient
ICD-9-CM	*International Classification of Diseases, Ninth Revision, Clinical Modification*
ICF	*International Classification of Functioning, Disability and Health*
ICU	intensive care unit
IQR	interquartile range
IRF	inpatient rehabilitation facility
IV	instrumental variable
KCF	key clinical finding (from MedisGroups)
LOS	length of stay
MAD	mean absolute deviation
MCBS	Medicare Current Beneficiary Survey

MCO	managed care organization
MDC	Major Diagnostic Category
MDS	Minimum Data Set
MedPAC	Medicare Payment Advisory Commission
MEDPAR	Medicare Provider Analysis and Review
MMPS	Medicare Mortality Predictor System
MPM	Mortality Probability Model
MSE	mean statistical error
NCH	National Claims History
NCHS	National Center for Health Statistics
NCQA	National Committee for Quality Assurance
NDC	National Drug Code
NHIS	National Health Interview Survey
NICU	neonatal intensive care unit
NSQIP	National Surgical Quality Improvement Program
OASIS	Outcome and Assessment Information Set
OLS	ordinary least squares
OSHPD	Office of Statewide Health Planning and Development (California)
PAI	Patient Assessment Instrument
PHC4	Pennsylvania Health Care Cost Containment Council
PICU	pediatric intensive care unit
PIP-DCGs	Principal Inpatient Diagnostic Cost Groups
PMCs	Patient Management Categories
PORT	patient outcome research team
PR	predictive ratio
PRISM	Pediatric Risk of Mortality Score
PTF	Patient Treatment File
RACHS	Risk Adjustment for Congenital Heart Surgery
RCT	randomized controlled trial
R-DRGs	Refined Diagnosis Related Groups
ROC	receiver operating characteristic
RRS	relative risk score
RUGs	Resource Utilization Groups
SD	standard deviation
SE	standard error
SF-20, SF-36	Short forms with 20 and 36 health status questions
SMR	standardized mortality ratio
SNAP	Score for Neonatal Acute Physiology

SNAPPE	Score for Neonatal Acute Physiology, Perinatal Extension
SNOMED	Systematized Nomenclature of Human and Veterinary Medicine
SSE	sum of squared errors
SSN	Social Security number
SST	sum of squares total
UB-82, UB-92	Uniform Bills promulgated in 1982 and 1992
UHDDS	Uniform Hospital Discharge Data Set
VA	Department of Veterans Affairs
VHA	Veterans Health Administration
WHO	World Health Organization

Index

About the Contributors

Lisa I. Iezzoni, M.D., M.Sc., is professor of medicine at Harvard Medical School and codirector of research in the Division of General Medicine and Primary Care, Department of Medicine, Beth Israel Deaconess Medical Center, in Boston. She received her degrees in medicine and health policy and management from Harvard University. Dr. Iezzoni has conducted numerous studies for the Agency for Healthcare Research and Quality, the Centers for Medicare & Medicaid Services, and private foundations on a variety of topics, including evaluating methods for predicting costs, clinical outcomes, and substandard quality of care. She has published and spoken widely on risk adjustment. A 1996 recipient of the Investigator Award in Health Policy Research from The Robert Wood Johnson Foundation, she is studying health policy issues relating to persons with disabilities. Dr. Iezzoni is a member of the Institute of Medicine in the National Academy of Sciences, serves on the editorial boards of major medical and health services research journals, and is on the board of directors of the National Quality Forum.

Arlene Ash, Ph.D., is a research professor at Boston University's schools of Medicine (Division of General Internal Medicine) and Public Health (Department of Biostatistics) and a cofounder and senior scientist at DxCG, Inc., a company that licenses risk-adjustment software. She is an internationally recognized expert in the development and use of risk-adjustment methodologies and an experienced user of national research databases, especially for Medicare, where her diagnostic cost group models have been adapted for use in HMO payment. Dr. Ash is a Fellow of AcademyHealth and of the American Statistical Association (ASA) and a recent Past Chair of ASA's Health Policy Statistics Section.

Dan R. Berlowitz, M.D., M.P.H., is associate director of the Center for Health Quality, Outcomes, and Economic Research at the Bedford VA Hospital and is associate professor at Boston University's schools of Public Health and Medicine. He is a graduate of the Albert Einstein College of Medicine and obtained his clinical and health services training at Boston Medical Center. Dr. Berlowitz has been principal or coinvestigator on more than 30 grants that have centered on his primary research interest of assessing and improving the quality of health care. He has particularly focused on long-term-care settings, where he has developed risk-adjustment models for a variety of clinical outcomes.

Jennifer Daley, M.D., is the chief medical officer and senior vice president of clinical quality at Tenet HealthSystem in Dallas, Texas. She is also an adjunct associate professor of community and family medicine at Dartmouth Medical School in Hanover, New Hampshire. From 1999 to 2002, Dr. Daley was the director of the Center for Health Systems Design and Evaluation in the Institute for Health Policy at Massachusetts General Hospital and Partners HealthCare System in Boston and associate professor of medicine at Harvard Medical School. From 1996 to 1999, Dr. Daley was the vice president and medical director of health care quality at the Beth Israel Deaconess Medical Center, a 600-bed teaching hospital. From 1990 to 1996, Dr. Daley was the recipient of a Senior Career Development Award in Health Services Research and Development from the Department of Veterans Affairs. Based at the West Roxbury Division of the VA New England HealthCare System, Dr. Daley's research and quality-improvement activities focused on access to care, patient satisfaction, utilization and outcomes in ischemic heart disease, and the development of an innovative, systemwide outcomes and quality improvement program in surgery for the VA National Surgical Quality Improvement Program.

Timothy G. Ferris, M.D., M.Phil., M.P.H., is a practicing general internist and pediatrician and a senior scientist in the Mass General Hospital Institute for Health Policy and the Center for Child and Adolescent Health Policy. He is an assistant professor of medicine and pediatrics at Harvard Medical School. His research has focused on the measurement and improvement of quality of health care for adults and children. In addition to conducting trials of quality improvement interventions, he has published studies on the effects of the organization and financing of care on the costs and quality of care. He has developed and deployed survey instruments designed to determine hospital safety characteristics for adults and children and investigated the role of risk adjustment in quality measurement. He was principle investigator for the development of the pediatrics-group-level CAHPS instrument, has served on a national advisory panel for the development of quality indicators for child health, and is a member of the Agency for Healthcare Research and Quality's Health Care Quality and Effectiveness Research study section.

Richard C. Hermann, M.D., M.S., is on the faculty of the departments of medicine and psychiatry at Tufts University School of Medicine–New England Medical Center, assistant professor of health policy and management at the Harvard School of Public Health, and director of the Center for Quality Assessment and Improvement in Mental Health. He has been granted funding by the National Institute of Mental Health, Agency for Healthcare Research and Quality, and U.S. Substance Abuse and Mental Health Services Administration to conduct research on variation and appropriateness of clinical practice, quality measurement, and quality improvement in mental health care. He developed and led a quality management program for a public mental health care system and serves on quality measurement committees for the Organization for Economic Cooperation and Development, American Psychiatric Association, Foundation for Accountability, National Committee for Quality Assurance, and Physician Consortium for Performance Improvement.

Karen Kuhlthau, Ph.D., is an assistant professor in the department of pediatrics at Harvard Medical School and associate director of the Center for Child and Adolescent Health Policy at the Mass General Hospital for Children. She is also an adjunct assistant professor at Boston University's School of Public Health in the social and behavioral sciences department. She received her doctoral degree from the University of Michigan, Ann Arbor, in the department of sociology. Dr. Kuhlthau is the recipient of the 2002 Health Services for Children Foundation Award for Child Health Services Research. Her research concerns health services use for children, issues relating to children with special health care needs, and quality-of-life studies. Dr. Kuhlthau is also interested in the pathways through which child health status and use of services affects family health and related outcomes.

Erol Peköz, Ph.D., is associate professor of operations management at Boston University's School of Management. Working in the area of quantitative methods, much of his research has focused on statistical models for understanding congestion and delay in service operations. Current research has focused on statistical models for geographical variations in health care usage and supply-induced demand for hospital beds. Other areas of interest include risk management, theory of rare events, and Monte Carlo simulation. His work appears in academic journals such as the *Journal of Applied Probability; Statistics and Probability Letters; Queueing Systems: Theory and Applications; Statistics in Medicine; and Probability in the Engineering and Informational Sciences.* Prior to coming to Boston University, Professor Peköz taught at the University of California, Los Angeles and the University of California, Berkeley and worked in the financial and information technology industries. He received his doctoral degree from UC Berkeley. He is the recipient of the 2001 Broderick Prize for Teaching at Boston University.

Amy K. Rosen, Ph.D., is an associate professor in the department of health services at Boston University's School of Public Health and a senior research scientist at the Center for Health Quality, Outcomes, and Economic Research, a Department of Veterans Affairs Health Services Research and Development Center of Excellence located at the Bedford VA Hospital in Massachusetts. She received her doctoral degree from the University of Maryland in sociology and social policy. Her research interests include the development of risk-adjustment methods for a variety of settings, including long-term care; acute and ambulatory care; large administrative databases, particularly VA and Medicare; quality assessment; and patient safety. She also continues to explore the use of episodes of care for quality assessment purposes.

Michael Shwartz, Ph.D., is professor of health care and operations management at Boston University's School of Management. He received his doctoral degree in urban and regional planning from the University of Michigan, Ann Arbor, and his M.B.A. from the University of California, Berkeley. He was the founding director of the Institute for Health Care Policy and Research within the Boston Department of Health and Hospitals. His research interests include the use of mathematical models of disease processes to analyze screening programs, studies of the relationship between severity of illness and hospital costs and outcomes, health care reimbursement, analyses related to quality of care, small area variations analyses, substance abuse program evaluations, and analyses of large databases.